IMPACT INJURY AND CRASH PROTECTION

IMPACT INJURY AND CRASH PROTECTION

Compiled and Edited by

ELISHA S. GURDJIAN, M.D.

Professor and Chairman
Department of Neurosurgery
Director, Bioengineering Research Center
Wayne State University
Detroit, Michigan

WILLIAM A. LANGE, M.D.

Associate Professor of Surgery
Wayne State University
Detroit, Michigan

LAWRENCE M. PATRICK, M.S.

Professor, Department of Engineering Mechanics
Wayne State University
Detroit, Michigan

and

L. MURRAY THOMAS, M.D.

Professor, Department of Neurosurgery
Wayne State University
Detroit, Michigan

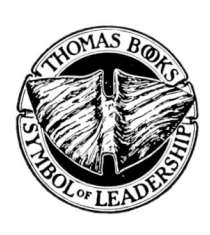

CHARLES C THOMAS • PUBLISHER
Springfield • Illinois • U.S.A.

Published and Distributed Throughout the World by
CHARLES C THOMAS • PUBLISHER
BANNERSTONE HOUSE
301–327 East Lawrence Avenue, Springfield, Illinois, U.S.A.
NATCHEZ PLANTATION HOUSE
735 North Atlantic Boulevard, Fort Lauderdale, Florida, U.S.A.

This book is protected by copyright. No part of it may be reproduced in any manner without written permission from the publisher.

© *1970, by* CHARLES C THOMAS • PUBLISHER

Library of Congress Catalog Card Number: 77–83988

With THOMAS BOOKS *careful attention is given to all details of manufacturing and design. It is the Publisher's desire to present books that are satisfactory as to their physical qualities and artistic possibilities and appropriate for their particular use.* THOMAS BOOKS *will be true to those laws of quality that assure a good name and good will.*

Printed in the United States of America

BB-14

CONTRIBUTORS AND DISCUSSANTS

JOHN E. ADAMS, M.D., Professor and Chairman, University of California, San Francisco Medical Center, Division of Neurological Surgery, San Francisco, California.

MAURICE S. ALBIN, M.D., M.Sc., Assistant Professor of Anesthesiology, Case Western Reserve University Medical School, Assistant Director of Anesthesiology, Cleveland Metropolitan General Hospital, Cleveland, Ohio.

DAVID L. BECKMAN, Ph.D., Associate Research Physiologist, Highway Safety Research Institute, The University of Michigan, Ann Arbor, Michigan.

CHARLES E. BRACKETT, M.D. (Discussant), Professor, Department of Surgery, Head, Section of Neurological Surgery, University of Kansas Medical Center, Kansas City, Kansas.

B. J. CAMPBELL (Discussant), Director, Highway Safety Research Center, The University of North Carolina, Chapel Hill, North Carolina.

CARTER COMPTON COLLINS, Ph.D., Senior Research Member, Institute of Medical Sciences, Presbyterian Medical Center, San Francisco, California.

F. GAYNOR EVANS, Ph.D., Professor of Anatomy, University of Michigan, East Medical Building, Ann Arbor, Michigan.

JOSEPH P. EVANS, M.D. (Discussant), Professor of Neurological Surgery, The University of Chicago Hospitals, Chicago, Illinois.

CHANNING L. EWING, M.D. (Discussant), Capt., MC, USN, Chief, Bioengineering Sciences Division, Naval Aerospace Medical Institute, Pensacola, Florida.

ELDON L. FOLTZ, M.D. (Discussant), Professor, Department of Neurological Surgery, University of Washington School of Medicine, Seattle, Washington.

VICTOR H. FRANKEL, M.D., Ph.D. (Discussant), Associate Professor of Orthopedic Surgery, Case Western Reserve University, Biomechanics Laboratory, Cleveland, Ohio.

CHARLES W. GADD (Discussant), Electro-Mechanics Department, General Motors Research Laboratories, Warren, Michigan.

DOMINGO GONZALEZ, M.D., Department of Neurosurgery, Wayne State University School of Medicine, Detroit, Michigan.

SAM W. GREENBERG, Research Assistant, Department of Neurosurgery, Wayne State University School of Medicine, Detroit, Michigan.

THOMAS J. GRIFKA, M.D., Assistant Professor, Department of Surgery, Wayne State University School of Medicine, Detroit, Michigan.

GEOFFREY GRIME, Research Group in Traffic Studies, University College London, London, England.
ELISHA S. GURDJIAN, M.D., Professor and Chairman, Department of Neurosurgery, Wayne State University, Detroit, Michigan.
JOSEPH L. HALEY, JR., Senior Project Engineer, AvSER Division of Flight Safety Foundation, Inc., Phoenix, Arizona.
ARTHUR E. HIRSCH, Senior Scientist, National Highway Institute, Bureau of Transportation, Washington, D.C.
CARL HIRSCH, Professor, Head of Department of Orthopedic Surgery, University of Göteborg, Göteborg, Sweden.
VOIGT R. HODGSON, Ph.D., Instructor, Department of Neurosurgery, Wayne State University, Detroit, Michigan.
JAAKKO K. KIHLBERG, Ph.D., Head, Data Processing and Statistics Section, Transportation Research Department, Cornell Aeronautical Laboratory, Inc., Buffalo, New York.
CHARLES K. KROELL, Senior Research Engineer, Electro-Mechanics Department, General Motors Research Laboratories, Warren, Michigan.
WILLIAM A. LANGE, M.D., Associate Professor of Surgery, Wayne State University School of Medicine, Detroit, Michigan.
RAYMOND R. McHENRY, Head, Engineering Mechanics Section, Transportation Research Department, Cornell Aeronautical Laboratory, Inc., Buffalo, New York.
RICHARD H. MAHONE, Personnel Protection Branch, Naval Ship Research and Development Center, Washington, D.C.
JOHN L. MARTINEZ, Professor of Mechanical Engineering, Assistant Dean, College of Engineering, Tulane University, New Orleans, Louisiana.
HAROLD J. MERTZ, JR., Ph.D., Assistant Professor, Department of Engineering Mechanics, Wayne State University, Detroit, Michigan.
AYUB K. OMMAYA, F.R.C.S., Associate Neurosurgeon, Surgical Neurology Branch, National Institute of Neurological Diseases and Blindness, National Institutes of Health, Bethesda, Maryland.
LAWRENCE M. PATRICK, Professor, Department of Mechanical Engineering Sciences, Wayne State University, Detroit, Michigan.
HEBERT E. PEDERSEN, M.D. (Discussant), Professor and Chairman, Department of Orthopedic Surgery, Wayne State University School of Medicine, Detroit, Michigan.
ROBERT H. PUDENZ, M.D., Associate Professor of Neurological Surgery, University of Southern California, School of Medicine, Pasadena, California.
ANTHONY J. RAIMONDI, M.D., Chairman, Cook County Hospital, Department of Neurological Surgery, Chicago, Illinois.
VERNE L. ROBERTS, Ph.D., Coordinator, Biomechanics Research, Institute

of Science and Technology, University of Michigan, Ann Arbor, Michigan.

DONALD SASS, M.D., Lieut., MC, USNR, Naval Medical Research Institute, Bethesda, Maryland.

TAKASHI B. SATO, Associate Professor, Division of Mechanical Engineering, Keio University, Tokyo, Japan.

RICHARD C. SCHNEIDER, M.D. (Discussant), Professor, Department of Surgery (Neurosurgery), University Hospital, The University of Michigan Medical Center, Ann Arbor, Michigan.

RICHARD G. SNYDER, Ph.D., Manager, Biomechanics Department, Office of Automotive Safety Research, Ford Motor Company, Dearborn, Michigan.

JOHN P. STAPP, Col. USAF, MC, Chief Scientist (Medicine), National Highway Safety Bureau, Federal Highway Administration, Washington, D.C.

L. MURRAY THOMAS, M.D., Professor, Department of Neurosurgery, Wayne State University, Detroit, Michigan.

F. J. UNTERHARNSCHEIDT, M.D. (Discussant), Chief, Division of Neuropathology and Experimental Neurosurgery, University of Texas Medical Branch, Galveston, Texas.

A. EARL WALKER, M.D. (Discussant), Professor of Neurological Surgery, The Johns Hopkins Hospital, Baltimore, Maryland.

ALEXANDER J. WALT, M.D., Professor and Chairman, Department of Surgery, Wayne State University School of Medicine, Detroit, Michigan.

ROBERT J. WHITE, M.D., Ph.D., Professor of Neurosurgery, Case Western Reserve University School of Medicine, Director of Neurological Surgery, Cleveland Metropolitan General Hospital, Cleveland, Ohio.

JACK K. WICKSTROM, M.D., Professor and Chairman, Department of Orthopedics, Tulane University School of Medicine, New Orleans, Louisiana.

ROGER D. WILLIAMS, M.D. (Discussant), Professor of Surgery, Department of Surgery, University of Texas Medical Branch, Galveston, Texas.

D. J. VAN KIRK, Research Assistant, Department of Mechanical Engineering Sciences, Wayne State University, Detroit, Michigan.

PREFACE

In this volume are published the papers given at the Wayne State University Symposium on "Impact Injury and Crash Protection." Discussions by selected participants are given after each paper. Because of the amount of material to be considered, there was not sufficient time to have open discussion of many of the topics presented.

The papers were given in four parts. Part I dealt with mechanisms of impact injury. Part II dealt with research methods in impact injury. Part III considered tolerance to impact, while Part IV dealt with principles of impact injury mitigation.

It is hoped that the publication of all this material in one volume will be welcome by many of those who are involved in research on impact injury and crash protection.

The editors thank the participants for their cooperation in providing their manuscripts in a form suitable for publication. This has materially accelerated the publication of this volume so soon after the presentation of the Symposium.

E. S. Gurdjian, M.D.
L. M. Patrick, M.S.
L. M. Thomas, M.D.
W. A. Lange, M.D.

CONTENTS

Page

Contributors and Discussants v

Preface

 E. S. Gurdjian, M.D., W. A. Lange, M.D., L. M. Patrick, M.D., and L. M. Thomas, M.D.

PART I

MECHANISMS OF IMPACT INJURY

Chapter

 I. MULTIPLICITY OF INJURY IN AUTOMOBILE ACCIDENTS
   Jaakko K. Kihlberg 5
   Discussion
    B. J. Campbell 25

 II. MECHANISMS OF HEAD INJURY
   L. Murray Thomas 27
   Discussion
    Friedrich J. Unterharnscheidt 43

 III. SPINE AND SPINAL CORD INJURY
   Robert J. White and *Maurice S. Albin* 63
   Discussion
    Richard C. Schneider 84

 IV. THE MECHANISMS OF CHEST INJURIES
   Verne L. Roberts and *David L. Beckman* 86
   Discussion
    Charles E. Brackett 99

 V. BLUNT ABDOMINAL INJURY: A Review of 307 Cases
   Alexander J. Walt and *Thomas J. Grifka* 101
   Discussion
    Roger D. Williams 124

Chapter	Page
VI. BIOMECHANICS IN ORTHOPEDIC SURGERY, An Account of Aims and Methods	
Carl Hirsch	125
Discussion	
Herbert E. Pedersen	141

PART II

RESEARCH METHODS IN IMPACT INJURY

VII. TELEMETRY IN BIOLOGICAL SCIENCES	
Robert H. Pudenz	145
Discussion	
Carter C. Collins	157
VIII. FINE STRUCTURE IN CEREBRAL DAMAGE: Toxic and Mechanical	
Anthony J. Raimondi, Fred Beckman and *Joseph P. Evans*	160
Discussion	
Joseph P. Evans	177
IX. IMPLANTED MONITORS	
John E. Adams and *Carter C. Collins*	180
Discussion	
Eldon L. Foltz	186
X. HIGH SPEED FLASH X-RAY AND CINEMATOGRAPHY IN INJURY RESEARCH	
John L. Martinez	196
Discussion	
Voight R. Hodgson	208
Discussion	
Donald J. Sass	210
XI. MATHEMATICAL MODELS FOR INJURY PREDICTION	
Raymond R. McHenry	214
XII. COMPARISONS OF RESEARCH IN INANIMATE AND BIOLOGIC MATERIAL: Artifacts and Pitfalls	
Elisha S. Gurdjian, M.D., D. Gonzales, M.D., Voigt R. Hodgson, M.S., L. Murray Thomas, M.D., and *S. W. Greenberg, B.S.*	234
Discussion	
A. Earl Walker	254

PART III

TOLERANCE TO IMPACT

XIII. METHODS OF ESTABLISHING HUMAN TOLERANCE LEVELS: Cadaver and Animal Research and Clinical Observations
    Lawrence M. Patrick and Takashi B. Sato 259
    Discussion
        L. Murray Thomas 274

XIV. PHYSICAL FACTORS RELATED TO EXPERIMENTAL CONCUSSION
    Voigt R. Hodgson 275
    Discussion
        Ayub K. Ommaya 303

XV. VOLUNTARY HUMAN TOLERANCE LEVELS
    John P. Stapp 308
    Discussion
        Channing L. Ewing 350

XVI. TOLERANCE OF SUBHUMAN PRIMATE BRAIN TO CEREBRAL CONCUSSION
    Arthur E. Hirsch, Ayub K. Ommaya, and Richard H. Mahone .. 352
    Discussion
        Elisha S. Gurdjian 370

XVII. TOLERANCE OF THORAX AND ABDOMEN
    Harold J. Mertz, Jr. and Charles K. Kroell 372
    Discussion
        F. Gaynor Evans 400

XVIII. IMPACT TOLERANCE OF HUMAN PELVIC AND LONG BONES
    F. Gaynor Evans 402
    Discussion
        Victor H. Frankel 418

PART IV

PRINCIPLES OF IMPACT INJURY MITIGATION

XIX. FUNDAMENTALS OF KINETICS AND KINEMATICS AS APPLIED TO INJURY REDUCTION
    Joseph L. Haley, Jr. 423
    Discussion
        Geoffrey Grime 442

Chapter	Page
XX. APPLICATIONS OF HUMAN TOLERANCE DATA TO PROTECTIVE SYSTEMS: Requirements for Soft Tissue, Bone and Organ Protective Devices	
Lawrence M. Patrick and *Geoffrey Grime*	444
Discussion	
Charles W. Gadd	474
XXI. THE EFFECTIVENESS OF CURRENT METHODS AND SYSTEMS USED TO REDUCE INJURY	
William A. Lange and *Donald J. Van Kirk*	475
Discussion	
Richard G. Snyder	494
XXII. OCCUPANT RESTRAINT SYSTEMS OF AUTOMOTIVE, AIRCRAFT, AND MANNED SPACE VEHICLES: An Evaluation of the State-of-the-Art and Future Concepts	
Richard G. Snyder	496
Discussion	
John P. Stapp	562
Index	565

IMPACT INJURY AND CRASH PROTECTION

PART I

MECHANISMS OF IMPACT INJURY

Chapter I

MULTIPLICITY OF INJURY IN AUTOMOBILE ACCIDENTS

JAAKKO K. KIHLBERG

INTRODUCTION

The concept of epidemiology of whole body area injury is not well defined. National injury data[1,2] are limited in quality and coverage, and are not directed toward answering questions on epidemiology of whole body area injury, or multiplicity of injury, as the concept may well be labeled.

The latest available data from the National Center of Health Statistics[1] indicate that in 1966 to 1967 (1-year period) 51.8 million persons in the United States were injured, and suffered 54.1 million injuries. The sources of the injuries were described as follows:

Moving motor vehicle accidents	3.5 million persons
Work accidents	10.3
Home accidents	22.6
Other accidents	17.4
Total	53.8*

According to the official source,[1] 1.04 injuries were suffered per injured person. Such an average is not indicative of much multiplicity of injury, but it can well be speculated that different types of accidents are quite different in this regard.

Work accidents, related to handling tools and operating machines, or to falling objects, appear to result in localized rather than multiple injury (hand injury with a press-punch being an example to the point). Falls

---

* This total is higher than the number of injured persons because the four accident classes are not mutually exclusive.

EDITORS NOTE: This research has been supported in part by Public Health Service Research Grant No. UI-00053 from the National Center for Urban and Industrial Health, and in part by the Automobile Manufacturers Association, Inc.

from height, as they do happen for example in the construction industry, are more conducive to multiple injuries, but their number is relatively limited. Similarly, a good portion of home accidents result in localized injuries only, like those from kitchen mishaps or from hitting one's thumb with the hammer. Yet there are falls from the ladder or down stairs in which multiple injuries are more likely. The category of "other" accidents primarily consists of accidents in public areas like department stores, schools, playgrounds, streets, community swimming pools and other recreation areas (including parks and camping areas), and many an injury suffered under those circumstances tends to be localized rather than general.

Moving motor vehicle accidents are those in which the vehicle occupant, or the pedestrian, motorcyclist, or cyclist involved is likely to suffer multiple injuries.[3,4,5] The Automotive Crash Injury Research program (ACIR) of the Cornell Aeronautical Laboratory, Inc. is in possession of a large volume of injury data on passenger car occupants who were involved in rural injury-producing motor vehicle accidents.

An examination of those data in regard to the multiplicity of injury is believed to contribute to the study of epidemiology of whole body area injury.

MATERIAL

For purposes of the present study, the ACIR computer tape was interrogated in December 1967, in search for information on incidence or nonincidence of injury among occupants of passenger cars which had been involved in an injury-producing accident (*i.e.* at least one occupant in each accident car was injured). Basically, the tape contains data accumulated through the past 15 years and from thirty-one different states, from primarily rural highway accidents investigated and reported by State Police or State Highway Patrol, with medical data obtained from the physicians and hospitals involved in care of the accident victims.

For inclusion in the present study, the following requirements on occupant data were set:

1. Occupants whose age is known to be 15 years or more
2. Occupants whose seat in the car is known to be one of the following:
    a. Driver without passengers
    b. Driver with one or more passengers
    c. Front (center or right)
    d. Rear (left, center, or right)
3. Occupants for whom it is known whether ejected from the car or not
4. Occupants who were in one of the four following types of impact:

a. Frontal: principal impact on the front-facing portion of the car
   b. Side: principal impact on fenders or other side structure
   c. Rear: principal impact on the rear-facing portion of the car
   d. Principal rollover: principal impact not assigned to a localized portion of the vehicle, but rather to rollover movements
5. Occupants for whom the incidence or nonincidence of injury is known for each of the six gross areas of the human body to be specified below
6. Occupants for whom the degree, or severity, of the "overall injury" is known

The six gross areas of the human body to be referred to throughout the study are the following:

1. Head (H): skull and other portions of head above the neck
2. Neck (N): neck in the common usage of the term, and cervical spine
3. Thoracic Area (T), or Upper Torso: torso below the neck, largely guarded by the rib cage, including dorsal spine, excluding upper limbs
4. Abdominal Area (A), or Lower Torso: torso below the Upper Torso, including lumbar spine and pelvis, excluding lower limbs
5. Upper Limbs (U): arms, forearms, hands
6. Lower Limbs (L): legs, feet

The letters H-N-T-A-U-L will be frequently used in the present report to refer to the injured main body areas, individually, or in combinations like HN, HNTAU, *etc.*

An injury scale for evaluation of severity, or degree, of injury has been developed by ACIR with the assistance of specialists and members of the staff of the New York Hospital—Cornell University Medical College.

Progressive degrees of injury are outlined in terms of simple key words and phrases. Examples of typical injuries are provided to serve as guides. It will be noted that many types of injuries are not included as examples; these injuries have not occurred with sufficient frequency to require specific listing. When exceptional types of injury occur, medical consultants have had no difficulty in assigning these to one of the injury categories.

As an example, guidelines for classification of head injury are given below; comparable guidelines have been established for all areas of the body.

1. *No Injury*

2. *Minor:*
   a. Contusions and abrasions, superficial lacerations
   b. Fractures, dislocations of nose

c. Mild concussion with no loss of consciousness
  d. Teeth loosened, broken or knocked out
  e. Whiplash (unqualified)
3. *Nondangerous:*
  a. "Deep" or "disfiguring" lacerations
  b. Extensive lacerations without dangerous hemorrhage
  c. Compound, comminuted fractures of nose
  d. Concussion with unconsciousness 5 to 30 minutes. No evidence of other intracranial injury
  e. Skull fracture without evidence of concussion or other intracranial injury
  f. Loss of eye
4. *Dangerous* (Survival not assured):
  a. Lacerations with dangerous hemorrhage
  b. Skull fracture with concussion as evidenced by loss of consciousness up to 2 hours
  c. Concussion as evidenced by loss of consciousness from 30 minutes to 2 hours without evidence of other intracranial injury or more than 2 hours without reference to possible intracranial injury.
  d. Depressed fractures of skull
  e. Evidence of critical intracranial damage
5. *Fatal* (Death within 24 hours)

The degree, or severity, of the "overall injury" is equal to the most severe degree of injury assigned to any one of the six body areas.

A total of 72,991 occupants from the ACIR computer tape met the study specifications and are included in the present study.

METHODS

Multiplicity of Injury

Being an inquiry into the multiplicity of injury in automobile accidents, the present study is concerned with the number of body areas injured, referring to the six gross areas of the human body already introduced. An occupant in an injury-accident car may not suffer injury in any of those areas, or he may be injured in all of the six simultaneously, or in any combination of a lesser number of body areas.

Measuring the multiplicity of injury only along a scale from one to six body areas, has its severe limitations, of course. For example, if the little finger of the left hand of the occupant is bruised, this is counted as an upper limb injury (U), but so is amputation of both his arms. Certain types of impacts may result in fractures of the skull and the cervical spine, the injury being listed as double (HN) although one impact only was responsible for the outcome. On the other hand, if a front passenger is hurled against the face of the instrument panel and suffers knee injury (L), hits the side vent handle with his hand (U), hits the instrument panel with both upper and lower torso (TA), is thrown skull first against the header or windshield frame (H), then through the windshield (H), and in backward motion suffers neck cuts from the hole in the windshield (N), the multiplicity of injury (HNTAUL) tells something about the complex nature of the impact.

Thus, the multiplicity measure adopted here sometimes does and sometimes does not describe the complexities of injury production in automobile accidents. It is believed, however, that even with such limitations the number of body areas injured is a useful measure, at least in some overall average terms.

With six body areas, there are $2^6 = 64$ possible combinations of no-injury or injury. First, *none* of the body areas may be involved, and there is no injury at all. Second, *one but no more* body areas may be injured (H, N, T, A, U, or L), giving six combinations. Third, *exactly two* body areas may be injured (HN, HT, ... TA, ... AL, UL), in fifteen combinations. For *three* body areas simultaneously, there are twenty possible combinations; for *four*, 15; for *five*, 6; and for *six*, of course 1. In the present study, the frequencies of all the sixty-three possible injury combinations have been taken under examination. The first combination, no injury, was omitted. The distribution into all the possible injury combinations is labeled as a six-factorial distribution.

Tabulation of the distribution of the occupants into the sixty-three theoretically possible injury combinations also provides material for summarization in terms of the relative involvement frequency of one, two, three, *etc.*, body areas.

Severity of Injury

Within the sixty-three injury combinations, distribution of injury by degree, or severity, was obtained, the evaluation being based on the degree of the "overall injury." The data allow for an examination of such distributions in various subcategories, or groups. The combined relative frequency of fatal and dangerous injury can be used as a summary figure to indicate the severity of injury in any particular group. Since many persons classified by ACIR into the "dangerous" injury category actually died, although not within 24 hours from the accident, this combined category of dangerous and fatal injuries can be labeled as *"high risk injuries."*

Lethality of High Risk Injury

As indicated already, ACIR does not follow up the accident victims, but classifies as fatalities only those who die within the first 24 hours. To be sure, a number of those classified as suffering "dangerous" injury die later, but the ACIR data collection system does not get observations or information on these cases.

A certain measure of the lethality of high risk injury is obtained, however, by calculating the percentage of nearly immediate deaths (deaths within 24 hours) among those so severely injured. This percentage serves as an additional index of severity of injury.

Injury Associations

A question of general interest, and of importance to those rendering medical emergency care, is to what extent and in what manner injuries to the several body areas are associated with or dissociated from each other. Examination of that question requires setting up a mathematical model which is able to describe and predict with what frequencies the various body area combination injuries would be expected to occur if there were no associations—meaning calculation of the expected frequencies under a Null Hypothesis of the common type.

If the observed body area combination frequencies of injury differ substantially from those expected, then it could be concluded that some two or three, *etc.*, body areas associate with each other more frequently than expected under the Null Hypothesis, or that some other body area combinations occur less frequently than expected.

In order to examine and identify such associations or dissociations, the model of the common multifactorial distribution was utilized in calculation of the expected frequencies of the various body area injury combinations.

If comprehensive data from all auto accidents were available, for each seated position separately, then it would be possible to estimate, say, the probability of a driver to suffer, in an accident, a head injury, p_H, or neck injury, p_N, or thoracic area injury, p_T, *etc.* Each of these probabilities would be equal to the ratio of the number of drivers injured in each particular area to the number of drivers exposed to such injury in an accident. Out of all drivers, a fraction equal to $(1-p_H)(1-p_N) \ldots (1-p_L)$ would escape injury to any of the six body areas.

In the past, the ACIR system did not assemble data on *all* drivers in accidents, and the present study data cannot provide information on quantities like p_H, or p_N, *etc.* Within the ACIR sampling areas, *lone* drivers (no passengers in the car) involved in accidents but suffering *no injury*,

Multiplicity of Injury in Automobile Accidents

never were included in the ACIR cases; on the other hand, *all injured lone drivers* were. Of the *lone* drivers in the ACIR sample, then, 100 per cent were injured (injury probability = 100%), in order to satisfy the ACIR requirement that at least one person in the car was injured.

Of the drivers with just *one* passenger, not all had to be injured in order that the accident car be included in the ACIR sample (injury frequency < 100%), because instead of the driver, the passenger alone could be injured (or both, for that matter). Of the drivers with *two* passengers, an even smaller percentage had to be injured in order that the accident car be included in the ACIR sample (injury frequency << 100%). And so on. The frequency of driver's injury in the ACIR sample is therefore a function of the car occupancy, that is, the number of other occupants in the car (and the seating of those occupants, as well).

Modified, the same consequence holds for injury frequencies for any other car occupants in the ACIR sample. For example, the frequency by which a center rear seat passenger will be found injured is also dependent on the occupancy pattern of the vehicle. All *injured* center rear seat occupants are observed and recorded by ACIR, to be sure; but the frequency of injury among the center rear seat occupants will be high if in addition to this passenger there was only the driver in the car, because then the required minimum of at least one injured person in the car would be "shared" between the driver and the rear center passenger. However, if there were four more passengers in the car, the rear center passenger would not have to "compete" for injury with the driver alone, but the "necessary" injury could be suffered by any one of the five others (driver and four extra passengers), leaving the rear center passenger with a smaller probability of injury.

Under these circumstances, it then is not possible to determine from the ACIR data the probability of escaping injury in all automobile accidents. Only the conditional probability of escaping injury, *given* at least one person in the vehicle was injured, can be determined, but that probability is not suitable for the purposes of the model building now in question.

For this reason, a specific procedure was developed for purposes of calculation of the expected frequencies of the various injury combinations. The procedure is described in technical terms in the Statistical Appendix; here it may suffice to state that the procedure makes it possible to estimate all the six parameters of a multifactorial distribution even if the observed frequency of one crucial injury combination—namely, no injury at all—out of all those possible (64 in the case of the six-factorial distribution) is missing. This means estimation of body area injury probabilities from data on *injured persons* only, excluding those escaping injury. For details, see the Statistical Appendix.

Once the necessary parameters of the six-factorial distribution were estimated, it became feasible to calculate the expected number of persons with any given injury combination such as H, NT, or HTAUL, *etc.*, and then compare the observed numbers with those expected. Such comparisons lead to an understanding of which injury combinations are more frequent in practice than in theory, and which are comparatively infrequent.

Also, data of this kind make it possible to identify associations among the six body areas in regard to injury. Some associations are *positive* in the sense that some two or more body areas tend to be injured simultaneously, some others are *negative*, in the opposite sense. The specific statistical techniques used in this analysis of association will be described in connection with the presentation of the findings.

RESULTS

In reviewing the results it must be kept in mind that the data given refer only to the totality of occupants as defined under "MATERIAL," that is, occupants in any of the specified seated positions, ejected or not, and in any of the specified types of accidents. Thus, the results will give only gross averages and no differentiation. It is known perfectly well that injury mechanism in automobiles is different for the different seated positions, that ejected persons are, in regard to injury, much worse off than those who are kept within the vehicle, and that injuries are different in different types of accidents.[6] Furthermore, it is known that there are interactions among these (and other) accident characteristics or factors.[7] Presenting only the overall average picture has been dictated by requirements of space, yet there is reason to believe that such a picture may be useful to those members of the medical profession, police officers, and others who have to deal with the overall situation. It is worth noting that the data largely reflect injuries to *front seat* occupants because nearly 80 per cent of the people in ACIR cases occupy the front seat. A separate study, to be published later, is being contemplated to deal with differential analysis which cannot be covered in the present report.

Multiplicity of Injury

Among the 72,991 occupants tabulated, 57,597 injured persons were discovered. The injured suffered a total of 130,525 injuries ("injury" meaning an injured body area), or about 2.3 injuries per injured person. Such an average suggests that there was a large number of persons with multiple injuries. That this was the case is seen from Table 1-I which gives the per cent distribution of the 57,597 injured persons into the sixty-three possible injury combination categories.

TABLE 1-I
PER CENT DISTRIBUTION AND RANKING BY FREQUENCY OF OCCURRENCE OF 57,597 INJURED PERSONS BY INJURY COMBINATION

Rank, Body Area Combination, and Per Cent Frequency

One Body Area:			Three Body Areas:			Four Body Areas:		
1	H	14.21	31	HNT	0.69	50	HNTA	0.19
18	N	1.30	47	HNA	0.22	42	HNTU	0.33
10	T	3.35	38	HNU	0.44	32	HNTL	0.64
15	A	1.41	30	HNL	0.72	56	HNAU	0.11
9	U	3.82	20	HTA	1.25	53	HNAL	0.14
4	L	5.95	11	HTU	2.86	33	HNUL	0.63
	Total	30.04	6	HTL	5.43	28	HTAU	0.73
			25	HAU	0.81	22	HTAL	1.19
Two Body Areas:			21	HAL	1.22	8	HTUL	5.11
24	HN	1.13	3	HUL	6.40	23	HAUL	1.14
5	HT	5.70	51	NTA	0.14	61	NTAU	0.05
16	HA	1.40	52	NTU	0.14	59	NTAL	0.09
7	HU	5.24	49	NTL	0.19	54	NTUL	0.14
2	HL	9.19	63	NAU	0.03	60	NAUL	0.06
34	NT	0.50	58	NAL	0.10	41	TAUL	0.37
45	NA	0.26	48	NUL	0.21		Total	10.92
44	NU	0.28	43	TAU	0.30			
40	NL	0.38	39	TAL	0.43	Five Body Areas:		
26	TA	0.78	19	TUL	1.30	57	HNTAU	0.11
17	TU	1.31	36	AUL	0.48	46	HNTAL	0.24
14	TL	1.88		Total	23.36	29	HNTUL	0.73
35	AU	0.48				55	HNAUL	0.12
27	AL	0.74				13	HTAUL	1.98
12	UL	2.74				62	NTAUL	0.05
	Total	32.01					Total	3.23
						Six Body Areas:		
						37	HNTAUL	0.45
						Grand Total		100.00

In the data, there was not a single combination of body areas which did not occur. Some combinations were quite frequent, some very rare. The full ranking of the sixty-three combinations in order of magnitude of the per cent frequency is also shown in Table 1-I. From Table 1-I, the five most frequent and the five least frequent combinations can be picked up:

COMBINATION	PER CENT FREQUENCY AMONG INJURED OCCUPANTS
The Five Most Frequent:	
H	14.21
HL	9.19
HUL	6.40
L	5.95
HT	5.70
The Five Least Frequent:	
NTAL	0.09
NAUL	0.06
NTAU	0.05
NTAUL	0.05
NAU	0.03

In part, the frequencies are determined by the basic probabilities of each body area's being involved. The head, an exposed part of the body, is easily involved, while the neck, not so much exposed and smaller in size, is not. Thus, in the data, head involvement appears readily at the top of the ranking, neck involvement at the bottom.

Table 1-I allows for calculation of the percentage (of injured persons) by which any given body area was involved. The results are as follows:

Head Involved	70.8)	
Neck Involved	10.8)	Per Cent
Thorax Involved	38.6)	of
Abdomen Involved	17.1)	Injured
Upper Limb Involved	38.9)	Occupants
Lower Limb Involved	50.4)	

The above percentages are so high that multiple injury can be expected to be a rule rather than an exception. Actually, if the percentages are added up, the sum equals to 226.6 which divided by 100 gives about 2.3 as the average number of injuries per injured person, as already indicated.

Table 1-I also provides data for calculation of the following distribution by the number of body areas (per injured occupant) involved:

One Body Area Only	30.0)	
Two	32.0)	Per Cent
Three	23.4)	of
Four	10.9)	Injured
Five	3.2)	Occupants
Six	0.5)	
Total	100.0	

Single body area injury is limited to 30 per cent of the number of injured occupants; at least two body areas are involved in 70 per cent, and more than two, in 38 per cent. *Multiplicity of injury, therefore, is a dominant feature for victims injured in automobile accidents.* This multiplicity is primarily governed by the high involvement rate of the head in the first place; of lower limbs, second; and of upper limbs and the thoracic region, third. The lower involvement rates for the abdominal area and the neck, on the other hand, help set limitations to the multiplicity of injury (in terms which in the present report are being used to measure multiplicity).

Severity of Injury

According to the ACIR classification, the severity of whole body (or "overall") injury was distributed as follows:

Minor	52.0)	Per Cent
Nondangerous	34.5)	of
Dangerous	7.6)	Injured
Fatal	5.9)	Occupants
Total	100.0	

Of these, High Risk Injuries = Dangerous or Fatal Injuries—13.5

The percentage of high risk injuries (including dangerous and fatal injuries) is shown and ranked in Table 1-II.

TABLE 1-II
PER CENT FREQUENCY AND RANKING BY FREQUENCY OF HIGH RISK INJURIES FOR THE VARIOUS BODY AREA COMBINATIONS

Rank, Body Area Combination, and Per Cent Frequency

One Body Area:			Three Body Areas:			Four Body Areas:		
52	H	7.0	9	HNT	41.7	2	HNTA	52.3
45	N	10.7	22	HNA	25.0	13	HNTU	36.1
47	T	10.1	18	HNU	28.1	8	HNTL	42.1
40	A	14.3	25	HNL	24.8	23	HNAU	25.0
61	U	0.4	7	HTA	43.4	17	HNAL	28.4
62	L	0.1	35	HTU	18.1	24	HNUL	24.9
	Total	5.9	37	HTL	17.0	12	HTAU	37.6
			36	HAU	17.2	10	HTAL	41.6
Two Body Areas:			32	HAL	19.4	28	HTUL	20.8
15	HN	31.6	53	HUL	6.7	26	HAUL	23.5
33	HT	19.0	38	NTA	16.2	43	NTAU	11.5
21	HA	25.0	39	NTU	14.6	14	NTAL	34.7
55	HU	5.6	41	NTL	13.9	34	NTUL	19.0
57	HL	5.3	27	NAU	22.2	42	NAUL	12.1
30	NT	19.7	59	NAL	5.2	29	TAUL	20.1
58	NA	5.3	44	NUL	11.4		Total	27.1
50	NU	8.1	31	TAU	19.7			
51	NL	8.1	20	TAL	25.1	Five Body Areas:		
19	TA	26.1	60	TUL	4.2	3	HNTAU	50.8
54	TU	6.1	48	AUL	9.0	4	HNTAL	49.6
56	TL	5.6		Total	16.3	6	HNTUL	45.2
46	AU	10.5				11	HNAUL	38.2
49	AL	8.4				5	HTAUL	47.2
63	UL	0.1				16	NTAUL	31.0
	Total	10.1					Total	46.5
						Six Body Areas:		
						1	HNTAUL	59.2
						Grand Total		13.5

The following five most severe and five least severe injury combinations were picked up from that Table:

COMBINATION	PERCENTAGE OF HIGH RISK OVERALL INJURY AMONG THOSE INJURED
The Five Most Severe:	
HNTAUL	59.2
HNTA	52.3
HNTAU	50.8
HNTAL	49.6
HTAUL	47.8

The Five Least Severe:

NAL	5.2
TUL	4.2
U	0.4
L	0.1
UL	0.1

It is seen that there are body area injury combinations (all six areas, HNTAUL, to start with) in which up to nearly 60 per cent of cases represent danger to life. The high risk injury patterns, as a rule, include simultaneously the head, the neck, the thoracic area, and the abdominal area, in some combinations, with a certain amount of extremity involvements (the latter mostly will not pose danger to life). On the other hand, injuries at the lowest end of the severity scale generally are not multiple and tend to involve the limbs rather than other parts of the body.

Table 1-II also allows for observation of severity of injury as a function of the number of body areas involved:

NUMBER OF INVOLVED BODY AREAS	PERCENTAGE OF HIGH RISK OVERALL INJURY AMONG THOSE INJURED
One Only	5.9
Two	10.1
Three	16.3
Four	27.1
Five	46.5
Six	59.2

If only one body area is involved, then the relative frequency of high risk injury is only about 6 per cent as contrasted to about sixty per cent if all the six body areas are involved. The dangerousness of whole body injury is well documented here. However, the issue is more complicated than that expressed only in terms of the number of body areas involved. For example, while of two-area injuries only 10.1 per cent are severe (high risk), on the average, of HN-injuries 31.6 per cent are severe as contrasted to 0.1 per cent of UL-injuries. Thus, detailed examination of Table 1-II is advisable.

Lethality of High Risk Injury

An additional measure of severity of injury is obtained by calculating the percentage of almost immediate deaths (death within 24 hours) among those suffering high risk injury. The results are given in Table 1-III.

Multiplicity of Injury in Automobile Accidents

TABLE 1-III
PER CENT FREQUENCY AND RANKING BY FREQUENCY OF IMMEDIATE DEATHS AMONG THOSE SUFFERING HIGH RISK INJURY

Rank, Body Area Combination, and Per Cent Frequency

One Body Area:			Three Body Areas:			Four Body Areas:		
15	H	55.0	6	HNT	66.3	36	HNTA	40.4
18	N	53.8	35	HNA	40.6	22	HNTU	50.7
43	T	30.8	21	HNU	52.1	3	HNTL	72.1
60	A	6.0	7	HNL	66.0	49	HNAU	25.0
63	U*	0.0	47	HTA	25.3	4	HNAL	69.6
41	L*	33.3	38	HTU	39.1	11	HNUL	60.0
	Total	43.6	30	HTL	46.2	44	HTAU	28.0
			53	HAU	18.8	40	HTAL	35.7
Two Body Areas:			46	HAL	25.7	17	HTUL	54.1
16	HN	54.4	29	HUL	46.6	45	HAUL	27.7
32	HT	43.2	19	NTA	53.8	5	NTAU*	66.7
54	HA	18.3	34	NTU	41.7	1	NTAL	82.4
37	HU	39.6	28	NTL	46.7	12	NTUL	60.0
23	HL	50.5	48	NAU*	25.0	26	NAUL*	50.0
10	NT	63.2	42	NAL*	33.3	50	TAUL	23.3
24	NA*	50.0	13	NUL	57.1		Total	47.0
51	NU	23.1	55	TAU	17.6			
39	NL	38.9	58	TAL	12.9	Five Body Areas:		
56	TA	13.7	31	TUL	45.2	27	HNTAU	48.4
57	TU	13.0	59	AUL	12.0	9	HNTAL	64.7
52	TL	20.0		Total	40.8	2	HNTUL	72.3
62	AU	3.4				20	HNAUL	53.8
61	AL	5.6				33	HTAUL	43.2
25	UL*	50.0				14	NTAUL*	55.6
	Total	38.5					Total	52.0
						Six Body Areas:		
* Less than 10 Occupants Suffering High Risk Injury.						8	HNTAUL	65.2
						Grand Total		43.7

From Table 1-III, the following combinations emerge as the five most frequently lethal and the five least frequently lethal ones:

COMBINATION	PERCENTAGE OF ALMOST IMMEDIATE DEATHS AMONG THOSE SUFFERING HIGH RISK INJURY
The Five Most Frequently Lethal:	
NTAL	82.4
HNTUL	72.3
HNTL	72.1
HNAL	69.6
NTAU	66.7
The Five Least Frequently Lethal:	
AUL	12.0
A	6.0
AL	5.6
AU	3.4
U	0.0

It is seen that the most frequently lethal high risk injuries involve several vital body areas simultaneously, while the least frequently lethal ones involve a lesser number of body areas with a preponderance of involvement of abdomen and extremities. These findings are in agreement with those presented in the above section on severity of injury.

Injury Associations

The method described in the Statistical Appendix made it possible to calculate the expected number of persons in each of the sixty-three potential injury combinations, and to compare the observed numbers with those expected. Calculation of the expected number was based on the assumption that injuries to the six body areas are independent of each other, and any deviations from the expectations, except within limits of random fluctuations, can be viewed as evidence of association, or nonindependence, among the body areas. If the observed number for any given injury combination is larger than expected, then the body areas involved have a *positive* association, and if the reverse is true, a *negative* association. For example, the injury combination HTAUL was expected in only 391 persons but found in 1,141, indicating a quite strong tendency for those five body areas to be simultaneously injured, or to be positively associated (which may mean that there is a substantial number of impacts of a type to favor the formation of this particular injury combination). For another example, the combination TL was expected in 1,652 cases but found only in 1,080. This negative association may indicate that there is a limited number of impact conditions in which only the thoracic area and legs are injured.

The observed and expected numbers for each injury combination are given in Table 1-IV.

Comparisons between the observed and the expected numbers can be made in various ways. If the observed number is given the symbol O and the expected the symbol E, then the difference O-E could be used as a measure of discordance. However, if any particular injury combination has a small expected number, the difference O-E simply could not be large and thus could not serve as an indicator of essential associations. The relative difference (O-E)/E could then be used to remedy the situation, except that this ratio may be either very large or very small with no statistical significance to the difference. A statistical approach is to calculate the quantity $(O-E)^2/E$ which is a chi-square with one degree of freedom. The larger the chi-square, the more important the difference, statistically. Again, it is quite possible that a difference becomes statistically very significant but is of little practical import. For example, the com-

TABLE 1-IV
OBSERVED AND EXPECTED FREQUENCIES

Body Area Combination, Observed Frequency (O) and Expected Frequency (E)

	O	E		O	E		O	E
One Body Area:			*Three Body Areas:*			*Four Body Areas:*		
H	8187	6345	HNT	398	424	HNTA	109	82
N	749	352	HNA	128	141	HNTU	191	250
T	1929	1786	HNU	253	430	HNTL	366	392
A	811	595	HNL	416	673	HNAU	64	83
U	2200	1809	HTA	719	717	HNAL	81	131
L	3427	2836	HTU	1649	2180	HNUL	361	397
			HTL	3126	3417	HTAU	418	423
Two Body Areas:			HAU	464	726	HTAL	687	663
HN	651	728	HAL	700	1138	HTUL	2942	2016
HT	3285	3695	HUL	3686	3461	HAUL	659	672
HA	809	1231	NTA	80	40	NTAU	26	23
HU	3020	3743	NTU	82	121	NTAL	49	37
HL	5292	5866	NTL	108	190	NTUL	79	112
NT	289	205	NAU	18	40	NAUL	33	37
NA	151	68	NAL	58	63	TAUL	214	189
NU	161	208	NUL	123	192			
NL	221	326	TAU	173	204	*Five Body Areas:*		
TA	449	347	TAL	247	320	HNTAU	61	49
TU	756	1054	TUL	746	974	HNTAL	137	76
TL	1080	1652	AUL	277	325	HNTUL	423	231
AU	275	351				HNAUL	68	77
AL	427	550				HTAUL	1141	391
UL	1577	1673				NTAUL	29	22

Six Body Areas:
HNTAUL   262   45

Total   –57597–

bination of all six body areas, HNTAUL, was expected only in forty-five cases but found in 262—this is statistically very significant, but materially not substantial if it is remembered that the total number of injured occupants is 57,597.

Originally, all three alternatives were used, but the statistical one was selected for presentation. In broad terms, each method actually resulted in about the same kind of ranking of the leading positive and negative associations.

Based on the chi-square statistic, shown in Table 1-V, the five leading positive associations and the five leading negative associations (these ten alone are responsible for about 75 per cent of the total chi-square calculated from the data) are given below:

INJURY COMBINATION	CHI-SQUARE
Positive Associations:	
HTAUL	1,438
HNTAUL	1,050
H	535
N	447
HTUL	426

Negative Associations:

TL	198
HAL	169
HA	145
HU	140
HTU	129

The above data and a careful examination of Table 1-V provide findings of some interest. First, the chi-squares for the leading positive associations are much larger than those for the leading negative associations. This seems to indicate that the tendency of certain body areas to cluster is

TABLE 1-V
LISTING OF CHI-SQUARES IN DESCENDING ORDER

Body Area Combination and Chi-Square

HTAUL	1438+*	HNTAL	49+	HN	8
HNTAUL	1050+	HT	46	AUL	7
H	535+	NTA	41+	UL	6
N	447+	NTL	35	TAU	5
HTUL	426+	NT	34+	HNAU	5
TL	198	NL	34	NTAL	4+
HAL	169	TA	30+	HNUL	3
HNTUL	159+	AL	28	TAUL	3+
HA	145	NUL	25	HNTAU	3+
HU	140	HTL	25	NTAUL	2+
HTU	129	HNAL	19	HNTL	2
L	123+	TAL	17	HNT	2
NA	100+	AU	16	HNA	1
HNL	98	HUL	15+	HNAUL	1
HAU	95	HNTU	14	HTAL	1+
U	84+	NTU	13	NAUL	0
TU	84	NAU	12	NAL	0
A	78+	T	11+	NTAU	0+
HNU	73	NU	11	HAUL	0
HL	56	NTUL	10	HTAU	0
TUL	54	HNTA	9+	HTA	0+
				Total	4642+
					1586(−)

* The +-sign identifies those combinations where the observed frequency is higher than the expected one; in others, the reverse is true.

stronger than the tendency of certain body areas *not* to cluster. This appears to be in line with the statement already made, namely, that automobile accident injury tends to be multiple; yet the issue is somewhat more complex. The leading negative associations are multiple injuries, too, but their negative sign is indicative of existence of a *pattern* to the multiplicity of injury: Combinations such as HTU, for example, are not seen as frequently as expected, for if the impact is of the type to involve HTU, it is quite likely to involve L as well, so as to result in HTUL which again is seen more frequently than expected, assuming independency among body area involvements.

Second, and not so obvious from the few leading associations shown above (and becoming obvious only after a detailed perusal of Table 1-V), the excess numbers (positive associations) are concentrated on either one body area injuries or on the truly multiple area injuries (four body areas at least), but not on the two or three area injuries. The negative associations, on the other hand, are primarily found among the two or three area combinations. In numbers from Table 1-IV, single area injuries were expected in 13,724 cases but found in 17,303; four or more body area injuries expected in 6,398 but found in 8,400; two or three body area injuries, on the other hand, were expected in 36,474 cases but found only in 31,894.

Interpretation of these findings is difficult on the basis of crude overall data only. The excess number of certain injury combinations may reflect some characteristics of the human body under impact conditions, but it may also be simply the result of a large number of accidents of a specific type which creates conditions suitable for those particular injury combinations. A thorough study of such relationships must take into account the type of impact—and other variables as well—but the present report is not designed to go into those details.

SUMMARY

The injury patterns of 57,597 injured passenger car occupants were examined in terms of six gross areas of the human body.

1. The head was most frequently involved, the neck least frequently.
2. Multiple injury was found to be a rule rather than an exception. In only 30 per cent of the injured persons was the injury limited to one body area only.
3. Large differences were demonstrated among injury combinations in regard to severity of injury. In general, the more body areas involved, the more severe the overall injury.
4. Similarly, large differences were demonstrated in regard to lethality of high risk injuries (fraction of nearly immediate deaths among those suffering high risk injury). Again the multiple injuries were generally classified as most frequently lethal.
5. A demonstration was given of how certain injury combinations occur more frequently and others less frequently than expected statistically. In general, either one body area or four or more body areas were involved more frequently than expected, two or three body areas less frequently.

REFERENCES

1. *Current Estimates From the Health Interview Survey.* United States—July 1966–June 1967. National Center for Health Statistics, Series 10, Number 43, Jan. 1968.
2. *Accident Facts,* 1967 ed. Chicago, National Safety Council, 1967.
3. BRAUNSTEIN, PAUL W.: Medical aspects of automotive crash injury research. *JAMA,* 163:249–255, 1957.
4. GÖGLER, EBERHARD: *Road Accidents.* Series Chirurgica Geigy No. 5, 1962.
5. SLĀTIS, PÄR: *Injury Patterns in Road Traffic Accidents.* Health Services Research of the National Board of Health, Finland, March 1967.
6. Reference is made to the dozens of ACIR technical reports from 1952 through 1967.
7. KIHLBERG, JAAKKO K.: Interaction of injury factors in automobile accidents. *Automobilismo e Automobilismo Industriale,* 2:1–31, 1967.

STATISTICAL APPENDIX 1-I

The statistical problem to be resolved is estimation of parameters of a multifactorial distribution from data which are incomplete (truncated) in that no information is given on the frequency in the "zero" (no injury) category. For simplicity, the situation will be exemplified by a three-factorial distribution; the solution can be generalized to the six-factorial as well as any multifactorial distribution.

The General Situation

Suppose that there are just three body areas A, B, and C (e.g., head, trunk, and extremities), and that the injury probabilities of each (parameters of the three-factorial distribution) are p_A, p_B, and p_C. If the assumption of independence is made, then the expected relative frequencies of the eight possible injury combinations are as follows:

INJURY COMBINATION	EXPECTED RELATIVE FREQUENCY
0 (No injury)	$(1-p_A)(1-p_B)(1-p_C)$
A	$p_A(1-p_B)(1-p_C)$
B	$(1-p_A)p_B(1-p_C)$
C	$(1-p_A)(1-p_B)p_C$
AB	$p_A p_B (1-p_C)$
AC	$p_A (1-p_B) p_C$
BC	$(1-p_A) p_B p_C$
ABC	$p_A p_B p_C$
Total	1

Adding up those components which contain A (body area A injured) yields the following:

$$p_A(1-p_B)(1-p_C)$$
$$+ p_A p_B (1-p_C)$$
$$+ p_A (1-p_B) p_C$$
$$+ p_A p_B p_C$$

$$= p_A$$

Obviously, the same holds for B and C.

Let now a sample of N observations be taken from the three–factorial distribution, and let the observed number in each injury combination be denoted as follows:

INJURY COMBINATION	OBSERVED NUMBER
0	n(0)
A	n(A)
B	n(B)
C	n(C)
AB	n(AB)
AC	n(AC)
BC	n(BC)
ABC	n(ABC)
Total	N

The total number of A-involvements is $n_A = n(A) + n(AB) + n(AC) + n(ABC)$, and similarly for B and C. The expected number of A-involvements is equal to $p_A N$, and therefore the sample estimator of p_A is equal to $p_A^* = n_A/N$. Similarly for B and C. Note carefully *that the expected value of n_A is proportional to p_A, that of n_B to p_B, and that of n_C to p_C.* This fact provided for straightforward estimation of the p's.

Truncated Data

Suppose now that the number of uninjured persons, n(0) is not known. Then the observer is in possession of only the following data:

INJURY COMBINATION	OBSERVED NUMBER
A	n(A)
B	n(B)
C	n(C)
AB	n(AB)
AC	n(AC)
BC	n(BC)
ABC	n(ABC)
Total	M

Since n(0) is not known, N cannot be determined either, and available is only M, the number of injured. Among these, the number of A-involvements still is $n_A = n(A) + n(AB) + n(AC) + n(ABC)$, and similarly for B and C, but $s_A = n_A/M$ is *not* an estimator of p_A: $s_A = n_A/M = n_A/(N-n(0)) \neq n_A/N$. However, the expected value of n_A is proportional to p_A, as is that of s_A, and these facts provide for a method of estimation.

DISCUSSION

B. J. CAMPBELL

Dr. Kihlberg's chapter very well documents the fact that the characteristic result of an automobile accident is victims who have serious injuries, who have multiple injuries, and who have head and leg injuries.

Dr. Kihlberg has shown, however, that certain patterns of injury occur with great regularity, and that certain other patterns of injury are quite unusual. He shows that these departures go far beyond what would be expected if only chance variation were at work.

No doubt it would also be shown that the characteristic type, patterns, and severity of the crashes themselves that produce these frequent and infrequent injury patterns differ greatly from one another. No doubt it is the case that the most frequent types of injuries accompany the most frequent types of accidents, etc.

One of the most interesting aspects of the chapter is Dr. Kihlberg's clever treatment of the data to avoid certain problems imposed by Cornell's sampling procedure. Cornell data are based on injury-producing rural accidents. Thus, since the criteria for admission into the sample is that an injury has occurred, it becomes difficult to relate these findings to those based on samples of all events—including those in which injury does not occur.

Dr. Kihlberg has used an ingenious approach in his estimates, and has developed a procedure that should be useful in other future studies. The statistical appendix merits careful review.

I would like to comment on another problem which faces Cornell or any other research project that depends on collecting large amounts of data from the field to study the highway accident or injury problem. This is the necessity for linking up and synthesizing medical information gathered at one place and under one set of circumstances, and relating these to antecedent information about accidents which was collected under other circumstances and by other people.

The Cornell project has met this problem through a sampling procedure in which physicians are asked to cooperate in filling out special forms. It seems worthwhile to consider alternate, supplementary approaches to that employed by Cornell. For example, there is now in existence a data processing system called "PAS" in which certain in-patient data are recorded. This includes diagnosis, treatment, etc. This information is entered into a central records system and is compiled nationally. Hundreds of hospitals now participate.

While the identity of these patients is not retained, there seems to be at least a small ray of hope that one day it will be possible to link sets of records such as these with other record banks.

It will be worth some considerable amount of effort to search for ways to link hospital data files on injuries and treatment with data files on accident events generated by the police. It would of course be possible to set up safeguards to protect patient identity. The fruits of such file linkages would be the ability to carry out an increased scope of research covering both the antecedent events and the proper medical diagnosis and treatment later on.

Chapter II

MECHANISMS OF HEAD INJURY

L. Murray Thomas

Much has been and more will be written about the mechanical factors involved in head injury. Ours is a highly mobile and mechanical culture, and the potential for head injury as a major cause of physical, psychological and economic crippling becomes greater each year. If we are to rationally discuss head protection, we must understand the mechanisms involved in all forms of head injury. A protection against one form of trauma may substantially lead to a greater risk from another.

Head injury may be considered under many headings as seen in Table 2–I.

TABLE 2–I
VARIETIES OF HEAD INJURIES

Scalp	Intracranial Clot
Laceration	Epidural
Subgaleal Hematoma	Subdural
Skull Fracture	Brain Injury
Linear	Contusion
Depressed	Laceration
Perforating	Intracerebral Clot
	Concussion

Each of these headings is a subject for extensive discussion. Much is known about causal factors—more is yet to be learned. It is the purpose of this presentation to discuss cerebral concussion: its definition, neuroanatomic and neurophysiologic basis and causal factors. The fact that skull fracture, intracranial hematoma and crushing injuries are not discussed is not to be considered as evidence that the author is unaware of their importance, but rather expresses the fundamental need to understand cerebral concussion.

CEREBRAL CONCUSSION

Concussion is defined by Dorland[5] as ". . . a violent jar or shock or a condition which results from it." More recently a committee of the Congress of Neurological Surgeons defined brain concussion as ". . . a clinical syndrome characterized by immediate and transient impairment of neural function, such as alteration of consciousness, disturbance of vision, equilibrium, etc., due to mechanical forces."[15] The same group further defined consciousness as ". . . a state of general wakefulness and responsiveness to environment."[15]

Our discussion is to be confined to that form of concussion known as cerebral concussion: ". . . that immediate post-traumatic unconscious state; not associated with macroscopic lesions of the brain; frequently reversible but potentially fatal; and associated, in the human, with amnesia." This is, in fact, the form of concussion under consideration by most of the recent authors on the subject, minor differences in semantics notwithstanding.

CONSCIOUSNESS

Consciousness is the expression and awareness of an *aroused* mind. Consciousness may be inferred in the experimental animal. As discussed by Plum and Posner[27] consciousness has two components: content and a crude on-off quality. It is to the latter that our attention should be directed in the understanding of cerebral concussion. Current evidence indicates that no single cortical lesion or combination of lesions confined to the cortex alone will alter the basic substrate of consciousness.[32] On the other hand, the central core of the brain, the brain stem (Fig. 2–1), is directly concerned with consciousness, particularly that portion called the reticular formation by Magoun.[23] This formation, the ascending reticular activating system (ARAS), does not possess homogeneous properties of control over the CNS throughout its length. Only the diencephalic and midbrain portions are capable of creating the rapid shifts in the reactivity of the central nervous system related to consciousness.[29] The caudal extent of the structures critical to consciousness does not appear to extend lower than the trigeminal nerve.[27] Batini,[1] Jouvet[20,21] and others report an alert appearance in animals with midpontine and retropontine brain stem transections.

The reticular formation in the lower pons and medulla is the site of the important activating and suppressor centers for respiratory and vasomotor control. Many other complex integrating, facilitating and suppressing areas interconnect the ARAS with all components of the CNS. Areas responsible for decerebrate posturing, extensor jerks and rigidity and flaccid paralysis exist in this complex structure. We shall confine ourselves to the crude dichotomy existing between the upper ARAS controlling the basic substrate of consciousness and the lower or medullary reticular system controlling the vegetative functions of blood pressure, heart rate and rhythm and respiration.

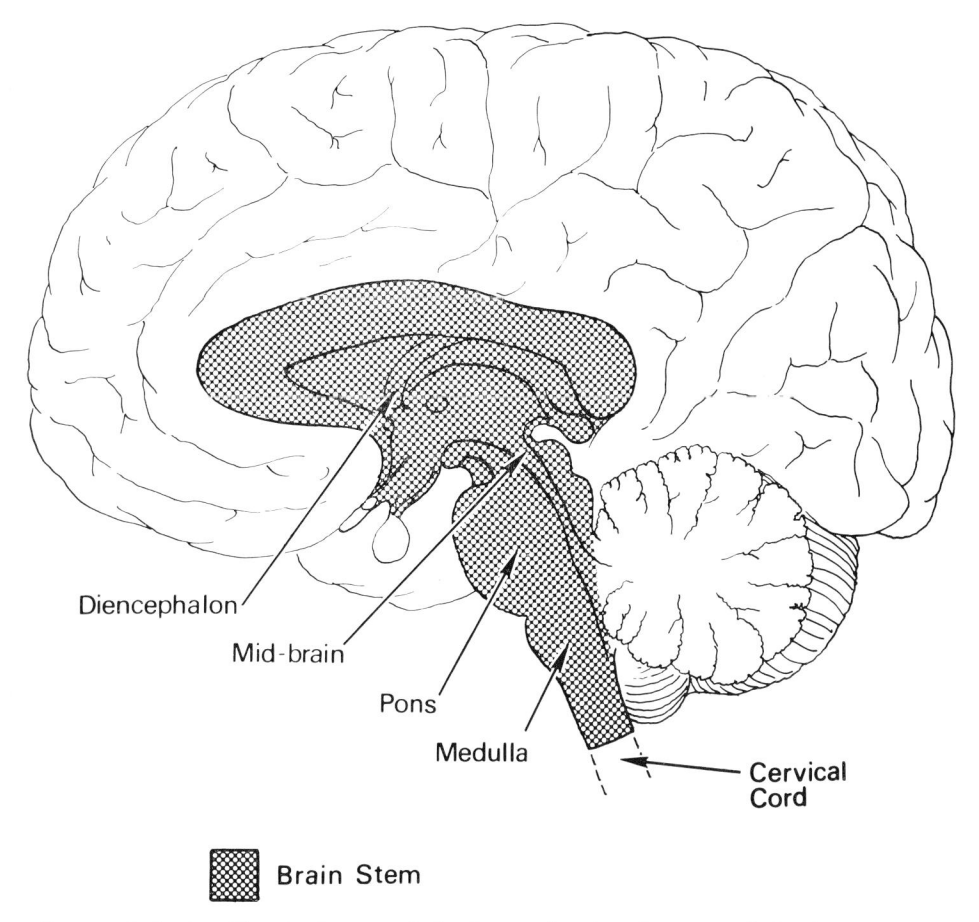

FIGURE 2-1. A midsagittal view of the brain showing the area of the brain stem.

What evidence exists that the upper reticular formation controls consciousness? Stimulation of this area causes arousal in the sleeping animal.[7] Destruction of the area produces a state of chronic unresponsiveness.[8] Evoked potentials, produced by stimulating a peripheral nerve, can be recorded along the classic pathways of touch to the cortex. A similar evoked potential, of longer latency, can be recorded in the ARAS. This latter evoked potential, in the reticular formation, is abolished following a concussive blow as shown by Foltz and Schmidt.[6]

CEREBRAL CONCUSSION VERSUS MEDULLARY CONCUSSION

It is necessary to realize that a localized lesion in the diencephalon can produce unconsciousness without changes in vasomotor control and respiration. It is just as important to realize that medullary and upper cervical cord lesions can produce apnea, blood pressure changes, loss of corneal reflex without loss of consciousness. In fact, as shown by Walker,[4] these symptoms can be produced by head injury in a decerebrate animal.

It is obvious that many, and possibly most, forms of "concussion" producing head trauma involve the entire brain stem. Early investigators[2,11] studied animals under light analgesia and were able to observe changes in conscious reaction. Denny-Brown and Russell[2] described ". . . an orderly succession of recovery of nervous function . . ." and defined experimental concussion therefore by its ". . . profound effect on respiration and blood pressure, on corneal and pinna reflexes. . . ." Denny-Brown, however, later implied that the corneal reflex was the most important criteria of concussion.[3] There is no question that the loss of the corneal reflex in their methodology was well equated to cerebral concussion but their criteria were, nonetheless, expressions of medullary involvement and could all be obtained without loss of consciousness in a decerebrate animal. As long as the method of producing concussion remained unchanged, it was proper to relate concussion to the medullary signs so carefully observed. It is unfair, however, to produce trauma in an entirely different manner, as reported by Hollister[19] and Friede[5,10] relative to stretching of the cervical cord in the cat, and deduce cerebral concussion on the basis of corneal reflex loss. Put another way, trauma which injures the medulla and medullary cervical function may produce the "classic symptoms" of experimental concussion in an anesthetized animal. It is possible that cervical stretch may produce unconsciousness but there is no good evidence for this as yet, in my opinion. Each new method of experimentally producing a concussion must be measured against loss of consciousness in the unanesthetized animal or by abolition of evoked potentials in the appropriate area of the reticular formation. Without this confirmation arguments regarding mechanisms of concussion are without merit.

THE FINAL COMMON PATH OF CEREBRAL CONCUSSION

Loss of consciousness, caused by upper or midbrain reticular system dysfunction, and vasomotor and respiratory changes from reticular system dysfunction in the pontine-medullary area may occur simultaneously and, in fact, usually do so. The mechanism most likely responsible for dysfunction in this area was deduced by Gurdjian and Webster in 1945.[12] This mechanism, the production of shear stress along the brain stem axis by the flow generated from intracranial pressure gradients was confirmed by birefringent dye studies.[13] (Fig. 2–2) Holbourn[17] pointed out that the ratio of the brain's compressibility to its elasticity rendered shear the damaging stress while compression was likely negligible.

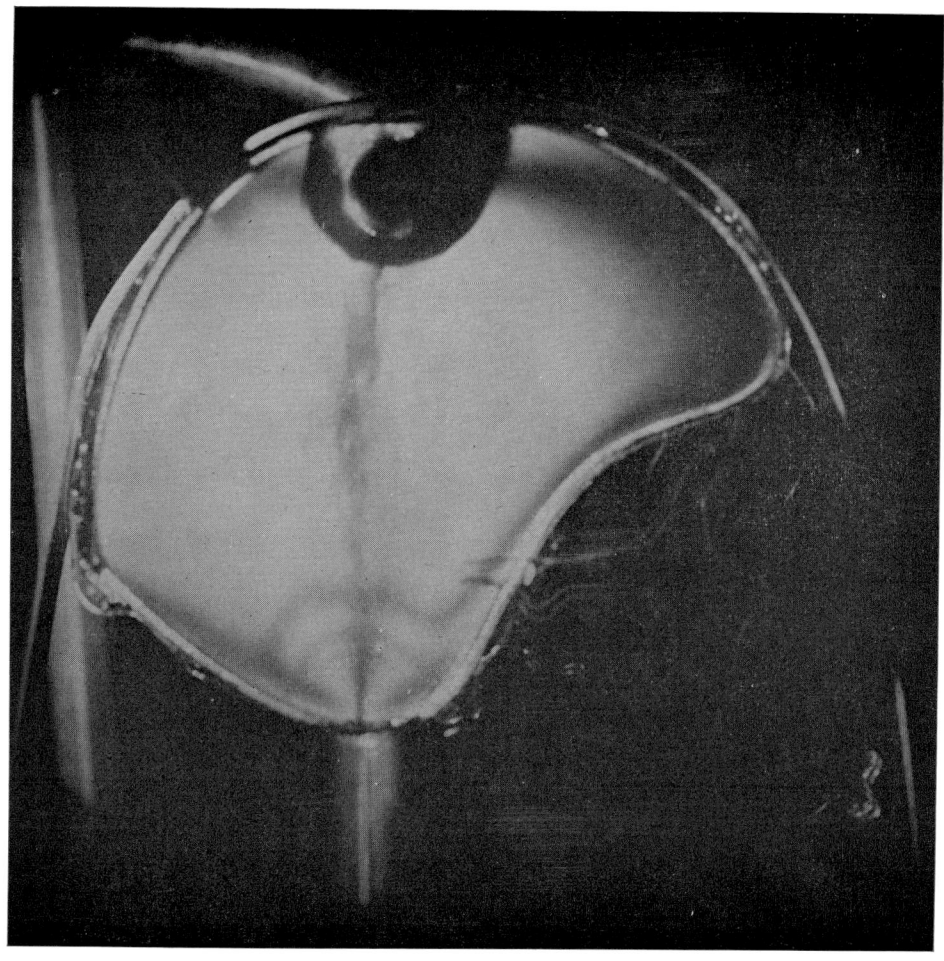

FIGURE 2–2. Stress concentration demonstrated by birefringent fluid in a sagittal skull model at impact.

We propose to present shear stress along the brain stem axis as the final common path of concussion and to point out that this shear stress is developed most easily by pressure gradient induced flow of the brain and brain stem from the cranial cavity through the tentorial incisura and foramen magnum. Stretching forces from below as inferred from Hollister[19] and Friede[10] may, theoretically at least, contribute to this effect.

The presence of such an elastic flow has been shown in our laboratories by high speed x-ray studies[16] (Figs. 2–3,4,5,6). The movement of the lead pellets placed across the brain stem and medulla is clearly time and pressure related and is developed by impact and by air blast to the dura. These studies confirm the deductions of Gurdjian and Webster, and Gurdjian

32   *Impact Injury and Crash Protection*

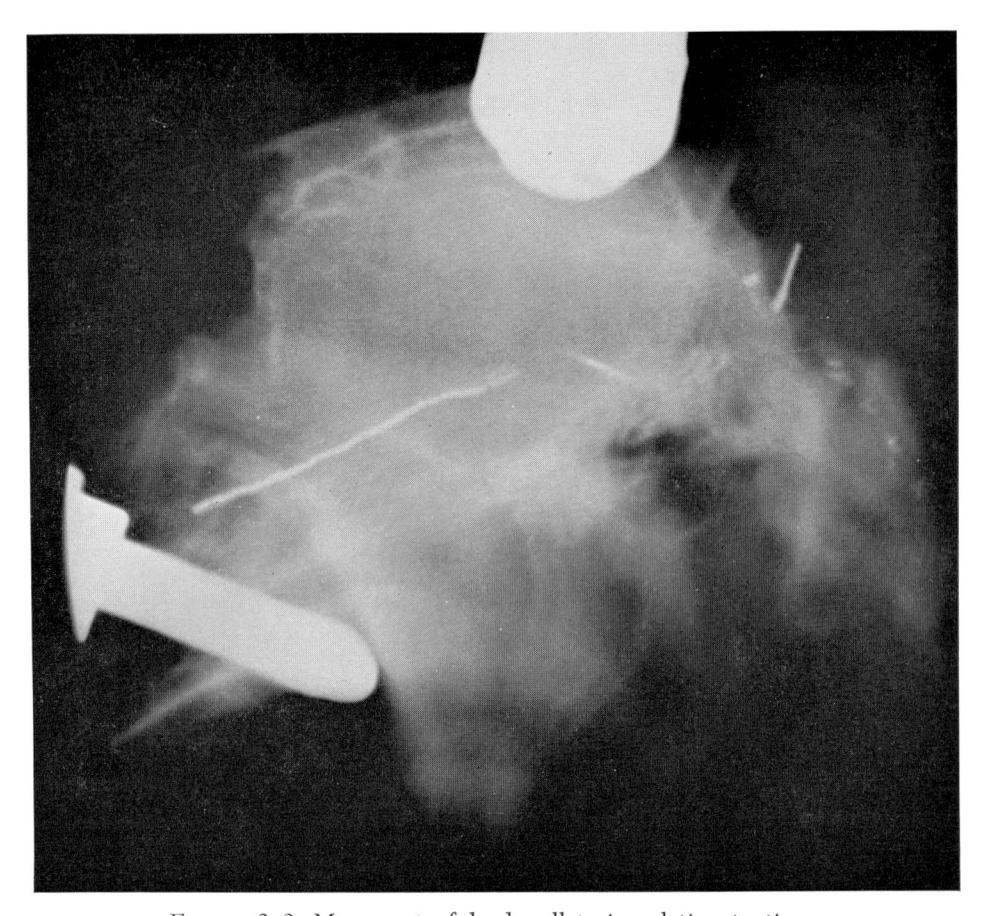

FIGURE 2–3. Movement of lead pellets in relation to time.

and Lissner, and correlate with the shear stress pattern shown by birefringent model studies.

I wish to point out to those who are not neurosurgeons that the physiologic changes seen in the phenomenon of concussion are mimicked, except in time span, by tumors and intracranial hematomas which increase cerebral pressure and force a downward herniation of the brain stem through the incisura and foramen magnum.

METHODS TO INDUCE PRESSURE GRADIENTS

In order for flow to take place in a rigid container, a portion of the wall must be elastic or otherwise deformable. Under these circumstances increased pressure within the container will cause a flow toward and through the opening. The skull represents a rigid container containing a noncom-

Mechanisms of Head Injury 33

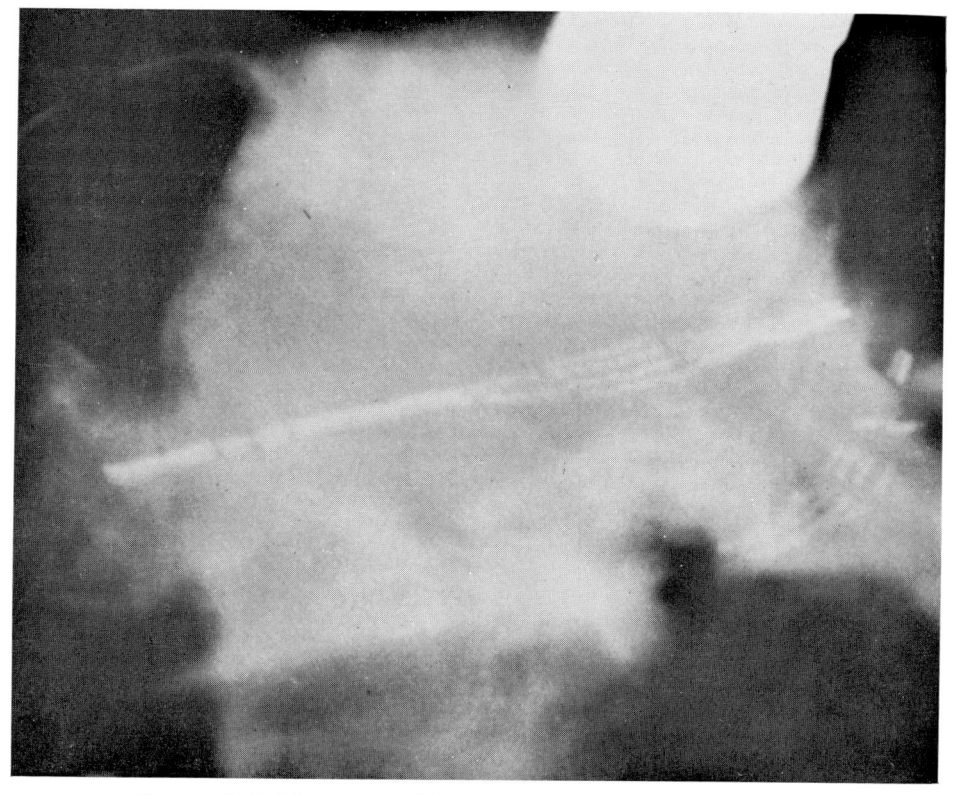

FIGURE 2-4. Movement of lead pellets in relation to pressure.

pressible material and the foramen magnum acts as the elastic portion of the container. (Fig. 2-7)

Obviously the simplest way to displace brain through the foramen magnum is to reduce the volume of the skull. The skull is an elipsoid, and volume may increase or decrease depending upon the axis of deformation as pointed out by Unterharnscheidt.[31] This has recently been confirmed in our laboratory by measuring skull volume during static deformation. (Fig. 2-8) When deformation occurs and decreases skull volume, the brain will tend to extrude through the incisura and foramen magnum. This is most pronounced in transverse axis deformation. In the A-P axis, the volume actually increases. The value to be assigned to a decrease in skull volume seems low. Our method of producing experimental concussion by an air blast against the intact dura[14] is an experimental model duplicating this situation and clearly produced brain stem signs, cellular damage in the brain stem (Fig. 2-9) and elastic deformation of the brain stem (Fig. 2-3).

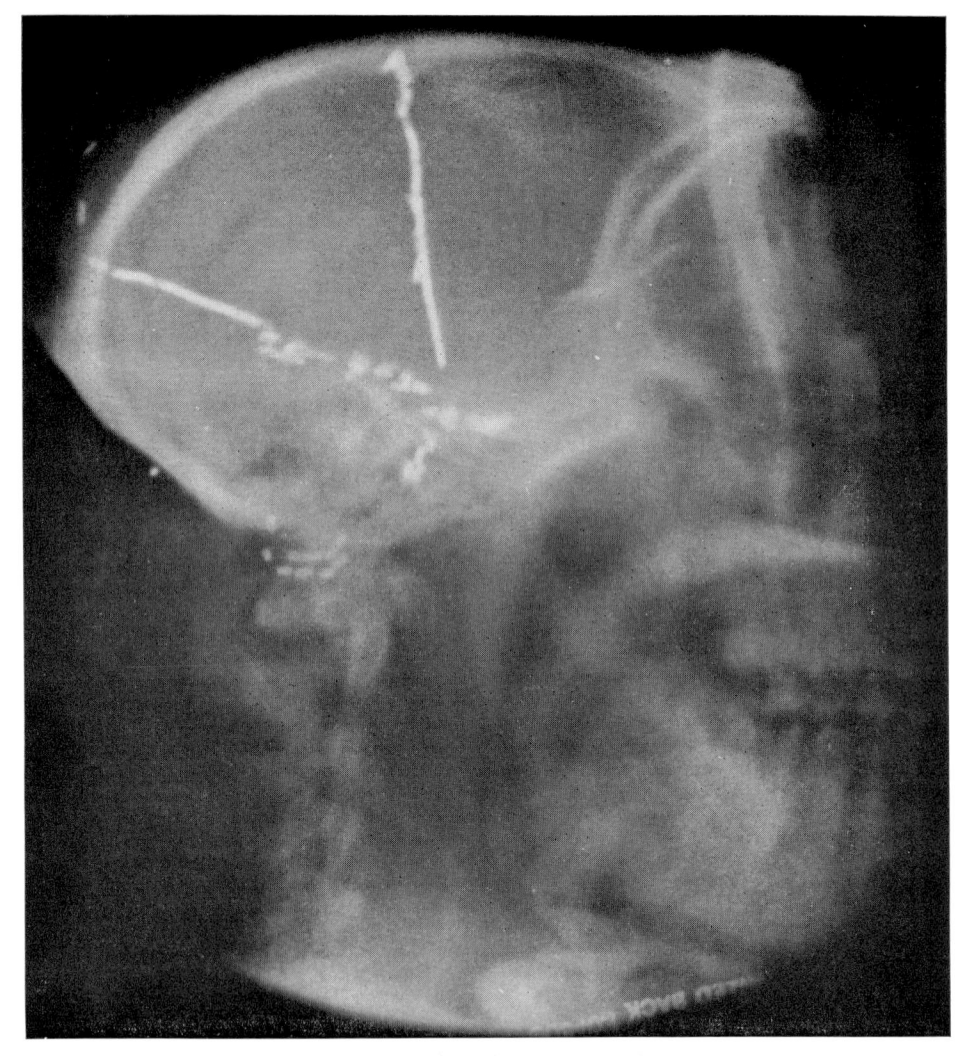

FIGURE 2-5. Movement of lead pellets in relation to impact.

ACCELERATION INDUCED PRESSURE GRADIENTS

It is manifestly impossible to strike a head without acceleration even though efforts are made to fix the head in space. High speed movies clearly confirm this observation. Acceleration of a fluid-filled container will induce a pressure gradient along the axis of acceleration. Such data has been presented by Sellier and Unterharnscheidt[28] and by Lindgren.[22] We have confirmed this in a water-filled skull measuring simultaneous pressures at five points along each of three axes in the skull. (Fig. 2-10) More recent studies utilizing a silastic-filled model have demonstrated cavitation at the

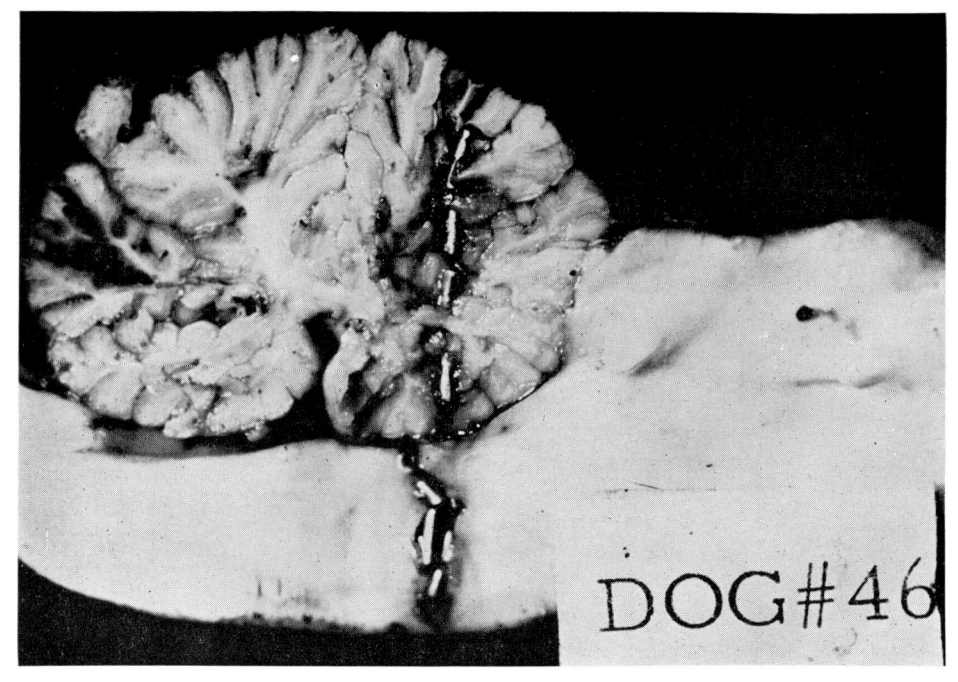

FIGURE 2-6. Gross anatomic view of lead pellets *in situ*.

antipole as predicted by Unterharnscheidt[28] and shown earlier by Gross[24] in a glass sphere.

The effect of this acceleration is twofold. The negative pressure at the antipole may easily reach −1 atmosphere and cavitation may result producing local lesions. Although the negative pressure may not exceed −1 atmosphere, the effect of this may reach greater depths with increasing levels of acceleration. This phenomenon is probably not related to cerebral concussion, as defined, although it may be of great importance in head injury.

When an acceleration induced pressure gradient develops in a container with an elastic opening the zero or nodal point will move toward that opening indicating flow (Fig. 2-10). It may be inferred that acceleration is a potent cause of increased intracranial pressure. It is our impression that acceleration of the head is a most important factor in concussion.

TRANSLATIONAL VERSUS ANGULAR ACCELERATION

Much attention has been directed by Ommaya *et al.*[24,25,26] regarding the importance of angular acceleration. Great emphasis has been placed on the theoretical proposal voiced by Holbourn.[17,18]

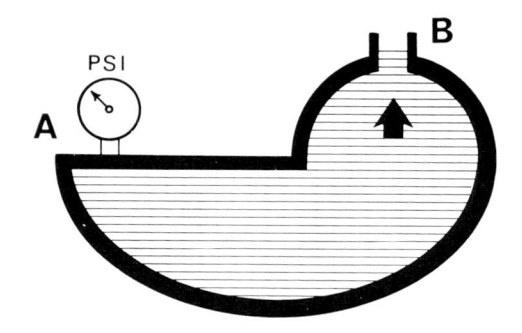

PRESSURE INCREASE AT A. WILL CAUSE A
RISE IN FLUID LEVEL AT B.

FIGURE 2–7. Schematic representation of rigid skull and elastic foramen magnum.

Holbourn postulated that translational or linear acceleration would have a negligible effect and that rotational acceleration would produce maximum shear. The elastic deformity possible at foramen magnum was apparently neglected. There is no question that angular acceleration is important. I believe that it functions in two ways. First, angular acceleration will cause a shear that is normal or perpendicular to the radius of rotation. This mechanism may clearly result in cortical and subcortical injuries of great magnitude as shown by Strich,[30] if the forces are great enough.

Secondly, and of more importance in concussion, is the effect of angular acceleration upon pressure gradients across the skull. Angular acceleration produces, at any point, an acceleration vector which can be resolved into components, one additive to the translational acceleration induced by the blow and the other perpendicular to it (Fig. 2–11). High speed movie studies show clearly that both linear and angular motion result from head impact. (Fig. 2–12).

We believe that this effect, i.e. increasing the acceleration induced pressure gradient, is the operative factor in concussion. When the head is free to move on the neck, angular acceleration occurs more readily and permits a greater pressure build-up. If similar accelerations are obtained when the neck is fixed, similar results may be expected. A careful study of Ommaya's results reported in 1964[21] confirms this postulate. (Fig. 2–12) Higher accelerations were derived from similar energy input with the neck free. However, when similar accelerations were recorded, concussion was reported in each group. The effect would therefore seem to be acceleration related rather than to movement per se at the craniospinal junction. It must be emphasized that all of these effects are time dependent.

FRONTAL LOADING

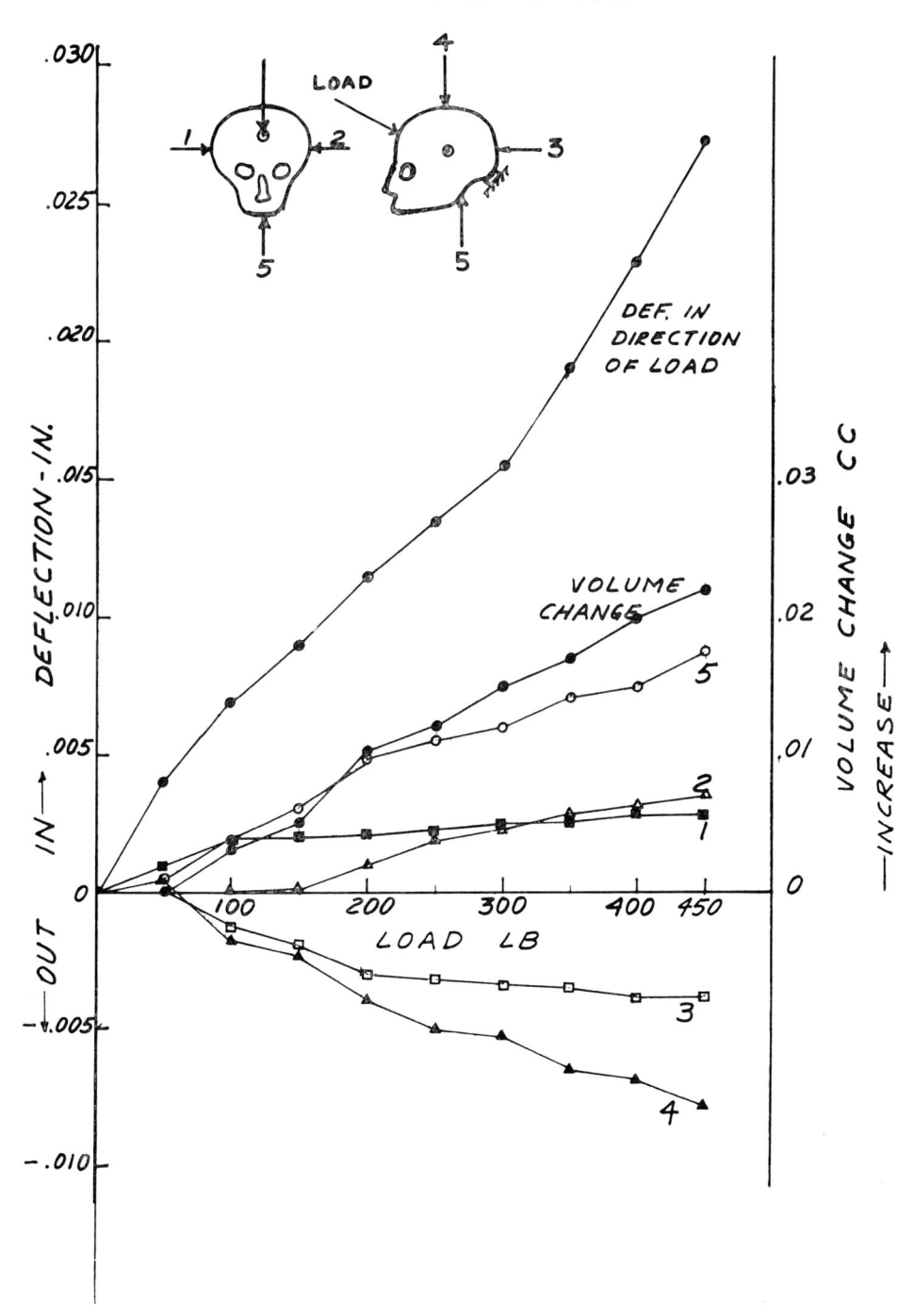

FIGURE 2–8. Skull deflection and volume change in relation to varying frontal loads.

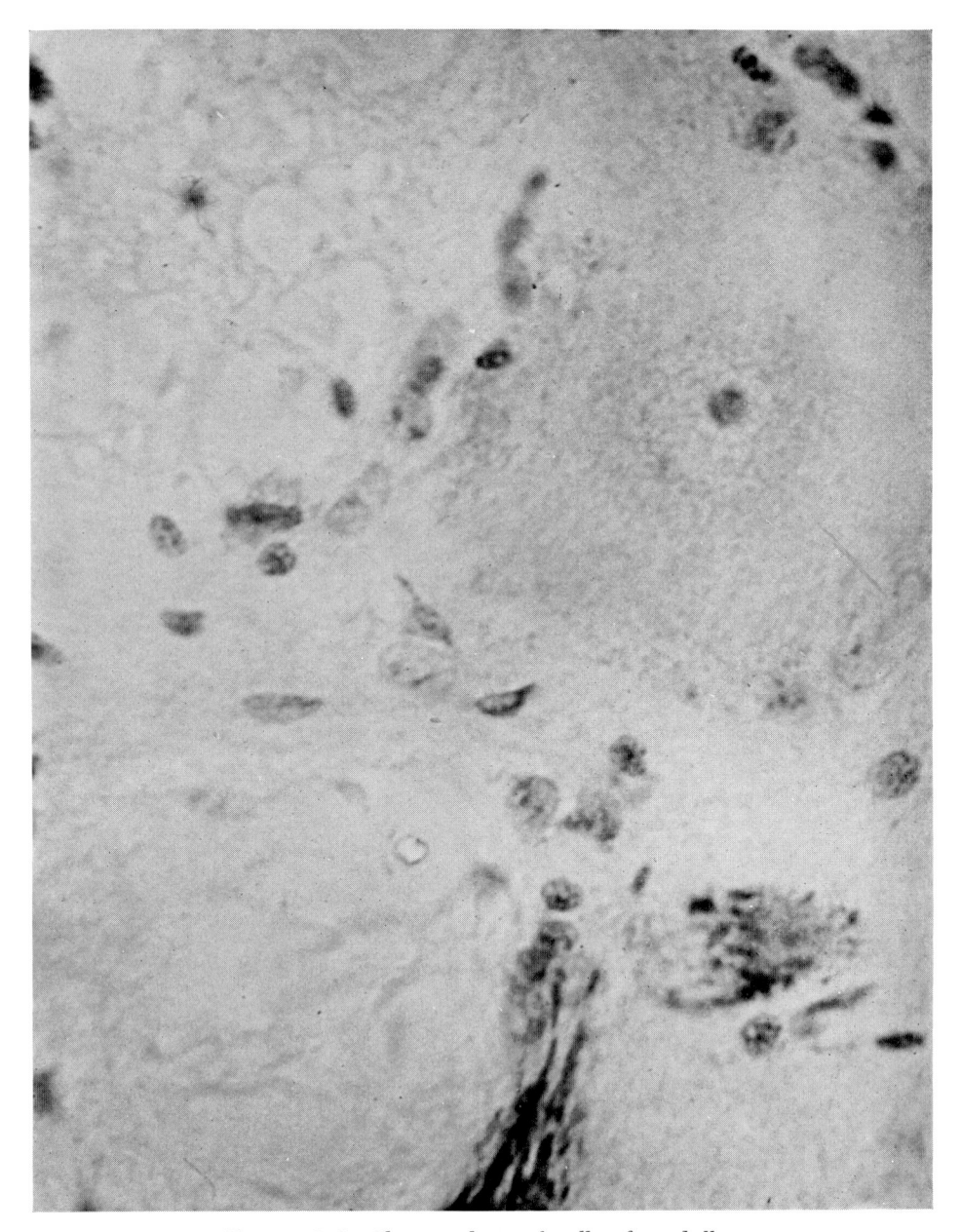

FIGURE 2-9. Chromatolysis of cells of medulla.

SUMMARY

Cerebral concussion is mediated through the brain stem reticular formation and conscious control is centered in the ARAS of the midbrain.

The final common path of cerebral concussion is in the shear stress

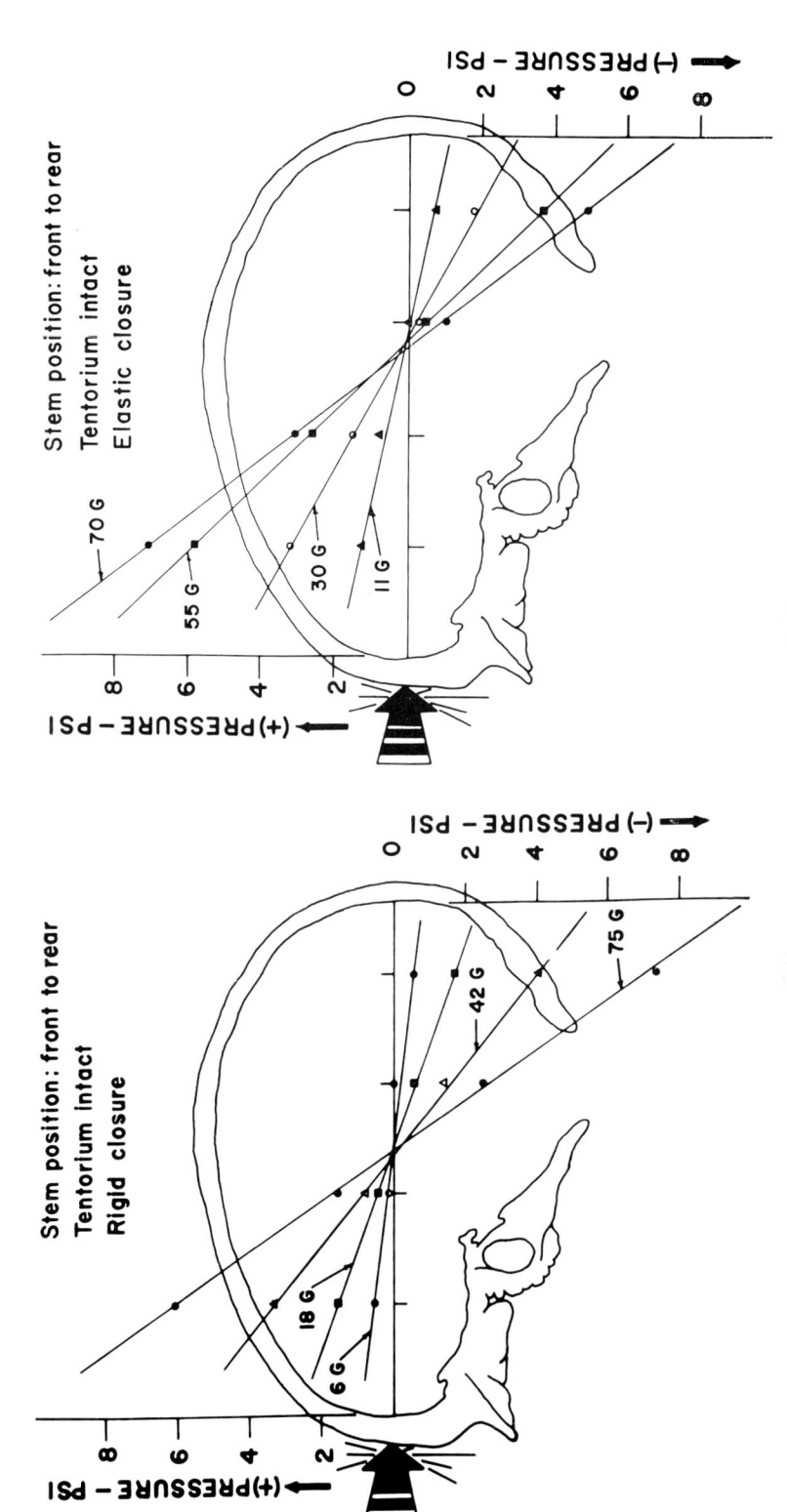

FIGURE 2–10. Impact induced pressure gradients across skull. Left, with rigid closure at foramen magnum; right, with an elastic closure.

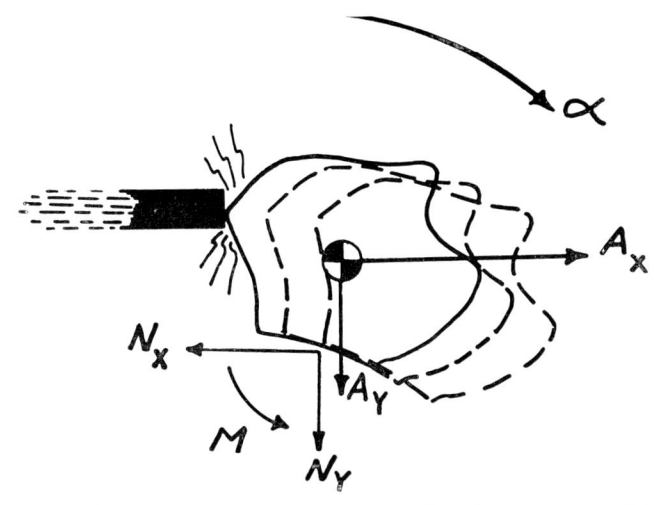

FIGURE 2-11. Schematic representation at accelerations generated by impact.

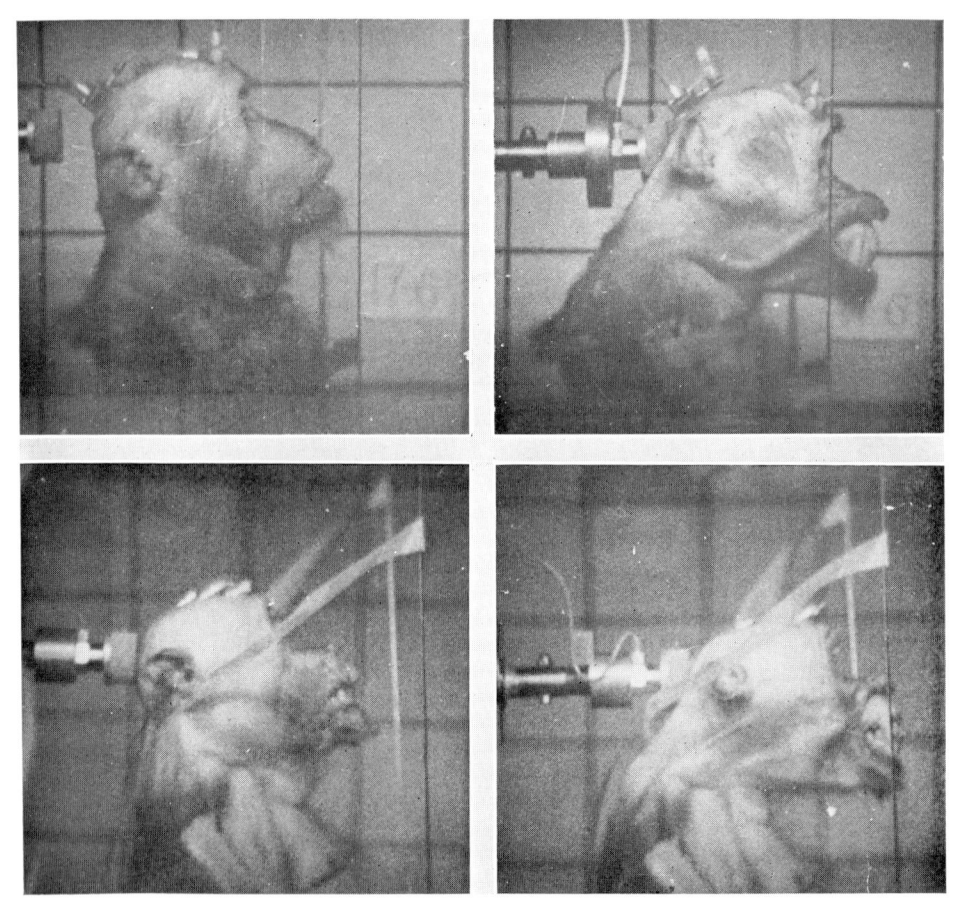

FIGURE 2-12. Selected frames from high speed movie to show head movements at impact.

developed in the brain stem as a result of elastic flow. This flow is produced by pressure gradients along the brain stem axis.

Acceleration, both translational and angular, appears to be the most powerful cause of increased intracranial pressure.

Unorthodox methods of producing concussion must be measured against loss of consciousness and not against the functions of the medullary reticular formation.

REFERENCES

1. BATINI, C., et al.: Effects of complete pontine transections on the sleep-wakefulness rhythm: the mid-pontine pretrigeminal preparation. Arch Ital Biol, 97:1–2, 1959.
2. DENNY-BROWN, D., and RUSSELL, W. RITCHIE: Experimental cerebral concussion. Brain, 64:93–164, 1941.
3. DENNY-BROWN, D.: Cerebral concussion. Physiol Rev, 25:296–325, 1945.
4. Discussion—Symposium on head injuries, Dr. A. Earl Walker. J Neurosurg, 15:157–158, 1958.
5. Dorland's Illustrated Medical Dictionary, 23rd ed. Philadelphia, Saunders, 1957.
6. FOLTZ, E.L., and SCHMIDT, R.P.: The role of the reticular formation in the coma of head injury. J Neurosurg, 13:145–154, 1956.
7. FRENCH, J.D.; VON AMERONGEN, F.K., and MAGOUN, H.W.: An activating system in the brain of the monkey. Arch Neurol Psychiat, 68:577–580, 1952.
8. FRENCH, J.D., and MAGOUN, H.W.: Effects of chronic lesions in the cephalic brain stem of monkeys. Arch Neurol Psychiat, 68:591–604, 1952.
9. FRIEDE, REINHARD: Biophysics of concussion. WADC Technical Report 58–193, Wright-Patterson Air Force Base, Ohio, Sept. 1958, pt. II.
10. FRIEDE, REINHARD: Specific cord damage at the atlas level as a pathogenic mechanism in cerebral concussion. J Neuropath Exp Neurol, 19:266–279, 1960.
11. GURDJIAN, E.S., and WEBSTER, J.E.: Experimental head injury with special reference to mechanical factors in acute trauma. Surg Gynec Obstet, 76:623–634, 1943.
12. GURDJIAN, E.S., and WEBSTER, J.E.: Experimental and clinical studies on the mechanism of head injury. In Trauma of the Central Nervous System. Baltimore, Williams & Wilkins, 1945, p. 48.
13. GURDJIAN, E.S., and LISSNER, H.R.: Photoelastic confirmation of the presence of shear strains at the craniospinal junction in closed head injury. J Neurosurg, 18:58–60, 1961.
14. HADDAD, B.F.; CHASON, J.L.; LISSNER, H.R.; WEBSTER, JOHN E., and GURDJIAN, E.S.: Alterations in cell structure following sudden increase in intracranial pressure. Surg Forum, 6:496–498, 1956.
15. CAVENESS, WILLIAM F., and WALKER, A. EARL (EDS.): Head injury glossary (appendix). In Head Injury Conference Proceedings. Philadelphia, Lippincott, 1966, pp. 571–576.
16. HODGSON, V.R.; GURDJIAN, E.S., and THOMAS, L.M.: Experimental skull deformation and brain displacement demonstrated by flash x-ray technique. J Neurosurg, 25:549–552, 1966.
17. HOLBOURN, A.H.S.: Mechanics of head injuries. Lancet, 2:438–441, 1943.

18. Holbourn, A.H.S.: The mechanics of trauma with special reference to herniation of cerebral tissue. *J Neurol,* 1:190–200, 1944.
19. Hollister, Nathaniel R.; Jolley, William P., and Horne, Robert G.: Biophysics of concussion. *WADC Technical Report 58–193,* Wright-Patterson Air Force Base, Ohio, Sept. 1958, pt. I.
20. Jouvet, M.: Telencephalic and rhombencephalic sleep in the cat. In Wolstenholme, G.E.W., and O'Conner, J., (Eds.): *The Nature of Sleep.* Boston, Little, 1961, p. 188.
21. Jouvet, M.: Recherches sur les Structures Nerveuses et les Méchanismes Responsables des Differentes Phases du Sommeil Physiologique. *Arch Ital Biol,* 100: 125–206, 1962.
22. Lindgren, S.O.: Experimental studies of mechanical effects in head injury. *Acta Chir Scand (Suppl. 360),* 1966.
23. Magoun, H.W.: *The Waking Brain.* Springfield, Thomas, 1958.
24. Ommaya, Ayub K.; Rockoff, S. David, and Baldwin, Maitland: Experimental concussion. *J Neurosurg,* 21:249–265, 1964.
25. Ommaya, Ayub K.; Hirsch, Arthur E., and Martinez, John L.: The role of whiplash in cerebral concussion. In *Proceedings of Tenth Stapp Car Crash Conference.* Society of Automotive Engineers, Inc., 1967, p. 314.
26. Ommaya, Ayub K.; Yarnell, P.; Hirsch, A.E., and Harris, E.H.: Scaling of experimental data on cerebral concussion in sub-human primates to concussion threshold for man. In *Eleventh Stapp Car Crash Conference.* New York, Society of Automotive Engineers, Inc., 1967, p. 47.
27. Plum, Fred, and Posner, Jerome B.: *The Diagnosis of Stupor and Coma.* Philadelphia, Davis, 1966.
28. Sellier, K., and Unterharnscheidt, F.: The mechanics of the impact of violence on the skull. In *Third International Congress of Neurological Surgery,* Excerpta Medica International Congress Series No. 110. Copenhagen, Excerpta Medical Foundation, 1965, p. 87.
29. Sharpless, S., and Jasper, H.H.: Habituation of the arousal reaction. *Brain,* 79: 655–680, 1956.
30. Strich, S.J.: Shearing of nerve fibers as a cause of brain damage due to head injury. *Lancet,* 2:443–448, 1961.
31. Unterharnscheidt, Friedrich, and Sellier, Karl: Closed brain injuries: mechanics and pathomorphology. In Caveness, W.F., and Walker, A.E., (Eds.): *Head Injury Conference Proceedings.* Philadelphia, Lippincott, 1966, p. 321.

DISCUSSION

Friedrich J. Unterharnscheidt

My contribution is to discuss Dr. Thomas'[53] chapter on cerebral concussion, and in this connection to point out some aspects of the superficial and central lesions of the CNS associated with violence of high intensity.

I fully subscribe Dr. Thomas' definition that cerebral concussion is ". . . that immediate post-traumatic unconscious state not associated with macroscopic lesions of the brain."[53] I should add "nor with any detectible histological lesions produced either mechanically or after a lapse of time as the result of reactive processes, such as cerebral edema and hypoxidosis." The whole process seems to be traceless, as Spatz[50,51] observed long ago. Our experiments on rabbits and cats showed that the single violence, or blow, while strong enough to produce an uncomplicated concussion, leaves no sign that would indicate histological alterations,[54-56,59-65] let alone permanent brain damage, when examined microscopically after criteria laid down by Nissl and Spielmeyer[52] for intravital alterations. This observation is again supported by new (unpublished) experiments on rats (Unterharnscheidt, Parsons, and Ruedenberg[58]). Our viewpoint is, therefore, opposed to that taken by Dey, Fox, Simmons, Groat, Magoun, Windle and others[5-7,67-69] who reported alterations such as cell shrinkage, hyperchromatosis, etc. Several of these authors, however, point out the absence of mesodermal glial reactions. Besides, their illustrations fail to show conclusively that the described alterations are intravital lesions.

Permanent brain damage results, as we now know, after a period of latency and in the absence of primary lesions, from recurrent violence in daily or weekly intervals, or from a number of successive blows. Alterations include ischemic neurons, which are found disseminated in all cortical layers; elective necroses of the parenchyma combined with glial reaction in the cerebral cortex; disseminated and focal loss of neurons in the various sections of the ammonshorn formation, along with consecutive glial proliferation and marked alterations in the cerebellum, such as serial loss of purkinje cells and proliferated Bergmann glia, as well as destruction of neurons in the granular cell layer (see Table).[54-56,59-65] Consequently, the histological alterations take place first of all in the neurons which we know to be particularly vulnerable to hypoxia (for literature, see W. Scholz 1957[37]).

In a word, brain concussion is a clinical diagnosis. We know from Denny-Brown[2] and Russell[3] the velocity, and from our own experiments the acceleration needed to produce cerebral concussion in animal experiments

Editors Note: Supported in part by U.S.P.H.S. Grant NB 07377-07, by the Research Foundation of Texas, and the Mary K. Petersen Foundation.

TABLE 2-II

Number of impacts	Intensity of impact				Behavior	Unconsciousness	Primary traumatic alterations	Secondary traumatic alterations
	in m/sec	in km/h	Acceleration					
Single blow	7,1	25,0	Cat ≈ 205 g Rabbit ≈ 190 g		Unremarkable	None	None	None
5 successive blows	7,1	25,0	Cat ≈ 205 g Rabbit ≈ 190 g		Reversible parapareses of front legs	None	None	None
10 successive blows	7,1	25,0	Cat ≈ 205 g Rabbit ≈ 190 g		Largely reversible parapareses of front legs	None	None	Secondary traumatic lesions in cerebellum and cerebrum
10 successive blows	7,5–	27,0–	Cat > 205 g Rabbit ≈ 260 g		Irreversible parapareses of front legs	None	None	Secondary traumatic lesions in cerebrum and cerebellum.
15 successive blows	8,3	30,0	Cat > 205 g Rabbit ≈ 280 g		Tetrapareses, irreversible in front legs, reversible in hind legs except for weakness.	Occurs in part of experiments after summation. "Summation type."	None	Secondary traumatic lesions. Cerebellum, severe. Cerebrum, moderate.
Single blow	8,3–9,4	30,0–34,0	Cat ≈ 315 g Rabbit ≈ 400 g		Unremarkable after regaining consciousness	General unconsciousness, lasting from several seconds to minutes.	None	None
Single blow repeated at daily and weekly intervals, resp.	8,3–9,4	30,0–34,0	Cat ≈ 315 g Rabbit ≈ 400 g		Unremarkable after regaining consciousness.	General unconsciousness. Its duration is reduced as the number of blows is increased. "Adaptation type."	None	Cerebrum: Disseminated ischemic alterations. Elective necroses of parenchyma. Loss of neurons and glia reaction in Ammonshorn. Cerebellum: Loss of Purkinje cells and granular cells.

Subconcussive strength. Subcommotio cerebri.

Concussive strength
Commotio cerebri = cerebal concussion.

Mechanisms of Head Injury

Single blow	10,5	37,0	Cat ≈ 360 g Rabbit ≈ 450 g	Rather long unconsciousness.	Epidural, subdural, subarachnoidal hemorrhages. So-called cortical contusion at impact and antipole. Rupture of extra and intracerebral vessels. Central hemorrhages.	Partial and total necroses, hemorrhagic necroses, edematous lesions.
Single blow	13,6	49,0	Cat ≈ 525 g	Long unconsciousness.	Most severe primary traumatic alterations of same quality as above.	Most severe secondary traumatic alterations of same quality as above.
Single blow	16,1	58,0	Cat	Severe primary traumatic alterations and lacerations which the cats survive in rare instances.
Single blow	17,2–18,3	62,0–66,0	Cat	Most severe lesions and disruptions, involving bones and dura (open injuries). Tissue destructions and lacerations which are not survived by the cats.

Primary-traumatic alterations. | Lethal intensities.

(Sellier and Unterharnscheidt[40-42,65]). We also know from these latter investigations[40] into trauma mechanics, what degree of acceleration will produce cerebral concussion in man, and what intensities are necessary to produce primary traumatic lesions, like the so-called cortical contusions which we have renamed cortical cavitation traumas.

Further, pursuing Dr. Thomas'[53] ideas on the "pressure-induced flow of the brain and brainstem from the cranial cavity through the tentorial incisura and foramen magnum," I should like to mention the central hemorrhages that occur with high intensity violence in the midbrain, pons and medulla. With the mechanogenesis of primary traumatic cortical lesions largely explained,[15,20,21,23,32-33,40,43-51,54-65] the primary and secondary traumatic central alterations were still awaiting their analysis. This has now been achieved. It has made available the intimate knowledge of these lesions.[30,31,36,40,56,65]

To explain the primary central hemorrhages in the subependyma of the ventricles and in portions of the corpus callosum situated near the ventricles, the effects of deformation must be considered in conjunction with those of negative pressure. In the most common case of sagittal impact, the impact axis is identical with the sagittal diameter of the skull, with the effect that by subsequent deformation the bitemporal axis is lengthened and the ventricles are dilated; their volume, therefore, is increased. Since the duration of the impact is too short for the cerebrospinal fluid to fill the suddenly enlarged ventricular space, negative pressure and cavitation occur in the ventricular system and walls in a way similar to that observed at the point opposite and across from the impact point. We have called this phenomenon "central cavitation effect."[40,65] According to the theory, the ventricular walls and portions of the corpus callosum placed next to the ventricles are particularly subject to the effects of negative pressure, a view confirmed by the observation that those structures are in fact the principal sites of the primary traumatic hemorrhages. These particular alterations were surnamed "butterfly lesions" in the Max Planck Institute for Brain Research at Munich (Unterharnscheidt, Peters, Schacht, Minauf, and E. Th. Mayer[30,31,36,40,65]). For, the lateral ventricles, outlined by the hemorrhages strung along their edges, recall the open wingpair of a butterfly. The secondary alterations, by contrast, are found disseminated in the entire region of the basal ganglia and the white substance of the cerebral hemispheres. They include partial and total necroses, hemorrhagic necroses, diapedetic hemorrhages, coagulation necroses due to fat embolism, among others. By considering the period of survival and analyzing the histological findings, the quality of central alterations as to their primary or secondary origin can be largely determined.

We distinguish arteriorhectic and venorhectic hemorrhages caused

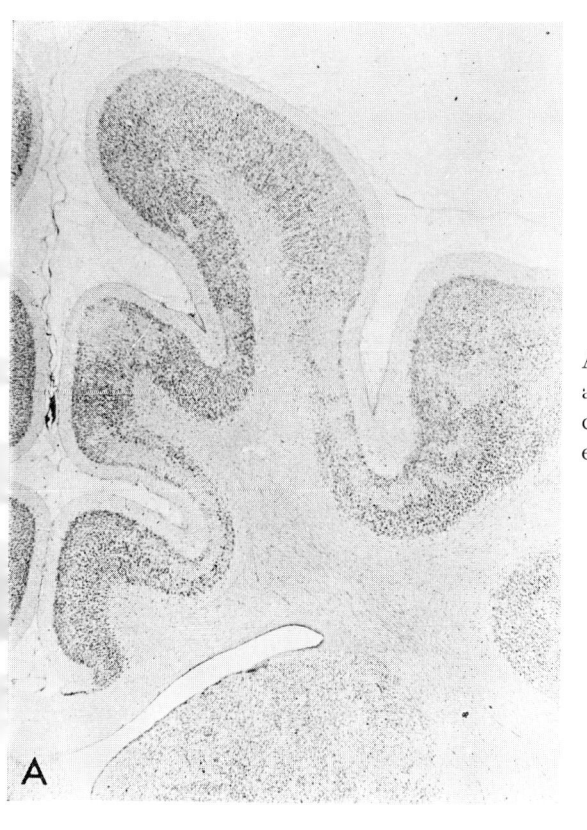

A. Cerebrum. Extensive focal and pseudolaminary elective necrosis of the parenchyma of the cortex. Glial proliferation in the white matter, especially of astroglia. (Nissl, 5:1.)

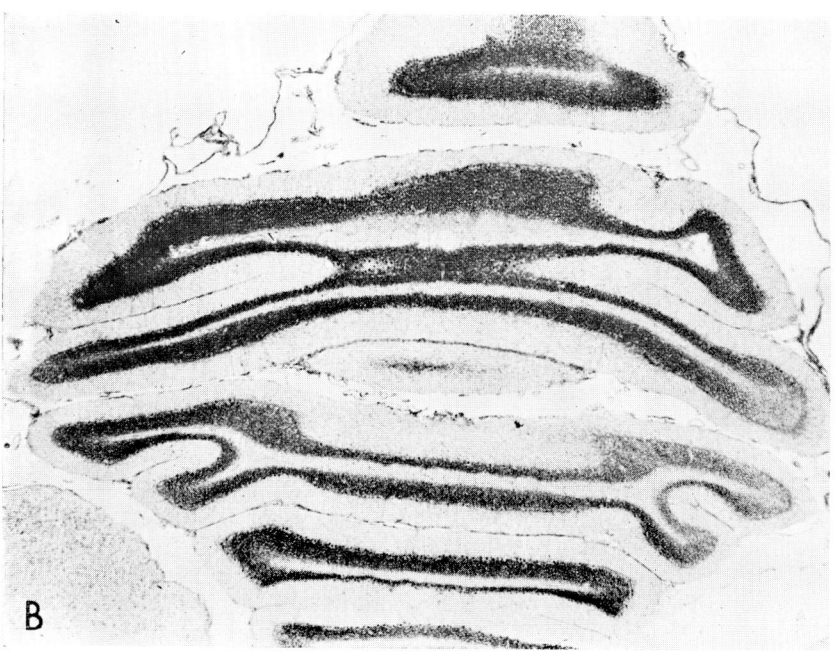

B. Vermis cerebelli. Serial loss of purkinje cells and proliferating Bergmann glia on the summits of the convolutions. Reduction of granular cell layer. Glial proliferation in the striae medullares and molecular layer. (Nissl, 20:1.)

FIGURE 2–13 A.-G. Successive blows administered in repeated series of subcommotio and commotio strength resulted in permanent brain damage, while no primary traumatic alterations like hemorrhages or so-called cortical contusions were found in the cats.

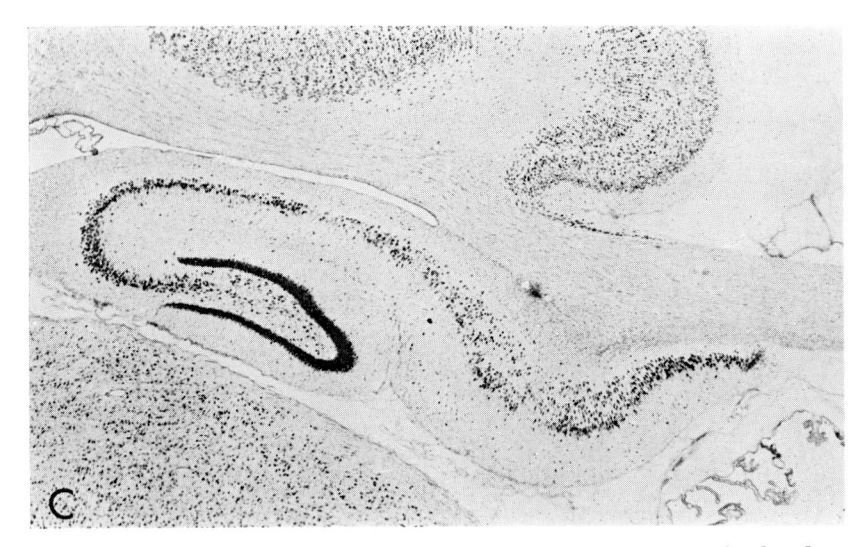

C. Left Ammonshorn formation. Disseminated loss of nerve cells in the band, mainly in section h_1, combined with microglial proliferation. (Nissl, 20:1.)

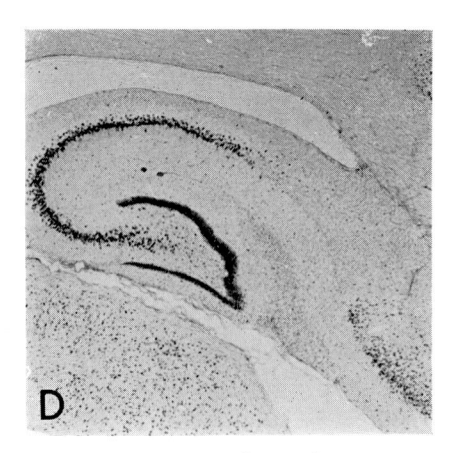

D. Left Ammonshorn formation. Topistic loss of neurons in Sommer's sector h_1, followed by glial proliferation. (Nissl, 16:1.)

FIGURE 2–13 A.-G. Successive blows administered in repeated series of subcommotio and commotio strength resulted in permanent brain damage, while no primary traumatic alterations like hemorrhages or so-called cortical contusions were found in the cats.

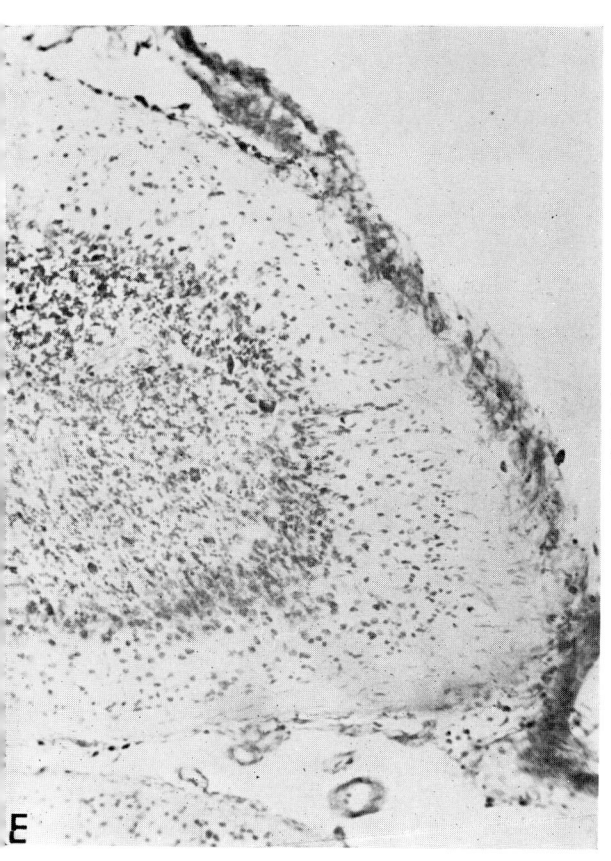

E. Cerebellum. Summits of the convolutions of the vermis. Reduced granular cell layer. Proliferated Bergmann glia. Proliferated micro and macroglia in the molecular layer. (Nissl, 128:1.)

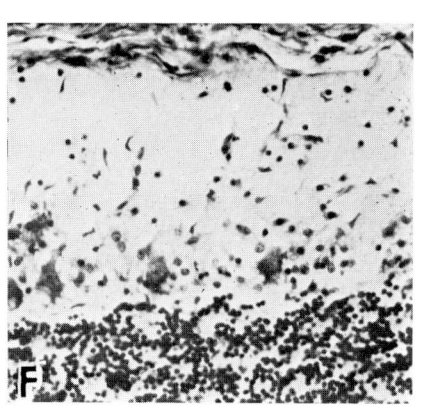

F. Cerebellum. Disseminated glial cell proliferation in the molecular layer. Irreversible alterations and loss of purkinje cells combined with proliferation of Bergmann glia in several places. (Van Gieson, 160:1.)

FIGURE 2–13 A.-G. Successive blows administered in repeated series of subcommotio and commotio strength resulted in permanent brain damage, while no primary traumatic alterations like hemorrhages or so-called cortical contusions were found in the cats.

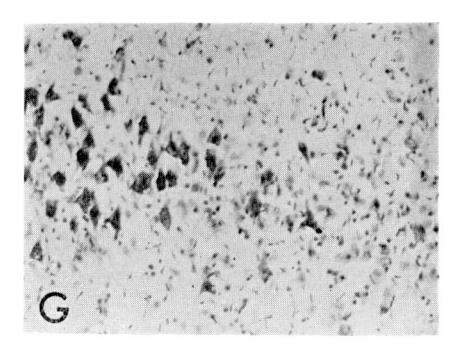

G. Ammonshorn formation. Enlargement showing transition from area with unaltered cells to area with complete loss of cells. Considerable proliferation of microglia, to a lesser degree also of astroglia. (Nissl, 128:1.)

FIGURE 2–13 A.-G. Successive blows administered in repeated series of subcommotio and commotio strength resulted in permanent brain damage, while no primary traumatic alterations like hemorrhages or so-called cortical contusions were found in the cats.

directly by the violence, from circulatory disturbances, such as necrosis, hemorrhagic necrosis and diapedetic hemorrhage, caused by the developing cerebral edema.[40,65] E. Th. Mayer[30] identified and classified these lesions according to their location in the various supporting areas of arteries and veins in the midbrain, pons and medulla.

With this knowledge, the use of the term Duret-Berner hemorrhages modeled on an erroneous concept of identity should be abandoned,—just as we can no longer speak of brain stem contusions. There are plainly no criteria for this diagnosis.

I also agree entirely with Dr. Thomas[53] that angular acceleration is important. Alterations that are related to extreme angular motion are essentially different from those seen in translatory traumas. According to our experiments (Unterharnscheidt and L. S. Higgins[57]), angular motions cause subdural hemorrhage due to the rupture of bridging veins, and produce scattered subarachnoid hemorrhages near the midline. They also cause the rupture and hemorrhage of the larger intra and extracerebral vessels, of vessels in cranial nerves, of smaller vessels of the medulla and cerebellum (mostly those situated in the midline), in the gray and, to some extent also in the white substance of the cervical, thoracic, and markedly the lumbar region, as well as, in the cauda equina. Figure 2–14c illustrates a rupture of the arteria basilaris in man after a trauma involving extreme angular motion. The rupture is followed by tearing of the elastica interna and by lamellar hemorrhaging, a process that leads eventually to aneurysma

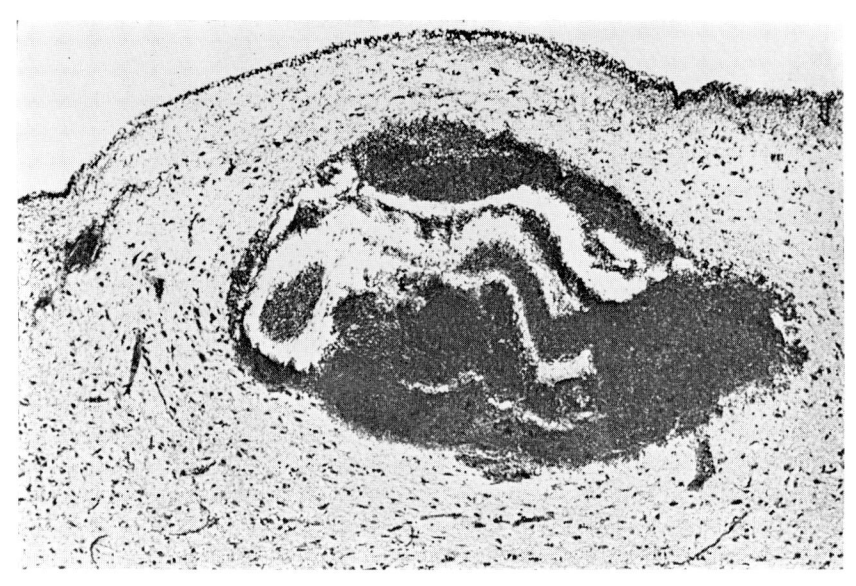

FIGURE 2–14A. Subependymal rupture of a vein, near the lateral ventricular wall. The spreading hemorrhage has caused a considerable compression of the vascular lumen. (Masson Goldner.)

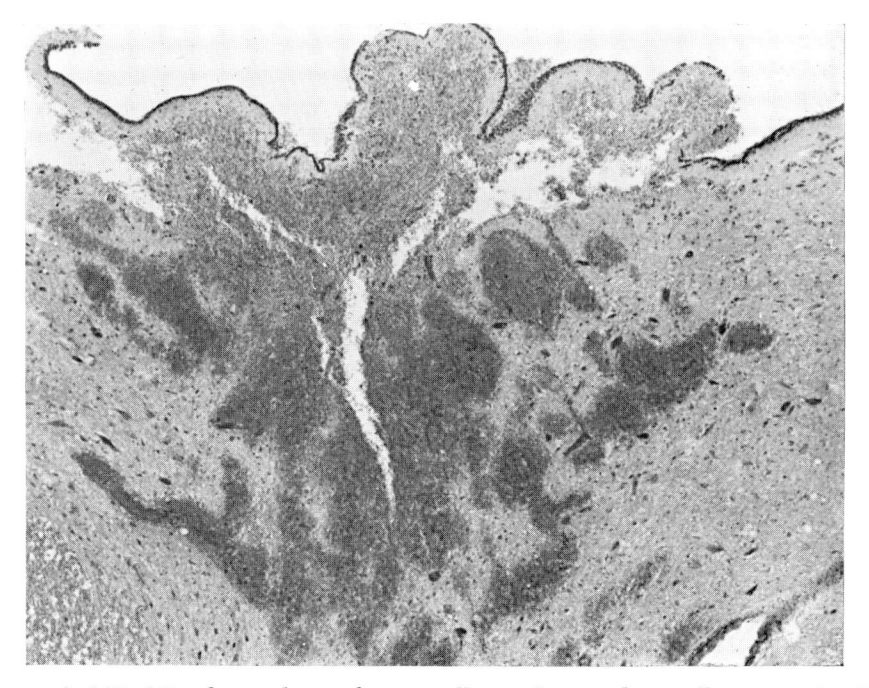

FIGURE 2–14B. Microhemorrhages from small vessels, mostly capillaries on the floor of the fourth ventricle, combined with lesions of the ependyma and erruption of microhemorrhages into the ventricle. (Van Gieson.)

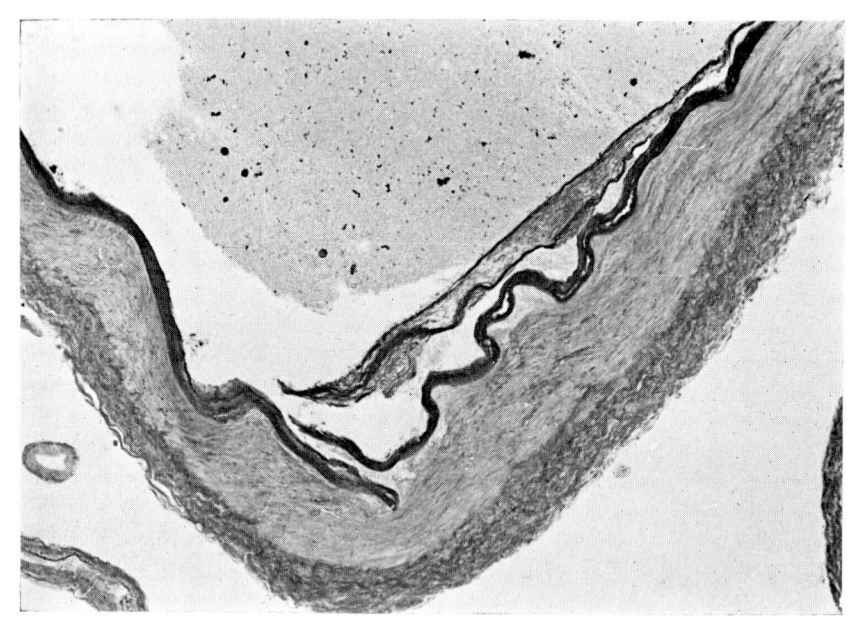

FIGURE 2–14C. Sectional enlargement of rupture of the intima of the Arteria basilaris. Disseminated and lamellar hemorrhages in the vessel walls. First stage of aneurysma dissecans. (Van Gieson-Elastica.)

disseccans. The same findings were reported by Roberts[34] after chest injuries in dogs.

With regard to the primary alterations associated with translatory traumas, we repeat that Holbourn's theory does not explain their origin. The pattern of distribution in conjunction with the analysis of histological details exhibited by the so-called cortical contusions both indicate that the discussed alterations cannot be retraced to angular motion, but must be produced by the effects of acceleration or deceleration, respectively. The mechanical origination and the pathomorphology of these particular lesions found in superficial layers of the cortex have been widely investigated and described by Spatz,[43-51] Peters,[32-33] Unterharnscheidt,[56] and by Bloomquist and Courville[1] (using a different terminology). The hitherto so-called cortical contusions in particular were seen only when the acceleration or deceleration trauma involved a freely moving skull, as Le Count and Apfelbach were first to observe. The lesions would be located at a point across from and opposite the impact site (Spatz[43,51] Peters,[32-33] Welte,[66] Bloomquist and Courville,[1] Unterharnscheidt,[56] Sellier and Unterharnscheidt[40,42] and others). Experiments with skull models (Sellier and Unterharnscheidt,[40,42] Edberg et al.,[4] Lindgren,[29] Gurdjian et al.[13,16,35] proved the existence of a negative pressure cone at the antipole. Gross[8,9] finally demonstrated by means of a glass sphere that sufficient acceleration or

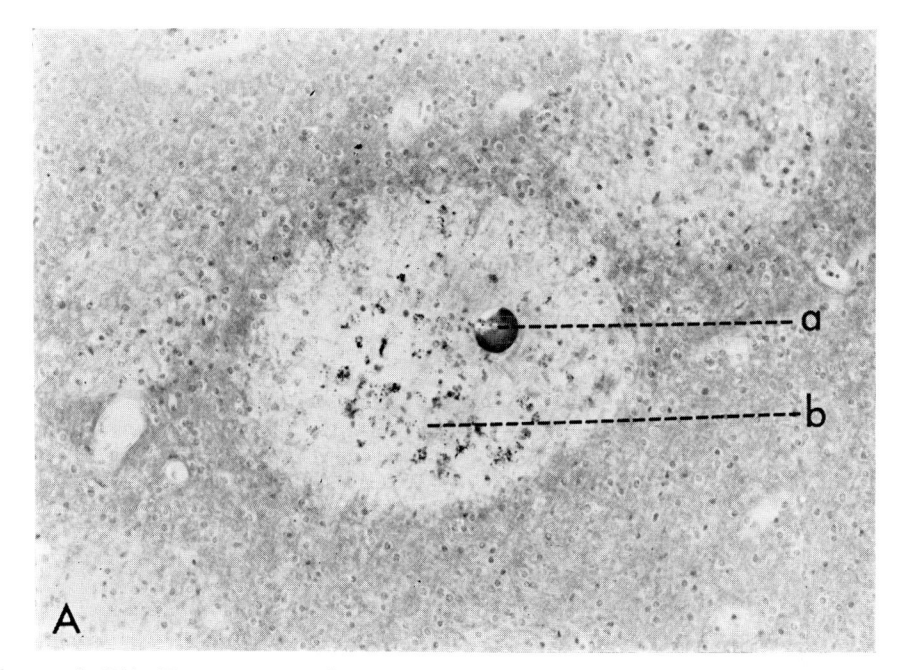

FIGURE 2–15A. Fat staining technique reveals vessel occluded by fat embolus at (a). The vascular walls are necrotic. Nearby is a coagulation necrosis, at (b) which is also visible in the Van Gieson preparation of Figure 2–15B. (Sudan III technique.)

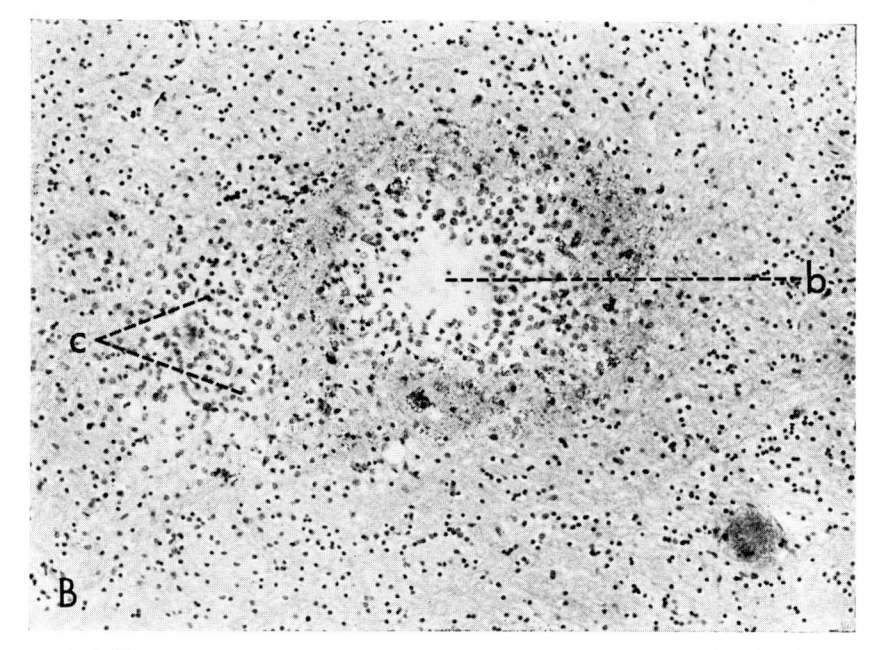

FIGURE 2–15B. The necrotic area contains macrophages, some with blood pigment, as well as, recent hemorrhages. The surrounding glia shows the onset of a reaction, most clearly on the left margin of the picture, at (c). Period of survival 7 days. (Van Gieson.)

FIGURE 2–15. Man. Fatty emboly. White matter of the cerebrum. Gross examination shows purpura cerebri.

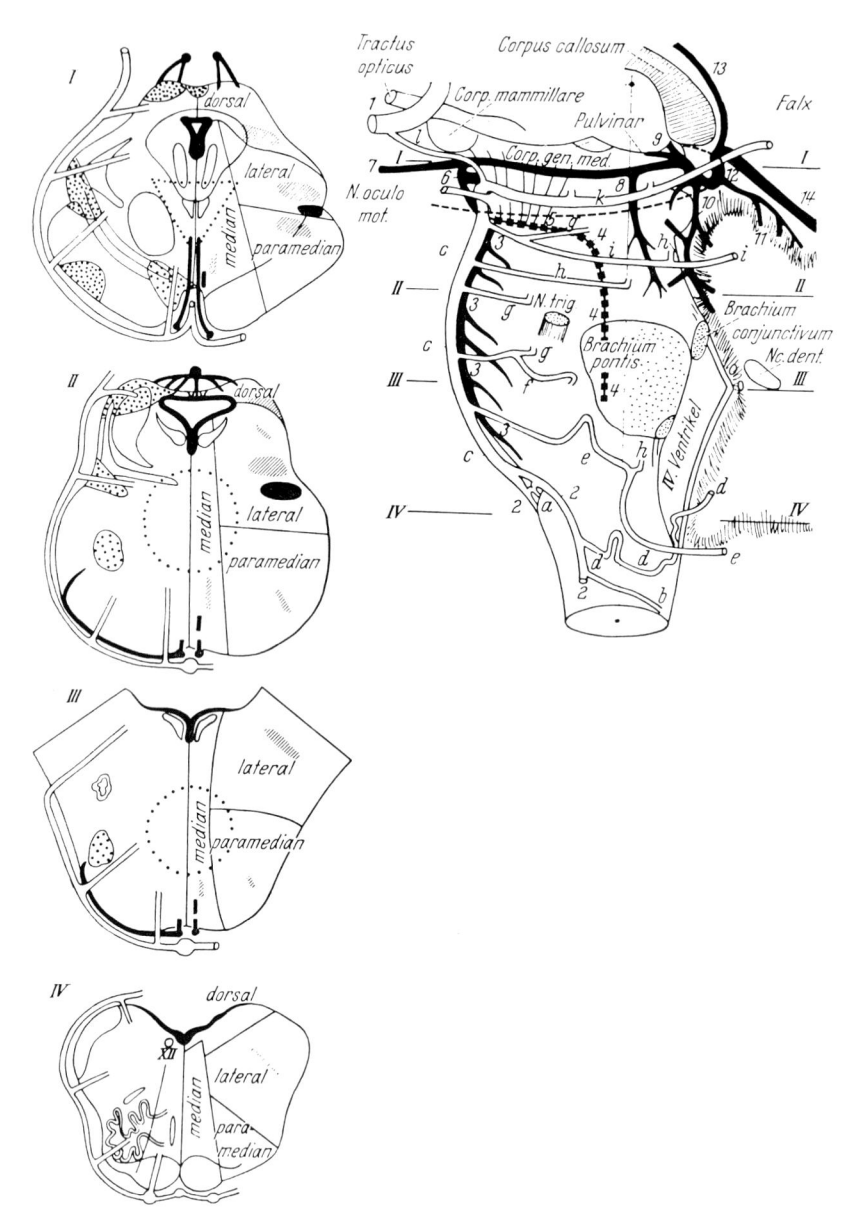

FIGURE 2–16. Diagram of a normal brainstem (above right), and four typical cross-sections I–IV (left column), drawn from E. Th. Mayer's anatomic preparations using Gillilans diagrams (1964). Roman numerals indicate levels of the brain stem sections and refer to the corresponding cross sections. The dotted line around the midbrain marks the edge of the tentorium slit. On the right side of cross-section I–IV, the arterial supply areas have been outlined, and locations typical of the hemorrhages found in Mayer's observations have been marked. These are hemorrhages due to arteriorhexis (cross-hatched), or venorhexis (black), target sites of secondary alterations (occlusive hemorrhages, black dotted areas), and so-called venous swamp (circled by black dots). Arabic numerals and roman minuscules indicate vessels. (1) A. carotis interna, (2) Aa. vertebrales, a: A. spinalis anterior, b: A. spinalis posterior,

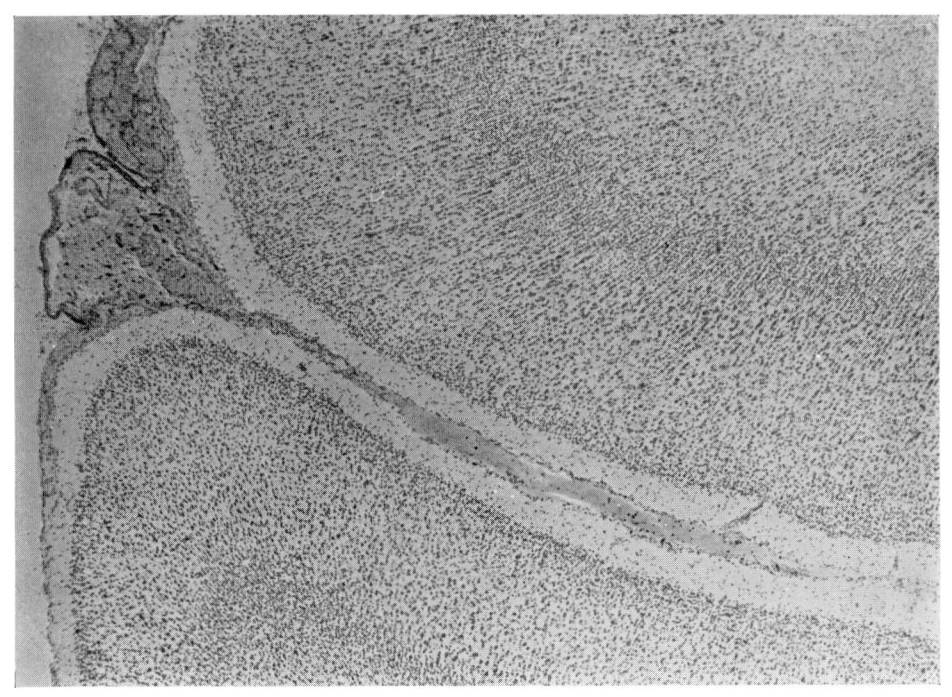

FIGURE 2–17. Squirrel monkey. Angular acceleration of the head. Occipital region. Scattered, recent subarachnoid hemorrhages. Unremarkable molecular layer. Stratification of the cortex is undisturbed. Neurons and glial elements show no morphological alterations. (*From* Nissl, 10:1.)

deceleration produced cavitations in the area of negative pressure. The morphological analysis of the resulting lesions which we have renamed cortical cavitation trauma to reflect their origination indicates that they present the effects of capillary ruptures due to cavitation. The last piece of evidence, for which contrast methods and highspeed cinematography will be employed, has not yet been furnished. Nevertheless, in my opinion

---

c: A. basilaris, d: A. cerebellaris posterior, e: A. cerebellaris inferior anterior, f: A. labyrinthi, g: A. circumferens brevis, h: A. circumferens longa, i: A. cerebellaris superior, k: A. cerebri posterior, l: A. communicans posterior, (3) Vv. pontis superficiales, (4) Vv. pontis centrales, (5) Vv. intercrurales (caudal group), (6) Vv. intercrurales (dorsal group), (7) Vena basalis Rosenthali, (8) Vv. sulcilaterales, (9) V. cerebri interna, (10) V. praecentralis cerebellaris, (11) Vv. cerebellares superiores, (12) Vena magna Galeni, (13) Sinus sagittalis inferior, (14) Sinus rectis.

In cross-section I, tiny veins draining into the venae cerebri internae are marked at the tegmentum, while the Vv. intercrurales (dorsal group) are indicated in the midbrain raphe. Cross-section II indicates tiny veins draining into the V. praecentralis cerebellaris, also at the tegmentum. Cross-sections II and III show veins draining into the Vv. pontis superciales. (From E. Th. Mayer.[30])

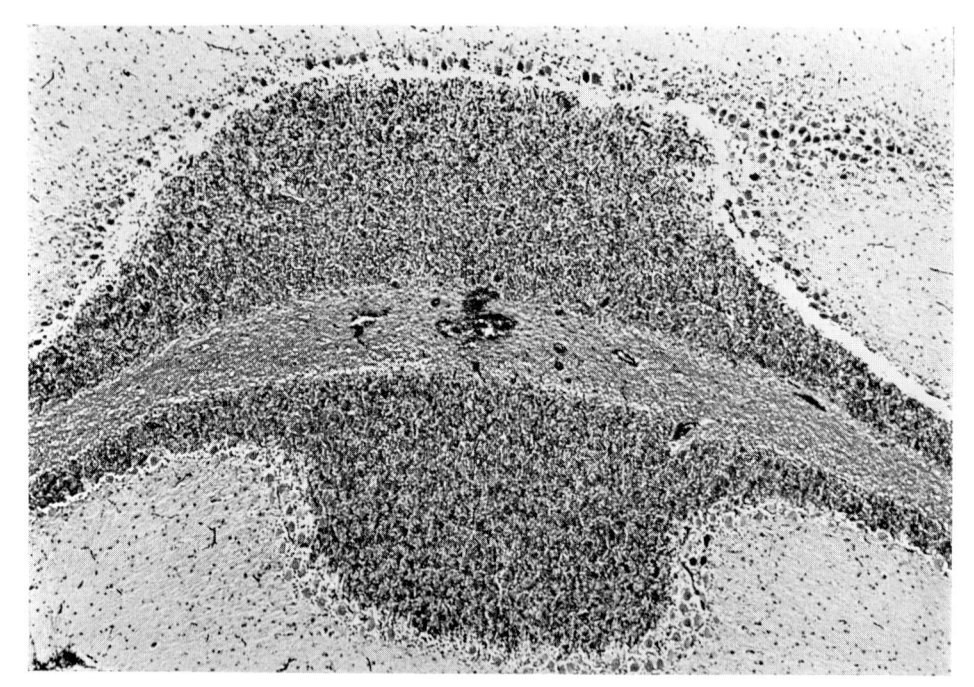

FIGURE 2–18. Squirrel monkey. Angular acceleration of the head. Vermis cerebelli. Minor recent rhectic hemorrhages in the striae medullares, due to vessel rupture after strain. Molecular, purkinje, and granular cell layers are all unremarkable. (*From* Masson-Goldner, 16:1.)

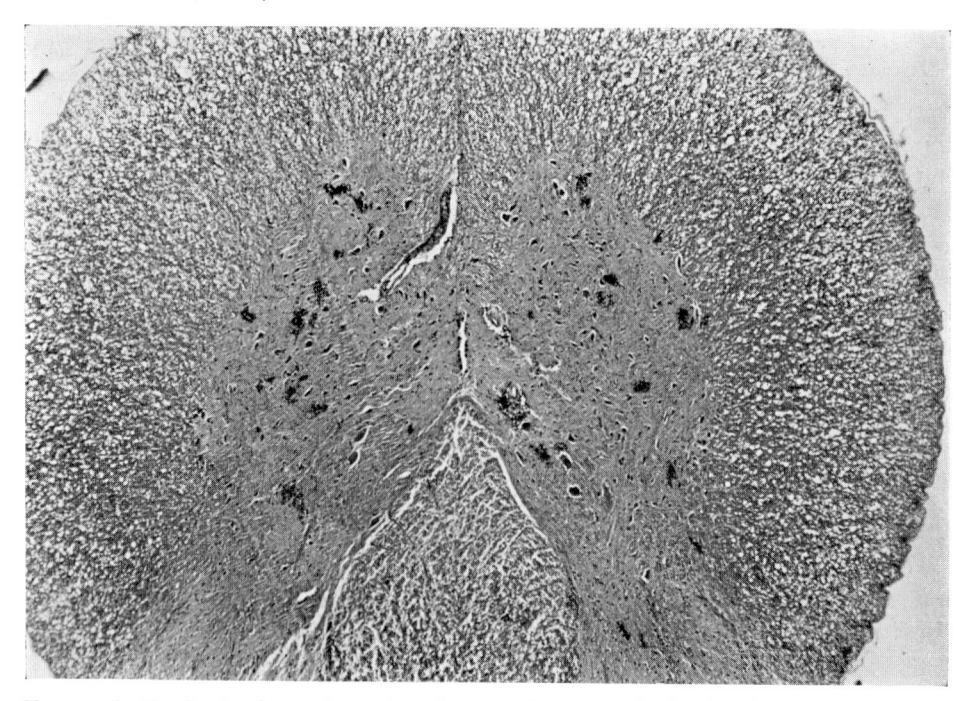

FIGURE 2–19. Squirrel monkey. Angular acceleration of the head. Lumbar region. Small recent rhectic hemorrhages in the gray matter due to vessel rupture after strain. (*From* Masson-Goldner, 10:1.)

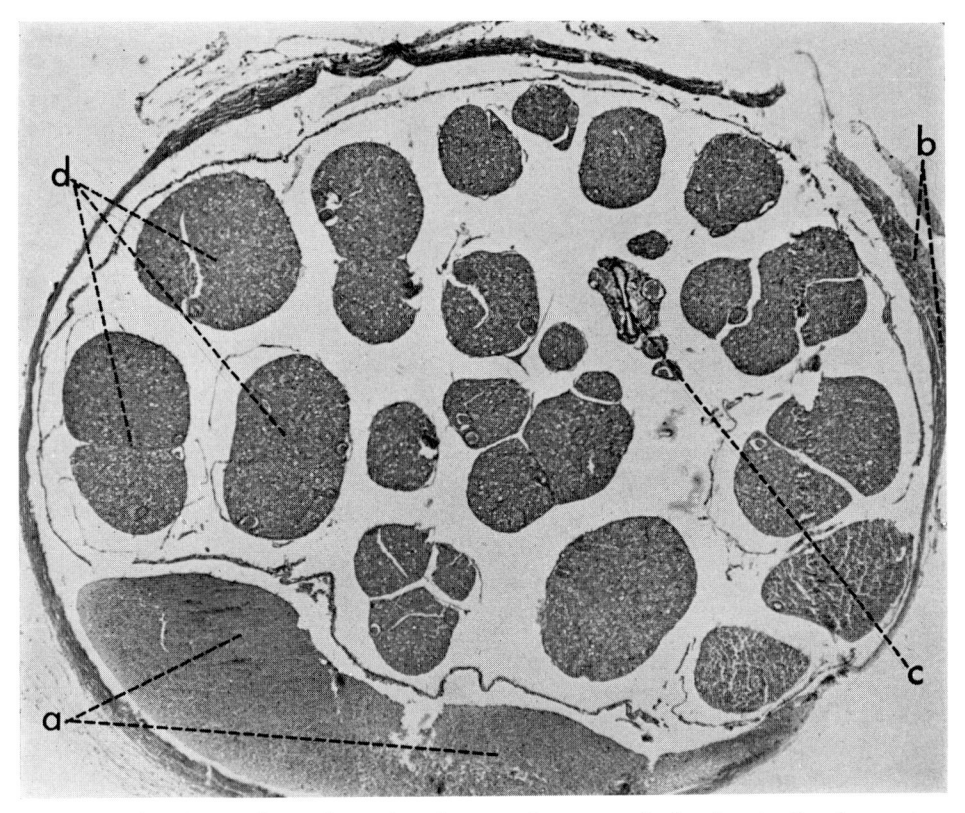

FIGURE 2–20. Squirrel monkey. Angular acceleration of the head. Cauda equina. Recent subdural hemorrhage at (a). The dura is seen at (b). Central canal in the filum terminale at (c). Nerve roots at (d). (*From* Van Gieson, 10:1.)

the existing evidence appears sufficiently strong to explain these primary traumatic lesions by cavitation.

Rotational traumas, on the other hand, produce both subdural hemorrhages and hemorrhages in superficial layers of the cortex by rupturing bridging veins and intracerebral veins, respectively. Typical antipole lesions, like the cortical cavitation trauma, do not occur in predominantly rotational traumas.

Dedication

I wish to dedicate this chapter to one of our founders of modern neuropathology and eminent scientist and teacher, the venerable Professor Dr. med. Dr. h. c. Hugo Spatz, on the event of his eightieth birthday.

REFERENCES

1. BLOOMQUIST, E.R., and COURVILLE, C.: The nature and incidence of traumatic lesions of the brain. A survey of 350 cases with autopsy. *Bull Los Angeles Neurol Soc*, 12:174–183, 1947.

58   *Impact Injury and Crash Protection*

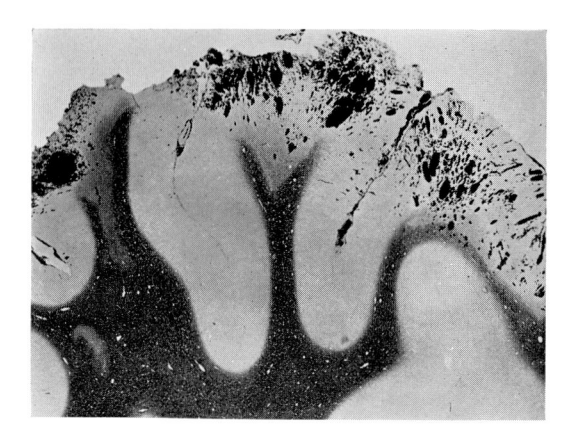

FIGURE 2-21-A. Man, closed brain injury. So-called cortical contusions on the summits of the convolutions, hemorrhagic stage (first stage). They are caused by the rupture of capillaries and veins. Paling of the surrounding brain tissue. The sulci, by contrast, appear histologically unaltered ("isolated sulci," Spatz). Period of survival 17 hours. Myelin technique according to Heidenhain.

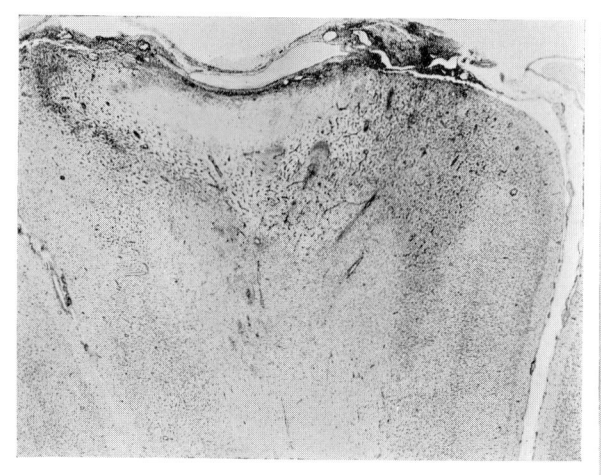

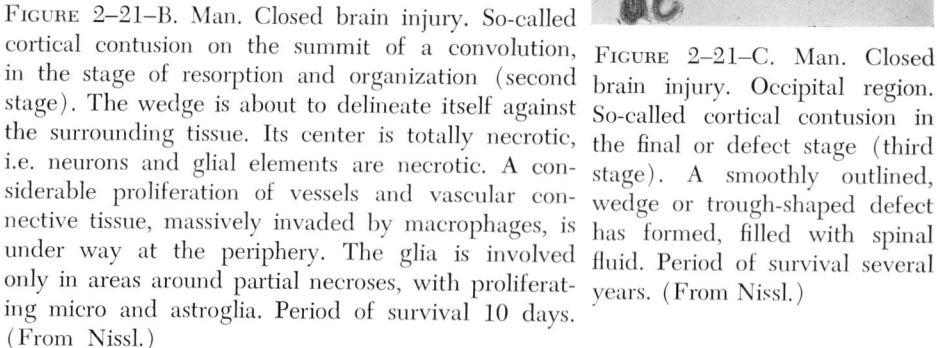

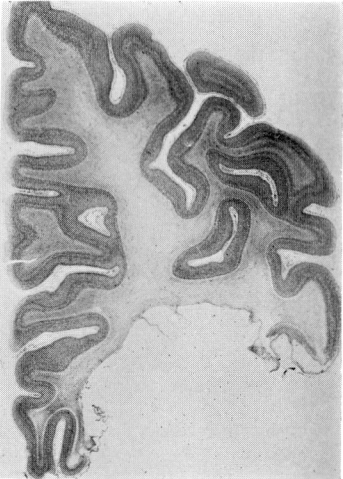

FIGURE 2-21-B. Man. Closed brain injury. So-called cortical contusion on the summit of a convolution, in the stage of resorption and organization (second stage). The wedge is about to delineate itself against the surrounding tissue. Its center is totally necrotic, i.e. neurons and glial elements are necrotic. A considerable proliferation of vessels and vascular connective tissue, massively invaded by macrophages, is under way at the periphery. The glia is involved only in areas around partial necroses, with proliferating micro and astroglia. Period of survival 10 days. (From Nissl.)

FIGURE 2-21-C. Man. Closed brain injury. Occipital region. So-called cortical contusion in the final or defect stage (third stage). A smoothly outlined, wedge or trough-shaped defect has formed, filled with spinal fluid. Period of survival several years. (From Nissl.)

2. DENNY-BROWN, D.: Cerebral concussion. *Physiol Rev, 25*:296-325, 1945.
3. DENNY-BROWN, D., and RUSSELL, W.R.: Experimental cerebral concussion. *Brain, 64*:93-164, 1941.
4. EDBERG, S.; RIEKER, B.A., and ANGRIST, A.: Study of impact pressure and acceleration in plastic skull models. *Lab Invest, 12*:1305-1311, 1963.

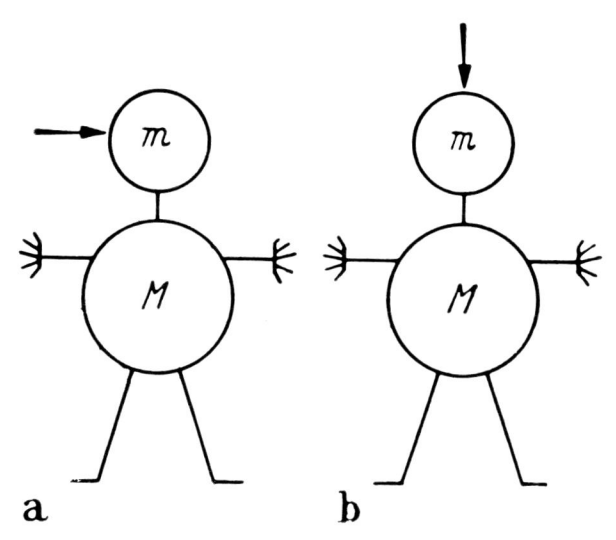

FIGURE 2-22. Different impact axes. (a) Frontal, occipital, temporal impact. The head may be considered unsupported during the collision (lasting only a few msec.). The spinal cord has no influence on the event. Acceleration trauma. (b) Impact in the direction of the axis of the spinal column. The head is "dynamically fixed" by the spinal column and the mass of the body.

5. GROAT, R.A.; MAGOUN, H.W.; DEY, F.L., and WINDLE, W.F.: Functional alterations on motor and supranuclear mechanisms in experimental concussion. *Amer J Physiol,* 141:117–127, 1944.
6. GROAT, R.A., and SIMMONS, J.A.: Loss of nerve cells in experimental cerebral concussion. *J Neuropath Exp Neurol,* 9:150–163, 1950.
7. GROAT, R.A.; WINDLE, W.F., and MAGOUN, H.W.: Functional and structural changes in the monkey's brain during and after concussion. *J Neurosurg,* 2: 26–35, 1945.
8. GROSS, A.G.: A new theory on the dynamics of brain concussion and brain injury. *J Neurosurg,* 15:548–561, 1958.
9. GROSS, A.G.: Impact thresholds of brain concussion. *J Aviat Med,* 29:725–732, 1958.
10. GÜTTINGER, W.: Der Stosseffekt auf eine Flüssigkeitskugel als Grundlage einer physikalischen Theorie der Entstehung von Gehirnverletzungen. *Z Naturforsch,* 5:622–627, 1950.
11. GURDJIAN, E.S., and LISSNER, H.R.: Mechanism of head injury as studied by cathode ray oscilloscope. *J Neurosurg,* 1:393–399, 1944.
12. GURDJIAN, E.S., and LISSNER, H.R.: Photoelastic confirmation on the presence of shear strains at the craniospinal junction in closed head injuries. *J Neurosurg,* 18:58–60, 1961.
13. GURDJIAN, E.S.; LISSNER, H.R.; EVANS, E.C.; PATRICK, L.M., and HARVEY, W.G.: Intracranial pressure and acceleration accompanying head impacts in human cadavers. *Surg Gynec Obstet,* 113:189, 1961.
14. GURDJIAN, E.S.; LISSNER, H.R.; LATIMER, F.R.; HADDAD, B.F., and WEBSTER, J.E.: Quantitative determination of acceleration and intracranial pressure in experimental head injury. *Neurology,* 3:417–423, 1953.

15. GURDJIAN, E.S.; LISSNER, H.R., and STONE, W.E.: Observations on the mechanism of brain concussion, contusion and laceration. *Surg Gynec Obstet, 101*:680–690, 1955.
16. GURDJIAN, E.S.; ROBERTS, V.L., and THOMAS, L.M.: Tolerance curves of acceleration and intracranial pressure and protective index in experimental head injuries. *J Trauma, 6*:600–604, 1966.
17. GURDJIAN, E.S.; STONE, W.E.; WEBSTER, J.E.; LATIMER, F.R., and HADDAD, B.F.: Studies on experimental concussion. Relation of physiological effect to time duration of intracranial pressure increase at impact. *Neurology, 4*:674–681, 1954.
18. GURDJIAN, E.S., and THOMAS, L.M.: Management of head injury in the United States. In Caveness, W.F., and Walker, E.A. (Eds.), *Head Injury*, Conference Proceed.: Philadelphia, Lippincott, 1966, chap. 13, pp. 168–171.
19. GURDJIAN, E.S., and WEBSTER, J.E.: Experimental head injury with special reference to the mechanical factors in acute trauma. *Surg Gynec Obstet, 76*:623–634, 1943.
20. GURDJIAN, E.S., and WEBSTER, J.E.: Experimental and clinical studies on the mechanism of head injury. In *Trauma of the Nervous System Research Publ. Ass. f. Research in Nervous and Mental Disease*. Baltimore, Williams & Wilkins, 1945, Vol. 24, pp. 48–97.
21. GURDJIAN, E.S., and WEBSTER, J.E.: Traumatic intracranial hemorrhage. *Amer J Surg, 75*:82–98, 1948.
22. GURDJIAN, E.S., and WEBSTER, J.E.: *Head Injuries—Mechanism, Diagnosis and Treatment*. Boston, Little, 1958.
23. GURDJIAN, E.S.; WEBSTER, J.E., and LISSNER, H.R.: Observations on the mechanism of brain concussion, contusion and laceration. *Surg Gynec Obstet, 101*: 680–690, 1955.
24. GURDJIAN, E.S.; WEBSTER, J.E., and LISSNER, R.M.: Biomechanics: brain concussion, contusion and laceration. In Glaser, von O. (Ed.): *Medical Physics*. Chicago, Year Book, 1960, Vol. III, pp. 84–88.
25. GURDJIAN, E.S.; WEBSTER, J.E.; LATIMER, F.R., and HADDAD, B.F.: Studies on experimental concussion. Relation of physiological effect to time duration of intracranial pressure increase at impact. *Neurology, 4*:674–681, 1954.
26. HOLBOURN, A.H.S.: Mechanics of head injury. *Lancet, II*:438–441, 1943.
27. HOLBOURN, A.H.S.: The mechanics of trauma with special reference to herniation of cerebral tissue. *J Neurosurg, 1*:190–200, 1944.
28. HOLBOURN, A.H.S.: The mechanics of brain injuries. *Brit Med Bull, 3*:147–148, 1945.
29. LINDGREN, ST. O.: Experimental studies of mechanical effects in head injury. *Acta Chir Scand* (Suppl 360), 1966.
30. MAYER, E. TH.: Zentrale Hirnschäden nach Einwirkung stumpfer Gewalt auf den Schädel. Hirnstammschäden. *Arch Psychiat Nervenkr, 210*:238–262, 1967.
31. MINAUF, M., and SCHACHT, L.: Zentrale Hirnschäden nach Einwirkung stumpfer Gewalt auf den Schädel. II. Mitteilung: Läsionen im Bereich der Stammganglien. *Arch Psychiat Nervenkr, 208*:162–176, 1966.
32. PETERS, G.: *Spezielle Pathologie der Krankheiten des zentralen und peripheren Nervensystems*. Stuttgart, Thieme, 1951.
33. PETERS, G.: Die gedeckten Gehirn- und Rückenmarksverletzungen. In Scholz, W. (Ed.): *Hdb. d. spez. pathol. Anatomie u. Histologie*. Berlin-Göttingen-Heidelberg, Springer, 1955, Vol. XIII, pt. 3, pp. 84–143.

34. ROBERTS, V.: Personal communication.
35. ROBERTS, V.L.; HODGSON, V.R., and THOMAS, L.M.: Fluid pressure gradients caused by impact to the human skull. Human Factors Conference, Washington, March 28–29, 1966. Amer. Soc. of Mechanical Engineers. *ASME publication.*
36. SCHACHT, L., and MINAUF, M.: Zentrale Hirnschäden nach Einwirkung stumpfer Gewalt auf den Schädel. I. Mitteilung: Balkenläsionen. *Arch Psychiat Nervenkr,* 207:416–427, 1965.
37. SCHOLZ, W.: Die Krampfschädigungen des Gehirns. *Monog Neurol Psychiat,* 1951, No. 75.
38. SELLIER, K., and UNTERHARNSCHEIDT, F.: Experimental studies on the mechanism of nonpenetrating brain injuries. IV. Internat. Congress of Neuropathology, Munchen, 4–8 September, 1961, Abstracts 82, Stuttgart, Thieme, 1961.
39. SELLIER, K., and UNTERHARNSCHEIDT, F.: Untersuchungen zur Mechanik der gedeckten Schädelhirnverletzungen. IV. Internationaler Kongress für Neuropathologie, Proceedings. Stuttgart, Georg Thieme, 1962, vol. 3, pp. 226–230.
40. SELLIER, K., and UNTERHARNSCHEIDT, F.: Mechanik und Pathomorphologie der Hirnschäden nach stumpfer Gewalteinwirkung auf den Schädel. *Hefte Unfallheilk,* 1963, pt. 76.
41. SELLIER, K., and UNTERHARNSCHEIDT, F.: Mechanik der Gewalteinwirkung auf den Schädel. IIIrd Congress of Neurolog. Surgery, Copenhagen, August 23–28, 1965. *Excerpta Medica Internat. Congress Series,* 93:55–61, 1965.
42. SELLIER, K., and UNTERHARNSCHEIDT, F.: The mechanics of the impact of violence on the skull. Proceed: Internat. Congress of Neurological Surgery, Copenhagen, August 23–28, 1965. *Excerpta Medica Internat. Congress Series,* 110:87–92, 1965.
43. SPATZ, H.: Kann man alte Rindendefekte traumatischer und arteriosklerotischer Genese voneinander unterscheiden? Die Bedeutung des "etat vermoulu." *Arch Psychiat Nervenkr,* 90:885–887, 1930.
44. SPATZ, H.: Über Entstehung und Bedeutung traumatischer Rindendefekte. *Allg Z Psychiat,* 94:218–221, 1931.
45. SPATZ, H.: Die Erkennbarkeit der Rindenkontusion im Endzustand in anatomischer und klinischer Hinsicht. *Zbl ges Neurol Psychiat,* 61:514–515, 1932.
46. SPATZ, H.: Pathologische Anatomie mit besonderer Berücksichtigung der Rindenkontusion. *Zbl ges Neurol Psychiat,* 78:615–616, 1936.
47. SPATZ, H.: Pathologische Anatomie der gedeckten Hirnverletzungen mit besonderer Berücksichtigung der Rindenkontusion. *Arch Psychiat Nervenkr,* 105: 80–83, 1936.
48. SPATZ, H.: Über die Bedeutung der basalen Rinde. Auf Grund von Beobachtungen bei Pickscher Krankheit und bei gedeckten Hirnverletzungen. *Z ges Neurol Psychiat,* 158:208–232, 1937.
49. SPATZ, H.: Gehirnpathologie im Kriege. Von den Gehirnwunden. *Zbl Neurochir* 6: 162–212, 1941.
50. SPATZ, H.: Brain injuries in aviation. In *German Aviation Medicine. World War II* Dept, of the Air Force, 1950, Vol. I, pp. 616–640.
51. SPATZ, H.: Die Pathologie der Hirnverletzungen. *Zbl ges Neurol Psychiat,* 113: 9–10, 1951.
52. SPIELMEYER, W.: *Histopathologie des Nervensystems.* Berlin, Springer, 1922.
53. THOMAS, L.M.: Mechanisms of head injury. In *Proceed. Impact Injury and Crash Protection.* Wayne State University, May 9 and 10, 1968.
54. UNTERHARNSCHEIDT, F.: Experimentelle Untersuchungen über die Schädigung des

ZNS durch gehäufte stumpfe Schädeltraumen. *Zbl ges Neurol Psychiat, 147*: 14, 1958.
55. UNTERHARNSCHEIDT, F.: Experimentelle Untersuchungen über gedeckte Schäden des Gehirns nach einmaliger und wiederholter stumpfer Gewalteinwirkung auf den Schädel, *Fortschr Med, 80*:369–378, 1962.
56. UNTERHARNSCHEIDT, F.: Die gedeckten Schäden des Gehirns. Experimentelle Untersuchungen mit einmaliger, wiederholter und gehäufter stumpfer Gewalteinwirkung auf den Schädel. *Monogr Neurol Psychiat*, 1963, pt. 103.
57. UNTERHARNSCHEIDT, F., and HIGGINS, L.S.: Unpublished data.
58. UNTERHARNSCHEIDT, F.; PARSONS, and RUEDENBERG: Unpublished data.
59. UNTERHARNSCHEIDT, F., and SELLIER, K.: Experimental studies on the pathomorphology of nonpenetrating brain injuries due to single and repeated application of blunt violence to the head. IV. Internat. Congr. of Neuropathology, München, September 4–8, 1961 Abstracts 82–83. Stuttgart, Thieme, 1961.
60. UNTERHARNSCHEIDT, F., and SELLIER, K.: Experimentelle Untersuchungen zur Pathomorphologie der gedeckten Hirnverletzungen nach einmaliger und wiederholter stumpfer Gewalteinwirkung auf den Schädel. IV. Internationaler Kongress für Neuropathologie, Proceedings. Stuttgart, Thieme, 1962, vol. 3, pp. 231–233.
61. UNTERHARNSCHEIDT, F., and SELLIER, K.: Mechanik und Pathomorphologie der gedeckten Schäden des Gehirns nach einmaliger, wiederholter und gehäufter stumpfer Gewalteinwirkung auf den Schädel. *Jap Arch Chir, 31*:687–713, 1962.
62. UNTERHARNSCHEIDT, F., and SELLIER, K.: Mecanismo y Anatomia patologica de las lesiones tramaticas cerradas del cerebro prducidas par la accion unica, repetida y seriada de agentes contundentes sobre el craneo. *Med Clin (Barcelona), 39*:200–215, 1962.
63. UNTERHARNSCHEIDT, F., and SELLIER, K.: Pathomorphologie der gedeckten Schädelhirnverletzungen. IIIrd Internat. Congress of Neurol. Surgery, Copenhagen, August 23–28, 1965. *Excerpta Medica Internat. Congress Series, 93*:62–73, 1965.
64. UNTERHARNSCHEIDT, F. and SELLIER, K.: Pathomorphology of nonpenetrating brain injuries. Proceed. IIIrd Internat. Congress of Neurol. Surgery, Copenhagen, August 23–28, 1965. *Excerpta Medica Internat. Congress Series, 110*:93–103, 1965.
65. UNTERHARNSCHEIDT, F., and SELLIER, K.: Mechanics and pathomorphology of closed brain injuries. *Conference: Head Injury Planning Committee, Chicago, February 7–9, 1966*. Chapt. 26, 321–341, Proceed. Philadelphia, Lippincott, 1966, Chap. 26, pp. 321–341.
66. WELTE, E.: Über die Zusammenhänge zwischen anatomischem Befund und klinischem Bild bei Rindenprellungsherden nach stumpfen Schädeltrauma. *Arch Psychiat Nervenkr, 179*:243–315, 1948.
67. WINDLE, W.F., and GROAT, R.A.: Disappearance of nerve cells after concussion. *Anat Rec, 93*:201–209, 1945.
68. WINDLE, W.F.; GROAT, R.A., and FOX, C.A.: Experimental structural alterations in the brain during and after concussion. *Surg Gynec Obstet, 79*:561–572, 1944.
69. WINDLE, W.F., and MAGOUN, H.W.: Functional and structural changes in the central nervous system during and after experimental concussion. *Trans Amer Neurol Assoc*, 1944, pp. 117–122.

Chapter III

SPINE AND SPINAL CORD INJURY

ROBERT J. WHITE and MAURICE S. ALBIN

INTRODUCTION

One approaches a presentation of the biomechanics of spinal injury with a considerable degree of trepidation for at least two reasons: first, the multiplicity and individuality of the various tissues which compose the spinal system and the complex relationships which exist between them render their conversion to engineering models and mathematical formulae a Herculean task, and second, the research so far conducted in elucidating the etiological factors responsible for spinal trauma is characterized by its emphasis on the osseous and ligamentous structures and its necessity of conduction on autopsy material. Perhaps the finality of the resulting lesion, when it involves the spinal cord and its catastrophic functional consequences, has tended to paralyze investigation in the important area of traumatology—in marked contrast, it should be added, to the intensive multi-disciplined investigative programs concentrating on cephalic-cerebral injury.

Our purpose in this presentation is to provide a limited review of the pertinent literature devoted to the biomechanics of spinal trauma and to emphasize the central role that the spinal cord and its nervous elements must be accorded regardless of the architectural change documented in the supporting tissues of the spine. We will also advance the thesis that the rheological factors operating in the circulation and in the spinal cord are more critical to the development of a significant lesion during trauma than previously supposed. Finally, to assist in clarifying the physiology of spinal cord damage, a review of the experimental work devoted to this subject, including our own subhuman primate studies, will be undertaken.

ANATOMICAL REVIEW

For convenience of description and to provide a basis for biophysical comparison, the spinal anatomy has been artificially separated into three broad anatomical categories. The first includes the vertebral bony column and its attendant ligaments and muscles (referred to as the "vertebral unit"); the second is composed of the spinal cord, its associated nerve roots and its membrane investments, including the dura (this has been termed the "cord unit"); and the third comprises the vasculature of the spinal cord (this is called "the spinal vascular unit"). Admittedly such a division is purely arbitrary, because of the intimate relationship that exists between all the tissues that compose the spinal system; however, the clinical significance of biomechanical distortion of the vertebral unit and the spinal vascular units is most meaningful in reference to its resultant effects on the cord unit.

The Vertebral Unit—Vertebral Bony Column; Ligaments and Muscles

The stability and mobility afforded the human body is the mechanical responsibility of this unit. All of the individual bony elements composing the spine articulate by virtue of the intravertebral discs and by posterolateral joints with the exception of the first two cervical and the sacral vertebrae. The very strong annulus fibrosis of the disc provides stability of the synarthroses between the vertebral bodies. The diarthrodial apophyseal joints are stabilized by their capsule as well as the intrasupraspinous ligaments and ligamentum flava. The ligamentous structures, as a result of their intrinsic tensile strength and elasticity, as well as the engineering design utilized in their points of origin and termination, provide an almost idealized structural unit for stability and mobility. The articular processes are flat and small in the cervical region; those in the upper thoracic region are directed downward and forward while in the lower thoracic spine they are directed upward and backward. In the lumbar regions the articular surfaces are large and point inward and outward. In all cases, the upper facets of the lower vertebrae articulate with the lower facets of the superior vertebrae.[1] Further stability is afforded the thoracic spine through the rigidity of the thoracic cage.

The Cord Unit—The Spinal Cord and Its Attendant Nerve Roots and Surrounding Membranes

The spinal cord is a cylindrical extension of the brain stem, suspended by means of a monotonous, repeating series of nerve roots and ligaments in a fluid-filled cavity confined by a relatively inelastic fibrous membrane (the dura). The true spinal dura is a continuous extension of the inner layer of the cranial dura, firmly attached circumferentially at the foramen magnum. Frequently, it is also in close apposition with the posterior surfaces of the first and second cervical vertebrae and more loosely associated with the posterolongitudinal ligament in both the lumbar and cervical regions. At the second sacral level, the dural investment is penetrated by the filum terminale, a direct extension of the pia mater in direct continuity with the inferior tapering spinal cord. The filum terminale and its covering of narrowed dura continue as a multiple layered structure to blend, finally, with the periosteum of the dorsal surface of the coccyx as the coccygeal ligament.[2]

The interface between the spinal dura and the vertebral column is a true space, known as the epidural space, containing numerous venous plexuses, fat and ligaments of the vertebral unit. Also through this space passes the entering and exiting nervous elements of the cord as well as significant numbers of vascular structures supplying the cord substance.

Within the dural sac, two additional membranes surround the spinal cord and collectively with the dura, they are known as the spinal meninges. One of these membranes, the pia mater, is intimately applied to the external surface of the cord. A loosely arranged structure, referred to as the arachnoid, is interposed between the dura proper and the pia, constituting the third element of the spinal meninges. The spinal dura and the leptomeninges, by virtue of their intimate relationship to the existing nerve roots, virtually cuff these structures as they terminate their association at the intervertebral foramen.[2]

The ligamentous suspensory elements of the cord itself are known as dentate ligaments. Twenty-one of these processes are attached to the inner surface of the dura and the lateral surface of the cord. The first dentate is just cephalad to the first cervical roots and the lowest ligament is found between the last thoracic or just above the first lumbar roots. While the significance of their supportive function to cord remains controversial,[3,4] these tough, small triangular ligaments securely anchor the cord to the dural surface.

The paired spinal roots present a constant reminder of the segmental arrangement present in the substance of the spinal cord. They are divided anatomically into the anterior (motor) and posterior (sensory) roots and are blended together to form the spinal nerves exiting through their cuff of spinal dura at the intervertebral foramena. Aside from their obvious neurophysiological function, they are also considered by some to provide mechanical fixation to the cord, especially at the cervical level in certain pathological states.[3]

The Spinal Vascular Unit

Anatomically, the substance of the spinal cord is supplied by branches from a number of major vessels including the vertebral and posterocerebellar arteries.[2] Regional perfusion is provided by branches from the thoracic and abdominal aorta as well as from the deep cervical, intercostal, lumbar and lateral sacral arteries.[2] Lateral spinal arteries, originating from all of these parent vessels, eventually terminate in the anterior and posterior radicular arteries. The anterior radicular artery entering at each side of the cord with each anterior root (only six to eight of these vessels are of significant caliber) joins with the anterior spinal artery which descends on the ventral surface of the cord after its formation from branches from both vertebral arteries.[2] Within the cranium, small branches of the vertebral or posterior-inferior cerebellar arteries continue caudally over the dorsal surface of the cord, usually as two small trunks known as the posterior spinal arteries. Only five to eight of the posterior radicular arteries are of sufficient size to provide meaningful perfusion to the cord.[2] The largest radicular arteries, both anterior and posterior branches, usually enter the cord circulation in the upper lumbar region.[2] The intracord vascular aborization is depicted in Figure 3–1. While the venous drainage of the spinal cord may be variable its anatomical pattern is similar to that of the arteries.[2]

THE BIOMECHANICS OF DAMAGE TO THE VERTEBRAL UNIT

Tissue deformity and destruction of the vertebral unit result from a variety of forces whose vectors of delivery produce the following altera-

SPINAL CORD VASCULAR UNIT

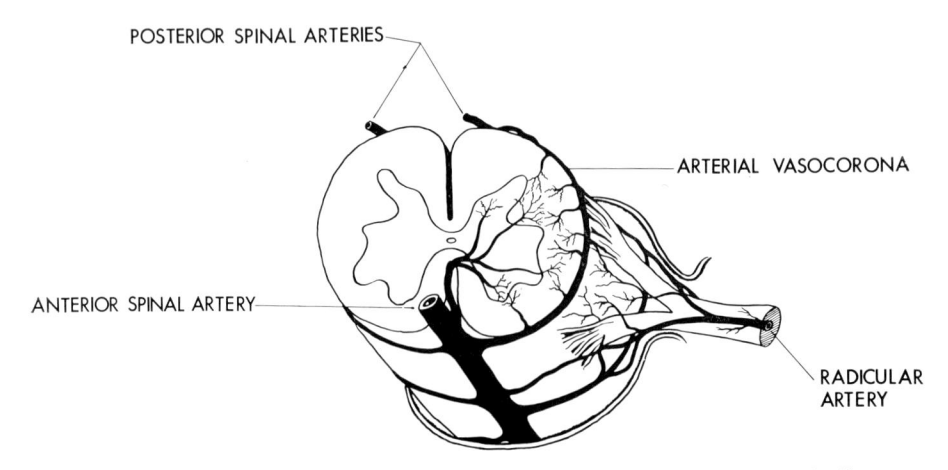

FIGURE 3–1. Artistic representation of a cross-section of the spinal cord illustrating the arterial pattern at the surface and within the substance of the cord.

tions in spinal architectural alignment: flexion, extension, compression, and rotation. While the energy of the force may be dissipated along the entire spinal axis, e.g., with compression, more frequently its impact is limited to a specific transverse (cross-sectional) area of the spine. The resultant extent of damage is further influenced by the anatomical modifications that characterize the various subdivisions of the vertebral unit. Thus, Walker[5] has recently reemphasized the poor mechanical stability of the cervical spine, necessitated by its function of providing support and mobility for the head, rendering it peculiarly susceptible to traumatic deformation.

Roaf,[6] in his carefully documented study of the mechanics of spinal injury, observed that compression forces were absorbed by the vertebral bodies, resulting in bulging of the vertebral end-plate and squeezing blood out of the cancellous bone of the body into the low pressure perivertebral sinuses. Increasing increments of compression produced end-plate rupture with vertical fracture which always preceded disc prolapse since the nucleus pulposus exists normally in a liquid state and, therefore, is incompressable. If the disc had lost its turgor (with age or disease) then prolapse of the annulus was easily accomplished with compression. This all-important channels in the physical matrix of nucleus pulposus with age has been ascribed by Horton[7] to degenerative alterations (documented by means of x-ray crystallographic and polarizing microscopic studies) causing loss of elasticity.

Hirsch[8] has investigated the physics of the intervertebral disc with particular reference to its performance characteristics under conditions of both static loading and dynamically applied stress. Under circumstances of an actively changing applied stress, he was able to record vibrations within the nucleus pulposus and if the dynamic force was added to an already applied static load, the vibratory deformation may exceed the rupture tolerance of the annulus or its attachment to bone. *In vivo* measurements of intradiscal pressure in the normal lumbar spine have demonstrated values ranging from 100 to 175 kg in the sitting position with lower pressure in the standing or reclining posture.[9]

Roaf's experiments[6] have demonstrated that hyperextension and hyperflexion deformation of the vertebral unit results in compression fracture of the bone before rupture of the spinal ligaments takes place, however, if rotational forces are added then production of ligamentous detachment and fragmentation are easily accomplished with associated dislocation. He[6] believes that clinically the commonly described hyperextension and hyperflexion injuries are, in reality, rotational injuries. In general, he[6] states, "Rotation forces produce dislocations whereas compression forces produce fractures." Holdsworth[1] has also emphasized the association of pure flexion forces with compression fractures of the vertebral body, particularly in the thoracic region where unusual stability is provided by the chest cage and in the lumbar area where the posterior ligament complex is strong. These fractures are stable since the bony fragments are impacted and the ligaments and articular processes are intact. With posterior ligament rupture, however (as seen in flexion-rotation injury), disengagement of the articular processes result with consequent bony dislocation. This is commonly observed in the cervical spine.[1] Extension forces generally cause rupture of the anterior spinal ligament with dislocation, but if the ligament remains unruptured then fractures of the lamina and pedicles will occur.[1] The former is a rare injury according to Holdsworth[1]; however, the latter (extension dislocation) is a frequent lesion in the cervical region.

While forceful deformation of the individual elements of the vertebral unit may cause architectural instability and challenging pain syndromes,[10] the main concern is the resulting effect that such traumatic injury has on the spinal cord. This is perhaps best exemplified in the cervical area where the uniqueness of the structure of the vertebral unit and the cephalic position of the spinal cord render injuries in this anatomical region frequent and devastating.[11]

Since the publications of Taylor,[12] and Taylor and Blackwood,[13] illustrating the production of cervical cord damage without vertebral fracture or dislocation in forcible extension, interest has centered on attempts to etiologically define such injuries in the absence of radiological evidence of bony deformity. These authors[12,13] have implicated the forward-bulging of the ligamentum flavum impinging on the cord. Previously these injuries were considered due to temporary dislocation with immediate reduction; the so-called "recoil injury of the cervical spine." The importance of the ligamentum flavum in reducing the cross-sectional area of the spinal canal during position change has been emphasized in the autopsy studies of Payne and Spillane,[14] Taylor,[12] and more recently by Stoltman and Blackwood[15] in cervical spondylosis.

Schneider,[16,17,18] in a series of classical papers published in the 1950's, has emphasized the anatomical factors including hypertrophic bony changes, ligamentous distortions and acute disc rupture which may produce both anterior posterior compression of the cervical cord during acute cervical trauma. Careful analysis of his case material has enabled him to establish specific neurological syndromes accompanying such injuries.[16,17,18]

Since the spinal cord is suspended in the hollow spinal canal, any reduction in its volumetric displacement renders the cord substance more susceptible to compression during abnormal movements of spine produced by externally imposed forces. The importance of these cross-sectional relationships in cord injury has been repeatedly emphasized in studies dealing with spondylosis. The average anteroposterior width of the normal cervical canal is 17 mm and if reduced to 10 mm, cord compression is likely.[14] Similar measurements made in spondylitic cervical spine demonstrated the cervical canal diameter was reduced to 14 to 15 mm,[14] indicative of the ease of compression of cord in this condition. It is reasonable to assume that the occurrence of cord injury in older persons is significantly influenced by the alterations in the vertebral unit, notably the reduction in spinal column diameter with age, favoring spinal cord compression.

A unique type of fracture-dislocation occurs in the cervical spine.[19] The results from a violent jerking of the head and neck, producing an acute forward displacement of the atlas on the axis. This pernicious fracture-dislocation frequently caused by fracture of the odontoid process of the axis or avulsion of the odontoid ligament[20] may produce sudden death[10] or conversely exhibit the extreme bony displacement possible in this region without compression or compromise of the spinal cord.

THE BIOMECHANICS OF DAMAGE OF THE CORD UNIT

In the final analysis, the extent of damage to spinal cord is really the core problem in spinal injury. Little imagination is required to appreciate the degree of destruction wrought on the soft matrix of cord when portions of fractured vertebrae are driven with piston-like force into the spinal canal, compressing and rupturing the tissue substance or when the extent of the dislocation is of such magnitude that the continuity of the cord is literally transected. It is in the more subtle injury states that careful evaluation of the stresses applied and the capacities of the cord unit to resist mechanical deformation must be undertaken to explain the resultant lesion.

Breig, in his monogram entitled "The Biomechanics of the Nervous System,"[3] documents the normal tissue deformation of the cord in relation to movements of the spinal column. The spinal cord does not move up and down axially in the canal as was formerly believed, but rather adapts itself to changes in canal length through the mechanism of plastic deformity of cord substance. For example, in flexion, the cord actually elongates while in extension the cord shortens, developing folds on its external surface. Biophysical studies[3] employing an isolated cord suspended in physiologic saline demonstrated a 1.0 cm elongation of a 20 cm cord segment resultant from the "apparent" weight of the cord (estimated at 0.3 gm) in liquid suspension. While it is obviously difficult to duplicate *in vitro* conditions in such experiments, attention has been paid to the restrictive and inertial forces of the pia mater resisting lateral compression of the cord, especially during flexion of the spine which is operant in the living person.[3]

The dentate ligaments, which offer stabilization to the human spinal cord, may undergo physical deformation during excessive movements of the spinal column.[3,22] Thus these ligaments are capable of stretching in flexion but not in extension, exhibiting slight elastic tension suggestive of providing a uniform distribution of tensile forces over the length of the cord.[3] Their fixation capabilities were originally implicated by Kahn[4] in the development of localized anterior cord lesion in spinal trauma.

The nerve roots are capable of tissue alteration allowing both elongation and shortening. In extension, the cross-sectional area of the nerve root increases and the nerve as a whole is converted into a series of gentle folds.[3] In flexion, the opposite occurs with elongation (straightening) of the root and its sleeve.[3]

Cord substance, without its pial casting, acts like a semifluid cohesive mass, offering little or no resistance to applied forces.[23] With the pia mater intact the cord is afforded protection from extreme deformation by virtue of the fact that it has a certain capability of movement within this tissue envelopment.[23,3,22]

Granting the above described biophysical properties of the cord unit, it is obvious that lesioning of the spinal nervous tissue results from exceeding the mechanical tolerances that are characteristic of these tissues and their interrelationships.

While it does appear that in the normal setting, the spinal cord is afforded both mechanical and hydraulic protection, the advantages of such protection are seriously reduced by pathological changes in both the vertebral and cord unit tissue matrixes with age, as evidenced by alterations in tissue elasticity,[7] narrowing of the spinal canal[14] and early structural fatigue of all structure elements.[24]

The precise biophysical changes that accompany injury to spinal cord tissue are not well understood. Extensive documentation is available referable to the resultant pathological lesions in spinal cord trauma,[25,26] however, little experimental work has been undertaken to elucidate the etiological factors implicated in acute injury. Recently, Breig and El-Nadi,[27] employing neuroradiological methods in the human subjects with cervical disc disease, analyzed the forces operating in spinal cord damage, indicating that flexion resulted in contact pressure and overstretching, while in extension true compression occurred. These same authors[27] emphasize the difficulty of extrapolating from histological data to the individual effects of the various forces operating within the cord substance with trauma, e.g., axial tension, radial tension and contact pressure. In addition, consideration must also be made for the variation in the mechanical properties of the two tissues (white and gray matter) that constitute the cord substance. Ommaya[28] has recently emphasized our ignorance of the mechanical properties of the spinal cord.

Coe et al.[29] and Ommaya et al.[30] have constructed ingenious models employing the subhuman primate to investigate the role of cervical cord-medullary injury to concussion. Coe et al.[29] were able to delineate significant instantaneous alterations in blood pressure, heart rate, respiratory rate and amplitude changes in spinal cord conduction and concussion-like state following measured flexion-compression of the cervical spine. Ommaya[30] has been able to construct mathematical models from his biological experiments characterizing cervical-cephalic displacement referable to cerebral concussion.

RHEOLOGICAL FACTORS IN SPINAL CORD INJURY

Generally, tissue damage in spinal cord trauma has almost universally been ascribed to compression forces. As early as 1939, Jefferson,[31] puzzled by the length of the lesions following spinal cord trauma attributed this phenomenon to associated vascular injury. Schneider[32,33] has recently ascribed this acute central softening of the cord to temporary anterior spinal arterial insufficiency resulting from reduction in flow in the vertebral arteries during spinal trauma. This is believed to occur in cases of cervical fracture-dislocations and hypertrophic cervical oeseophytes.

Symonds,[34] and Mair and Druckman[25] have implicated the same hydraulic mechanism of vascular insufficiency to explain myelopathy of cervical spondylosis. Breig[27] has also suggested reduction in arterial blood flow in the vessels supplying the cervical cord in spondylosis, thereby rendering the cord extremely vulnerable to ischemia if abnormal mechanical stresses are applied to the vessels in the cord substance. Drake,[11] after reviewing the available literature on the subject of vascular insufficiency of the cord in traumatic injury, was inclined to dismiss the evidence for anterior spinal involvement because of the immediateness of the neurological dysfunction. In autopsy material, Breig[27] has observed straightening of the course of radicular arteries as well as disappearance of some of the vessels on the surface of the cord in extreme flexion. Allen[35] has noted a pale appearance of the cord in flexion at surgery and has presumed that the blood supply is reduced.

In our experimental work,[36] we have documented an immediate reduction in flow in the posterior surface vessels of the monkey cord following direct impact trauma. This rheological change is potentiated by increasing flattening and narrowing of the vessels under direct vision as tissue edema develops (Fig. 3–2). Flurocein injections have further indicated reduced

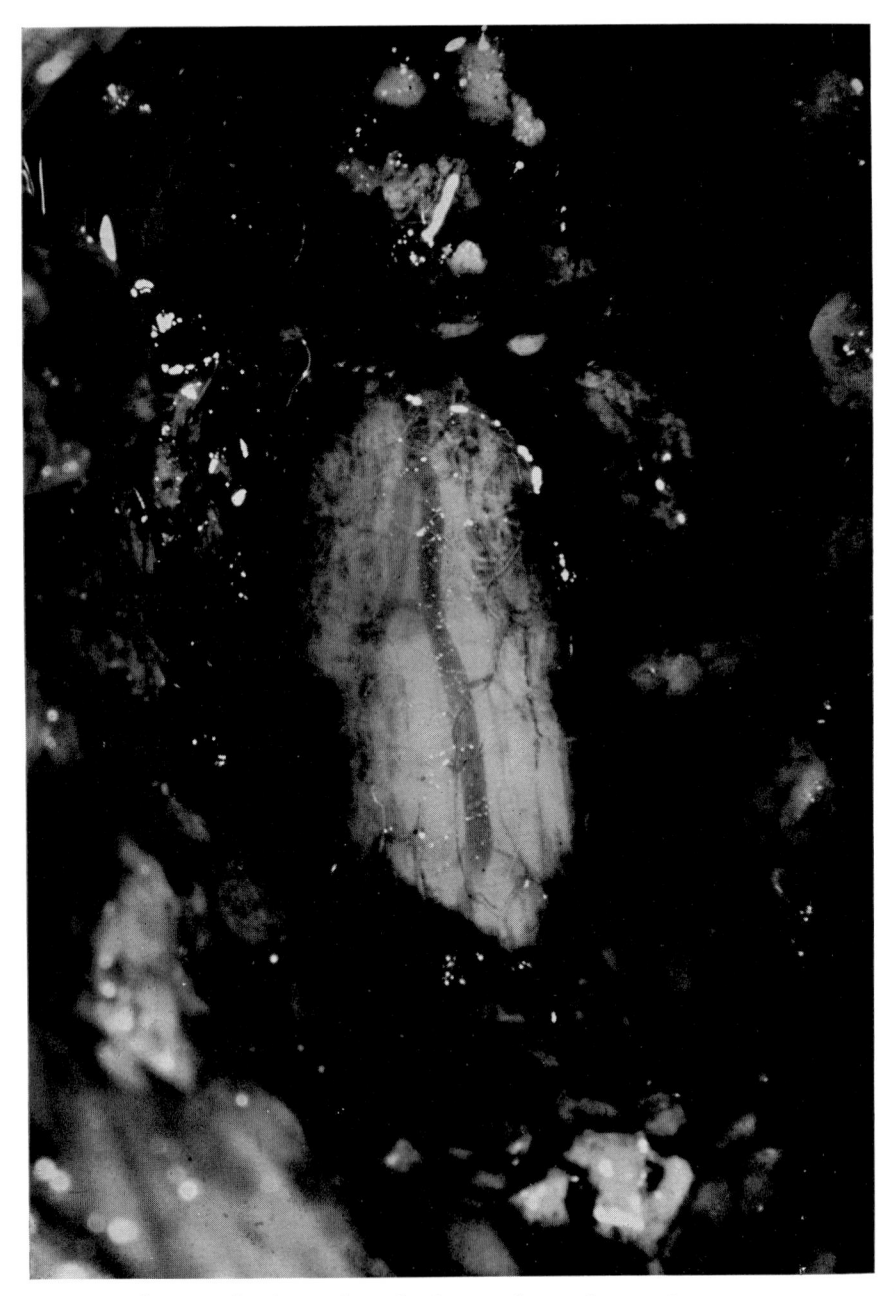

FIGURE 3–2. Photograph of spinal cord of a monkey 4 hours after impact injury with 300 GCF (impact velocity 170 cm/sec.). The cord is swollen against the transparent dura with diminution of its normal surface vasculature except for the posterior spinal artery and its major branches which evidence physical flattening and marked reduction of flow.

blood flow in the segmental area of injury with retarded circulatory movement at the borders of the lesion.

Our investigative work and review of the literature has led us to postulate that rheological factors are significant in traumatic lesioning of the spinal cord for the following reasons: (1) The arterial circulation to the spinal cord is marginal under normal circumstances, having a minimum of potential vascular anastomoses[37] as well as a unique architectural distribution from its surface, causing it to be vulnerable to compression forces; (2) Direct observation of the posterior surface circulation suggests early reduction in flow resulting from vascular spasm and interstitial edema[36]; and (3) The dependency of the intrinsic cord circulation on changes in flow and pressure in major arterial systems, e.g., vertebral, which may be compromised in injury and which may adversely affect cord tissue perfusion.[32]

EXPERIMENTAL INVESTIGATION OF SPINAL CORD INJURY

Historical Review

It is to be noted that with rare exception, experimental work dealing with the problems of spinal cord injury prior to the World War II were evaluated in terms of the development of clinical symptomatology and the description of the histological findings. It is only since World War II that some light has been focused on the biomechanical factors involved in spinal cord injuries, a good part of this direction being undoubtedly stimulated by the pioneering work of Gurdjian, Webster and Lissner[38] followed by the investigations of Breig[3] and Schneider.[18]

As will be noted, and as emphasized by Wolman[39] and Groat[40] et al., much of the early experimental work on spinal cord injury dealt with the pathology resulting from "concussion," a word that is used to cover a "multitude of sins." This has included according to Wolman[39] ". . . functional disturbance without microscopic change, mildness, reversibility, remoteness from the original site of injury and cord damage in the absence of any fracture or dislocation of the vertebrae." Schmaus[41] in 1890 was probably among the first to study the effect of concussion on the development of spinal cord injury when he found foci of softening, areas of necrosis, cavity formation and systemic degeneration after beating on wooden boards attached to the vertebral columns of dogs and rabbits. Schmaus felt that the spinal cord lesions in the animals were caused by the transmission of force from the vertebral column to the cerebrospinal fluid causing sufficient pressure on the spinal cord to rupture the walls of the blood vessels giving rise to hemorrhage or parenchymal lacerations. Spiller[42] produced spinal cord injury by squeezing a kitten with a heavy swinging door and finding degenerative changes in the white matter of the anterolateral and ventral columns. Kirchgasser,[43] in 1899, showed that considerable degeneration of the medullary sheaths in the rabbit resulted from severe blows to the back without injuring the vertebrae or causing hemorrhage into the vertebral canal or spinal cord. Schterbach,[44] in 1907, produced changes in the spinal cord using a vibrating apparatus, and found small areas of necrosis of the grey matter. D'Abundo,[45] in 1916, caused changes in the spinal cord by centrifuging small animals. He found localized necrosis in the posterior columns where the histologic lesions evidenced swelling of the axis cylinder, fragmentation, degeneration of the myelin sheath, and minute focal hemorrhages.

Mairet and Durante,[46] in 1919, reported on the effects of high explosives in causing hemorrhagic lesions of the medulla and spinal cord in the rabbit and thought these lesions were caused by changes in air pressure. Roussy, Lhermitte and Cornil,[47] in 1920, injured guinea pigs and one rabbit by blows to the back in the thoracic region. They purported to demonstrate that direct trauma to the vertebral column affects mainly the myelinated fibers of the white matter, while indirect trauma to the vertebrae produces less injury, with cellular lesions becoming more prominent. Ferraro,[48] in 1927, utilized the technique of hitting the vertebral region of the unanesthetized rabbit with an iron rod and examining the spinal cords within 6 days after injury. By 90 hours, he found diffuse and intensive degeneration in white matter and a pronounced neuroglial reaction. Anterior horn cells were also found to be involved. Like Schmaus, Ferraro speculated that the pathogenesis in this type of injury could be due to the transmission of shock waves by the cerebrospinal fluid (CSF) upon the spinal cord and also to the passage of vibration from the bony vertebra to the CSF and medullary parenchyma.

The difficulties involved in evaluating these earlier experimental procedures is obvious because of the lack of reliability of the methodology involved. Probably the best study delineating the effects of concussion was reported by Groat, Rambach and Windle[49] in 1945. Using freely suspended cats, injury was accomplished with a single blow against the back using a blunt wooden bar on a horizontal plane. Chalk applied to bar allowed for accurate placement of the blow site. Some animals were also injured after midthoracic cord section. Using electrophysiological parameters, they found that the severity of the concussion and longitudinal extent of spinal cord involvement was directly proportional to the strength of the blow. They concluded that uncomplicated concussion of the spinal cord causes a complete functional block of the spinal cord at the level of an adequate force to the nervous parenchyma. They noted that long ascending and descending fiber tracts were involved as well as the interneurons. Histologically evident cell alterations occurred, and frank chromatolysis was noted in the post-concussion period.

Allen[49] in 1911, was probably among the first to directly injure the spinal cord, and more importantly, developed a technique to produce a standardized type of injury. After laminectomy at low thoracic levels, he subjected dogs to trauma from a known weight dropping a calculated distance on the spinal cord with its investing membranes intact. This low velocity type of injury was accomplished by the weight falling on the cord through a metal dropping tube, with the force calculated in gram-centimeters (GCF). In his control groups, he found that animals subjected to less than 340 GCF made a complete functional recovery, while as the magnitude of impact forces were increased, more serious symptoms developed. At 340 GCF the animals evidenced a spastic paraplegia which cleared within 10 days. Most animals traumatized with 420 GCF showed complete spastic paraplegia with scissor crossing of the hind limb and fecal and bladder incontinence as well or trophic ulcers. At impact injury forces of 420 GCF, Allen found symptoms of complete cord transection with death resulting in all the animals in this group. He theorized that save for a spinal cord that was literally transected, the etiology of the symptom-complex of transverse lesions of the spinal cord in fracture dislocation of the spinal column was either due to destruction of axis cylinders due to impact or else the development of high intramedullary pressures due to hemorrhage and edema. Allen reasoned that it might be possible to relieve the edema and hemorrhage by doing a medial longitudinal myelotomy in animals who would be normally rendered paraplegic after high impact injury forces were implied. Five dogs were then subjected to 540 GCF and a medial longitudinal incision about 1.0 to 1.5 cm in length was made directly through the impact level passing through the cord as well. Allen states that the animals made an uneventful recovery, some of the dogs showing only slight spasticity in the hind limb. In a review of the histological findings after impact injury with 540 GCF, Allen[50] noted the development of hemorrhagic and edematous changes within the substance of the spinal cord starting as early as 15 minutes after impact injury. By four hours after injury he found numerous swollen axis-cylinders in the white matter of the lateral and posterior columns, the edema and hemorrhage reaching its peak at this time period.

Using dogs, McVeigh,[51] in 1923, produced lesions by compressing the spinal cord with a fingertip after laminectomy at the T^7 and T^8 vertebral level. He noted the striking development of edema involving the perivascular spaces and nerve sheaths located preponderantly in the lateral white columns, although the lateral and anterior columns were also affected. This edema started to appear eight hours after injury, and increased in amount of area involved for at least two days. He also described the presence of hemorrhage most marked in the dorsal white columns presenting itself above and below the site of injury and also appearing in the central grey matter. Thompson,[52] in 1923, working with and using the same technique as McVeigh, injured the spinal cords of dogs by digital compression and noted that the cone shaped areas of destruction above and below the lesion was in many ways similar to the lesions described in gunshot wounds of the spinal cord. Thompson also noted the contribution of the rapidly developing spinal cord edema to the pathogenesis of injury.

Freeman and Wright,[53] in 1953, applied Allen's method to produce standardized impact injury to the spinal cords of rats and dogs. Using paired controls, they tried to evaluate the effect of incision of the pia mater followed by the passage of a blunt probe halfway into the cord between the dorsal columns down logitudinally for a distance of 1.5 cm. They noted that functional improvement occurred in the animals who had been subjected to myelotomy when compared to the control. The authors speculated that after injury, functional damage occurred as a result of edema and hemorrhage; with the cord swelling against the pial barrier, the intrinsic segmental capillary circulation would fail because of this high pressure and ensuing ischemia would result.

Tarlov, et al.,[54,55,56] starting in 1953, pioneered studies on the effect of compressive stresses on the spinal cord. Using a sophisticated hydraulic apparatus to inflate a balloon placed extradurally, Tarlov and co-workers found that when small compressive forces were used to produce a total sensorimotor block, recovery ensued after compression periods of up to two hours. When large compressive forces were used, recovery occurred if the compression was released within one to five minutes. Combining this study, using electrophysiological and histological parameters, it was thought that the mechanical deformation caused by the pressure on the spinal cord was the primary mechanism. Although the factor of anoxia secondary to ischemia was ruled out, in the animals that did not recover, the pathological picture revealed extensive cord destruction and tissue vacuolation at the site of compression with extensions above and below. No qualitative histological differences could be ascertained in cords subjected to acute and gradual compressive forces.

Spinal Cord Injury In The Subhuman Primate

That the mammalian spinal cord is in itself exquisitely vulnerable to injury is attested to by the elaborate system of coverings, hydraulic dampening barriers, bony investments, muscular coatings as well as subcutaneous and cutaneous pads. All this may serve to dissipate energy that can cause structural damage and deformation resulting from externally applied as well as inertial forces.

To gain more insight on the direct effect of impact forces on the spinal cord, and in order to work with a standardized injury model, we have used a modified version of the simple technique first developed by Allen in 1911.[49] Under general anesthesia, and after laminectomy at T_{10}, a known weight is dropped a calculated distance on a metal impounder sitting on the spinal cord through a Teflon℗ dropping tube. Thus, a specific area of the spinal cord can be subjected to both compressive and shear strains at lesion site, the response of the cord to such injury can be studied immediately after onset and the force calculated in GCF. After our study in dogs[57] confirmed the feasibility of producing a standardized impact injury model patterned after the experiments of Allen[49] and Freeman and Wright,[53] we then moved to the experimental animal more closely related to man, the Rhesus monkey.[58] It was demonstrated that the minimal force necessary to cause irreversible paralegia in the monkey was 300 GCF (a 20 gm weight dropping 15 cm) and that the velocity of impact was indeed low, reaching 170 cm per second. Within seconds after injury, the circular imprint (0.5 mm diameter) of the impounder could often be noted on both dural and pial surfaces, and there developed a red-blueish discoloration with the spinal cord often becoming nonpulsatile. Within 15 minutes after injury, the cord appeared swollen, this edema becoming maximal generally within 3 to 6 hours after impact injury. In a neurophysiological study,[59] we demonstrated that conduction across the injured cord was blocked within one minute after a paraplegic producing threshhold force was used. It is interesting to note that the role of spinal cord edema as being an important factor in progressive spinal cord injury was cited by Allen[50] who stated that edema became maximal about 4 hours after injury. Ferraro,[48] McVeigh,[51] Thompson,[52] Freeman and Wright,[53] and Scarf,[60] have described spinal cord swelling after injury. One may then theorize that the resultant experimental impact injury affected the vascular irrigation of the damaged area and that with edema developing, ischemia would result. Thus, after laminectomy at T_{10}, the application of 300 GCF followed by a four hour delay and dural opening rendered thirteen control monkeys irreversibly paraplegic.

We then asked the question whether there was any agent or method that was effective in protecting the spinal cord from developing ischemia, that would help decrease the rapidly developing edema, would allow for a reduction in metabolic activity of the affected area, and would also allow for adequate blood flow through a vascularly compromised region. The clinical and experimental use of hypothermia in cardiovascular and neurological surgery during the past decade [61,62,63,64,65,66,67,68,69] led us to evaluate its effect on traumatic injury to the spinal cord. Since we felt that it was opportune to work in the specific area of injury, it was decided to utilize the surgical incision as a reservoir and cool the traumatized cord locally by continuously recirculating sterile, cold saline (3 to 5°C) with a roller pump through a Mayo Pediatric heat exchanger. Physiological studies in both dogs,[57,70] and monkeys,[58] allowed for intrinsic spinal cord temperature reductions from 37°C to 10°C within 30 minutes or less. Brain and esophageal temperatures, heart rates, EKG, and blood pressure showed little change from preperfusion levels. To allow for an analagous clinical situation, it was decided to wait 4 hours after injury before beginning the 3 hours of localized spinal cord cooling.

Fourteen monkeys subjected to laminectomy at T_{10}, 300 GCF, 4-hour delay, dural incision, and 3 hours of cooling, manifested functional recovery by the end of the first month, with one monkey having bilateral leg weakness and slight impairment in placing after that period of time.

Upon termination of the cooling, the cords revealed themselves to be pulsatile, the edema decreased, with the superficial vessels showing visible evidence of perfusion (Fig. 3–2, Fig. 3–3). While it is known that cerebral arterioles constrict during surface cooling to 30°C,[71] we have found from our studies on the donor perfused isolated brain,[72] that the normal autoregulatory cerebrovascular mechanisms were abolished when 12°C were reached; and flow rates through this isolated brain equalled and at times exceeded the normothermic baseline flows. Apart from the temperature reduced metabolic demand and a more adequate blood flow through marginally injured areas, it is possible that another mechanism to explain the effect of localized cooling on spinal cord injury exists on the cellular-membrane level. Electron microscopic techniques have showed[73,74,75] the existence of tubelike cytoplasmic structures that are cryoreactive. The microtubules (or neurotubules in nerve) are thought to make up a key axial structure in most if not all cystoplasmic gel formations by forming an elastic framework or cytoskeleton in order to give directional guidance for particle flow (in both dendrite and axon). Interestingly enough, these structures depolymerize under low temperature conditions and repolymerize on rewarming. Thus, the depolymerization of the neurotubule by cooling might help to stabilize the cell membrane and prevent abnormal metabolic shifts.

As we stated above, localized spinal cord cooling in the experimental animal was helpful in reversing the paraplegia producing effects of 300 GCF of impact injury to the Rhesus monkey spinal cord, after a 4-hour delay.

In six control, (not cooled) and six experimental, (cooled for 3 hours) animals doubling the delay period to eight hours after injury had no effect on the spinal cord and the animals in both groups remained paraplegic.[76] This seems to signify within the terms of our experimental method and

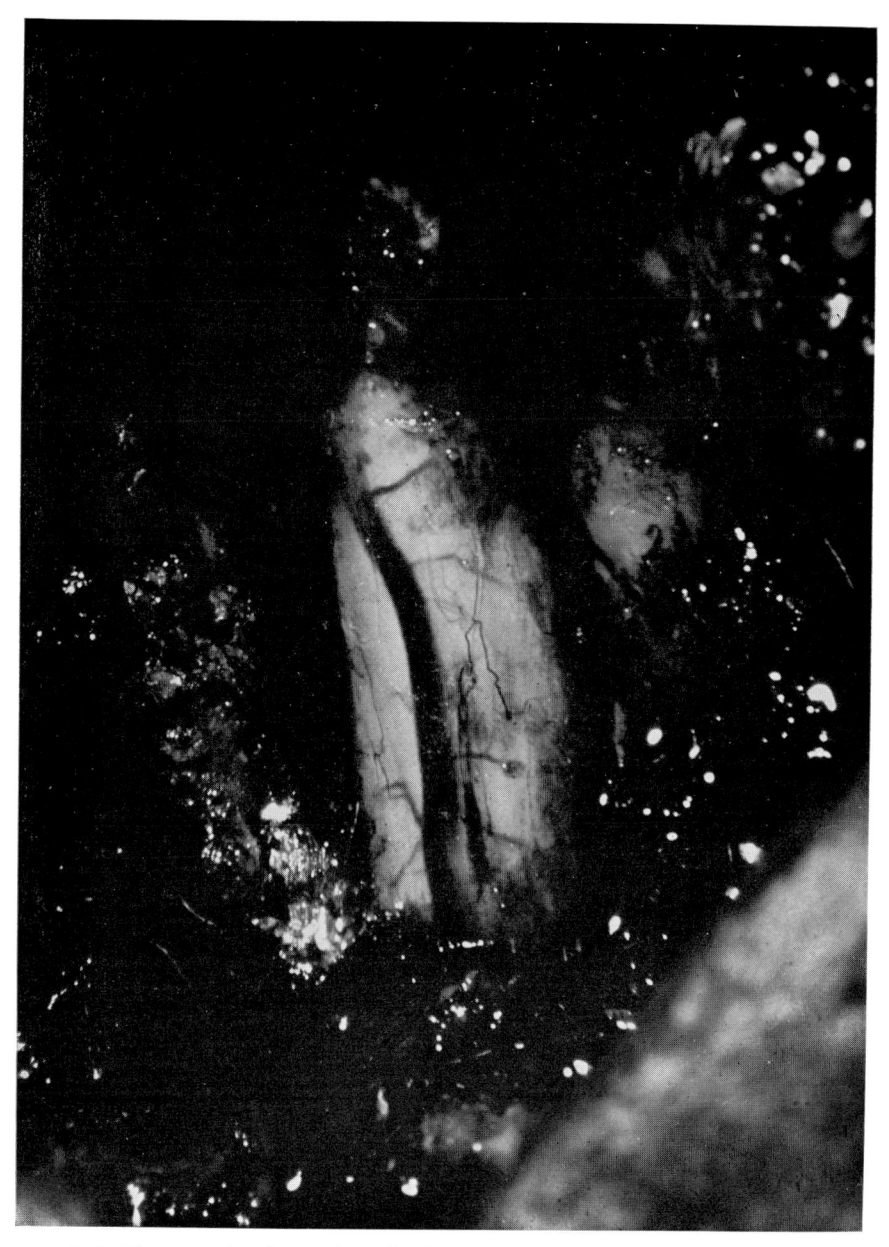

FIGURE 3–3. Photograph of spinal cord of monkey shown in Figure 3–2 after 3 hours of localized spinal cord cooling. The spinal cord volume is visually reduced and the large surface vessels demonstrate increased perfusion.

design that localized spinal cord cooling (for 3 hours) is effective in impact injury to the spinal cord if instituted earlier than eight hours after injury.

SUMMARY

Spinal injury continues as a major cause of disability and death in trauma. Central and critical to the complex problem of spinal injury is the production of specific lesions in the cord substance by the forces of violence. It is the finality and irreversibility of this catastrophic tissue damage which argues for research into its causes and prevention. The carefully reasoned studies of Schneider, Breig, and others, documenting some of the clinical and pathophysiological correlates of spinal trauma, are most significant. The investigations of Ommaya and Coe are especially exciting because of their development and utilization of living models anatomically similar to the human in elucidating the biophysical and physiological principles of mechanical stress to the spine. Yet, in spite of the work of the past, unless an accelerated and in-depth research program, national in scope, and similar to that for head injuries is developed, it will be decades before preventive and therapeutic techniques are at hand to scientifically manage spinal injury.

REFERENCES

1. HOLDSWORTH, F.W.: Fractures, dislocations and fracture-dislocations of the spine. *J Bone Joint Surg*, 45B:7, 1963.
2. PEELE, T.L.: *The Neuroanatomical Basis for Clinical Neurology*. New York, McGraw, 1954.
3. BREIG, A.: *Biomechanics of the Central Nervous System*. Stockholm, Almqvist and Wiksell, 1960.
4. KAHN, E.A.: The role of the dentate ligaments in spinal cord compression and the syndrome of lateral sclerosis. *J Neurosurg*, 4:101, 1947.
5. WALKER, E. A.: The neurosurgeon's viewpoint. *J Bone Joint Surg*, 46A:1806, 1964.
6. ROAF, R.: A study of the mechanics of spinal injury. *J Bone Surg.*, 42B:810, 1960.
7. HORTON, W.G.: Further observations on the elastic mechanism of the intervertebral disc. *J Bone Joint Surg*, 40B:552, 1958.
8. HIRSCH, C.: The reaction of intervertebral discs to compression forces. *J Bone Joint Surg*, 37A:1188, 1955.
9. NACHEMSON, A., and MORRIS, J.M.: Measurements of intradiscal pressure. *J Bone Joint Surg*, 46A:1077, 1964.
10. GOFF, C.W.; ALDEN, J.O., and ALDES, J.H.: *Traumatic Cervical Syndrome and Whiplash*. Philadelphia, Lippincott, 1967.
11. DRAKE, C.G.: Cervical spinal cord injury. *J Neurosurg*, 19:487, 1962.
12. TAYLOR, A.R.: The mechanism of injury to the spinal cord in the neck without damage to the vertebral column. *J Bone Joint Surg*, 33B:543, 1951.
13. TAYLOR, A.R. and BLACKWOOD, W.: Paraplegia in hyperextension cervical injuries with normal radiographic appearances. *J Bone Joint Surg*, 30B:245, 1951.

14. PAYNE, E.E., and SPILLANE, J.D.: The cervical spine—an anatomicopathological study of seventy specimens (using a special technique) with particular reference to the problem of cervical spondylosis. *Brain 80:*571, 1957.
15. STOLTMAN, H.F., and BLACKWOOD, W.: The role of the ligamenta flava in the pathogenesis of myelopathy in cervical spondylosis. *Brain,* 87:45, 1964.
16. SCHNEIDER, R.C.: A syndrome in acute cervical injuries for which early operation is indicated. *J Neurosurg,* 8:360, 1951
17. SCHNEIDER, R.C., CHERRY, G., and PANTEK, H.: The syndrome of acute central cervical spinal cord injury. With special reference to the mechanism involved in hyperextension injuries of cervical spine. *J Neurosurg,* 11:546, 1954.
18. SCHNEIDER, R.C.: The syndrome of acute central cervical spinal cord injury. *J Neurol Neurosurg Psychiat,* 21:216, 1958.
19. KAHN, E.A.; BASSETT, R.C.; SCHNEIDER, R.C., and CROSBY, C.E.: *Correlative Neurosurgery,* Springfield, Thomas, 1955.
20. MIXTER, S.J., and OSGOOD, R.B.: Traumatic lesions of the atlas and axis. *Ann Surg,* 51:193, 1910.
21. REID, J.D.: Effects of flexion-extension movements of the head and spine upon the spinal cord and nerve roots. *J Neurol Neurosurg Psychiat,* 23:214, 1960.
22. KEY, A., and RETZIUS, G.: Studien in der Anatomie des Nerven Systems. *Folio,* 166:1, Stockholm, P.A. Norstedt and Söner, 1875.
23. WHITE, R.J.: Unpublished data.
24. SMITH, F.P.: Experimental biomechanics of transvertebral disc rupture. *J Neurosurg,* 19:594, 1962.
25. MAIR, W.G.P., and DRUCKMAN, R.: The pathology of spinal cord lesions and their relation to the clinical features in protrusion of cervical intervertebral discs (a report of four cases). *Brain,* 76:70, 1953.
26. DAVIDSON, C.: Pathology of the spinal cord as a result of trauma. *Res Publ Assoc Res Nerv Ment Dis,* 24:151, 1945.
27. BREIG, A., and EL-NADI, A.F.: Biomechanics of the cervical spinal cord. *Acta Radiol,* 4:602, 1964.
28. OMMAYA, A.K.: Mechanical properties of tissues of the nervous system (manuscript kindly provided by the author).
29. COE, J.E.; CALVIN, T.H.; RODENBERG, R.H., and YEW, C.H.: Concussion-like state following cervical cord injury in the monkey. *J Trauma,* 7:512, 1967.
30. OMMAYA, A.K.; HIRSCH, A.E., and MARTINEZ, J.L.: The role of whiplash in cerebral concussion. *Proc Tenth Stapp Car Crash Conf.,* Holloman A. F. Base, New Mexico, Nov. 8–9, New York, 1966, p. 197.
31. JEFFERSON, G.: Discussion on fractures and dislocation of the cervical vertebrae. *Proc Roy Soc Med,* 33:657, 1940.
32. SCHNEIDER, R.C., and CROSBY, E.C.: Vascular insufficiency of brain stem and spinal cord in spinal trauma. *Neurology,* 9:643, 1959.
33. SCHNEIDER, R.C., and SCHEMM, G.W.: Vertebral arterial insufficiency in acute and chronic spinal trauma. With special reference to the syndrome of acute central cervical spinal cord injury. *J Neurosurg* 18:348, 1961.
34. SYMONDS, C.: The interrelation of trauma and cervical spondylosis in compression of the cervical cord. *Lancet,* 264:45, 1953.
35. ALLEN, K.L.: Neuropathies caused by bony spurs in cervical spine with special reference to surgical treatment. *J Neurol Neurosurg Psychiat,* 15:20, 1952.
36. WHITE, R.J., and ALBIN, M.S.: Vascular factors operating in experimental trauma to the spinal cord. (to be published).

37. Suh, T.H., and Alexander, L.: Vascular system of the human spinal cord. *Arch Neurol Psychiat, 41*:660, 1939.
38. Gurdjian, E.S.; Webster, J.E., and Lissner, H.R.: Observations and mechanism of brain concussion, contussion and laceration. *Surg Gynec Obstet, 101*:680, 1955.
39. Wolman, L: The neuropathology of traumatic paraplegia. *Paraplegia, 1*:233, 1964.
40. Groat, R.A.; Rambach, W.A., and Windle, W.F.: Concussion of the spinal cord —an experimental study and a critique of the use of the term. *Surg Gynec Obstet, 81*:63, 1945.
41. Schmaus, H.: Beitrage zue pathologischen Anatomie des Ruckenmarkserschutterung. *Virchow Arch Path Anat, 122*:326, 1890.
42. Spiller, W.G.: A critical summary of recent literature on concussion of the spinal cord with some original observation. *Amer J Med Sci, 118*:190, 1899.
43. Kirchgasser, G.: Experimentalle Untersuchungen über Ruckenmarkserschutterung. *Deutsch Z Nervenk, 2*:400, 1897.
44. Schterbach, H.: Des alterations de la moelle épinière chez le lapin sous l'influence de la vibration intensive. *Encephale, 2*:521, 1907.
45. D'Abundo, G.: Alterazioni del sistemo nervoso centrali consecutive a particolari commozioni traumatische. *Riv Ital Neuropat, 9*:145, 1916.
46. Mairet, A., and Durante, G.: Contribution a l'étude experimentale de lesions commotionneles. *Presse Med, 25*:478, 1917.
47. Roussy, G.; Lhermitte, J., and Cornil, L.: Etude experimentale des lesions commotionneles de la moelle épinière. *Ann Med, 8*:335, 1920.
48. Ferraro, A.: Experimental medullary concussion of the spinal cord in rabbits. *Arch Neurol Psychiat, 18*:357, 1927.
49. Allen, A.R.: Surgery of experimental lesion of the spinal cord equivalent to crush injury of fracture dislocation of spinal column. *JAMA, 57*:878, 1911.
50. Allen, A.R.: Remarks on the histopathological changes in the spinal cord due to impact. An experimental study. *J Nerv Ment Dis, 41*:141, 1914.
51. McVeigh, J.F.: Experimental cord crushes, with special references to the mechanical factors involved and subsequent changes in the areas of the cord affected. *Arch Surg, 7*:573, 1923.
52. Thompson, J.E.: Pathological changes occurring in the spinal cord following fracture dislocations of the vertebrae. *Ann Surg, 78*:260, 1923.
53. Freeman, L.W., and Wright, T.W.: Experimental observations of concussion and contusion of the spinal cord. *Ann Surg, 137*:433, 1953.
54. Tarlov, I.M., and Klinger, H.: Spinal cord compression studies. 2. Time limits for recovery after acute compression in dogs. *Arch Neurol Psychiat, 71*:271, 1954.
55. Tarlov, I.M.: Spinal cord compression studies. 3. Time limits for recovery after gradual compression in dogs. *Arch Neurol Psychiat, 71*:588, 1954.
56. Tarlov, I.M.: *Spinal Cord Compression—Mechanism of Paralysis and Treatment.* Springfield, Thomas, 1957.
57. Albin, M.S.; White, R.J.; Locke, G.E., and Kretchmer, H.E.: Spinal cord hypothermia by localized perfusion cooling. *Nature, 210*:1059, 1966.
58. Albin, M.S.; White, R.J.; Acosta-Rua, G., and Yashon, D.: Functional recovery after spinal cord injury in primates using delayed spinal cord cooling. *J Neurosurg,* 1968 (accepted for publication).

59. GOSSMAN, M.; WHITE, R.J.; TASLITZ, N., and ALBIN, M.S.: Electrophysiological responses immediately after experimental injury to the spinal cord. *Anat Rec, 160*:473, 1968.
60. SCARF, J.E.: Injuries of the vertebral column and spinal cord. In Brock, Samuel (Ed.): *Injuries of the Brain and Spinal Cord and Their Coverings*. New York, Springer, 1960.
61. ROSOMOFF, H.L., and GILBERT, R.: Brain volume and cerebrospinal fluid pressure during hypothermia. *Amer J Physiol, 183*:19, 1955.
62. ROSOMOFF, H.L.: A study of experimental brain injury during hypothermia. *J Neurosurg, 16*:177, 1959.
63. ROSOMOFF, H.L.: Hypothermia and cerebral vascular lesions. Experimental interruption of the middle cerebral artery during hypothermia. *J Neurosurg, 8*:332, 1956.
64. SHULMAN, G. and ROSOMOFF, H.L.: Effect of hypothermia on mortality in experimental injury to the brain. *Amer J Surg, 98*:704, 1959.
65. SEDZIMIR, C.B.: Therapeutic hypothermia in cases of head injury. *J Neurosurg, 16*:407, 1959.
66. WALKER, A.E.: The heroic treatment of acute head injuries: a critical analysis of the results. *Amer Surg, 26*:184, 1960.
67. WHITE, R.J.; ALBIN, M.S.; VERDURA, J., and LOCKE, G.E.: Differential extracorporeal, hypothermic perfusion and circulatory arrest to the human brain. *Med Res Engin, 6*:18, 1967.
68. PONTIUS, R.G., and DEBAKEY, M.E.: Hypothermia and clinical observation on the use of hypothermia to prevent ischemic damage to the central nervous system. In Dripps, R.D. (Ed.): *Physiology of Induced Hypothermia*. Washington, D.C., National Academy of Sciences, National Research Council, Publication 451, 1956, pp. 264-270.
69. PARKINS, W.M.; BEN, M., and VARS, H.M.: Tolerance of temporary occlusion of the thoracic aorta in normothermic and hypothermic dogs. *Surgery, 38*:38, 1955.
70. ALBIN, M.S.; WHITE, R.J.; LOCKE, G.E., and KRETCHMER, H.E.: Localized spinal cord hypothermia-anesthetic effects and application to traumatic injury. *Anesth Analg, 46*:8, 1967.
71. MEYER, J.S., and HUNTER, J.: Effects of hypothermia on local blood flow and metabolism during cerebral ischemia and hypoxia. *J Neurosurg, 14*:210, 1957.
72. WHITE, R.J., and ALBIN, M.S.: Perfusion Characteristics of the Isolated Brain. 1968 (To be submitted for publication).
73. PORTER, KEITH R.: Cytoplasmic microtubles and their functions. In Wolstenholme, G.E.W. (Ed.): *Principles of Biomolecular Organization (Ciba Foundation Symposium)*. Boston, Little, 1966.
74. BEHNKE, O.: Incomplete microtubules observed in mammalian blood platelets during microtuble polymerization. *J Cell Biol, 34*:697, 1967.
75. TILNY, L.G., and PORTER, K.R.: Studies on the microtubles in heliozoa. II. The effect of low temperature on these structures in the formation and maintenance of axopodia. *J Cell Biol, 34*:327, 1967.
76. ALBIN, M.S.; WHITE, R.J.; YASHON, D., and MASSOPUST, JR., L.: Functional and Electrophysiological Limitations of Delayed Spinal Cord Cooling. 1968 (Submitted for publication).

DISCUSSION

Richard C. Schneider

This chapter has been a fine review of the experimental and human anatomical material related to spine and spinal cord injuries. As is customary in Dr. White's and Dr. Albin's excellent presentations, they have provided an innovation in the treatment of such experimental injuries which has stimulated further work by other investigators.

One of our neurosurgical residents from the University of Michigan, who is now, shall we say on leave to the Armed Forces, at the Walter Reed Medical Center, Capt. Thomas B. Ducker in collaboration with Col. Harold F. Hamit has endeavored to repeat Dr. White's and Dr. Albin's work employing their technique using a 375 GCF in dogs. They had a total of forty-eight beagles which were subjected to this treatment. The animals were divided into four groups: (1) a control group with only laminectomy, opening of the dura, and application of the force, (2) another group similarly prepared but treated with local hypothermia protection for 3 hours of direct cooling by saline circulated at 50 to 100 ml per minute, (3) a third group given Decadron® .24 m per k for 24 hours for 2 days followed by 1.3 m per k per day for 7 days, (4) a fourth group had intrathecal steroid administration 3 hours after injury, a single dose of Depomedrol® 8 m per k. From their work it would appear that local hypothermia employing Drs. White and Albin's technique and the use of Decadron had achieved almost identical results in the treatment of such types of experimental spinal cord injuries.

I wonder whether Drs. White and Albin have subsequently used a series of animals treated with Decadron? Would they be somewhat concerned about using this drug in cervical spinal cord injury patients who are prone to develop gastrointestinal problems?

One cannot help but wonder about the rather minimal severity of trauma to the spinal cords of these animals. A comparatively minor degree of force has been applied to the cord compared to that which occurs in most patients who sustain spinal cord injuries. I would like to present the slides of two cases. One of these patients had a cervical spondylosis and suffered a hyperextension injury of the cervical spine without any fracture or dislocation. He had an acute central cervical spinal cord injury with minimal movement of the lower extremities, and complete paralysis of the arms and hands. During the ensuing few weeks, he had some slight recovery of motor power in the lower extremities, but suddenly had a pulmonary embolus and expired. At autopsy, the external surface of the cord appeared normal but three transverse sections through the C_4–C_5 spinal cord levels demonstrated progressive degrees of destruction. Although this was an incomplete lesion of the spinal cord, and the cord appeared grossly normal, hypothermia would have been of little value in treatment in this instance. In the second case, there was a fracture-dislocation of the spine resulting in a complete transverse myelitis. The patient succumbed within 36 hours, and at autopsy one can see on this slide the site of injury at the C_4–C_5 intervertebral space. Multiple transverse sections across the cord show the major area of damage at the fracture-dislocation site with areas of lesser damage at C_7 and T_1 levels; but the T_4 section, six segments below the site of injury, exhibits a zone of central necrosis. This is due to vascular insufficiency to the cord at the T_4 level, a zone which has poor collateral blood supply from the anterior spinal artery. Hypothermia would be of little value in such a case.

Therefore it would be necessary to select cases very carefully for local hypothermia treatment. It would seem to be most valuable in the incomplete cord lesion—namely, the acute anterior cervical spinal cord injury syndrome described in 1951. Such patients have an immediate complete paralysis with hypalgesia to the level of the lesion and preservation of motion, position, and touch. However, in these cases it will be difficult to demonstrate the value of the hypothermia technique, for decompressive laminectomy alone with section of the dentate ligaments may lead to recovery.

The authors have indicated that local hypothermia treatment was started on their animals within 4 hours after the traumatic insult. If this is a time factor which we must consider, then patients will have to be operated upon much earlier than is usually the case in our hospitals in order to achieve comparable results, even in the individual with relatively slight damage to the spinal cord.

There is no doubt that the photographs, which are to be published, suggest a definite increase in the caliber of the blood vessels in the spinal cords of the contused animals when one compares their condition prior to cooling and after local hypothermia. These observations will certainly bear further investigation.

Chapter IV

THE MECHANISMS OF CHEST INJURIES

Verne L. Roberts and David L. Beckman

INTRODUCTION

In terms of mortality, thoracic injuries occupy a position second only to head injury as a leading cause of death. In spite of the relative importance of thoracic injury, there has been a significantly smaller amount of research oriented toward understanding, describing, and preventing injuries to the heart, the great vessels, and the lungs. Despite the lack of work in this field, it is possible to describe rather explicitly some of the mechanisms responsible for thoracic injury.

HEART

Injury to the heart is a common result of blunt forces applied directly to the thorax or, in a large number of cases described in the clinical literature, forces applied to the abdomen or the lower extremities. Heart injuries appear to be devisable into two general groups: those which involve complete destruction of a localized area of muscle as typified by the blowout injuries of the various chambers of the heart, and those in which localized muscle damage may result in subsequent softening of the heart muscle or scarring resulting from tissue damage. Gross injury to the heart as indicated by sudden and immediate failure may take the form of extensive damage reported to divide the heart completely from the base to the apex with little or no tissue to hold the two halves together. In other cases, the failure is more localized and appears as a hole directly through the muscle itself with all the chambers as well as the divisions between them appearing to have equal potential for injury (Bright and Beck, 1935.) The mechanism of the total disruption of the heart can probably be ascribed to the impingement of the sternum against the vertebrae with the heart pinched between them. This extreme case must destroy any tissue caught between the uncompromising surfaces of the vertebrae and the sternum.

It has been speculated in the literature that there is an increased tendency for cardiac rupture if the heart is full of blood, i.e. at the end of diastole and the beginning of systole. This conclusion has recently been confirmed by an experimental study, (Life and Pince, 1968) which showed that the amount of blood present in the heart has a pronounced effect on the degree of injury, and that blowout failures of the heart are directly related to the heart cycle in terms of the potential for the injury. The marked friability of heart muscle has not been studied in such a manner as to indicate, in quantitive terms, the relative differences in mechanical properties.

The second class of heart injury is that impact which produces localized damage in the myocardium which may develop as a scar or which may produce softening and subsequent rupture. The physiological changes which are related to muscle injury are often used as indicators of the extent of the damage. Primary among these is the Electrocardiogram (EKG). EKG changes, due to thoracic impact, have been reported primarily in clinical studies which consistently emphasize alterations in the T wave, S-T segment, and the QRS complex. The incidence of cardiovascular injury following thoracic impact may be far greater than commonly thought. Many cases of injury may go unnoticed because of an absence of overt symptoms. Sixty-seven cases (Lasky et al., 1968) of cardiothoracic injuries from automobile collisions are cited, and EKG changes are commonly cited such as an altered S-T sequence, T wave, P wave, QRS complex, extrasystoles, paroxysmal tachycardia, and right or left bundle branch block. Ferré and Steward (1967) have reemphasized the point that myocardial contusions apparently go unobserved in many automobile accidents. In a study of ninety-two cases of thoracic impact, the initial serial EKG's were reported abnormal in all but five cases and these five subsequently developed abnormalities. EKG changes reported consisted of altered T waves, RS-T complex, Q waves, and slurring and notching of the QRS complex.

Barber (1942) reported eight abnormal EKG's out of thirty-three records obtained from hospital accident cases examined within 2 days of injury from impact. Common changes included partial heart block, and exaggerated or altered T-waves. In other studies, EKG changes in the voltage and appearance of the QRS complex, left axis deviation and frequent alterations in the T-wave were reported (Sigler 1942, 1945). In a report on clinical cases of cardiac rupture and studies of cardiac contusions in dogs produced by striking the exposed heart, the most frequent EKG changes were reportedly an altered S-T segment and T-wave and an exaggerated QRS complex (Bright and Beck, 1935).

Cardiovascular changes in correlation with thoracic injuries in animals include reports of bradycardia and hypotension (Slomka, 1934). Extrasystoles and occasional ventricular fibrillation occurred at the time of impact. Trauma to the precordia in the dog produced various forms of arrhythmic changes in the T-wave, the QRS complex and S-T interval (Kissane, Fidler and Koons, 1937).

The results of experimental and clinical studies indicate tears and pericardial and epicardial hemorrhages to be frequent injuries produced by blows administered to the anesthetized dog. Similar results were found in a study of fifty-eight autopsy cases of moderate chest trauma with severe extracardiac injury. There was reportedly subpericardial hemorrhage in fifty-five cases, pericardial hemorrhage in twenty-one, and small pericardial or epicardial tears in ten cases. Cardiac lesions were generally considered to be related to the point of compression against the spinal column. Severe trauma produced bursting of the myocardium or extensive adhesive pericarditis with frequent complete obliteration of the sac (Kissane, 1952).

Direct trauma to the myocardium in the dog produced extrasystoles, an altered Q deflection, and frequent T-wave inversion (Bright and Beck, 1935; Beck, 1935; Moritz and Atkins, 1940; and Moritz, 1958). Boyd and Scherf (1940) showed that after traumatization to the endocardium of a dog heart there was a temporarily altered T-wave and a reduced S-T segment. Hellstroem (1965) reported on EKG changes in dogs exposed to multiple closed liver trauma. Ectopic heart rhythms were observed immediately after impact, either in the form of ventricular extrasystoles, when the impact occurred during the diastolic phase, or in the form of supraventricular extrasystoles with impact during the systolic phase. The occurrence of extrasystoles was found to increase with higher impact velocities; there were EKG changes in the form of inverted T-waves, reduced take-off to the S-T segment and splitting of the QRS complex. Bradycardia was consistantly present after trauma.

The misconception that nonpenetrating trauma to the heart is relatively rare is probably due to the fact that myocardial contusion or traumatic pericardial lesions are usually well tolerated and the clinical findings transient and difficult to recognize. Demuth and Lissner (1965) discussed problems with recognizing serious nonpenetrating cardiac injuries indicating chest pain and tachycardia as the most prevalent symptoms of injury and that electrocardiography is the most reliable and objective diagnostic tool.

A report on 250 cases of nonpenetrating chest injuries indicated that the severity of chest injury and the injury to the myocardium do not necessarily correspond (Arenberg, 1943). Fracture of the ribs may, in fact, diminish the force of the blow on the heart thereby causing less damage.

The degree of elasticity of the chest wall and the type of blow are significant in determining the amount of resulting cardiac injury.

AORTA AND GREAT VESSELS

Aortic injury resulting from blunt trauma to the thorax commonly takes the form of partial or complete tears of the ascending aorta immediately above the heart, the descending aorta at the isthmus and the great vessels.

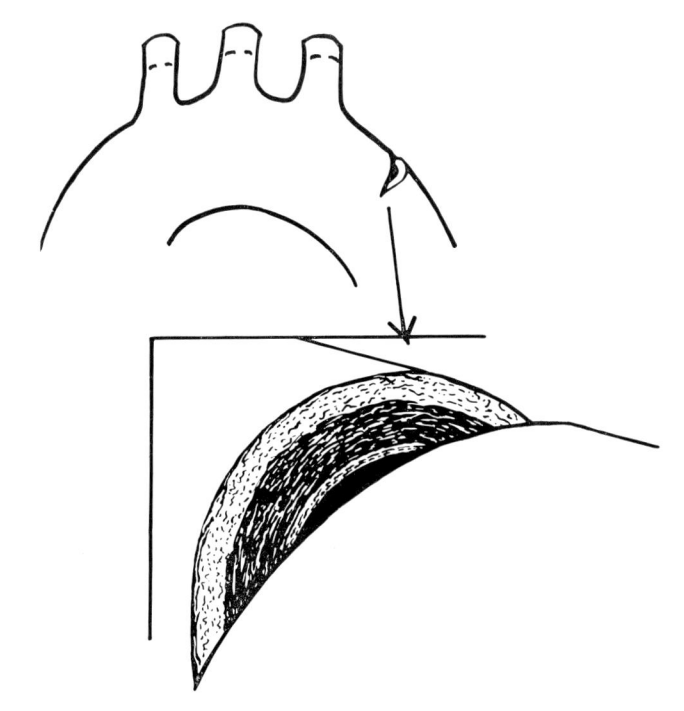

FIGURE 4–1. Illustration showing the location of aortic tears at the isthmus. The insert indicates the tears frequently extend through all three layers of the vessel including the intima, media and adventitia.

A variety of mechanisms have been proposed for these injuries including pressure effects, congenital weakness, displacement of the heart or aorta within the thorax and diseases which affect the structure of the vessels thus rendering them more susceptible to injury.

The mechanism cited most frequently in the literature (Klotz and Simpson, 1922; Strassman, 1947) is that of increased intra-aortic pressure at impact. It has been proposed that the compression of the heart between the sternum and spinal column or the hydrodynamic effects of acceleration on the intact column of blood produce an increase in pressure of sufficient magnitude to produce rupture. Pressure as the single mechanical

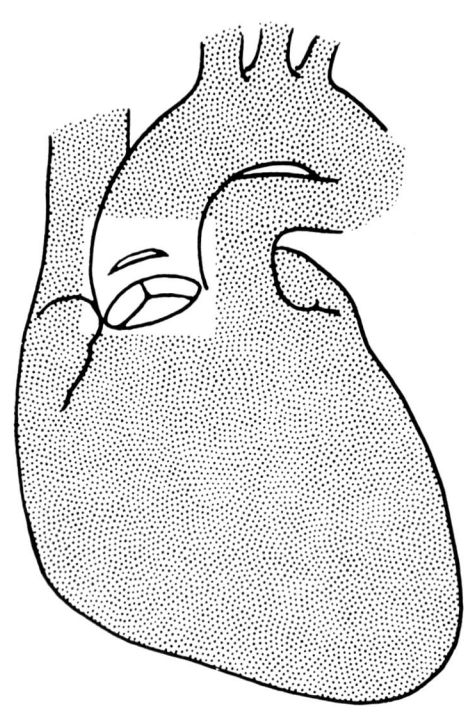

FIGURE 4–2. Location of the intra-aortic tears immediately adjacent to the heart.

phenomenon responsible for the injury can be rejected for two reasons. First, an elementary analysis of the stresses present in a thin walled vessel shows that they take the form of a hoop, or circumferential stresses, and longitudinal tensile stresses. The analysis shows that the circumferential stresses are always at least twice the magnitude of the longitudinal stresses. The tears which occur are always transverse to the vessel axis and, as the result, not the result of stresses due to internal pressure because they would produce tears along the vessel axis. Since pressure is nondirectional, any tears which resulted should be randomly dispersed with respect to their location. This is not the case either clinically or experimentally. Arteries are known to be pre-stressed in tension as evidenced by the fact that they shorten when cut. Techniques have recently been developed (Janicki and Patel, 1968) which allow the measurement of these stresses. Due to a lack of knowledge of the material properties of the aortic wall or the mechanism of failure, a complete analysis to predict failure cannot be accomplished. Second, a series of experiments performed in the Biomechanics Laboratory at Wayne State University in conjunction with staff from the Department of Surgery (Roberts et al., 1967) demonstrated that the lesion still occurred in animals whose blood volume had been reduced by $5/6$ of the total. The experiments were performed with canines which have a different vascular structure than man; however, the choice of experimental model does not negate the fact that in the absence of the fluid medium to transmit pressure, that it would be impossible to cite pressure as the single responsible mechanical parameter causing the injury.

Several authors (Abbott, 1928; Lasky et al., 1968) have cited congenital weakness (ligamentum arteriosum) in the aorta at the isthmus as being the factor responsible for the injury. A study of the mechanical properties of the aorta (Lundevall, 1964) did not indicate, however, that one section of the aorta was more susceptible to failure than any other. These experiments, were not performed at high rates of loading, and they lacked a great deal of technical expertise in properly defining the physical characteristics of the aorta; however, before congenital weakness can be said to be the sole mechanism, an extensive laboratory study of the vessel properties should be performed. Such a study should include whole vessels, as well as isolated strips, to completely define the variation in physical characteristics which occur throughout the thoracic aorta both in the longitudinal and circumferential directions, and should be accompanied by analysis to predict the site of the lesion on the basis of mechanics rather than pure speculation predicted only on anatomical grounds.

Large displacements of the heart and aorta during impact have also been suggested as the possible mechanism (Cammack et al., 1959; Roberts, et al., 1966; Moffat et al., 1966). A study performed at Holloman Air Force Base utilizing high speed radiological techniques showed that the canine heart, during caudocephalad impact, behaves in a manner very similar to a damped, spring, mass system (Hanson, 1967). The investigators were able to calculate the effective spring rate and damping characteristics of the heart, the aorta, and the great vessel system, and to suggest that the displacement of the heart toward the diaphragm during impact might play a role in the production of the injury. Simultaneous studies (Roberts et al., 1967) utilizing similar equipment were conducted with canines in an upright position which were struck at midstream by a moving impactor. The animals in the series were injected with a radio-opaque medium via a cannula inserted into the aorta during impact to define the outline of the heart and aorta. The roentgenograms which resulted showed a significant amount of distortion of the heart as well as displacement downward and into the left chest. This characteristic pattern of displacement was further reinforced by the typical pattern of injury observed in the vessel walls. The tears were characteristically found on the posterior wall of the vessel, more frequently on the right than the left and, with the exception of those vessels which were completely avulsed, never appearing on the anterior vessel wall.

The consistent pattern of injury, which agreed with those seen clinically,

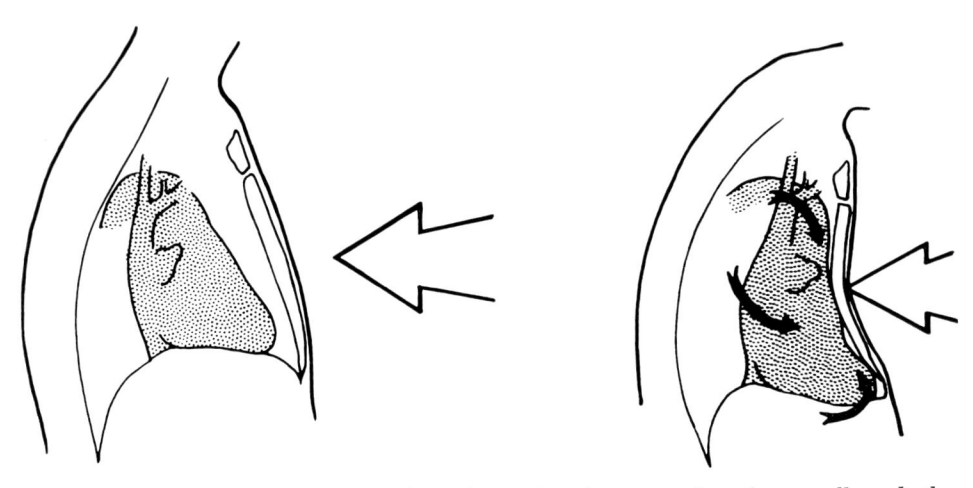

FIGURE 4–3. Illustration showing the relationship between the chest wall and the heart upon impact with distortions similar to those observed experimentally.

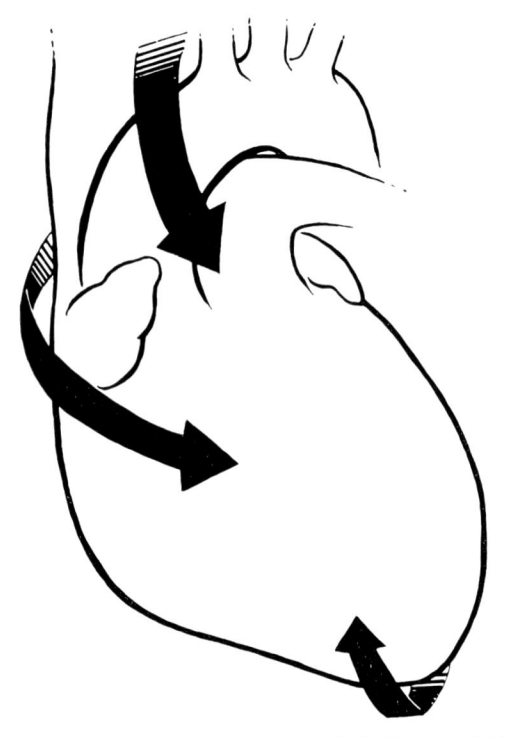

FIGURE 4–4. Illustration indicates the movement of the heart which takes place during thoracic impact with the components downward into the left chest and the rotation of the base of the heart.

coupled with the visualization of the heart during impact allows the prediction of a state of stress in the vessels which would produce failure at similar points. The displacement which is downward, to the left and accompanied by the rotation of the base of the heart anteriorly will deform the vessels in such a manner as to produce increased stress in the points which consistently failed. Thus the hypothesis may be made that displacement rather than pressure or cogenital weakness is the primary mechanism of injury. Increased intravascular pressure and localized disruptions in the vessel walls may also play a role in the etiology of the injury. However, they cannot be considered to be the major factors.

The relative fixation of the aorta at the isthmus has also been cited as a contributory factor in the production of the injury (Hass, 1944). It has been speculated that this fixation would allow the thoracic aorta to move anteriorly and create a high stress at the point of fixation contributing to failure. The validity of the mechanism is still open to question because of the lack of experimental evidence to support it as well as the lack of evidence regarding quantification of the "fixation." Therefore until proved otherwise, it must stand as a potential additional mechanism.

The effects of aging and disease on the injury process is unknown. However, it is reasonable to say that with increasing age and subsequent loss

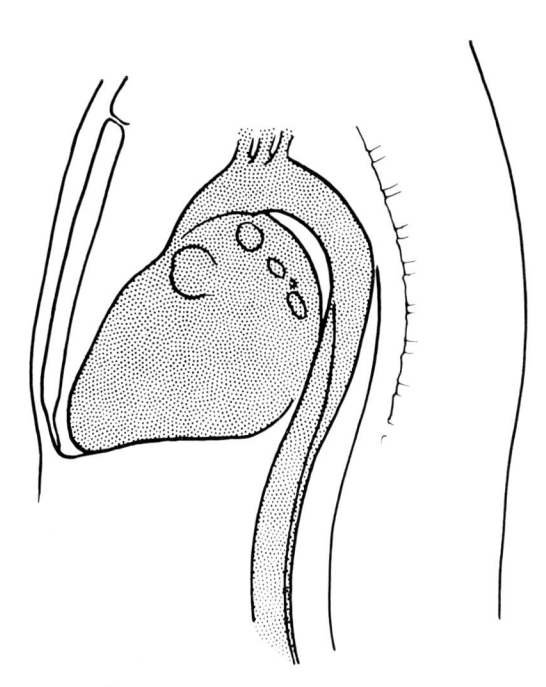

FIGURE 4–5. Illustration indicates the relative motion of the thoracic aorta anteriorly during impact as postulated in the literature.

of vessel distensibility that the ultimate stress required for failure will decrease. Any disease process which acts in such a manner as to change the structural properties of the vessel would also enhance the potential for injury.

BRONCHUS

The only definitive study described in the literature pertaining to the mechanism of bronchial rupture is that of Loyd et al., 1958. They found that rupture is more easily produced when the bronchus is stretched at right angles to the trachea than when the force acts along the trachea.*

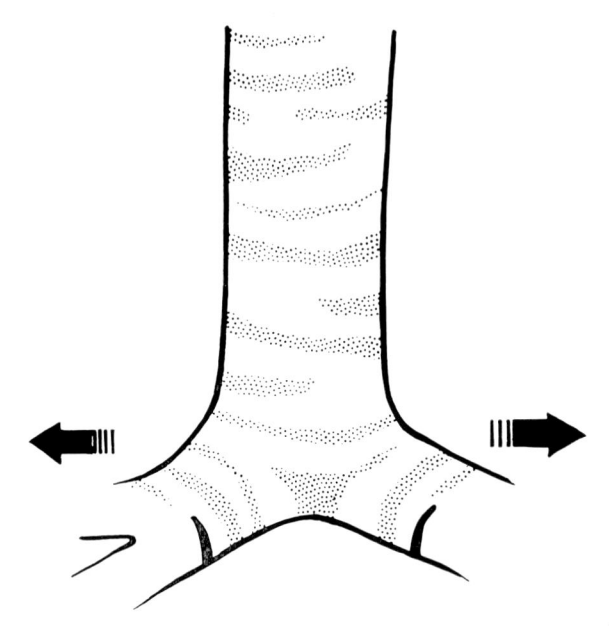

FIGURE 4-6. Illustration indicates the lateral movement of the bronchi which when combined with fixation at the carina enhances the potential for bronchial rupture.

They believed that such a force environment could occur if the carina were fixed between the sternum and the vertebra and thus prevented from moving laterally. This state of fixation is further complicated by the fact that in the absence of a pneumothorax, the negative pressure existing in the thorax will act in such a manner as to cause the lungs to follow the lateral motion of the chest wall.

The closed glottis was also shown to enhance the potential for injury. The prevention of deflation on the part of the lung also helps to spread

*3 kg force as opposed to 11 kg force (Values apply for canine bronchi only).

the bronchi at the carina and apply the forces at the structurally weakest part.

PULMONARY DAMAGE ASSOCIATED WITH HEAD INJURY

Another injury which pertains to the thorax comes about as the result of head injury rather than impact directly to the thorax.

There are several clinical reports on man indicating a relationship between head injury and lung damage such as edema, hemorrhage, and congestion, but there is apparently little duplication of this work in animals. The type of injury and the interval between impact and the first signs of pulmonary damage are not established nor is the mechanism producing damage. Major reports on man of pulmonary damage indicate a clear relationship between skull fracture, intracranial hemorrhage, lung congestion and edema (Weisman, 1939; Henneman, 1946; and Swann, 1960). These clinical reports indicate a further need for study of this aspect with experimental animals.

It is well established that a very large number of conditions can produce lung damage in terms of pulmonary edema, alveolar and interstitial hemorrhage, increased lung stiffness and congestion. Pulmonary edema is found routinely in such conditions as hypertensive disease, nephritis, coronary obstruction, cerebral hemorrhage, mitral stenosis, fractured skull, and multiple fractures (Cameron, 1948). It has been shown that hyperbaric oxygen exposure results in pulmonary edema (Bean, 1945), which can be prevented by the prior injection of a variety of sympathetic blocking agents (Johnson and Bean, 1957); it also has been shown that vibrations produce pulmonary edema which sympathetic blocking agents can prevent (Roberts and Aston, 1967). It is with these studies in mind that preliminary experiments have been started at the University of Michigan, Biomechanics Department, Highway Safety Research Institute on the value of sympathetic blocking agents on protection from the pulmonary involvement in experimental head injury (Beckman and Bean, 1969).

In these experiments, it was found that head injury in rats usually resulted in fatalities within a few minutes after the impact and that every fatality showed significant gross pulmonary damage as evidenced by patchy or wide spread hyperemia with translucency, petechiae, congestion, frothy fluid in the bronchi, pulmonary enlargement and increased lung weight body weight ratios. It was found also that drugs possessing sympatholytic, antiepinephrine, or general anesthetic action administered to the experimental animals prior to the cerebral traumatization prevented or very appreciably decreased the severity of this pulmonary damage. These changes would appear to be due, in part at least, to the involvement of the autonomic centers, their influence on their endocrine counterparts, on the cardiovascular system and possibly also more directly on the lungs themselves. That this may be so is suggested by the definite protective influence which is afforded by various antiepinephrine and autonomic blocking agents.

SUMMARY

The current research literature pertaining to thoracic injuries resulting from blunt forces yields only limited insight into the mechanism of the injuries involved. Only aortic injuries have been studied in sufficient detail to allow positive statements supporting or dismissing the proposed mechanisms. The sole conclusion which may be drawn is that much additional research is required to put the field of thoracic research on a level equal to that of other traumatic research areas.

BIBLIOGRAPHY

ABBOTT, M.E.: Coarctation of the aorta of the adult type. *Amer Heart J*, 3:574, 1927.

ARENBERG, H.: Traumatic heart disease: a clinical study of 250 cases of non-penetrating chest injuries and their relationship to cardiac disability. Ann Med, 19:326–346, 1943.

BARBER, H.: Electrocardiographic changes due to trauma. *Brit Heart J*, 4:83–90, 1942.

BECK, C.S.: Contusions of the heart. *JAMA, 104*:109–114, 1935.

BECKMAN, DAVID, L., and BEAN, JOHN W.: Pulmonary damage and head injury. *Proc Soc Expl Biol Med, 130*:5–9, 1969.

BLADES, B.: Management of injuries to the thorax. *JAMA, 159*:419–421, 1955.

BOAS, E.P.: Angina pectoris and cardiac infarction from trauma or unusual effort. *JAMA, 112*:1887–1892, 1939.

BOYD, L.J., and SCHERF, D.: The electrocardiogram mechanical injury of the inner surface of the heart. *Bull NY Med Coll*, 3:1–5, 1940.

BRIGHT, ERNEST F., and BECK, CLAUDE S.: Nonpenetrating wounds of the heart. *Amer Heart J*, 10:293–319, 1935.

CAMERON, G.R.: Pulmonary edema. *Brit Med J*, 1:965–972, 1948.

CAMMACK, K., RAPPORT, L., PAUL, J., and BAIRD, W.C.: Deceleration injuries of the thoracic aorta. Arch Surg, 79:244, 1959.

DEMUTH, W.E., and ZINSSER, H.F.: Myocardial contusion. *Arch Intern Med, 115*:434–442, 1965.

ELKIN, D.C.: Traumatic lesions of thorax with three cases of cardiac contusion. *Southern Med J*, 28:4–11, 1935.

FERRÉ, GEORGE A., and STEWARD, DEAN: *Cardiac Contusion Clinical Orthopaedics and Related Research*, Philadelphia, Lippincott, 1967, pp. 123–130, No. 53.

GORE, I.: The question of traumatic heart disease. *Ann Intern Med*, 33:865–878, 1950.

HALL, H.W., and MARTIN, J.W.: Myocardial contusion. *Amer J Surg*, 93:558–564, 1957.

HALTER, B.L.: Nonpenetrating trauma to the heart. *Amer J Surg*, 90:237–240, 1955.

Hanson, P.G.: Radiographic studies on cardiac displacement during abrupt deceleration. *Proc. Tenth Stapp Conf.*, 1967, pp. 227–241.

Hass, G.M.: Types of internal injuries of personnel involved in aircraft accidents. *J Aviat Med*, 15:77, 1944.

Hatcher, C.R. and Bahnson, H.T.: Cardiac contusion, puncture and tamponade. *Amer J Surg*, 105:485–491, 1963.

Hecht, H.H.: Heart trauma: myocardial involvement (contusion) following a non-penetrating injury to the chest (airplane accident). *Ann Intern Med*, 27:126–134, 1947.

Hellstroem, G.: Electrocardiographic, blood pressure, respiratory and electro-encephalographic responses to closed liver injury. An experimental study in dogs. *Acta Soc Med Upsal*, 70:167–190, 1965.

Henneman, H.: Acute pulmonary edema, with special reference to experimental studies. *New Eng J Med*, 235:590–596, 1946.

Janicki, Joseph S., and Patel, Dali J.: A force gauge for measurement of longitudinal stresses in a blood vessel *in situ*. *J Biomechanics*, 1:19, 1968.

Johnson, P.C.: Coronary occlusion. *JAMA*, 180:903, 1962.

Johnson, P.C., and Bean, John W.: The effects of sympathetic blocking agents on the toxic action of oxygen at high pressure. *Amer J Physiol*, 188:593, 1957.

Kissane, R.W.: Traumatic heart disease: nonpenetrating injuries. *Circulation*, 6:421–425, 1952.

Kissane, R.W.; Fidler, R.S., and Koons, R.A.: Electrocardiographic changes following external chest injuries to dogs. *Amer Intern Med*, 11:907–935, 1937.

Klotz, O., and Simpson, W.: Spontaneous rupture of the aorta. *Amer J Med Sci*, 184:455, 1932.

Lasky, Irving I.; Siegel, Arnold W., and Nahum, Alan M.: Automative cardiothoracic injuries: a medical–engineering analysis. *Society of Automotive Engineers 680052*, 1968.

Levy, H.: Traumatic coronary thrombosis with myocardial infarction—postmortem studies. *Arch Intern Med*, 84:261–276, 1949.

Life, Jeffry S., and Pince, Bruce W.: Response of the canine heart to thoracic impact during ventricular diastole and systole. *J Biomechanics* (in press).

Lloyd, J.R.; Heydinger, D.K.; Klassen, K.P., and Roettig, L.C.: Rupture of the main bronchi in closed chest injury. *Arch Surg*, 77:597, 1958.

Lundevall, Jon: The mechanism of traumatic rupture of the aorta. *Acta Path Microbiol*, 62:34, 1964.

Moffat, R.C.; Roberts, V.L., and Berkas, E.M.: Blunt trauma to the thorax: development of pseudoaneurysms in the dog. *J Trauma*, 6:666–679, 1966.

Moritz, A.R.: Trauma, stress and coronary thrombosis. *JAMA*, 156:1306–1309, 1954.

Moritz, A., and Atkins, J.P.: Cardiac contusion. An experimental and pathologic study. *Arch Path*, 25:445–562, 1938.

Parmley, L.F., and Manion, W.C.: Nonpenetrating trauma to the head. *Circulation*, 18:371–396, 1958.

Roberts, V.L.; Moffat, R.C., and Berkas, E.M.: Blunt trauma to the thorax-mechanism of vascular injuries. *Proc. Ninth Stapp Conf.*, 1966, pp. 3–12.

Roberts, V.L.; Jackson, F.R., and Berkas, E.M.: Heart motion due to blunt trauma to the thorax. *Proc. Tenth Stapp Conf.*, 1967, pp. 242–248.

Schlomka, G.: Influence of blunt injuries on heart in sensitized animals: experimental studies. *Z Fig Ges Exp Med*, 92:522, 1934.

SIGLER, L.H.: Traumatic injury to the heart. Incidence of its occurrence in forty-two cases of severe accidental bodily injury. *Amer Heart J, 30:*459–478, 1945.

SIGLER, L.H.: Trauma to the heart due to non-penetrating chest injuries. *JAMA, 199:* 855–861, 1942.

STRASSMAN, G.: Traumatic rupture of the aorta. *Amer Heart J, 33:*508, 1947.

SWANN, HENRY E., JR.: Occurrence of pulmonary edema in sudden asphyxial deaths. *Arch Path, 69:*557–570, 1960.

WEISMAN, SYDNEY J.: Edema and congestion of the lungs resulting from intracranial hemorrhage. *Surgery, 6:*722–729, 1939.

DISCUSSION

Charles E. Brackett

The lung has the function of adding oxygen to the blood to prevent tissue hypoxia and the removal of CO_2 to prevent tissue acidosis. Delivery of oxygenated blood depends on an adequate cardiac pump, blood volume, and vessel to cell transport mechanism. Just as lung injury leads to hypoxic brain damage, so brain injury may lead to secondary lung damage. The evaluation of adequacy of pulmonary ventilation or arterial oxygenation is not possible by clinical observation and direct monitoring of these parameters is required. Fortunately, easy to use and reliable instruments are now available for this type of assessment.

As Dr. Roberts points out, cardiac injuries secondary to chest injuries are common; it is fortunate their clinically significant consequences are rather uncommon. Cardiac tamponade with reduced cardiac output may be most significant. Rupture of the aorta and bronchial tree from thoracic displacements are uncommon but of such serious clinical significance that every effort at immediate diagnosis and treatment must be made. Traumatic asphyxia from severe superior vena cava obstruction may cause cerebral edema or paraplegia but has a characteristic clinical picture and is not usually fatal.

Reduction in vital capacity by pneumo or hemothorax, flail chest, upper airway trauma or obstruction, or simple unconsciousness, leads to the syndrome of hypoventilation, recognized by low arterial PO_2 and elevated PCO_2. If uncorrected, tissue hypoxia and secondary metabolic acidosis follows.

Distal pulmonary obstruction due to bronchial trauma, secretions, pulmonary contusion, or more especially fat embolization, leads to patchy atelectasis and inappropriate ventilation-perfusion ratios or so-called pulmonary shunting. This is recognized by low PO_2 and normal or low PCO_2. Tissue hypoxia results.

The patient made unconscious by a head injury may suffer secondary pulmonary changes, some man-made. The most common and serious is aspiration, either of blood from facial injury or gastric contents from vomiting. Immediate asphyxia or severe tracheobronchitis results, which may make oxygenation of the patient impossible. This injury results from transportion in the supine position. Unconscious patients should be transported prone or semiprone, preferably after the stomach has been emptied by nasogastric tube.

A second important cause of difficulty is failure to maintain adequate mechanical ventilation during transportation. Many ambulances have oxygen bottles but few have an Ambu bag or personnel to use it. These patients need mechanical ventilation. The simple use of the prone position and Ambu bag would go far toward reducing morbidity and mortality.

Many persons with chest trauma, or unconscious with head injury, require respiratory assistance and many injuries may result from such assistance. Pontopipidan has indicated the unpredictably high and possibly toxic concentrations of oxygen unknowingly achieved with pressure cycled respirators. High positive ventilation pressures decrease venous return and cardiac output. When the respirator is used in the assist mode, exhaustion may result from intolerable respiratory energy expenditure. Inappropriate hyperventilation leads to serious respiratory alkalosis with secondary cerebral hypoxia. Inadequate humidification leads to obstruction from secretions and infection. These secondary injuries can only be recognized and avoided by careful monitoring of ventilation and arterial gases.

Finally, Dr. Roberts has reviewed the interesting association of head injury and pulmonary edema. Very recent experimental work by Ducker would suggest that the mechanism central to the diverse etiologies of pulmonary edema is the sequence of elevated systemic pressure, left heart failure, pulmonary venous hypertension and finally pulmonary arterial hypertension; all leading to increased hydrostatic pressure in the low pressure pulmonary bed.

Pulmonary injuries interfere with brain oxygenation in a number of ways. The unconscious patient is deprived of normal protective reflexes. He may develop a number of pulmonary injuries secondary not only to his head and chest injuries but also to his medical care.

References

Ducker, T., and Simmons, R.: Increased intracranial pressure and pulmonary edema. 2. The hemodynamic response of dogs and monkeys to increased intracranial pressure. *J Neurosurg*, 28:118, 1968.

Pontopipidan, H., and Berry, P.: Regulation of the inspired oxygen concentration during artificial ventilation. *JAMA*, 1967, vol. 201.

Chapter V

BLUNT ABDOMINAL INJURY:
A Review of 307 Cases

ALEXANDER J. WALT and THOMAS J. GRIFKA

INTRODUCTION

The increased speed and frequency of automobile crashes is reflected in the rising incidence of serious abdominal injuries. The impact forces from acute frontal deceleration after an automobile accident may be as high as 2,000 pounds; the force generated in falls or direct kicks, although less, may still be considerable. The abdominal cavity, unprotected on its anterior surface, and containing a great variety and concentration of organs, is potentially susceptible to a wide spectrum of injury. The clinical picture may be equally variegated depending upon whether the solid, hollow or supporting tissues are damaged, either singly or in combination. The overall mortality rate for blunt abdominal injury ranges between 8 to 28 percent of those reaching the hospital. The incidence rises markedly with the number of intra-abdominal organs injured, and the occurrence of concomitant damage to the extra-abdominal organs.

The purpose of this paper is to review briefly the mechanism of the injuries encountered in blunt abdominal trauma, the protean nature of the clinical picture, the potential difficulties in diagnosis and some of the more obvious pitfalls to be avoided in management. No special attempt is made to discuss surgical technique.

MATERIALS

Three hundred and seven patients with blunt abdominal trauma, necessitating laparotomy in 249, were admitted to the Wayne State University Surgical Service at Detroit General Hospital, (303 cases) and the Allen Park Veterans Administration Hospital (4 cases) between January 1, 1962, and December 31, 1967. The anatomical distribution of the 487 abdominal injuries is presented in Table 5-I. Of the 307 patients, seventy-seven (25%) had concomitant head injuries, eighty-two (26.7%) thoracic

TABLE 5-I
CASES OF BLUNT TRAUMA REQUIRING EXPLORATORY LAPAROTOMY
AND/OR UROLOGICAL RADIOGRAPHIC STUDY

Total Number of Injuries (487):	
Stomach	5
Spleen	91
Duodenum	20
Jejunum	15
Ileum	28
Colon	17
Bladder	36
Liver	57
Kidney	73
Retroperitoneal hematoma	61
Gallbladder	3
Common bile duct	2
Mesentery	34
Pancreas	28
Diaphragm	7
Sup. mesenteric vessel injuries	6
Others	4

injuries and 112 (36.5%) fractures of the large bones. In about two-thirds of the patients only a single organ was injured; in the remaining one-third, between two and eight organs were injured, with an average of 1.5 to 2. Fifty patients died, representing a mortality rate of 16.2 percent.

The physical forces responsible for the lesions, seen as a result of blunt abdominal trauma, are summarized in Table 5-II. Various authors have

TABLE 5-II
TYPES OF ABDOMINAL INJURY

Solid Viscera	Direct Compression (Crush) Shearing (Inertial or Decelerative)
Hollow Viscera	Increased Intraluminal Pressure Shearing Compression
Supporting Structures	Shearing Compression Compression Expansile

attempted to relate individual lesions to specific physical forces in blunt abdominal trauma, both on clinical and laboratory observation.[1,2,3,4,5] A knowledge of the mechanism of injury aids in the appreciation of potential lesions, but each patient must be evaluated as an individual. The mechanism of injury may be one of the following:

1. Direct compression with disruption of tissues due to pressure from without, either direct or shearing in nature, seen especially in midline structures caught between the abdominal wall and the vertebral column.
2. Rupture of the hollow viscus due to increased intraluminal pressure which exceeds bursting wall tension, whether or not a closed loop is present.

Blunt Abdominal Injury

3. Shearing by torsional forces of relatively fixed and inelastic supporting ligaments, mesenteries or vessels.
4. Tearing of the diaphragm following sudden marked increase in the pressure of the intra-abdominal cavity.
5. Direct perforation by fragments of fractured bones which form part of the wall of the abdominal cavity, especially the pelvic area.

Many of these mechanisms of injury are observed simultaneously in "the stomped patient," who is both trampled upon and kicked forcibly in the abdomen. While there are no predictable constellations of injury, there are certain associations which should be looked for, such as the following:

1. The association of pelvic fractures and rupture of the urinary tract. It is extremely uncommon to have damage to the lower urinary tract in the absence of pelvic fracture or separation of the symphysis pubis.
2. Concomitant hepatic and splenic injuries following steering wheel injuries to the upper abdomen.
3. Rupture of the small intestine and its mesentery with or without lumbar fractures in the so-called "seat belt syndrome." These are sufficiently frequent to merit special attention and may present deceptively mild symptoms and signs in the early stages.

CLINICAL ASPECTS

Surgeons with a wide experience of intra-abdominal trauma soon lose their capacity for surprise by the lesions they may find (Fig. 5–1). These are frequently bizarre, multiple, anatomically unpredictable and out of proportion to the severity of the wounding force. The types of clinical pictures seen in blunt abdominal trauma are summarized in Table 5-III.

TABLE 5-III
BLUNT ABDOMINAL TRAUMA

Acute	Symptoms Immediately Apparent
Delayed Acute	Symptoms Appearing up to 72 hrs.
Chronic	Symptoms Appearing Days to Months Post Injury (eg: Pancreatic Pseudocyst Rupture of Spleen)
Late Effects	Symptoms Appearing Yrs. Later (Rupture of Diaphragm; Hypertension)

Some simple but often neglected facts merit emphasis:

1. The accompanying extra-abdominal injury may sometimes dominate the picture in the early stages and may indeed require the most

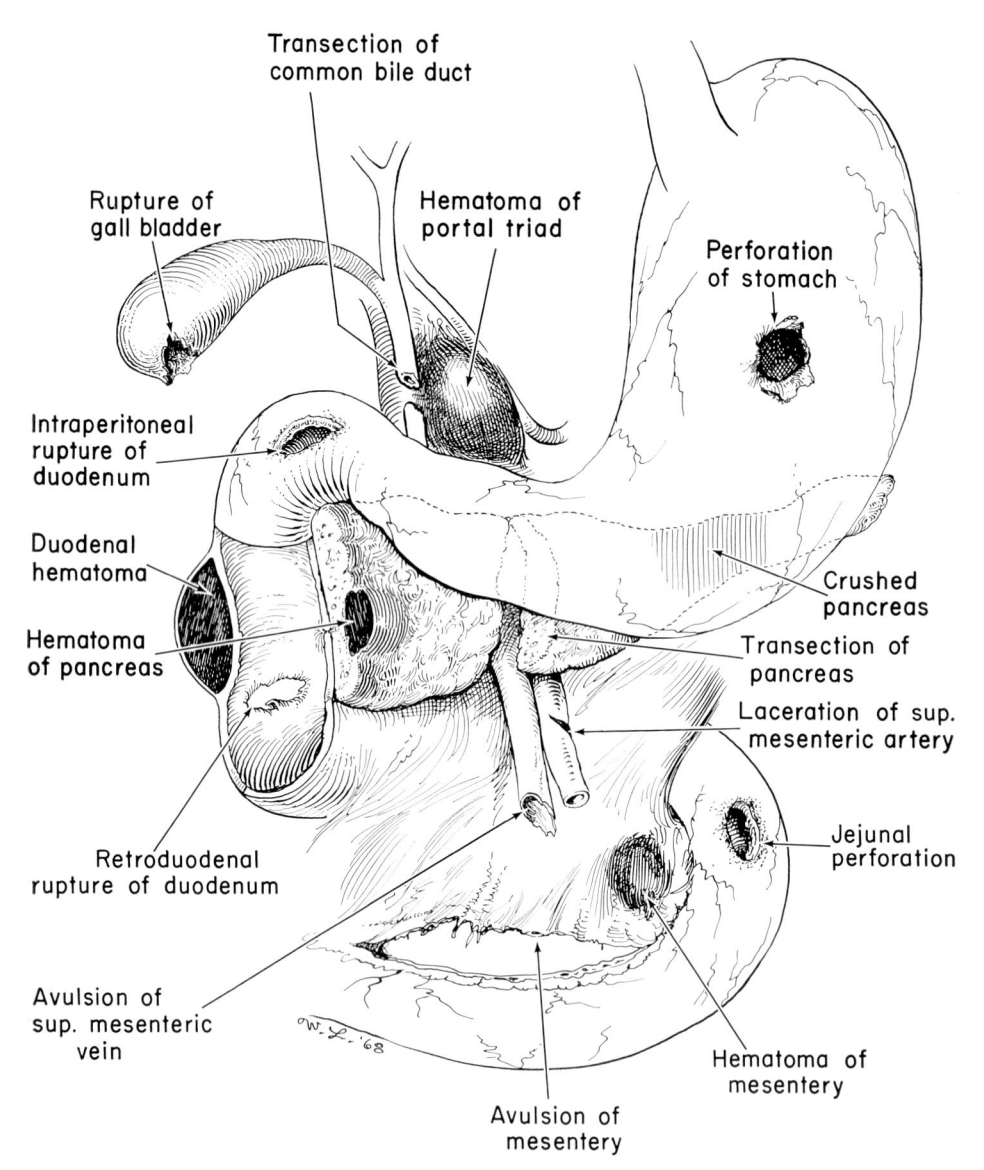

FIGURE 5–1A. Types of injuries observed in the pancreatic-duodenal areas secondary to blunt trauma.

urgent treatment, especially in the case of thoracic injuries. However, most closed chest injuries only require closed treatment such as the insertion of a thoracotomy tube, whereas closed abdominal injuries often require laparotomy.
2. Head injury, present in about 30 per cent of the cases, is for practical purposes, never the cause of shock. If shock is present, the cause

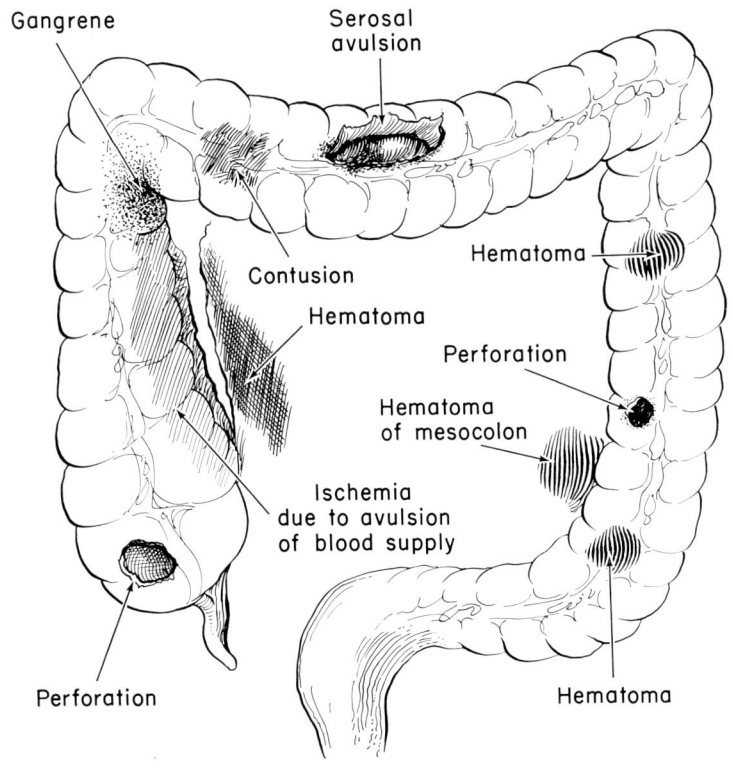

FIGURE 5–1B. Types of injuries to the colon due to blunt trauma.

will be found in the chest, in the blood loss associated with fracture, or in injuries to intra-abdominal structures.

3. A patient with life-threatening intra-abdominal injury may be apparently well for long periods of time; hours may pass before a ruptured liver becomes manifest (Case 1), days may pass before a transected bowel is confirmed (Case 2), months may elapse before a ruptured spleen declares itself (Case 3), while a ruptured diaphragm might not become apparent for years (Case 4). These features are well illustrated in the following case reports:

Case #1. R.C. #564543

This 36-year-old male, involved in an auto accident was given emergency care at another hospital, observed and discharged. Approximately 24 hours after injury, he developed abdominal pain which radiated into the left chest and shoulder. He denied nausea, vomiting, or bleeding. Forty-eight hours after injury, because of progressively increasing abdominal pain, the patient again sought medical help. On admission to Detroit General Hospital, the patient had generalized tenderness of the abdomen with marked

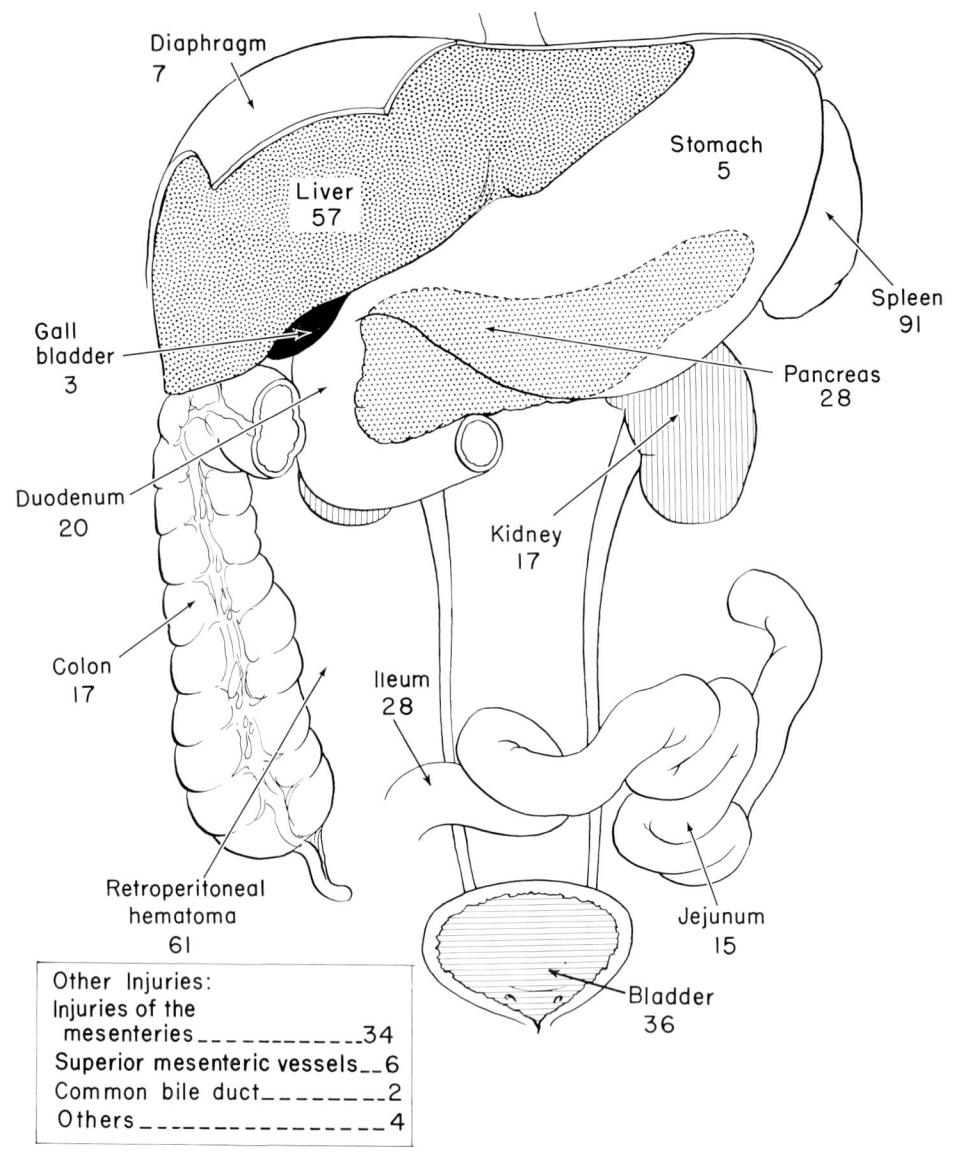

FIGURE 5–1C. Distribution of 427 injuries in 249 patients explored for blunt abdominal trauma.

left upper quadrant tenderness and rebound. The abdomen was flat. Temperature was 101°. With the preoperative diagnosis of a ruptured viscus, the patient had an exploratory laparotomy which revealed a fracture-laceration of the left lateral lobe of the liver with necrosis of the fractured segment. Contusion of the stomach, large bowel and kidney were also noted. Hepatic resection and biliary decompression by a cholecystostomy tube was carried out. Postoperatively, the patient did well and returned to work as a truck driver.

LESSONS LEARNED—CASE #1: *This case demonstrates, as have other cases involving hepatic fracture, that evidence of so significant an injury may not manifest itself for many hours.*[6]

Case #2. C.K. #1537604

This 48-year-old male was admitted to the hospital after having been struck in the left upper quadrant of the abdomen by a steel beam with sufficient force to knock him down. The patient did not lose consciousness. Initial physical examination revealed a slightly obese patient in no acute distress, complaining of tenderness in the left anterior abdominal wall, right flank pain and left buttock. Normal bowel sounds were present and no deep abdominal pain could be elicited. Vital signs were normal and routine admission laboratory studies were unremarkable. The roentgenogram revealed a fractured left eleventh rib; abdominal films showed a pattern of ileus but no free air. Initially the patient was given a clear liquid diet. Intravenous fluids and nasogastric suction were started on the second day after the patient began vomiting with persistent abdominal pain. By the eighth hospital day, the patient seemed considerably better, tolerating oral feedings and having semiliquid bowel movements. On the tenth hospital day, he ceased to pass flatus, had diminished bowel sounds and developed abdominal distention. Roentgenograms again showed a pattern of ileus. A gastrografin study, on the fourteenth hospital day, showed contrast material in the small bowel only, consistent with complete obstruction of the distal small bowel. The patient was then operated upon and found to have complete rupture of the terminal ileum with an associated abscess. An ileostomy was performed, subsequently closed, and the patient discharged completely recovered.

LESSONS LEARNED—CASE #2: *Although this is a very unusual type of injury, transection of the bowel usually presenting symptoms very early after injury, the bowel in this case was completely transected and the gastrointestinal continuity provided by the wall of the contiguous abscess. It points up the fact that in the presence of ileus and abdominal distention, frequent reevaluation is necessary if a satisfactory result is to be obtained.*

Case #3. R.K. #68135971

This 26-year-old male was admitted to the hospital complaining of abdominal pain, which radiated to the left shoulder, and intermittent vomiting for 2 weeks. The patient was a heavy drinker, but had no unusual past history except that he had been in a motorcycle accident about 3 months prior to admission, sustaining blunt trauma to the abdomen for which he sought no medical advice. Physical examination revealed an alert cooperative male in no acute distress. Temperature 100°; Pulse 100/min.; B.P. 128/70. Except for some left upper quadrant and rebound tenderness, the physical examination was unremarkable. No visceromegaly was detected. Laboratory studies: Hemoglobin, 9.9 grams%; WBC 10,900 cu./mm; amylase 106 Somogyi units. Subsequent hemoglobin determination was 8.8 grams%. Chest roentgenogram: Pleural reaction over the left lateral costophrenic angle, blunting of the costophrenic angle, and small pleural effusion. Abdominal roentgenogram showed no abnormality. An upper gastrointestinal series did not show any evidence of an intrinsic organic lesion. There was, however, an opacity in the left upper quadrant which was displacing the stomach to the right and the splenic flexure of the colon downward. Exploratory laparotomy revealed delayed rupture of spleen which had been leaking slowly, forming a large perisplenic hematoma.

LESSONS LEARNED—CASE #3: *(a) The importance of obtaining the past medical history, especially with reference to trauma, even though hospitalization has not been required. (b) Abnormal laboratory findings frequently help substantiate possible underlying injury—in this case, the abnormally low hemoglobin in a young man with no history of hematemesis, melena, or gross blood in the stool. (c) The value of the upper gastrointestinal series in demonstrating the displacement of the stomach and colon by an abnormal, clinically impalpable, left upper quadrant mass (Fig. 5-2).*

Case #4. E.M. #46123574

A 50-year-old male was admitted complaining of left flank pain which radiated into the left hemithorax after ingestion of food. The pain was more severe if a large meal had been eaten. Relief was obtained by induced vomiting. During the past year, the patient had lost 23 pounds. Past history: 9 years prior to admission, while driving a truck, the patient was involved in a head-on collision. He sustained fractures of the skull, the clavicle and the wrist and was unconscious for 2 days. Physical examination on the present admission was unremarkable. Admission chest x-rays were interpreted as showing an elevated left leaf of the diaphragm and gas shadows in the chest. An upper gastrointestinal series showed "a cascade stomach." On exploration of the abdomen, a 10 x 7.5 cm defect was noted in the left leaf of the diaphragm. The entire stomach, spleen, tail of the pancreas, and splenic flexure of the colon were herniated into the left thoracic cavity. A thin peritoneum-like membrane separated the abdomi-

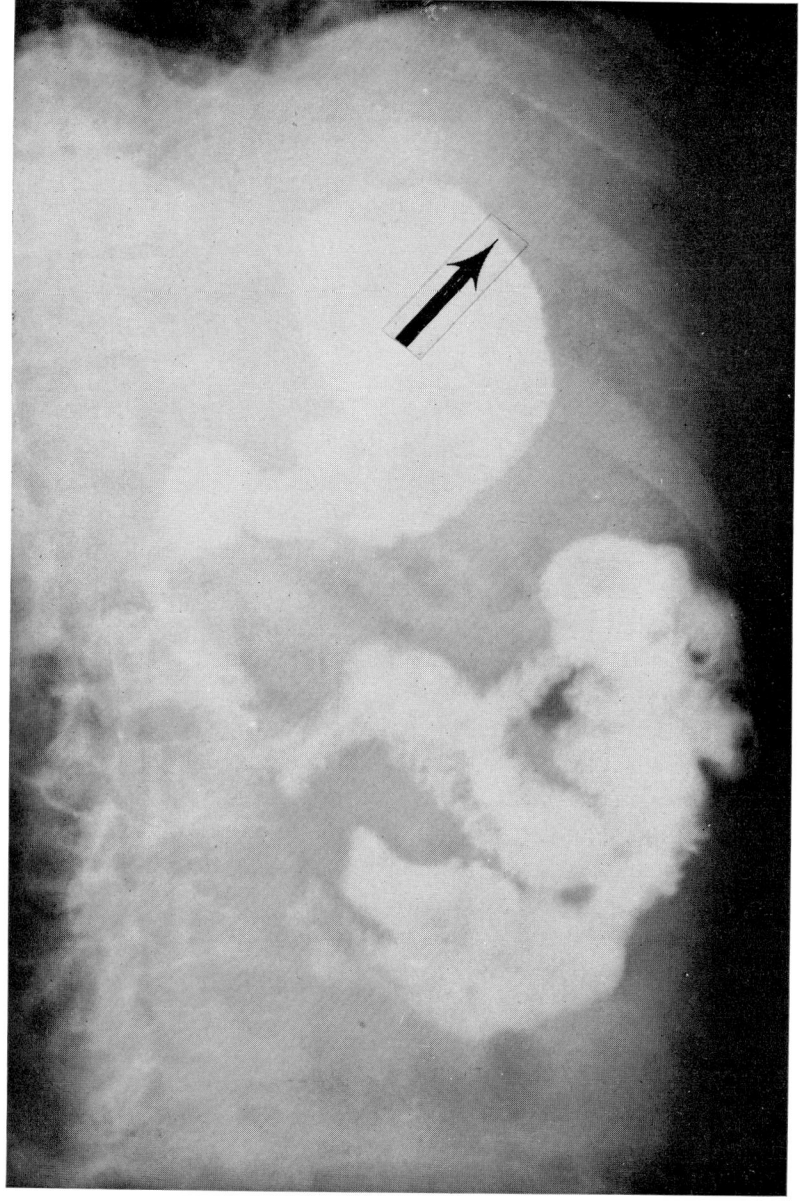

FIGURE 5-2: Case #3. Barium study 3 months after injury demonstrating displacement of the stomach to the right by the splenic hematoma.

nal organs from the lungs. The diaphragm was repaired and postoperatively the patient did well.

LESSONS LEARNED—CASE #4: (a) *Rupture of the diaphragm and herniation of several intra-abdominal organs may only become symptomatic for the first time many years after the injury.*[7] *(b) Visceral incarceration through such a defect must be relieved without delay before strangulation occurs. (c) The presence of an abnormally elevated diaphragm with intrathoracic gas shadows must be evaluated for diaphragmatic rupture.*

There are other obvious pitfalls.

1. The diagnosis of an injured organ may elude the physician who fails to take a careful history with special regard to seemingly trivial trauma.
2. Failure to examine the patient carefully.
3. Reliance on clinical acumen rather than dogged reexamination including periodic measurements of abdominal girth, changes in hematocrit, WBC, electrolytes, blood gases and enzymes.
4. Neglect to use paracentesis if in doubt and to repeat this when necessary. This is especially pertinent in patients who are very ill or unconscious in whom the surgeon is naturally reluctant to consider laparotomy which would add further insult to the patient.
5. Excessive reliance on roentgenograms. Other obvious pitfalls may be illustrated by some typical examples encountered in the series.

THE PLACE OF THE RADIOLOGICAL EXAMINATION

The diagnostic yield expected from radiological examination of the abdomen is often grossly overestimated. Established injury is revealed by roentgenography in only about 50 per cent of the patients with blunt abdominal trauma. Ruptures of the small bowel, for example, may not show free air for many hours (Case #5), leading to false optimism. Furthermore, a negative gastrografin swallow does not insure integrity of the gastrointestinal tract. Large perihepatic, perisplenic and retroperitoneal hemorrhages (Case #6), may also be present without radiological signs. On the other hand, roentgenograms may be invaluable to delineate the genitourinary tract (Case #7) and to reveal fractured bones. This latter feature may in fact alert the clinician to an injury of an underlying organ which may otherwise be temporarily overlooked, such as the spleen or liver in fractures of the lower ribs, the bladder or urethra in fractures of the pelvis or separation of the symphysis pubis (Case #8). While the demonstration of viscera in the chest or air under the diaphragm is of obvious diagnostic value, it is important to remember that roentgenography will often not disclose the presence of a ruptured diaphragm or hollow viscus.

Case #5. J.D. #535196

This 39-year-old male, a known epileptic, who was a chronic alcoholic, entered the emergency room with abdominal pain of approximately 8 hours duration. Prior to admission, the patient had been consuming a fifth of whiskey each day for many days. Twelve to 14 hours prior to admission, the patient claimed to have been kicked in the abdomen several times. Vomiting of a greenish material began approximately 6 hours prior to admission. There was no hematemesis. The pain was generalized throughout the abdomen, but was most severe in the midepigastric region, and the patient only obtained relief by doubling up. On the initial physical examination of the abdomen, there was mild generalized discomfort without rebound tenderness. The abdomen was soft and no distention was present. Roentgenograms of the chest and abdomen showed no evidence of traumatic injury. A tentative diagnosis of pancreatitis was made. While being observed, the patient developed increased abdominal pain, rebound tenderness, abdominal distention and finally profound shock with anuria despite receiving intravenous fluids. Repeat roentgenograms at this time revealed free air under the diaphragm. At the time of laparotomy, a 3 cm perforation of the jejunum was noted on the antimesenteric border approximately 6 inches from the ligament of Trietz. Generalized peritonitis and early saponification of the omentum were present. More than two liters of sanguinopurulent fluid were evacuated from the peritoneal cavity. Despite a very stormy postoperative course, the patient ultimately did well and was discharged from the hospital in good health.

LESSONS LEARNED—CASE #5: *(a) Seemingly inconsequential trauma may cause potentially lethal intra-abdominal injury. (b) Significant contusions and ecchymosis of the abdomen are easily overlooked in dark-skinned individuals. (c) The fact that the patient had a pronounced odor of alcohol and a striking history of alcoholism reinforced in the admitting physician's mind the diagnosis of pancreatitis. Alcoholic patients may be too easily labeled as having pancreatitis when in fact their pain is due to other causes. (d) Repeated radiological studies and paracentesis may be invaluable in atypical cases.*

Case #6. S.M. #528581

This 20-year-old female fell out of an automobile approximately 26 hours prior to coming to the emergency room with complaints of left shoulder and left upper quadrant pain. She denied nausea or vomiting and stated that she had struck the left side of the abdomen and left shoulder. She claimed to be approximately five months pregnant. Physical examination on admission demonstrated left upper quadrant tenderness and guarding. The uterus was thought to be compatible with a two month pregnancy. Admission roentgenograms of the chest failed to demonstrate any abnormality. The hemoglobin was 7.5 grams%; urinalysis showed 30 to 40

112   *Impact Injury and Crash Protection*

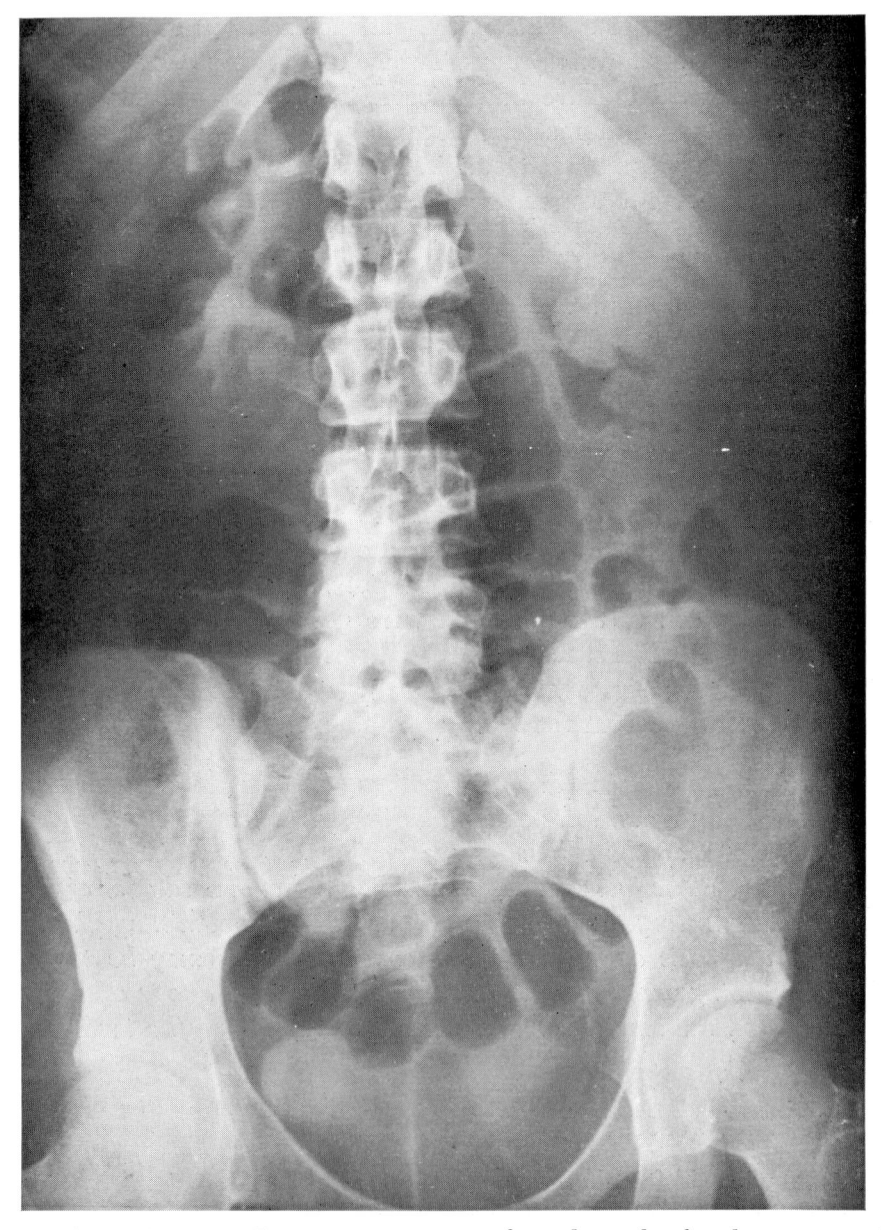

FIGURE 5–3A: Case #6. Excretory urogram performed on the fourth post-operative day to determine renal function, shows nonvisualization of the left kidney.

RBC's per high power field. Because of the possibility of early pregnancy an excretory urogram was not performed. With a preoperative diagnosis of a ruptured spleen, the patient was taken to the operating room where the ruptured spleen was removed. In addition, there was a large retroperitoneal hematoma extending downwards in the area of the left kidney.

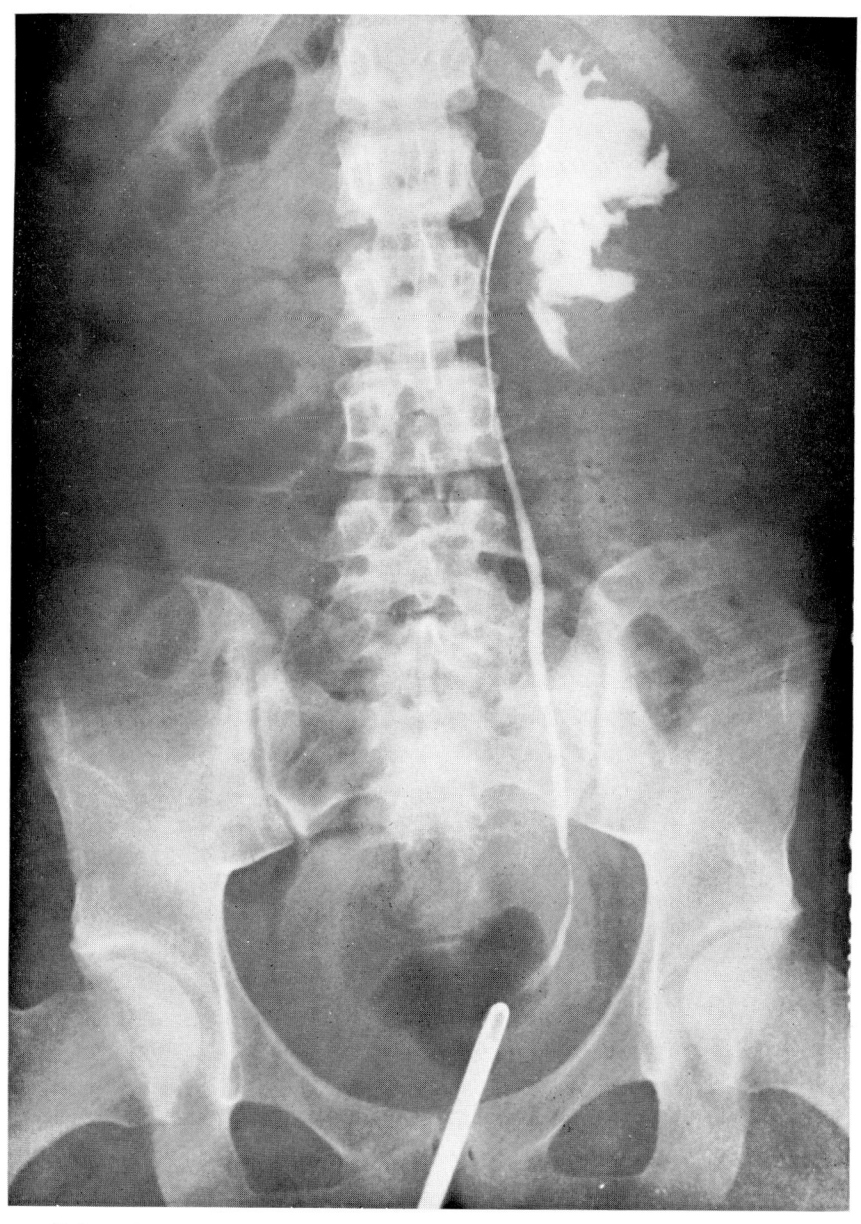

FIGURE 5–3B: Case #6. Retrograde pyelogram on the left side, fifth-operative day, demonstrates disruption of the calyceal pattern with extravasation of contrast material.

As it did not expand during the splenectomy or involve the paraduodenal area, it was elected not to open the retroperitoneal area. The right kidney was normal to palpation. The uterus was small and thought to be nongravid. Postoperatively, an excretory urogram failed to visualize the left kidney and arteriography showed no filling of the left renal artery (Fig.

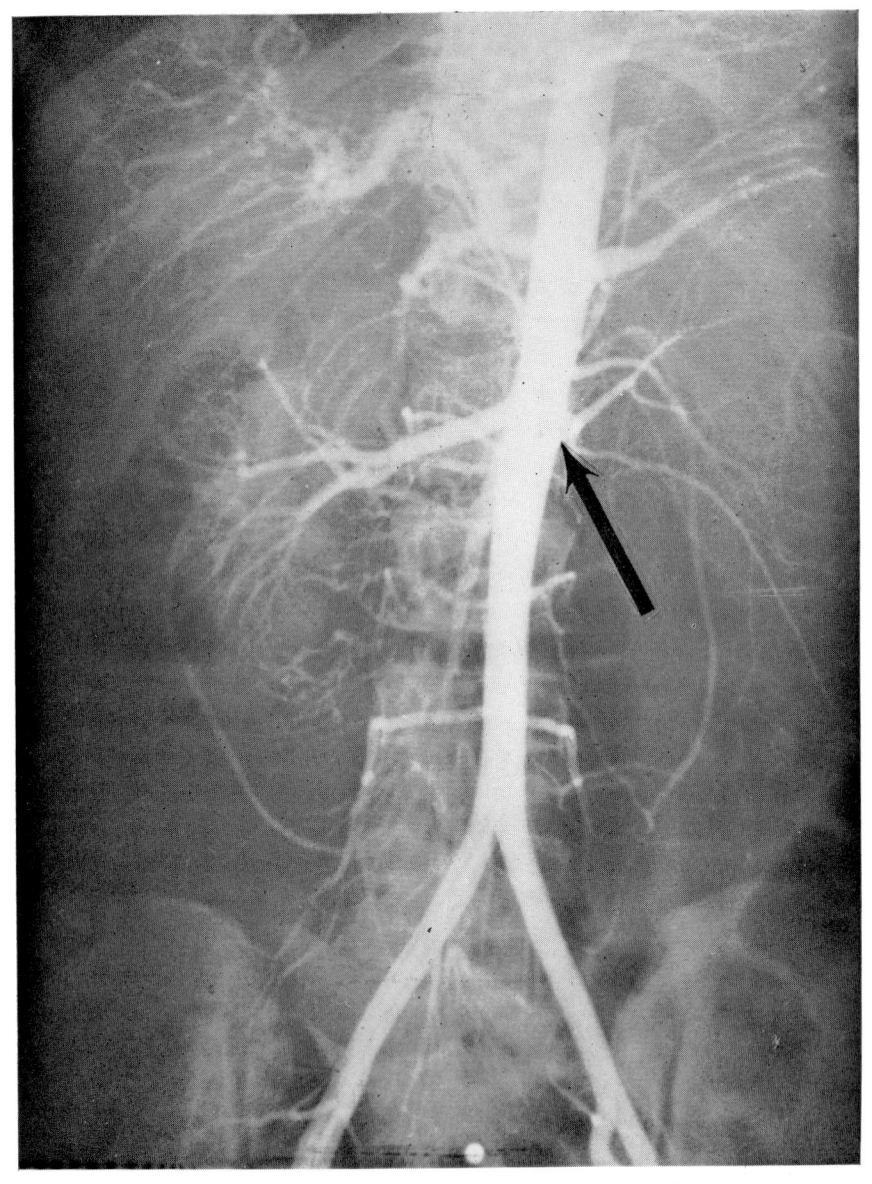

FIGURE 5–3C. Case #6. Transfemoral aortography on the sixth post-operative day reveals nonfilling of the left renal artery. (An excretory pyelogram 2 months later showed return of function of the left kidney. Aortography was not repeated).

5–3A,B,C). The kidney lesion was treated nonoperatively showing slow restoration of kidney function on later excretory urograms.

LESSONS LEARNED—CASE #6: (*a*) *Potentially lethal lesions may be present in an injured patient for a long period without major overt clinical signs.*

(b) *A low hemoglobin and severe hematuria in conjunction with nonvisualization of a kidney on excretory pyelogram may in the presence of a retroperitoneal hematoma—and even without one—be an indication for a renal arteriogram or an aortogram. The results of this study may indicate the need for a direct surgical approach to the renal artery. (c) Despite apparent occlusion of a renal artery, function of the ipsilateral kidney may return in time, presumably due to recanalization of a thrombus or the development of collaterals.*

Case #7. A.M. #583894

This 44-year-old female struck her flank when she fell against her bed approximately 15 hours prior to admission. Twelve hours later, she developed right flank pain and gross hematuria. She had no previous history of genitourinary disease. On physical examination at time of admission, the abdomen was markedly tender in the right upper quadrant and right flank which contained a tender palpable mass. Active bowel sounds were present. Admission roentgenograms of chest were negative; abdominal films showed obliteration of the right psoas shadow. Urinalysis revealed gross hematuria. Hemoglobin was 8.6 grams%. An excretory urogram showed delayed function of the kidney. Selective renal arteriography demonstrated a normal arteriographic pattern with a large perinephric hematoma (Fig. 5-4). The patient was treated conservatively with resolution of the hematoma.

LESSONS LEARNED—CASE #7: *(a) Contrasting this patient with the previous case (Case #6) the large tender mass in the flank led to an excretory urogram (which showed no function on the right side), followed by selective arteriogram which demonstrated that the renal artery was intact and the renal vasculature to be essentially normal. Arteriography, therefore, saved this patient from an unnecessary laparotomy (there have been numerous articles in the recent literature which deal with the important role of arteriograms in blunt trauma).*[8]

Case #8. N.P. #362118

This 72-year-old female was driving an automobile on the freeway and struck the rear end of a vehicle. She suffered injuries as a result of direct trauma to the chest from the steering wheel, and from hitting her face against the windshield. No seat belt had been employed. The patient was brought to the emergency room in obvious distress with multiple ecchymoses on the face, chest, abdomen and extremities. She had marked abdominal pain and severe respiratory distress. Examination revealed multiple fractures including ribs, pelvis and femur. Because of gross hematuria, a cystogram was performed which demonstrated a ruptured

116 *Impact Injury and Crash Protection*

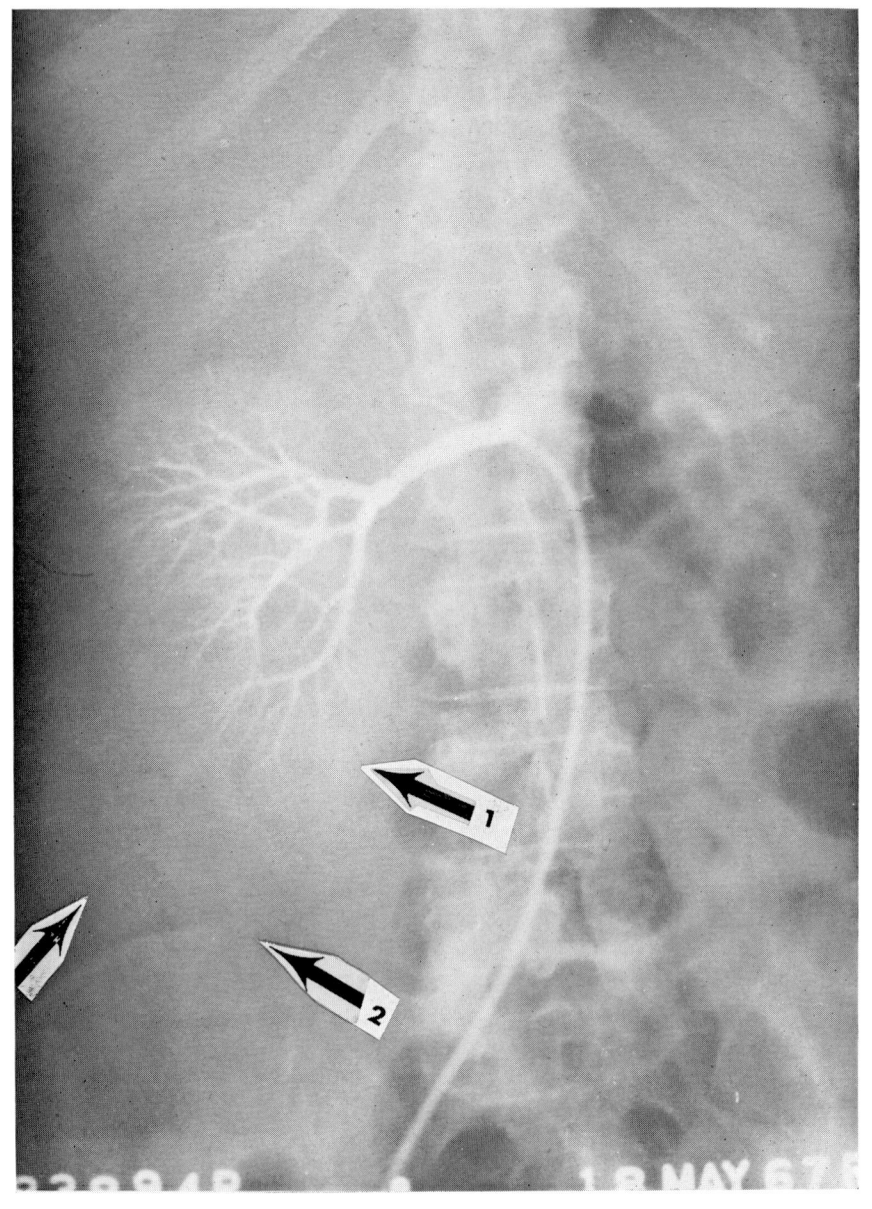

FIGURE 5-4. Case #7. Selective right renal arteriography shows intact renal vasculature and the presence of a large perinephric hematoma. This resolved gradually and completely.

bladder. Initial chest x-rays showed some elevation of the left diaphragm. Chest x-rays in the supine position showed a mass in the left pleural space (Fig. 5-5). The patient was taken to the operating room where a traumatic rupture of the diaphragm was repaired. Abdominal viscera, including

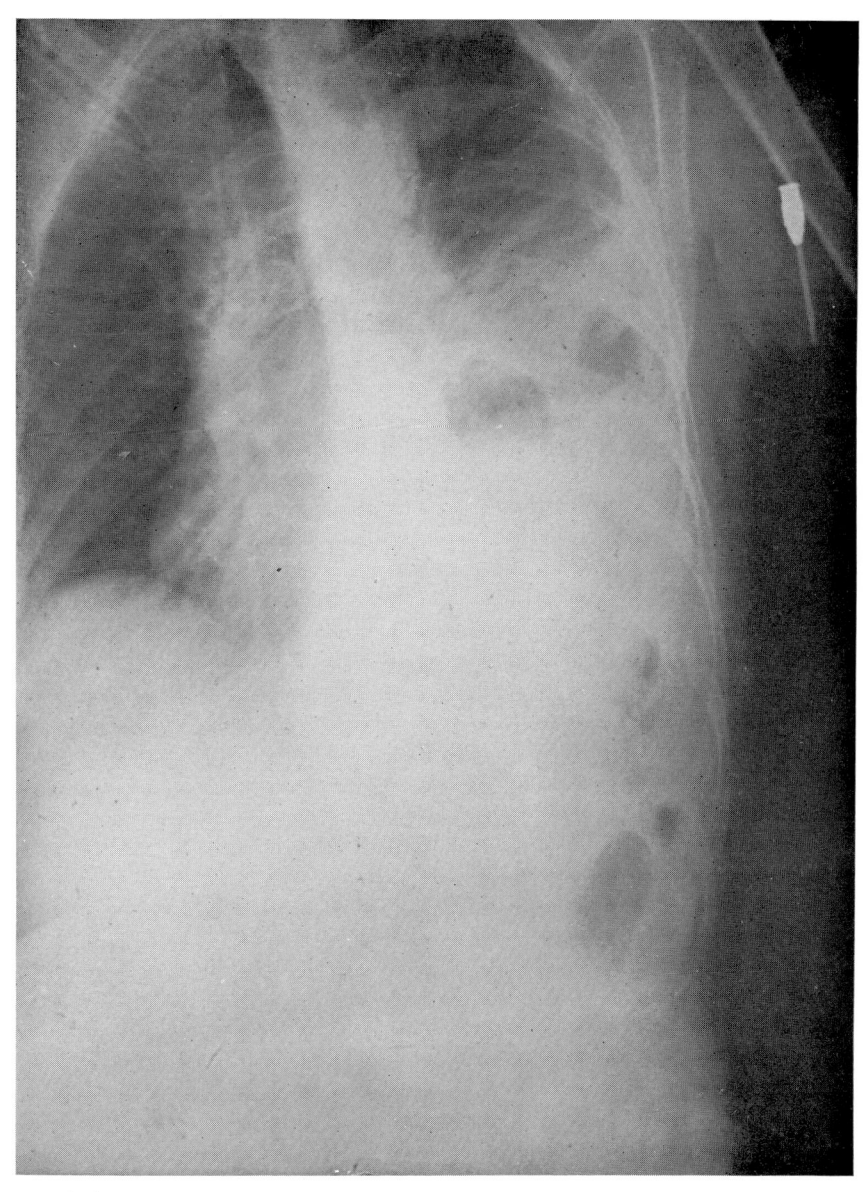

FIGURE 5–5A. Case #8. Roentgenograms in supine position taken at time of admission shows presence of gas-filled organs in the left hemithorax.

the left lobe of the liver, the spleen, and the stomach and the transverse colon and most of the small bowel were reduced into the peritoneal cavity from the left chest. The diaphragmatic defect was approximately 10 cm in length. There were no other peritoneal injuries except for a 6 cm transverse laceration in the dome of the urinary bladder. Postoperatively the patient ultimately did well and was discharged in good condition.

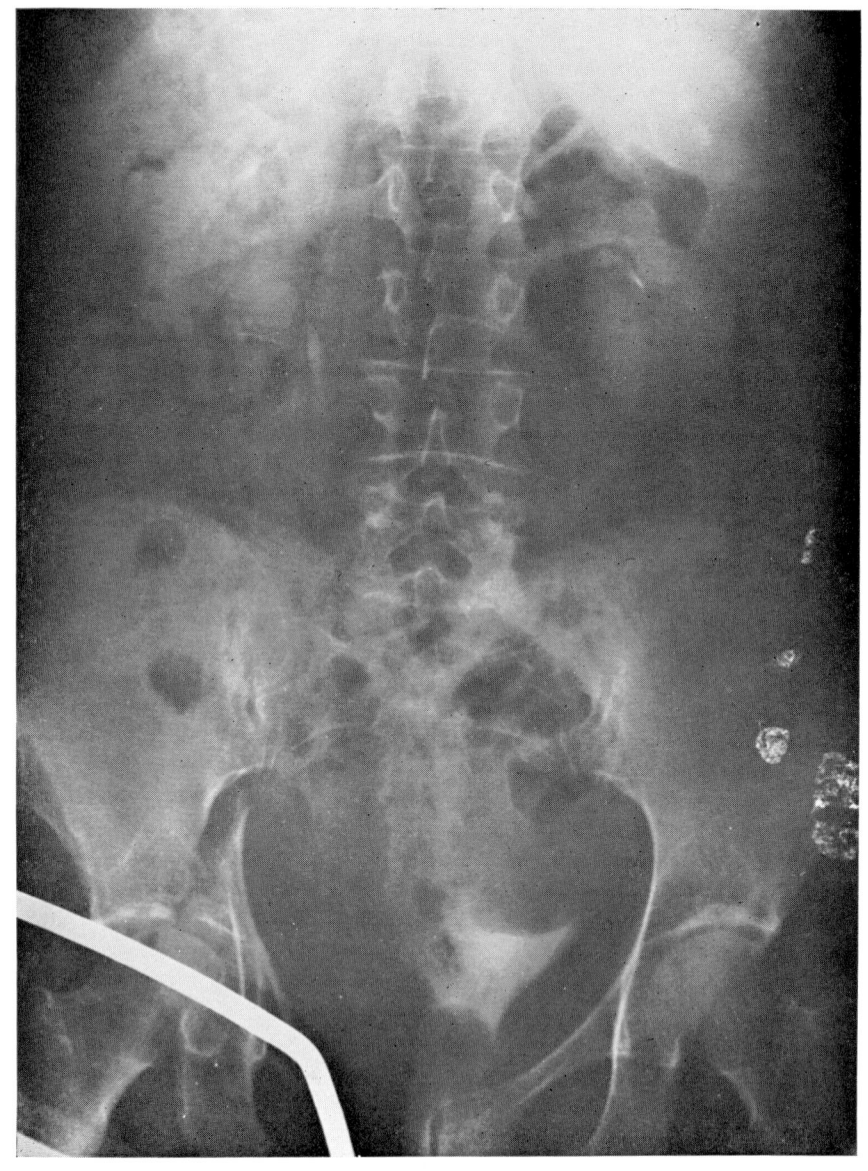

FIGURE 5–5B. Case #8. Cystogram demonstrating extravasation of contrast medium from the bladder. Note the multiple pelvic fractures.

LESSONS LEARNED—CASE #8: (a) *Upright chest films which are of greatest value in detecting free air in the peritoneal cavity and which are certainly the best diagnostic films of the chest, may fail to show the presence of a diaphragmatic defect. X-rays taken in the supine position and including the diaphragm may be required to demonstrate abdominal viscera in the thoracic cavity.* (b) *Cystography in the evaluation of hematuria is invalu-*

able in demonstrating the presence and location of the bladder injury. (c) Vigorous treatment of even elderly individuals, in this instance a 72-year-old female, with a multitude of severe injuries may save life if due regard is given to respiratory support, restoration of blood volume and the reduction of shock to the shortest possible period.

BRIEF NOTES ON SPECIFIC UNCOMMON INJURIES:

While much has been written on injuries to solid organs, notably the spleen, liver and kidney, which account for about 60 per cent of the injuries in blunt abdominal trauma, an important number of less well appreciated patterns of injury are encountered on any busy accident service and should be looked for. We wish to draw specific attention to the wide spectrum of injuries to the following:

1. The biliary-pancreatic apparatus
2. The area of the duodeno-jejunal flexure
3. The colon

1. The biliary-pancreatic injuries.

The mechanisms of these injuries have been discussed elsewhere.[9] Large hematomas of the retroperitoneal region and also the area of the portal triad and the head of the pancreas may obscure an underlying tear of the extrabiliary apparatus or the duodenum. In this situation, edema, crepitus and bile staining of the tissues may indicate the underlying lesion, making thorough exploration imperative.

Case #9. H.H. #377159

This 48-year-old Negro male entered the emergency room after suffering injury to the epigastric area in an automobile accident. Although epigastric tenderness was initially present, it was elected to admit and observe the patient as vital signs remained stable. Approximately 20 hours after admission, however, the patient began having severe abdominal pain and rigidity. At operation, the patient had a ruptured spleen, some minor hematoma in the right upper quadrant and slight discoloration in the pancreaticoduodenal area. After mobilizing the duodenum with a Kocher maneuver, a laceration of the second portion of the duodenum involving nearly three-fourths of its circumference and situated about 2 cms distal to the ampulla of Vater was found. The injured bowel was repaired with a single layer of 4–0 silk and a gastroduodenostomy was added. The patient did well postoperatively and returned to his job as a truck driver.

LESSONS LEARNED—CASE #9: *(a) Retroperitoneal ruptures of the duodenum may fail to demonstrate free air on the roentgenogram. (b) Even though the patient's symptoms could have been accounted for on the basis of the ruptured spleen alone, and the injury in the pancreatic-duodenal area did not appear to be extensive, the decision to visualize these areas directly was crucial to the patient's recovery.*

Case #10. L.K. #503834

This 34-year-old male sustained a steering wheel injury to the epigastrium in an automobile accident. Because of rather pronounced epigastric tenderness and rebound, exploration was carried out despite a normal roentgenologic report. At the time of laparotomy no bleeding was noted. Grossly, the liver, bowel and spleen were intact. However, bile was noted in the right upper quadrant with bilious staining of adjacent tissue. On mobilizing the gallbladder, a "blowout" laceration of its wall was found to be the source of the escaping bile. A cholecystectomy was performed and a T-tube was inserted into the common duct. Profuse irrigation was carried out. The patient did well postoperatively.

LESSONS LEARNED—CASE #10: *(a) Although only fifty-one cases of rupture of the gallbladder have been reported in the world literature, two were encountered in our series; death from bile peritonitis may well have occurred if the principle of exploring bile-stained areas had been ignored. (b) Rupture of the gallbladder may occur as an isolated lesion.*

2. Injuries in the area of the duodenojejunal flexure (Fig. 5–6).

Injuries in the area of the duodenojejunal flexure may involve the duodenum, upper jejunum, mesenteric vessels, and/or the pancreas. There may be frank rupture of the bowel, slow ischemia due to laceration of subtended vessels or obstruction due to intramural hematoma (Fig. 5–2). Although somewhat uncommon, we have encountered five injuries of the superior mesenteric vessels; four involved only the vein, one involved both the vein and the artery. Perforation of the jejunum was described in Case #5.

Case #11. P.F. #512589

This 34-year-old female was involved in an automobile accident. A ruptured spleen was removed at time of laparotomy and a ruptured contused duodenum close to the ligament of Treitz was found in a very large retroperitoneal hematoma in this area. It was felt that primary closure was not possible and formal resection undesirable. Consequently, a loop of jejunum was applied to the margins of the traumatized duodenum with interrupted silk sutures, closing the defect. The patient did well postoperatively.

LESSONS LEARNED—CASE #11: *(a) In this patient, who had been transfused with 10 units of blood, an extensive resection of duodenum and pancreas was circumvented by use of a serosal patch to repair the defect.*

Case #12. L.M. #376764078

This 25-year-old male was beaten up and kicked in the abdomen 10 days prior to admission. On the day following his trauma, the patient was seen in the emergency room complaining of nausea and vomiting. He was not admitted to the hospital at that time because of a paucity of clinical findings. In the 10-day interim, the patient had epigastric pain and following a heavy alcoholic intake he had persistent nausea and vomiting for the last 4 days. On admission, there was tenderness of the left upper quadrant and mild generalized abdominal tenderness. No masses could be palpated on abdominal examination. Bowel sounds were diminished. Admission roentgenograms were unremarkable. Laboratory investigations: WBC 20,850 per cu mm; Hgb. 14.1 gm%; Amylase 400 Somogyi units; Sodium 139 mEq/L; Potassium 3.2 mEq/L; CO_2 46 mEq/L; Creatinine 3.1 mg%. The patient was admitted to the hospital with the diagnosis of duodenal obstruction, probably secondary to a pancreatic pseudocyst and was placed on nasogastric suction and intravenous fluid therapy. An upper gastrointestinal series revealed obstruction of the second portion of the duodenum compatible with either a pancreatic pseudocyst or a hematoma of the duodenum. Failing to respond to conservative therapy, the patient had an exploratory laparotomy on the ninth hospital day. At operation, a subserosal hematoma compressing the entire second portion of the duodenum was found. There was no evidence of pancreatic trauma. A gastrojejunostomy was performed. The patient did well postoperatively and was discharged in good condition.

LESSONS LEARNED—CASE #12: (*a*) *Hematoma of the duodenum (due to blunt trauma) may give a picture of complete gastrointestinal obstruction.* (*b*) *Failure to respond to a reasonable period of conservative therapy necessitates laparotomy when obstruction persists.*

3. Colonic injuries.

It is often not recognized that the colon may be seriously injured as a result of blunt trauma.[10,11] Of the seventeen colon injuries in this series, three were of such extent that colectomies were required and, in another two, diverting colostomies were thought to be necessary. A typical case is reported.

Case #13. E.S. #180261

This 29-year-old white male, after having been involved in an automobile accident, suffered fractures of the transverse processes, lumbar vertebrae 1–4, and several ribs on the right. He had a right hemopneumothorax. Initially, no abnormal abdominal signs were present. On the fourth day after admission, when progressive abdominal distention and tenderness developed, the patient was taken to the operating room. At laparotomy, it was noted that loops of ileum were adherent to the cecum in the area of cecal perforation and that there was also a perforation of the right colon just below the hepatic flexure. The entire right colon was badly contused, very ecchymotic and presented numerous thinned-out areas. Because of the marked compromise of blood supply of the right colon, a right colectomy was performed with an ileotransverse colostomy. Despite some postoperative chest and wound complications, the patient was ultimately discharged in good condition.

LESSONS LEARNED—CASE #13: *(a) Constant close observation of the severely injured patient with a continuous review of all systems is mandatory. (b) Symptoms and signs may be delayed. In this patient, the severely contused colon was initially intact, but due to localized severe ischemia, necrosis and free perforation developed. Laparotomy became imperative on the fourth day and any significant delay might have resulted in the patient's demise. (c) A primary right colectomy and anastomosis may be safely performed in the presence of an unprepared bowel.*

SUMMARY

The experience, with a consecutive series of 307 patients with blunt abdominal trauma, seen on the surgical services of Wayne State University, over the past 6 years, has been reviewed. Fifty (16.2%) of these patients died. The mechanisms, varieties and clinical aspects of these injuries have been outlined. Problems encountered in patients with these injuries have been illustrated in a series of case studies. Stress has been laid on the many pitfalls in diagnosis and treatment, and the approach by which these may often be avoided. With an increasing incidence of abdominal injury due to automobile and other trauma, it is imperative that the deceptive and variegated nature of these injuries, both anatomical and clinical, is appreciated if the present high mortality rate is to be substantially reduced.

REFERENCES

1. BAXTER, C.F., and WILLIAMS, R.D.: Blunt abdominal trauma. *J Trauma*, 1:241, 1961.
2. WILLIAMS, R. D., and SARGENT, F.T.: The mechanism of intestinal injury in trauma, *J Trauma*, 3:288, 1963.
3. DESFORGES, G.; STRIEDER, J.W.; LYNCH, J.P., and MADOFF, I.M.: *Traumatic* rupture of the diaphragm. Clinical manifestations and surgical treatment. *J Thorac Surg*, 34:779, 1959.

4. FLETCHER, W.S.; MAHNKE, D.E., and DUNPHY, J.E.: Complete division of the common bile duct due to blunt trauma. Report of a case and review of the literature. *J Trauma, 1*:87, 1961.
5. BURRUS, G.R.; HOWELL, J.F., and JORDAN, G.L., Jr.: Traumatic duodenal injuries: an analysis of 86 cases. *J Trauma, 1*:96, 1961.
6. KINDLING, P.H.; WALT, A.J., and WILSON, R.F.: Hepatic trauma: with particular reference to blunt injury. (In press)
7. ARBULU, A.; READ, R., and BERKAS, E.M.: Delayed symptomatology in traumatic diaphragmatic hernia with a note on eventration. *Dis. Chest, 47*:527, 1965.
8. FREEARK, R.J.; LOVE, L., and BAKER, R.J.: The role of aortography in the management of blunt abdominal trauma. *J Trauma, 8*:557, 1968.
9. THAL, A.P., and WILSON, R.F.: A pattern of severe blunt trauma to the region of the pancreas. *Surg Gynec Obstet, 119*:773, 1964.
10. HAYNES, C.D.; GUNN, C.H., and MARTIN J.D., Jr.: Colon injuries. *Arch Surg, 96*:944, 1968.
11. NANCE, F.C., and CROWDER, V.H.: Intramural hematoma of the colon following blunt trauma to the abdomen. *Amer Surg 34*:85, 1968.

DISCUSSION

Roger D. Williams

Because of the varying opinions with little proof regarding the mechanisms of injury to abdominal viscera, we became interested several years ago in physical factors which might cause specific injuries. Anesthetized dogs whose sacrifice was scheduled were struck upright or supine with a force of about 300 to 400 foot-pounds. The injuries were similar to those in patients, but splenic injury was more frequently found in our sacrificed animals. Renal injury was more common in a large series of patients who had the injury often diagnosed from bloody urine, but such injury was unconfirmed if surgery was not performed. The location of the trauma was important, flank blows producing more renal and liver injuries than a blow to the anterior abdomen. The force used produced twice as many injuries as we saw in patients, yet is only equivalent to a 150-pound man striking the steering column when his automobile moving at 7 mph suddenly stops.

We have also used transducers in various parts of the gut and peritoneal cavity to measure pressure changes associated with blunt trauma. Although pressure varied in each animal, the intraperitoneal pressure always exceeded that in the gut lumen. If Pascal's law holds here, which I believe it does, rupture of the intestine can hardly be explained from acute pressure changes. We found the injuries occurring mostly in the midline and fixed segments of the gut over the spine. Injury could be prevented only when the striking force prevented approximation of the anterior abdominal wall and the spine.

Since someone may someday claim that sudden decompression of an astronaut can rupture the intestine, we performed rapid decompression experiments with a parasite chamber attached by a large window to a high altitude chamber. The pressure differential, when the plastic diaphragm between the two chambers was ruptured, was of the same magnitude, though negative, as that with blunt trauma. Again, the intraperitoneal pressure gradient was greater than that in the gut lumen and occurred in about $\frac{1}{50}$ of a second. We exposed the intestine of rats, even distended and occluded segments with air, yet we could not rupture it with acute decompression, although I suppose that a more chronically dilated gut would rupture. I must conclude, therefore, that a shearing force, rather than pressure, causes most gut injuries.

Finally, though we don't really know why the diaphragm ruptures, we have always found that with blunt trauma as well as explosive decompression, the intrathoracic pressure is higher above the diaphragm than in the abdomen.

Chapter VI

BIOMECHANICS IN ORTHOPEDIC SURGERY
An Account of Aims and Methods

CARL HIRSCH

INTRODUCTION

The locomotor system consists to a great extent of collagen structures and supporting tissues which have a mechanical function. Lesions occur when forces exceed the strength of the material. Diseases may change the physical properties of collagen.

Reconstructive orthopedic surgery often faces problems where the mechanical characteristics of collagen have to be considered.

In this presentation, ways are illustrated by which forces have been measured in the hip joint and the lumbar spine. As these anatomical units consist of bone, cartilage, capsules, ligaments and tendons, the understanding of how forces affect various parts must consider the properties of material of different morphological nature. Therefore, attempts have also been made to investigate different collagen tissues with regard to their material characteristics.

Collagen shows viscoelastic behavior which can be described by rheological models and correlated to morphological and chemical data.

The aim of these studies is to widen the background for further discussions in such orthopedic problems where knowledge of material properties is essential.

CLINICAL PROBLEMS

In everyday practice, there is an increasing demand of development and improvement of surgical techniques in orthopedic surgery, so that the function of various injured joints can be retained. There is an increased frequency of conditions where such procedures are desirable. Due to the intensity of traffic accidents, a great many young people are victimized. The number of aged people is increasing and their skeletal tolerance against mechanical strains is decreased. Consequently, geriatric fractures occur more often. Degenerative changes in joints (osteoarthritis) have also become more common as there is a change in the age distribution of the population and this is very often accompanied by invalidating conditions. The risks, with large surgical interventions, have nowadays decreased considerably due to the development of surgical techniques, and this has offered possibilities to remove large tumor masses, which at the same time creates problems of reconstructive surgery. Rheumatoid arthritis also represents a desire to substitute injured tissues in more advanced stages which have stimulated further progress.

As regards all above-mentioned clinical concepts, prophylactic measures must be pursued. At the same time, however, it is realistic to have a therapeutic aim, the object of which is to restitute or to compensate pathologically changed sectors within the locomotor system.

Operative techniques have for long been characterized by the art to remove organs or parts thereof. As for orthopedic surgery, this has been synonymous with resection or with amputation. Reconstructive orthopedic surgery nevertheless has old traditions. The skeleton with its tendons, ligaments, capsules and muscles has always been regarded as mechanically purposeful. Therefore, the experiments are numerous which have been designed to describe the connection between anatomical form and function. It has become evident that there are disturbances of differing origin which might be altered by a change in the mechanical function. On the whole, orthopedic surgery of today is characterized by procedures which redistribute the transmission of forces. Among the most usual operations, the elimination or transposition of muscle powers, osteotomy or arthrodesis are included. There is great experience behind this type of orthopedic surgery, and it is impossible today to be without the clinical effects of this reconstructive work.

If a procedure has an expected effect, it certainly meets with its aim and therefore most probably has a biological background of importance for further exploitation. Many of the procedures which are used are mechanically interpreted. It might now be more appropriate to inveigle us to obtain qualitatively and quantitatively registerable information about what actually happens in both normal and diseased skeletal system. The technical development has, in a very short time, given us an equipment which can well be adjusted to biologic concepts.

BIOMECHANICAL PROBLEMS

It is obvious that there would be great value in knowing how great forces act in joint systems and how they vary under different forms of activity and also how the different components of these anatomical systems behave during mechanical strains and further where the limits of tolerance are and so on. Experience from daily clinical work does not offer any difficulties in finding problems. When great forces exceed the tensile strength of collagen fractures and soft tissue, injuries ensue. How can we then protect ourselves? Increased speeds give more complicated lesions. What margins of safety do we have to surround ourselves by? How does it come about that in older people certain regions are more vulnerable like e.g., the femoral neck? Is this due to inferior properties of the material or reduced amount of osseous substance? When destructive changes occur in cartilage with increasing age, a series of peri- and subchondral reactions arise. Some of these are so painful and limit motion that patients find great difficulties in moving around. What then are the physical properties of cartilage which is so changed that an osteoarthritis ensues. In the near future, we plan to make long journeys to other planets. Is there a risk that the inactivity which follows the fixation during the transport creates injuries in the collagenous system, and what are the biomechanical problems we might meet in surroundings where gravitation is different?

EXPERIMENTAL PROBLEMS

In many biological contexts, animal experiments are suitable preambles for clinical information. Of course, this is also the case as regards the problems which have been mentioned above. The difference in form and function of the locomotor system is, however, so great that there are many good reasons to start model experiments on fresh autopsy material. This opinion has been based upon the desire to find a technique of measurement which would reproduce special clinical problems.

It is possible to apply strain gauges on the cortical shell of the femoral neck in hip joints secured postmortem. Muscular forces can be simulated and applied and the region can be loaded via the sacrum (Fig. 6–1). If the interaction of increasing loads and muscular tension is permitted to act on the upper part of the femur, the different types of fractures are obtained which are known from clinical experience. People above 60 years of age stand less strain; there is a distinct connection between type of fracture, loading and muscular response. Calculations can also be made of the engagement of very different parts of the cortical shell of the femoral neck and the trabecular system.[1,4,5]

Model experiments have also been carried out on the lumbar back. The anatomical form, the complex arrangement of the muscles, and the presence

Measuring Bridge   **Strain Gauge**

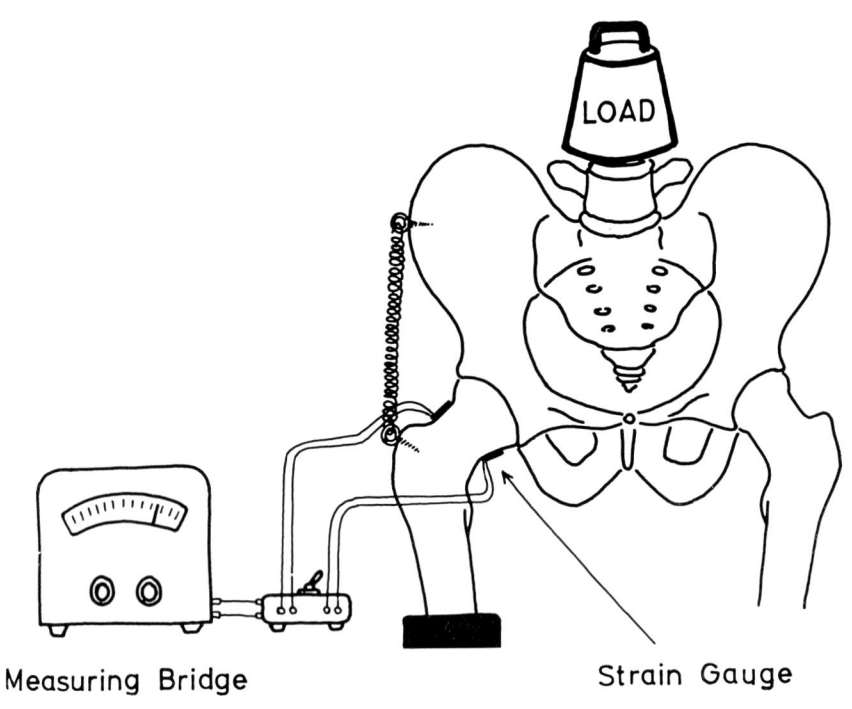

FIGURE 6–1. Drawing of model experiment on autopsy specimen. Strain-gauges have been attached to the neck of the femur. Muscles have been replaced by adjustable springs (in the picture gluteus medius is simulated). Body weight is put on the fifth lumbar vertebra. Movements in the superficial cortical layers of the femoral neck are recorded on a measuring bridge.

of other structural elements, give reason to register deformations in specially selected skeletal regions in another way. In, for example, the intervertebral discs, small cannulae were introduced with small polyethylene-covered openings. The cannula which was occluded in its inner part was filled with physiologic saline. When the membrane reacted to the inner pressure of the disc, the aqueous movements in the cannula were registered by a pressure transducer on measuring bridges.[12] The deformation of the intervertebral discs and vertebral bodies was plotted out with extensometers.[15] By using these measuring methods, it could be proved that the lumbar back forms a flexible system in which not only the discs represent the deformed parts but also the skeletal contribution to this deformation is greater than had previously been believed.

The hip joint and the lumbar back have been briefly mentioned above, but model experiments have also been carried out on feet, knees and wrists in order to establish the connection between trauma and injurious effect.[2,7,11,19]

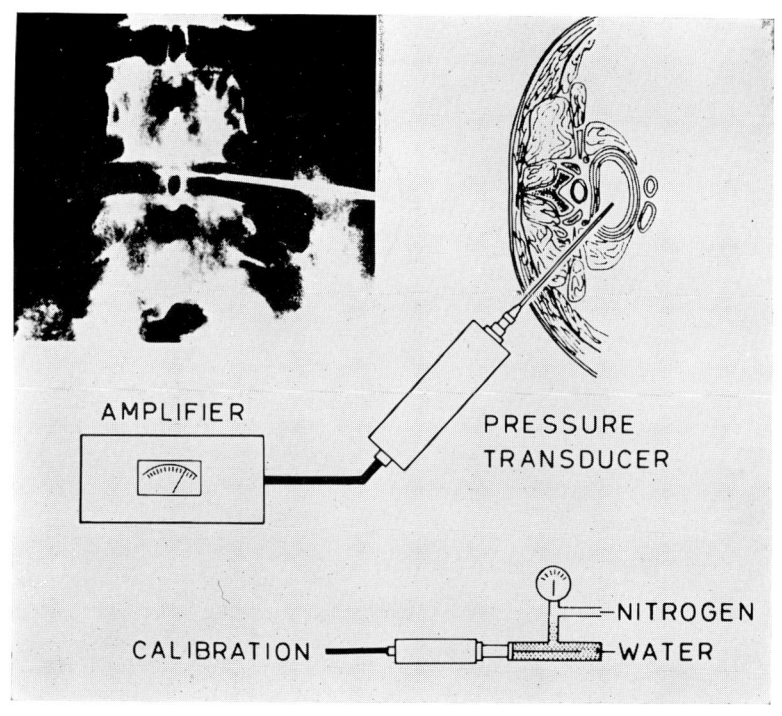

FIGURE 6–2. A cannula has been introduced in a lumbar disc and the intradiscal pressure is recorded.

INTRAVITAL MEASUREMENTS

It is obvious that the described models only give indications of possible mechanical reaction modes but hardly any information of what actually happens intravitam. The neural regulation, circulation, and metabolic events, with their combined influence on the tested object, have been put out of play. For this reason, experiments have been carried out by introducing measuring devices in the hip joint,[16] and lumbar back,[13] in patients where an indication for surgical intervention has been present. In two cases, the femoral head and neck have been removed following severe accidents and a substitute of metal has been implanted—hip joint prosthesis—in which strain gauges have been inserted in the neck following preliminary studies in model experiments (Fig. 6–3). The system was arranged in such a way that every force that was transferred to the femoral head could be registered by the metal substitute and recorded via connecting wires to measuring bridges. In this way, a series of information was obtained. The direction, the magnitude, the pressure region of the femoral head and the friction between the prostheses and acetabulum could be estimated.

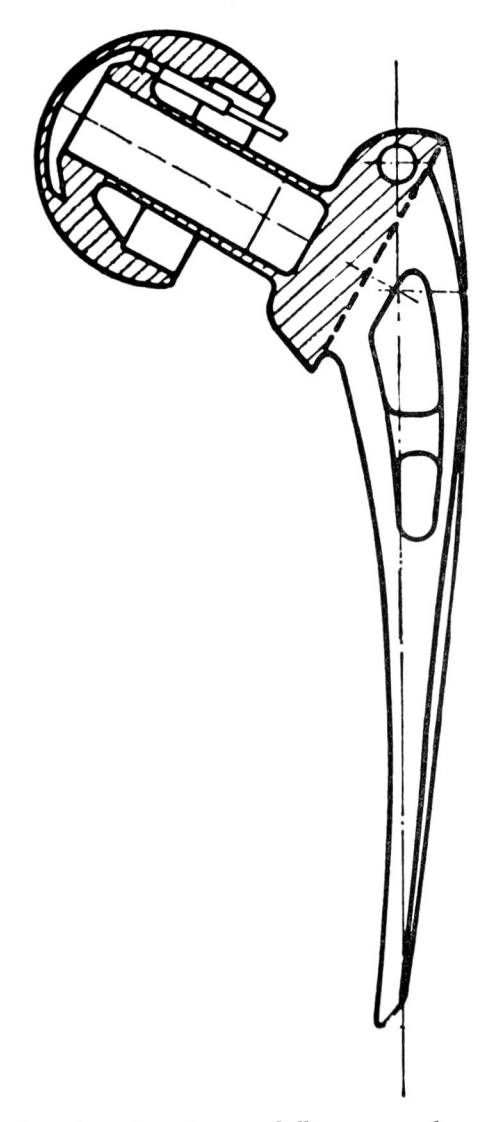

FIGURE 6–3A. Drawing of an intramedullary upper femoral replacement.

The introduction of pressure-registering organs of the same type used in autopsy models presented information of the magnitude of the interior pressure of the lumbar intervertebral discs and calculations were made of the tensile properties in the annulus fibrosus of these discs in different postures and loads.[14]

Strain gauges were also used partly to determine the force that the laminae in the thoracic and lumbar region could tolerate when scolioses were corrected by the introduction of metal rods, partly for direct measurement of the strains which were transferred to the metal rods during the

Biomechanics in Orthopedic Surgery 131

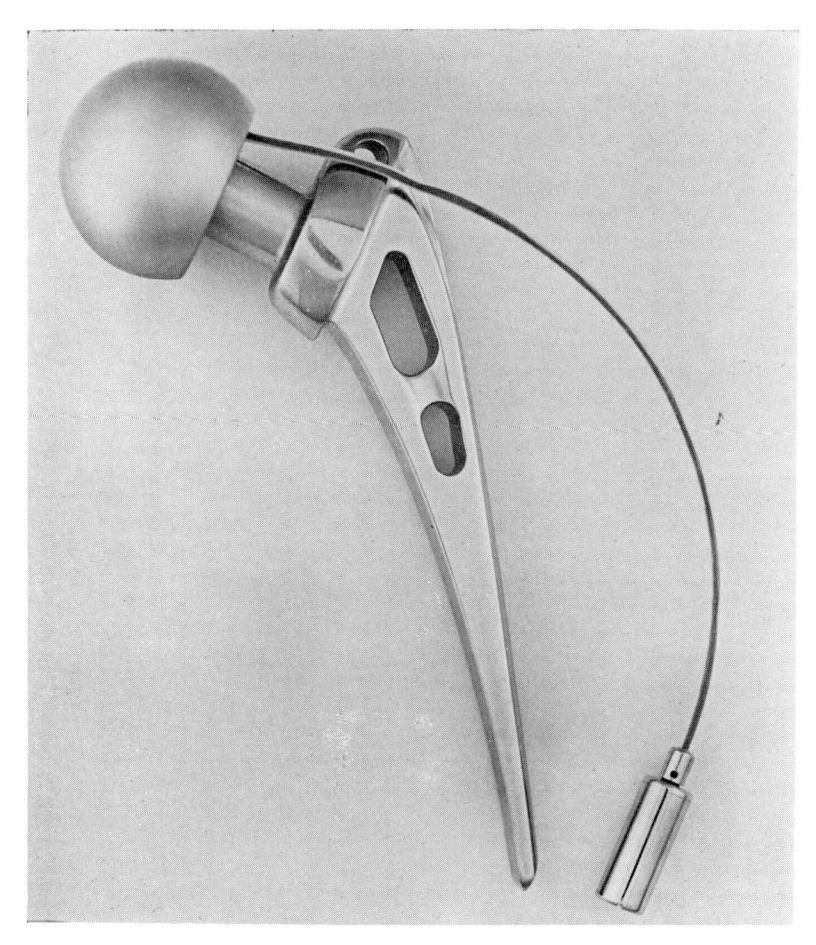

FIGURE 6–3B. Protheses to be used clinically. The wire connection from the prosthetic head and the box is left covered by the skin after surgery is completed. Six months later when the patient can walk normally the box is exteriorized and connected to a measuring bridge and recordings taken.

first few days after the operation in connection with mobilization of the patient who was also permitted to carry out different back movements (Fig. 6–4).[10,22]

All this information about the magnitude and direction of forces within regions of clinical interest has a great value when discussing the mechanical function of the locomotor system and what various interventions may stand from a mechanical point of view but data of this type eventually prove to be insufficient even if interesting. In order to estimate the effect of forces on biological material it is essential that we have knowledge of the mechanical characteristics of different collagenous structures.

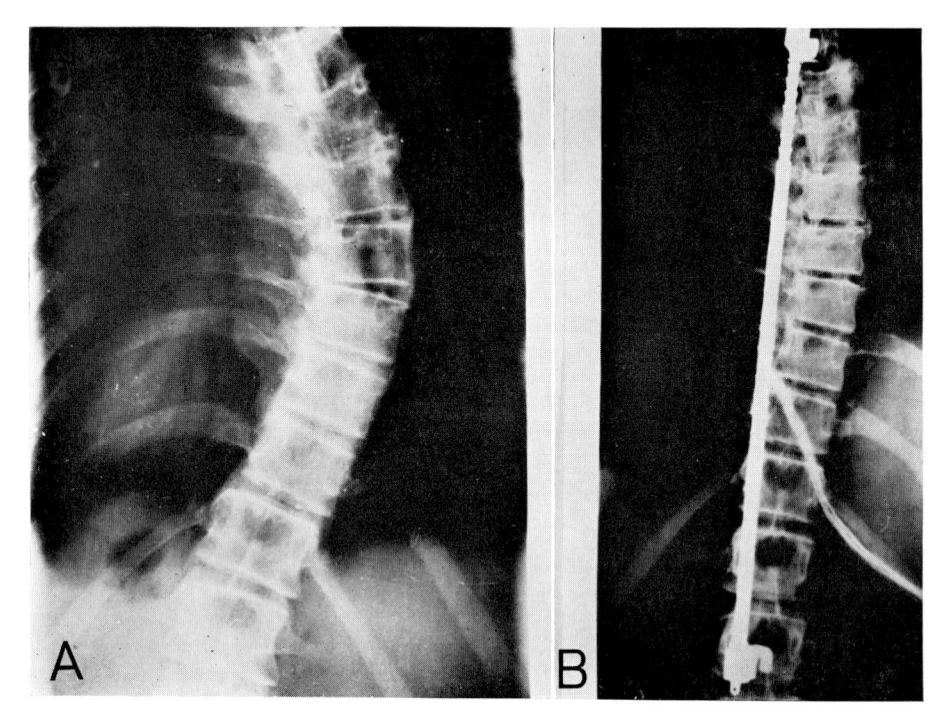

FIGURE 6–4A. Scoliosis with a thoracic curvature to the right.
FIGURE 6–4B. The same patient after instrumental correction. A rod has been introduced to hold the spine erect. Strain-gauges have been attached to the rod and wire connected with measuring bridges.

EVALUATION OF PROPERTIES OF MATERIAL

What material properties do biologic structures have? What actually happens when a given quantity of bone, tendon or ligament is subjected to a mechanical force? Only by knowing the properties of the material under normal and pathological conditions can the importance of the information which has been obtained in the previously described vital experiments be estimated. If, for example, an articular component or a complete anatomical system should be substituted and made to function, one has to avoid creating new problems by introducing constructions which do not fit in with the play of biologic forces, which appear between different materials. The experience of later years in metal and plastic prostheses in reconstruction shows the necessity of increased knowledge of the physical properties of collagen.

It is natural to attempt to find methods by which the mechanical properties of collagen might be plotted under vital conditions. However, technical difficulties are encountered in this context which at present have not been solved. At the moment when the test material had been removed from its biologic surroundings, a series of errors have been introduced, the importance of which cannot be neglected. It is therefore essential that laboratory conditions are systematically mapped out when dealing with problems of this kind in order to avoid large errors of method.

MEASURING TECHNIQUE

Preparation

Instruments have been constructed in which bone can be ground so that constant dimensions are obtained.[17,18] Soft collagenous tissues can be punched out to desired proportions.[3,8] Skeletal parts are often built so that different collagenous components are present in one and the same place, e.g., in a joint. It is therefore difficult to isolate a special material and there is a demand for working with small dimensions.

Tension and bending experiments have shown that a material obtained during operation or at autopsy rapidly can change its properties by the loss of fluids or uptake of the same. On the other hand, the mechanical characteristics remain constant in high aerial humidity (about 95%) and constant temperature (as a rule room temperature is used). In order to diminish autolytic processes, the material has to be frozen and stored in closed vessels provided of course, that the material is not used immediately. All preparations have to be carried out in high humidity; this is especially necessary during the experiments of tensile properties.[8,18]

Instruments of Registration

Our instrument for registration of tensile properties is composed of parts which are commercially obtainable. There are many systems to choose from. None of them, however, are intended for biologic purposes. After a series of experiments with different equipments, we have found the one in Figure 6-5 to be the most suitable. It consists of an instrument for testing tensile properties (Alwetron) in which the material is subjected to a force which can be regulated. The speed with which the force acts can also be adjusted and repeated with intervals at will. One of the difficulties has been to hold collagenous tissues without the fastened ends giving way or fracturing. For this purpose, special holding arrangements have been constructed.[6,8,18,20] The distance between these indicate the elongation during the experiments. In order to further follow the course of events and to check that no gliding influences the distance, extensometers have been applied.

The deflexion of the material has been registered on an xy-recorder and also with an oscilloscope with a Polaroid® camera. The information can

134 Impact Injury and Crash Protection

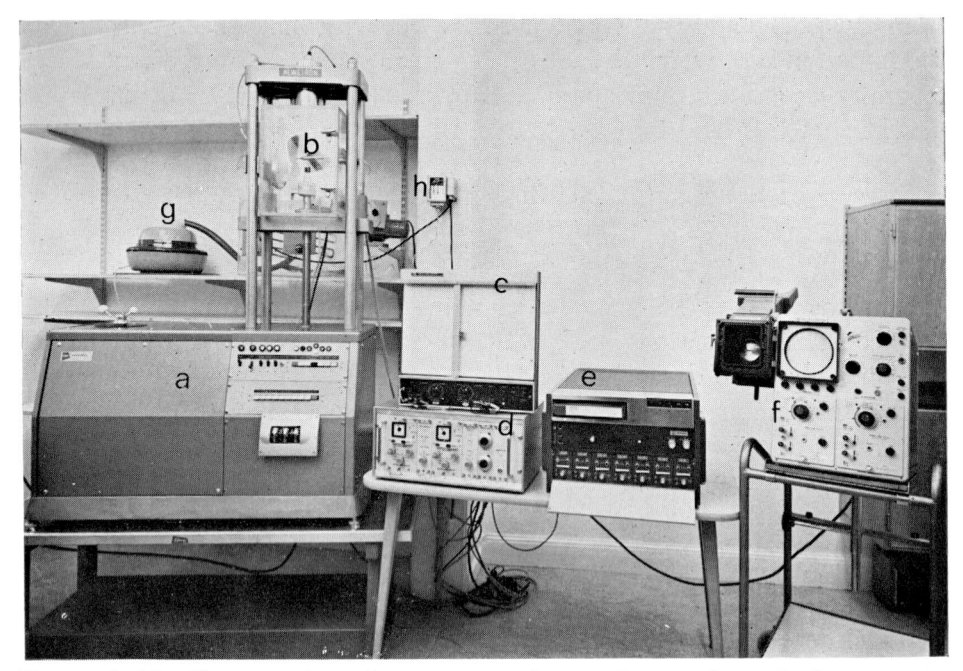

FIGURE 6–5A. Close-up view of equipment determining mechanical characteristics of collagen tissues.
a. Materials testing unit
b. Chamber for tensile tests
c. Xy-recorder
d. Amplifier
e. Tape-recorder
f. Oscilloscope
g. Humidifier
h. Temperature sensors

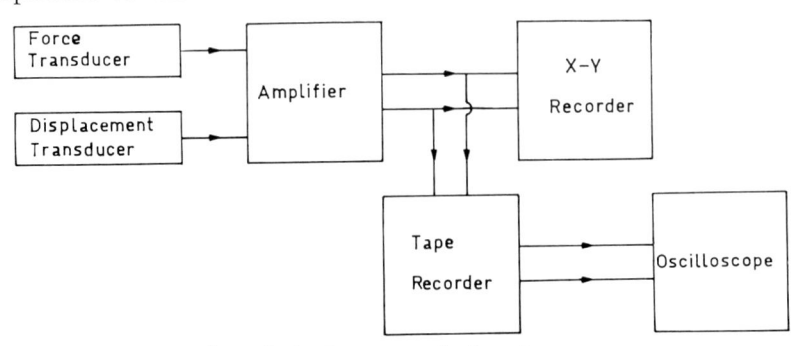

FIGURE 6–5B. Block diagram of the electronic system.

be transferred to a tape-recorder. Data from this can later be replayed and visualized on the xy-recorder. It is also possible to computerize the tapes after digital handling. As the properties of material are influenced by humidity and temperature, the loading experiments are carried out in

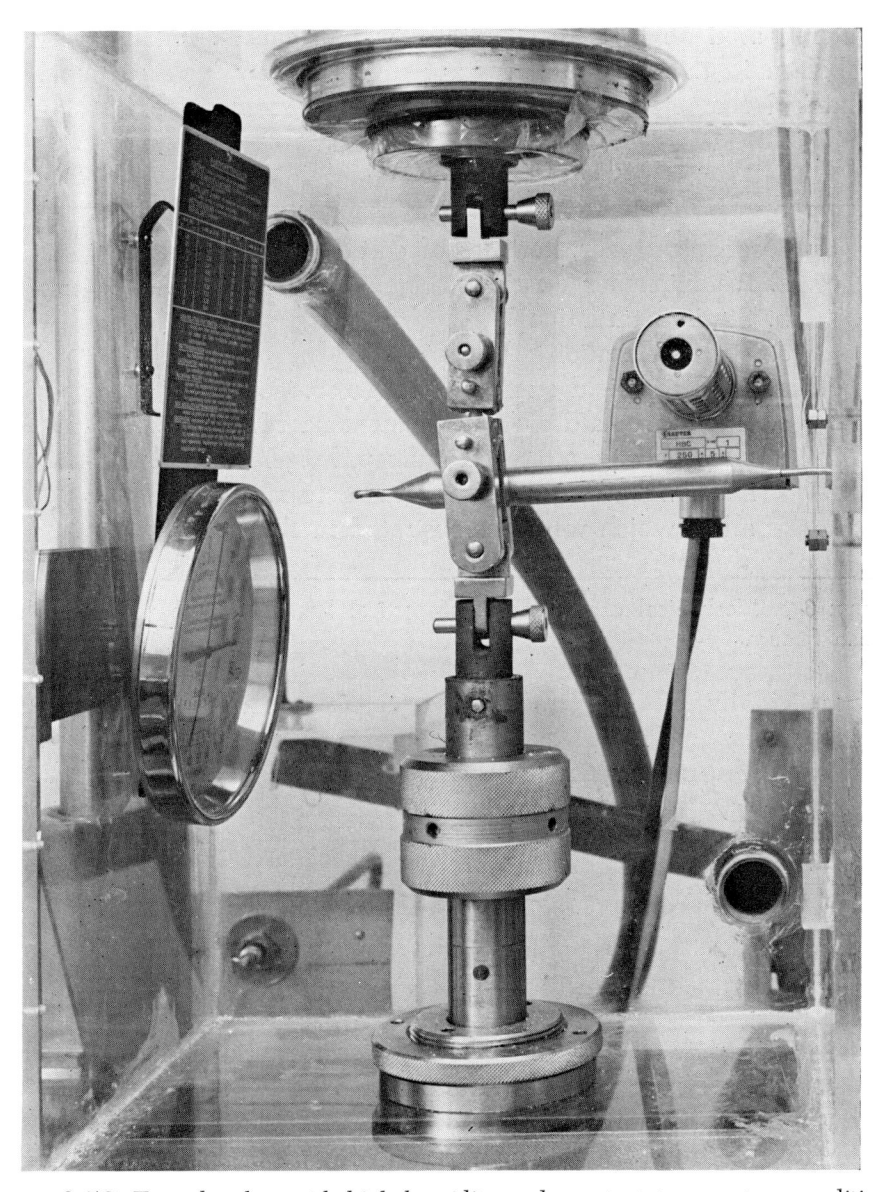

FIGURE 6–5C. Test chamber with high humidity and constant temperature conditions.

95 per cent relative humidity, and as a rule in 20°C, with the specimens in a chamber with walls of translucent plastic material. The humidity and temperature are checked and the values are kept constant with automatic regulators.

Properties of Material

Vital measurements have not yet been performed with sufficient precision in bone, tendinous and ligamentous tissues. Our knowledge is therefore based on *in vitro* conditions which, considering the very low metabolism in these tissues, does not divert in any higher degree. The mechanical characteristics of bone have been summarized.[17]

FIGURE 6-6.

> Mechanical characteristics of cortical bone
> a. Instantaneous elasticity
> b. Strain retardation
> c. Stress relaxation
> d. Multiple yield stresses
> e. Implicit in a-d are the phenomena of: elastic fore-effect, elastic after-effect, creep, hysteresis, and non-linear behavior on a usual load-deformation diagram, all of which were demonstrated in this study.

FIGURE 6-6. Mechanical characteristics of cortical bone from the proximal part of human femurs.

If an initially flaccid ligament is subjected to tension, the elastic limit is exceeded by small loads and under *in vitro* conditions, there is never a complete return to the original form. If, on the other hand, the ligament is subjected to preliminary stretching corresponding to the heating up of muscles in athletes, every cycle of loading is reproducible to high values, at least half the breaking load.

It is doubtful if there is an elasticity level for these materials as a whole. If the load exceeds a certain limit, injuries arise by ruptures of fibers in the specimen, which from a geometrical point of view is always unevenly loaded.

Figure 6-7 shows a typical sequence where a tendon or a ligament is subjected to a tensile test. The difference between the ascending curve (a) and the descending (b) is the hysteresis and represents the viscous moderation of the material. The curves in Figure 6-8 show the influence of speed on the material. Fast speeds give steeper curves, that is, more rigid tissues, which rupture at higher loading but at lower values of deformation.

The properties of collagenous materials can be summarized in a viscoelastic pattern, e.g., the course of events can be described with symbols where the elasticity is demonstrated by springs and the plasticity with fluid moderators.[3,9,16,21] It comes in handy to ascribe to the collagenous fiber the elastic property, and to the interfibrillar substance, e.g., mucopolysaccharides and intercellular fluids, the viscous effect. This explanation of sequences in symbols simplifies the interpretation of what really happens.

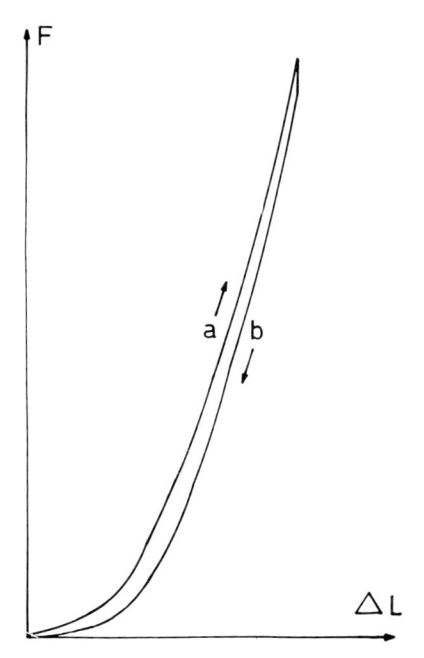

FIGURE 6-7. Diagram obtained from tensile tests on ligaments. The difference between a and b represents the viscous influence of the material.

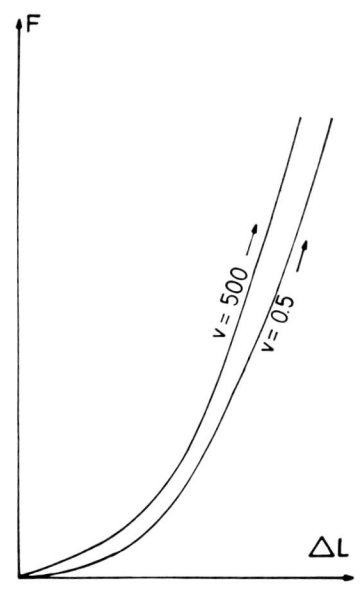

FIGURE 6-8. Time dependence upon the tensile pattern of ligament. Fast acting forces give steeper curves, e.g., rigid tissue response. The breaking load increases but the degree of deformation decreases.

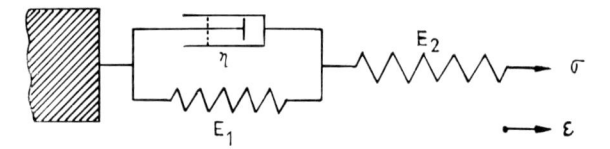

FIGURE 6–9. Model of viscoelastic properties in collagen material.

At the same time, it makes it easier to systematize those problems which are essential when comparison is to be made between normal and pathologic condition in which the definitions as a rule are based on morphologic and histochemical descriptions.

The morphologic structure which signifies the test object influences the deformation properties. It is therefore necessary to relate the viscoelastic sequences to the geometry of collagen. One can anticipate that the different components of the material change their mutual conditions during the course of strain, and that the appearance of the diagram also demonstrates this. In normal tissues, the morphologic picture is rather constant, and the mechanical characteristics, which are a function of the structure of material, remain constant. In pathologic conditions, the divergences are often considerable and more difficult to interpret.

It is of certain importance that the morphologic picture of the material is followed not only before and after tensile strength test has been carried out, but that the whole course of events or parts of the same can offer information about the behavior of the fibrillary structure. For this reason, a built-in microscope belongs to the above-mentioned equipment, and there are possibilities to carry out histologic work.

CLINICAL APPLICATION

The identification of the physical properties of collagenous structures is of importance in clinical reconstructive work. When a fracture has been sustained, it is reasonable to combine the parts so that they will be retained in their original place, and in a way that the organ part in question can start functioning as soon as possible. Interior nailing, and screwing of fragments or metal plates which bridge the fragments, have been used for a long time. Lately, the stability of these metal connections has been increased by the development of a technique permitting compression in the actual direction of the skeletal part. Often, such rigid fixations offer a faster healing while the patient can be mobilized. Knowledge of the properties of the biological material facilitates the technique of fixation but unfortunately also creates complications because mechanical disturbances may arise between metal and bone because of the mechanical discrepancies between the materials. It is therefore important to find suitable osteosynthetic materials which suit the play of biologic forces. Even if the metals of today have many advantages, it is obvious that other internal fixations of material with physical properties equal to those of bone should be a desirable aim. Frequently, a joint is injured to a degree that reconstruction with remaining osseous components is impossible. During a number of years, attempts have been made to substitute whole or parts of joints with plastic or metal or combinations of these. Difficulties are, however, encountered in obtaining a permanent stable fixation and to avoid mechanical injuries in the surrounding tissues because of differences in the material properties, it should theoretically be possible to find a substitute that carries properties more similar to the tissues which are substituted. It is possible that increased knowledge of the mechanical behavior of joint structure might lead us to constructions which are better tolerated in biologic surroundings than those obtainable at present. In these efforts, data of tensile properties and information of the magnitude of loads and strains are part of an attempt which should be possible to materialize.

At times it may appear as if biomechanical problems in the repair of injuries and diseases in the locomotor system have not given a good enough therapeutic response. This is however, not the case. We have learned to understand the material that we work with, and even if all clinical measures do not come up to the expectations of today, we can nevertheless exhibit greater effectivity in the work which is being carried out. We now have shorter times of hospitalization and better end-results than previously; in this way marked socioeconomic gains have been made. Finally, we carry a continuous debate where at least principles and aims appear more outlined than before.

REFERENCES

1. FRANKEL, V.: *The Femoral Neck. Function Mechanism, Internal Fixation.* An experimental study. Sweden, Almqvist & Wiksell, 1960.
2. FRYKMAN, G.: Fracture of the distal radius including sequelae—shoulder-hand-finger syndrome, disturbance in the distal radio-ulnar joint and impairment of nerve function. A clinical and experimental study. *Acta Orthop Scand* (Suppl. 108), 1967.
3. GALANTE, J.: Tensile properties of the human lumbar annulus fibrosus. *Acta Orthop Scand* (Suppl. 100), 1967.
4. HIRSCH, C., and FRANKEL, V.: Analysis of forces producing fractures of the proximal end of the femur. *J Bone Joint Surg*, 1960, vol. 42B, No. 3.
5. HIRSCH, C., and FRANKEL, V.: *The Reaction of the Proximal End of the Femur to Mechanical Forces. Biomechanical Studies of the Musculo-Skeletal System.* Springfield, Thomas, 1961.
6. HIRSCH, C., and EVANS, G.: Studies on some physical properties of infant compact bone. *Acta Orthop Scand*, XXXV:300–313, 1965.

7. HIRSCH, C., and LEWIS, J.: Experimental ankle-joint fractures. *Acta Orthop Scand*, 36:408–417, 1965.
8. HIRSCH, C., and GALANTE, J.: Laboratory conditions for tensile tests in annulus fibrosus from human intervertebral discs. *Acta Orthop Scand*, 38:148–162, 1967.
9. HIRSCH, C., and SONNERUP, L.: Macroscopic rheology in skeletal structures. *J Biomechanics*, 1968, No. 1.
10. HIRSCH, C., and WAUGH, T.: The introduction of force measurements guiding instrumental correction of scoliosis. *Acta Orthop Scand*, 39:1, 1968.
11. HIRSCH, G., and SULLIVAN, L.: Experimental knee-joint fractures. *Acta Orthop Scand*, 36:391–399, 1965.
12. NACHEMSON, A.: Lumbar intradiscal pressure. *Acta Orthop Scand* (Suppl. XLIII), 1960.
13. NACHEMSON, A.: The effect of forward leaning on lumbar intradiscal pressure. *Acta Orthop Scand*, XXXV:314–328, 1965.
14. NACHEMSON, A.: The load on lumbar disks in different positions of the body. *Clin Orthop*, 1966.
15. ROLANDER, S.: Motion of the Lumbar Spine with Special Reference to the Stabilizing Effect of Posterior Fusion. An experimental study on autopsy specimens. Tryckeri AB Litotyp, 1966.
16. RYDELL, N.: Forces Acting on the Femoral Head-Prosthesis. A study on Strain Gauge Supplied Prostheses in Living Persons. Tryckeri AB Litotyp, 1966.
17. SEDLIN, E.: A rheological model for cortical bone. A study of the physical properties of human femoral samples. *Acta Orthop Scand* (Suppl. 83), 1965.
18. SEDLIN, E., and HIRSCH, C.: Factors affecting the determination of the physical properties of femoral cortical bone. *Acta Orthop Scand*, 37:29–48, 1966.
19. THORÉN, O.: Os Calcis Fractures. Orstadius Boktryckeri AB, 1964.
20. VIIDIK, A.: Biomechanics and functional adaption of tendons and joint ligaments. In Evans, F.G. (Ed.): *Studies on the Anatomy and Function of Bone and Joints*. Heidelberg, Springer, 1966, pp. 17–39.
21. VIIDIK, A.: Experimental evaluation of the tensile strength of Isolated rabbit tendons. *Biomed Engineering*, 2:64–67, 1967.
22. WAUGH, T.: Intravital Measurements During Instrumental Correction of Idiopathic Scoliosis. Tryckeri AB Litotyp, 1966.

DISCUSSION

HERBERT E. PEDERSEN

This chapter briefly describes the several techniques which Dr. Carl Hirsch has used in his laboratory, such as his adherence to the scientific method, and the objectivity of his observations and conclusions. These are pioneer efforts that apply engineering methods to that most inconstant and variable of research objects: the human organism. Care must be taken in the application of simple facts, gathered in the engineering laboratory, to the solution of clinical problems, which are usually very complex. I think it important to point out that the initial establishment of Dr. Hirsch's laboratory and his stimulus and training of other investigators to work in this area was at least as important as his currently reported results. He has trained other investigators who have established laboratories in many other areas, and have contributed extensively.

So far as orthopedic surgery is concerned, there probably is no other medical discipline which lends itself so well to the application of engineering principles. The supporting and the locomotive apparatus must behave according to established mechanical principles. So far as fractures of long bones are concerned, our basic research has given us much information. The strength of materials, the organization of these materials, and their response to stress are somewhat known. That bone can resist compression better than it can resist tension is a fact. The efficient nature of long-bone construction, namely the organization as a tube is recognized. These long bones behave and have mechanical properties of the tube. It's usually possible, by the inspection of long-bone fractures, to determine how the force was applied. While it's true that the mechanism of injury, under clinical circumstances, is much more complicated than can be devised in the laboratory, these studies do supply sufficient information so that the consequences of most injuries can be predicted.

In the treatment of long-bone injuries, much from engineering has aided us. Many things have been learned about the usefulness of available metals: which ones are suitable for internal support, and which ones are not. Metals cannot be mixed in their application for internal support. Many important lessons have been learned in the design of these structures, plates and screws and rods. The application of those devices to most efficiently resist stress has been discovered.

I am particularly interested in Dr. Hirsch's efforts to study the prosthetic replacement of the femoral head, where, characteristically, he begins by studying stress and strain *in vivo*. For those who don't already recognize it, the prosthetic replacement of the femoral head has been available for many years, and there are now a multitude of prostheses of varying designs which are available. Each one of these uses a perfect sphere to replace what was not a perfect sphere to begin with. To date, there is no real evidence which will suggest whether the prosthetic replacement should have a diameter which is the same, which is larger, or which is smaller than the one which was originally removed. No evidence exists to prove that a perfect sphere is the ideal shape, and that it's any better than any other possible design that we can consider. There is nothing to tell us exactly how long this prosthesis should be. Normal joints involve the apposition of two incongruent surfaces, each of which is covered by a compressible articular cartilage. The lubrication of this joint uses the wedge principle of lubrication. There is considerable room for expanded and continued research in this area.

PART II

RESEARCH METHODS IN IMPACT INJURY

Chapter VII

TELEMETRY IN BIOLOGICAL SCIENCES

Robert H. Pudenz

Biological telemetry is defined as the transmitting and receiving of bioelectrical information at points geographically distant from each other. With the advent of space exploration, the term is associated with the use of miniaturized sensors and transmitters that provide physiological and behavioral data on animals and man subjected to the stressful environments of space. Telemetering equipment developed in space technology is now being employed with increasing frequency in biology and medicine. For the first time, the physician and the biologist are able to study physiological mechanisms in hitherto inaccessible locations for long periods of time under dynamic, rather than static, conditions. In this report, we are concerned with the current uses of these techniques in modern biology and medicine.

It is now recognized that electrical phenomena are associated with the biological processes of all living plant and animal cells, irrespective of their size or function. The cell is comparable to a battery in which the negative pole, or cathode, is enclosed within the cell membrane. Intracellular recordings with microelectrodes have shown that the interior of a cell is from -20 mv to -100 mv negative to its external environment. In excitable cells such as nerve and muscle cells, the potential gradients are subject to change depending on whether the cell is polarized, depolarized or hyperpolarized. These voltage differences are the result of ionic migration, hydrogen ion concentration, the activity of oxidation-reduction systems, as well as other biological phenomena. In addition to polarizability, the cell has other electrochemical properties such as resistance and capacitance; and it can be altered metabolically by electrical stimulation. Were it not for these basic electrical properties of the cell, modern telemetry could not exist.

HISTORICAL BACKGROUND

Developments in the science and technology of electrophysiology and biotelemetry are intimately bound and inseparable from each other. Continuous refinements in electronics have enabled the physiologist to study bioelectrical phenomena with increasing detail. A review of the subject could not be complete without paying tribute to the pioneers.

Our knowledge of the electrical properties of tissues begins with Luigi Galvani in the latter part of the eighteenth century. Galvani, a physician and physiologist of the University of Bologna, has been called the "Father of Modern Neurology." There are fascinating tales about his observations on the twitching of frogs' legs suspended on copper hooks in a butcher shop. However, his essential contribution was his awareness of the action of the nerve on muscle which established one of the most important facts of biology, namely, the electrical basis of nerve action.

In 1850, Helmholtz began his investigation of conduction in the sciatic nerve of frogs. In 1856, von Kölliker and Müller discovered that an electrical current was generated by the frog's heart when it contracted. However, it was not until 1903 that electrocardiography really began with the introduction of the string galvanometer by Einthoven.[38]

In 1875, Caton demonstrated electrical activity in the exposed brain of an animal. Subsequently, this was confirmed by other workers. However, the development of modern electroencephalography dates back to Hans Berger who, in 1929, published the first work on electrical activity of the brain recorded through the unopened skull.[38]

Discoveries in the first decade of this century set the stage for the exciting developments that have now occurred in physiology, electronics and telemetry. In 1904, Fleming patented the first diode, and 2 years later, de Forest introduced the triode. Thus began the era of electronics, the application of electrical conduction *in vacuo.*

The year 1906 also marks the beginning of medical telemetry. It was at this time that Einthoven transmitted electrocardiograms over the lines of the Leyden Telephone Company. Shortly thereafter, attempts were made to develop central stations for cardiac monitoring in hospitals; but the techniques were impractical and soon abandoned.

Following Einthoven, and particularly during World War I, there was a steady improvement in the techniques of thermionic emission. However, a major breakthrough in electronics occurred when Bardeen, Brattain and Shockley, the Nobel Laureates in Physics in 1956, introduced the transistor. The transistor made possible the miniaturization of all electronic equipment. More recently, we have seen the development of "molecular electronics" so that presently, a small disc less than 1 cm in diameter can replace the radiofrequency and audio sections of a television set.[13]

As noted previously, the greatest impetus for the development of telemetering equipment has come as a result of the space program. For the first time, it became mandatory to monitor continuously the physiological and psychological responses of man exposed to the stressful environment of a vehicle orbiting in space. From space technology has come high performance equipment which is being used with increasing frequency and application in terrestrial biology and medicine.

INSTRUMENTATION

In any telemetering system, two essential groups of equipment are necessary.[8,9] One group of instruments must reside with the subject under investigation, and the other resides with the observers receiving and evaluating the data. Between these transmitting and receiving components is the communication link. This link may be by direct-wire transmission, the so-called hard-wire telemetry, by suitably modulated radiofrequency carriers, by light beams with either intensity or pulse modulation, or even by sound waves where frequency and amplitude can convey the desired information.

The biological telemetering system is divisible into six parts. First of all, there is the information source consisting of the patient and the appropriate pick-up equipment, that is, the sensing device or transducer and the associated signal amplifiers. Second, a modulation section which operates on the message permitting it to be transmitted over the channel. This process is often referred to as "coding the message." Third, a noise source must always be considered even though it is an unwelcome part of the transmission. Fourth, the telemetry section or carrier which is the medium used to transmit the signal and, as noted above, consists either of wires, electromagnetic waves or radio frequency, light beams or sound. The fifth component is the receiver and modulator section which converts the signal back to the original message, a process known as decoding. Finally, the sixth component is the data recording section. This displays the data in such a way that it can be acted upon by the person or the computer monitoring the patient. The ultimate goal of all telemetering systems is distortionless transmission which, in the absolute sense, is never achieved.

One of the most important aspects of telemetry is transduction, which converts the biological signal into useful information. This may involve the conversion of biological energy into electrical energy, but this is not necessarily true if the signal is electrical to start with, for example, an electrocardiogram or electroencephalogram. Conversion from biological into electrical energy requires a transducer, a device that converts chemical, mechanical, thermal or light energy into electrical energy or vice versa. For example, a pressure level is electromechanically converted into an electrical signal by the use of a strain gauge or a piezoelectric crystal. This signal, in turn, is amplified, modulated and transmitted over the telemetry channel.

The communication link in telemetry is generally direct connection by wire or by radiotelemetry using frequency modulation. Both systems have certain advantages and disadvantages. For example, if hard-wire telemetry is used, not the least of the problems is a shock hazard. It is absolutely necessary to have the subject isolated from the AC power source as well as grounded. Radio transmission can be easily interfered with in the usual hospital environment by a myriad of interference sources such as relays, motors, switching circuits, pulse circuits, cauterizing machines, x-ray equipment and short wave diathermy. The development of a telemetering system in any laboratory or hospital environment should have the services of a qualified design engineer. Only by this means can one develop a relatively noise-free system with the necessary reliability and freedom from hazard.

By the use of modern electronic components, small radiotransmitters no larger than a large vitamin capsule can transmit information continuously for as long as 2 years. These instruments, called endoradiosondes, can be swallowed or surgically implanted in animals or men for both medical and biological research. Some of the values that have been transmitted include local values of pressure, temperature, pH, oxygen tension, blood pressure, radiation intensity, motion, site of bleeding and bioelectrical potentials associated with the electrocardiogram and the electroencephalogram. Miniature motors have been built into intestinal endoradiosondes which propel the transmitter along a previously swallowed nylon string.[14] This endomotorsonde has two pressure-sensitive membranes, as well as two electrodes designed to record the local hydrogen-ion concentration. More recently, transmitters small enough to pass through a trocar or a large hollow needle have been built. It is now possible to implant circuits in relatively inaccessible areas that produce little or no disturbance to the host.

A significant obstacle in the development of miniaturized telemetering equipment for implantation in the organism has been the size of the power source.[43] One solution is the development of the passive sensor,[47] which is energized by an outside power source, for example, an encircling antenna. Other systems enable the batteries of the implant to be recharged by inductively coupled power. Currently, efforts are being made to utilize the electrochemical reactions of tissue fluids or the cyclic contraction of muscles to furnish power.[43] Energy derived from aortic pulsation has been used to power cardiac pacemakers.

USES OF TELEMETRY AND BIOLOGY IN MEDICINE

Telemetering techniques have many advantages for the physician and biologist. Their chief advantage is that they permit the monitoring of biological processes in a continuous, rather than discontinuous, manner.

This is particularly important in observing stressed individuals in whom changes in physiological processes often occur with amazing speed. For example, patients under observation after myocardial infarction may develop arrhythmias that herald serious trouble unless they are promptly treated. Such changes could be missed by serial electrocardiography.

Another advantage of biotelemetry is that it permits observation of individuals who are inaccessible, mobile, or under quarantine. Finally, the use of implanted telemetering devices enables the observer to obtain information from the otherwise inaccessible internal milieu of the organism.

Space Biology

Monitoring in space began with the development of jet aircraft and became mandatory when man ventured into space in supersonic aircraft and space vehicles. A considerable amount of information has been obtained by observation of pilots in the X-15 Program.[7,23] By 1965, this space probe had attained altitudes in excess of 350,000 feet and speeds exceeding 4000 mph. Bratt and Helvey and his associates have described the biomedical monitoring equipment used in this program. Lightweight telemetering equipment has been developed which monitors such data as the electrocardiogram, pressure differentials in the space suit and cabin, Korotkoff sounds, the partial pressure of oxygen in the breathing space, electroencephalography, electromyography, galvanic skin resistance, temperature, and respiration. Two-way-wave communication is possible between the subject and observer. The design of the apparatus permits interchangeability of channels for the various sensors. Data so obtained has not only provided information on the changes in physiological processes under stress, but has contributed to the design of protective equipment and other safety measures.

Cardiology

Telemetering of biological information has come into its most widespread use in cardiac monitoring. Throughout the country, intensive care units in hospitals are now monitoring patients with cardiac disease, particularly those with myocardial infarction. In most instances, this monitoring is by hard wire, although radiotelemetry is used in some circumstances.

Constant cardiac monitoring enables the medical team to recognize the arrhythmias that herald disaster unless they are promptly treated. More serious conditions such as ventricular fibrillation and asystole can be likewise recognized and death prevented by prompt intervention. Statistics are now available to show that continuous monitoring in coronary care units has affected a significant reduction in mortality and morbidity.

Transmission of the electrocardiographic data by telephone has been recommended by some individuals.[28] Telephone telemetry permits transmission over longer distances than are generally available for radiotelemetry. It has the advantage of avoiding transport of a disabled patient as well as continuous monitoring and speed of data collection and reduction.

Radiotelemetry provides a technique for cardiac monitoring of individuals at work and play. Cerkez et al.,[10] have monitored their patients engaged in their ordinary daily activities. They comment that the technique has proved extremely useful in the detection and diagnosis of cardiac arrhythmias, intermittent conduction disturbances, latent coronary artery disease and asymptomatic heart disease.

Norland and Semmler,[35] and Corday et al.,[11] have used monitoring equipment employing a tape recorder in their ambulatory cardiac patients. This technique permits the recording of more than 50,000 electrocardiographic impulses which can be analyzed in 10 minutes with a scanner. When the electrocardiographic tracings were correlated with the patient's diary of his symptoms, the changes indicative of cardiac ischemia could be documented. Similarly, phantom arrhythmias and other evanescent cardiac abnormalities could be detected.

Hinkle and his colleagues,[43] at Cornell University Medical College, recorded the electrocardiograms of three hundred ostensibly healthy individuals varying from 20 to 60 years of age. In this group, changes indicative of impending serious cardiac disease were found in some of the individuals and preventative measures were then instituted.

Radiotelemetry has been used to distinguish real from simulated Adams-Stokes seizures. Ira et al.[25] described the cardiac findings in four patients with syncopal episodes. All these individuals were scheduled for surgical implantation of a cardiac pacemaker. Only two of the patients were demonstrated to have a conduction block associated with their syncope. The third patient had a myxoma of the atrium and the fourth had hyperventilation attacks. They commented that continuous cardiac monitoring saved the last two patients from having unnecessary surgery.

Cardiac radiotelemetry has been used to evaluate the physical fitness of athletes Goldwin,[18] Hanson and Tabakin,[22] Rose,[40] Rothfeld, E.L. et al.,[41] and in fetal electrocardiography.[1,27]

Anesthesiology

Continuous monitoring of the patient's vital functions is standard practice in the operating room. Complex cardiopulmonary, neurosurgical and other formidable surgical procedures, particularly if hypothermia and the heart-lung machines are used, have required elaborate instrumentation. In some institutions[15] where these procedures are carried out, equipment is available to monitor pulse rate, rectal temperature, esophageal temperature, brain and skin temperature in multiple locations, multichannel electrocardiography, venous and arterial pressure, arterial and venous pCO_2 and pO_2, blood loss, electroencephalography and electrocorticography.

Currently, most of these techniques use hard-wire telemetry but anesthesiologists employing extensive monitoring believe that in the future radiotelemetering techniques will be used. The advantage of these techniques is that there is a reduction of the explosion hazard in the operating room and that the instrumentation can be transferred to the recovery and intensive care rooms with the patient, so that monitoring can continue until the vital measurements have stabilized.

Neurology

Telemetering equipment has been developed to monitor the signals originating from all areas of the nervous system. Continuous monitoring of the cerebral cortical potentials is particularly useful in patients with convulsive disorders where short-term monitoring might not detect the abnormal cortical impulses associated with the clinical seizure. Radiotelemetry has been used to evaluate the neurophysiological wakefulness of airline pilots during flights,[5] a technique designed to promote safety in air travel. The continuous monitoring of the brain waves of humans and animals under observation for behavioral changes has been described.[21,44]

Radiotelemetric techniques have been used by physiologists to stimulate various areas of the brain of the conscious animal. A most ingenious telestimulator, using a solar power supply, has been described by Robinson and his associates.[39]

The electromyogram has been observed by radiotelemetry. This has permitted the observers to teach functional anatomy and therapeutic exercise as well as to determine if abnormalities might occur under more dynamic conditions.[19,33] Currently, electrical impulses originating in normally functioning muscles are being used to trigger externally powered orthotic devices attached to paralyzed limbs.[24]

Many hard-wire and radiotelemetry systems have been developed to monitor intracranial pressure.[36] Currie and his associates[12] have used a ventricular catheter attached to an endoradiosonde fitted in a burr hole. The aerial receiving the signal is placed under the patient's pillow and this, in turn, is connected to a radio receiver and potentiometric recorder placed at the patient's bedside. Pressure recordings can be made for a considerable period of time and require only slight repositioning of the aerial to compensate for the loss of signal strength due to movement of the patient. Atkinson and his associates[2] have used radiotelemetry to monitor the intracranial pressure of patients with hydrocephalus without recourse to repeated puncture of the cerebrospinal fluid system. In our laboratory, we have monitored the ventricular pressures of animals with experimental hydrocephalus using a pressure transducer 1.5 × 3.0 mm in size, which is attached to an implantable telemetering system.

A report on the uses of telemetry in neurology would not be complete without comment on the classical head injury studies of Drs. Gurdjian, Webster, Lissner, Patrick, and their associates here at Wayne State University.[20,29,37] Systems devised by these observers have thrown considerable light on our knowledge of the forces involved in the production of skull fracture and cerebral concussion, contusion, and laceration. Information obtained from this research has enabled design engineers to improve the safety standards of automobiles and other vehicles.

Further applications in the neurological sciences include transmission of baroreceptor impulses from the carotid sinus of dogs[26] and of action potentials in peripheral nerves.[34]

Urology

Radiotelemetric methods have been used to record pressures in the urinary bladder as well as to stimulate its contraction in paraplegic animals and patients. Bradley and his associates[6] have produced satisfactory emptying of the urinary bladder in paraplegic dogs. Their device employed stainless steel electrodes attached to the bladder wall. These were connected to a receiving unit implanted beneath the abdominal wall. The receiving unit was activated by a detached external radiotransmitter. Although this system functioned well in animals, difficulties were found during its trial in one human patient.

Gleason and his associates[17] described a telemetering capsule which can be inserted into the urinary bladder for continuous monitoring of pressure. They comment that this system will give more accurate measurements than the use of a catheter which impedes urinary outflow. Their system employed a passive radiosonde which was activated by a power transmitter, in this case, an antenna surrounding the patient which generated a charge within the capsule.

Biology

Telemetry has come into increasing use in the monitoring of physiological changes in free roaming animals and a voluminous bibliography has resulted. Among the more interesting studies are those of Van Citters and his associates.[47,48] In one of their investigations, they monitored the carotid arterial blood pressure of giraffes by inserting a small blood pressure transducer into the artery and connecting this, in turn, to a telemetry pack which was attached to the animal's neck with adhesive tape. This technique permitted them to study blood pressure changes associated with the position of the animal's head with relationship to its body as well as during rest and activity. They determined that the perfusion pressure at the base of the giraffe's skull when upright was maintained at a satisfactory level and compared favorably with the known values of many other species, including man. They furthermore noted that the giraffe has excellent collateral circulation because no neurological deficit was sustained as a result of approximately 10 minutes of arterial occlusion necessitated by implanting the transducer. Finally, they observed that during the carotid artery occlusion, the pressure above the occlusion was identical to that below it.

In another study, Van Citters et al. implanted ultrasonic Doppler flowmeters in the major arteries in captured baboons which were then released and monitored with radiotelemetry techniques. By this method, they noted a marked variation in the renal blood flow which was usually minimal during the pre-dawn hours in the sleeping animal, became higher during arousal. Higher transients were observed in these animals during ordinary physical activity such as tree-climbing. Stattleman and Cook[45] have used radiotelemetry to study motion patterns involved in walking, trotting, eating, flying and breathing in animals and humans. Mackay has recorded the body temperature of active dolphins, tortoises and marine iguanas with an ingested radiotransmitter. He comments that the system is adaptable for telemetering heartbeat, movement, as well as other physiological variables.

Miscellaneous Applications

Telemetering techniques have been used for many other purposes in medicine and biology. In man, endoradiosondes have been employed to measure gastric pH[14] and to monitor gastrointestinal pressures.[7,14] Ovarian physiology has been studied by this technology[3,4] and information has been gathered on the circadian rhythm.[49] In animals, complex systems have been built to monitor a broad spectrum of physiological data.[30,31,32]

As noted previously, a voluminous literature has accumulated. Many of the reports describe the details of instrumentation, while others are concerned with biological measurements. The interested reader is referred to the volume on biomedical telemetry edited by Caceres and the bibliography compiled by Geddes.[16]

SUMMARY

It is evident that biotelemetry has provided the physician and the biologist with techniques for acquiring new knowledge of biological processes. Shipp[42] comments that the biological advances tied to electronics will compare with those resulting from the discovery of x-ray and the introduction of the heart-lung machine. Miniaturized telemeters implanted in the living organism will provide continuous data which have heretofore been unobtainable by conventional methods. This data will be evaluated by computers and by the use of Baye's theorem, a probability formula, the diagnosis of disease will be enhanced.

The treatment of disease will also be improved. The signals resulting from physiological processes can be used to operate servomechanisms that will supply quantitative amounts of biologically active substances to the diseased organism. A mechanism to regulate blood sugar levels has already been developed.

Slater[43] predicts that biotelemetry will start to invade medicine by force in 1970. He visualizes that by this time, hospitals will use sophisticated monitoring systems for patients both during and after surgery. Patients who need constant observation will be monitored both at home and at work and play. Two-way telecommunication with artificial organs and various prosthetic devices will be perfected.

Progress in biotelemetry will require the close collaboration of the design engineer with the physician and the biologist. From our current vantage point, the possibilities presented by electronics, in general, and biotelemetry, in particular, seem limitless.

REFERENCES

1. Asa, M.M.; Crews, A.H., Jr.; Rothfeld, E.L.; Savel, L.E.; Zucker, I.R., and Bernstein, A.: High fidelity fetal radioelectrocardiography. *Amer J Cardiol,* 14:530–532, 1964.
2. Atkinson, J.R.; Shurtleff, D.B., and Foltz, E.L.: Radio telemetry for the measurement of intracranial pressure. *J Neurosurg,* 27:428–432, 1967.
3. Balin, H.; Busser, J.H.; Fromm, E.; Wan, L.S., and Israel, S.L.: Biotelemetry as an adjunct to the study of ovarian physiology. *Fertil Steril,* 16:1–15, 1965.
4. Balin, H.; Wan, L.S., and Israel, L.: Ovarian biotelemetry. *Surg Forum* 16: 404–406, 1965.
5. Blanc, C.; Lafontaine, E., and Medvedeff, M.: Radiotelemetric recordings of the electroencephalograms of civil aviation pilots during flight. *Aerospace Med,* 37:1060–1065, 1966.
6. Bradley, W.E.; Wittmers, L.E.; Chou, S.N., and French, L.A.: Use of a radio-transmitter receiving unit for the treatment of neurogenic bladder. *J Neurosurg,* 19:782–786, 1962.

7. BRATT, H.R.: Biomedical aspects of the X-15 program. *Milit Med*, 130:404–413, 1965.
8. BYFORD, G.H.: Medical radiotelemetry. *Proc Roy Soc Med*, 58:795–798, 1965.
9. CACERES, C. (Ed.): *Biomedical Telemetry*. New York and London, Academic, 1965, 392 pp.
10. CERKEZ, C.T.; STEWART, G.C., and MANNING, G.W.: Telemetric electrocardiography. *Canad Med Assoc J*, 93:1187–1199, 1965.
11. CORDAY, E.; BAZIKA, V.; LANG, T.W.; PAPPELBAUM, S.; GOLD, H., and BERNSTEIN, H.: Detection of phantom arrhythmias and evanescent electrocardiographic abnormalities. Use of prolonged direct electrocardiocording. *JAMA*, 193:417–421, 1965.
12. CURRIE, J.C.M.; RIDDLE, H., and WATSON, B.W.: The measurement of intracranial pressure using the pressure endoradiosonde. *J Physiol (London)*, 189:22P–23P, 1967.
13. DAVIS, D.A.: The monitoring of hospital patients with remarks on radio techniques. *Clin Pharmacol Ther*, 5:546–552, 1964.
14. D'HAENS, J.P.: The endomotorsonde. A new device for studying the gastrointestinal tract. *Amer J Med Electronics*, 3:158–161, 1964.
15. FARRIER, R.M.; FINK, B.R.; HARMEL, M.H.; STEEN, S.N., and WELKOWITZ, W.: Patient monitoring in the hospital. *Ann NY Acad Sci*, 118:384–438, 1964.
16. GEDDES, L.A.: A bibliography of biological telemetry. *Amer J Med Electronics*, 1:294–299, 1962.
17. GLEASON, D.M.; LATTIMER, J.K., and BAUXBAUM, C.: Bladder pressure telemetry. *J Urol*, 94:252–256, 1965.
18. GOODWIN, A.B., and GORDON, R.C.: Radiotelemetry of the electrocardiogram, fitness tests and oxygen uptake of water polo players. *Canad Med Assoc J*, 95:402–406, 1966.
19. GROTZ, R.C.; YON, E.T.; LONG, C. II, and KO, W.H.: Intramuscular FM radio transmitter of muscle potentials. *Arch Phys Med*, 46:804–808, 1965.
20. GURDJIAN, E.S.; WEBSTER, J.E., and LISSNER, H.R.: Observations on the mechanism of brain concussion, contusion and laceration. *Surg Gynec Obstet*, 101:680–690, 1955.
21. HAMBRECHT, F.T.; DONAHUE, P.D., and MELZACK, R.: A multiple channel EEG telemetering system. *Electroenceph Clin Neurophysiol*, 15:323–326, 1963.
22. HANSON, J.S., and TABAKIN, B.S.: Electrocardiographic telemetry in skiers. Anticipatory and recovery heart rate during competition. *New Eng J Med*, 271:181–185, 1964.
23. HELVEY, W.M.; ALBRIGHT, G.A., and AXELROD, A.E.: A review of biomedical monitoring activities and report of studies made on F-105 pilots. *Aerospace Med*, 35:23–27, 1964.
24. HIRSCH, C.; KAISER, E., and PETERSEN, I.: Telemetry of myopotentials. A preliminary report on telemetering of myopotentials from implanted microcircuits for servo control of powered prostheses. *Acta Orthop Scand*, 37:156–165, 1966.
25. IRA, G.H.; FLOYD, W.L., and ORGAIN, E.S.: Syncope with complete heart block. Differentiation of real and simulated Adams-Stokes seizures by radiotelemetry. *JAMA*, 188:707–710, 1964.
26. KEZDI, P., and NAYLOR, W.S.: Telemetry system to transmit baroreceptor nerve action potentials. *Amer J Med Electronics*, 4:153–155, 1965.
27. LEPESCHKIN, E.: Electrocardiographic instrumentation. *Progr Cardiovasc Dis*, 5:498–520, 1963.

28. LEVINE, I.M.; JOSSMAN, P.B.; TURSKY, B.E.; MEISTER, M., and DE ANGELIS, W.: Telephone telemetry of bioelectric information. *JAMA, 188*:794–798, 1964.
29. LISSNER, H.R.; LEBOW, M., and EVANS, F.G.: Experimental studies on the relation between acceleration and intracranial pressure changes in man. *Surg Gynec Obstet, 111*:329–338, 1960.
30. MACKAY, R.S.: Deep body temperature of untethered dolphin recorded by ingested radio-transmitter. *Science, 144*:864–866, 1964.
31. MACKAY, R.S.: Galapagos tortoise and marine iguana deep body temperatures measured by radiotelemetry. *Nature (London), 204*:355–358, 1963.
32. MACKAY, R.S.: A progress report on radiotelemetry from inside the body. *Biomed Sci Instrum, 2*:275–292, 1964.
33. MOORE, M.L.; FARRAND, S., and THORNTON: The use of radiotelemetry for electromyography. *J Amer Phys Ther Assoc, 43*:787–791, 1963.
34. MORRELL, R.M.: Amplitude-modulation radiotelemetry of nerve action potentials. *Nature, 184*:1129–1131, 1959.
35. NORLAND, C.C., and SEMLER, H.J.: Angina pectoris and arrhythmias documented by cardiac telemetry. *JAMA, 190*:115–118, 1964.
36. OLSEN, E.R.; COLLINS, C.C., and LOUGHBOROUGH, W.F.: Intracranial pressure measurement with miniature passive implanted pressure transensor. *Amer J Surg, 113*:727–729, 1967.
37. PATRICK, L.M.; LANGE, W.A., and HODGSON, V.R.: Facial injuries—causes and prevention. *Seventh Stapp Car Crash Conference Proceedings.* Springfield, Thomas, 1965, chapt. 42, pp. 541–568.
38. PESSAR, T.; KROBATH, H., and YANOVER, R.R.: The application of telemetry to industrial medicine. *Amer J Med Electronics, 1*:287–293, 1962.
39. ROBINSON, B.W.; WARNER, H., and ROSVOLD, H.E.: Brain telestimulator with solar cell power supply. *Science, 148*:1111–1113, 1965.
40. ROSE, K.D., and DUNN, F.L.: Telemeter electrocardiography; a study of heart function in athletes. *Nebraska Med J, 49*:447–456, 1964.
41. ROTHFELD, E.L.; BERNSTEIN, A.; PARSONNET, V.; ZUCKER, I.R., and ALINSONORIN, C.A.: Telemetric monitoring of the electrocardiogram in acute myocardial infarction. *Dis Chest, 51*:193–198, 1967.
42. SHIPP, L.M.: Electronics and medicine. *J Occup Med, 7*:423–430, 1965.
43. SLATER, L.E.: Biotelemetry and the physician. *New York J Med, 65*:2893–2901, 1965.
44. SPERRY, C.J., JR.; GADSDEN, C.B.; RODRIGUEZ, C., and BACH, L.M.N.: Miniature subcutaneous frequency modulated transmitter for brain potentials. *Science, 134*:1423–1424, 1961.
45. STATTLEMAN, A., and COOK, H.: A transducer for motion study by radiotelemetry. *Proc Soc Exp Biol Med, 121*:505–508, 1966.
46. TOLLES, W.E.: Telemetry in medical research and patient care. *Progr Cardiovasc Dis, 5*:595–609, 1963.
47. VANCITTERS, R.L.; KEMPER, W.S., and FRANKLIN, D.L.: Blood pressure responses of wild giraffes studied by radiotelemetry. *Science, 152*:384–386, 1966.
48. VANCITTERS, R.L.; SMITH, O.A., JR., and FRANKLIN, D.: Renal blood flow responses of wild baboons in habitat (radiotelemetry techniques). *Circulation, 36*(Supp. 11L):155, 1967.
49. WINGET, C.M., and FRYER, T.B.: Telemetry system for the acquisition of circadian rhythm data. *Aerospace Med, 37*:800–803, 1966.

DISCUSSION

Carter C. Collins

Dr. Pudenz has given us an excellent review of the history, methods and capabilities of biotelemetry in medical research. His major emphasis has been on bioelectrical phenomena, particularly electrocardiography. Further comments may be in order covering recent instrumentation of other physical quantities

I want to underscore Dr. Pudenz' emphasis on the importance of long-term continuous records rather than intermittent sampling measurements. As he has stated, continuous records are now made possible by implanted or attached telemetering monitors. As you are well aware, significant physiological data is contained in the nature of the temporal patterns, and changes, which characterize the state of health of an organ or organism. Signs are sometimes of an intermittent nature, showing up in their early phases only once for a brief instant and possibly not being manifest again for hours. In such cases, long-term continuous records can certainly lend valuable diagnostic aid to the physician.

In the field of ophthalmology, we have recently found an occasional transient departure from equality of the pressure in the two eyes of experimental animals by means of implanted pressure transensors. The physiological mechanism and significance of this observation is still under investigation.

In impact injury studies, biological transducers and measuring systems should be acceleration insensitive in order to eliminate undesirable artifacts. The design of such systems can profitably incorporate low mass, high stiffness, and especially an acceleration balanced mechanical force bridge configuration for pressure measurements.

A miniature implantable acceleration-balanced pressure transensor employing these principles has been devised.[1,2] It employs two spiral coils each with a mass of only 2 mg supported on two parallel stiff diaphragms (200 g/mm) which are displaced differentially by pressure changes but show negligible differential displacement due to acceleration. The mechanical resonance of the system is over 1,000 Hz.

Transensors only 3 μl in volume have been made which is two orders of magnitude smaller than anything heretofore available. They require no batteries and only one electronic part which is considered the minimum possible configuration.

Telemetry is especially pertinent to tissue displacement and pressure studies during impact. We are making spinal fluid dynamic investigations

Editor's Note: Much of the new work outlined here was supported by Public Health Service Grants NB 04669, NB 06038 and NIH General Research Support Grant FR-05566.

in the monkey relating to acceleration effects on the intracranial pressure. These indicate a rather rigid craniospinal sac without significant compliant communication with the rest of the body.[3] These investigations also indicate that the various cranial compartments enjoy rather free compliant intercommunication. The various separating membranes such as the falx cerebri and tentorium do not significantly impede pressure variations of physiological magnitude throughout the brain. However, these supporting and dividing membranes are expected to be responsible for significant intracranial pressure gradients, limiting the maximum transient pressures that might otherwise develop during impact.

Atkinson and Foltz are now using the transensor system to measure intracranial pressure in hydrocephalic children. A glass transensor is incased in a rigid plastic box mounted near the surface. A short tube extending into the ventricle allows continuous records of intraventricular pressure to be made.

Telemetry has allowed long-term studies in alert and responsive animals. Ophthalmological investigations indicate that the salient feature of intraocular pressure is its extreme lability. The pressure has been seen to exceed 70 mm Hg during a blink. Variations of a few mm Hg can be measured during eye movements, presumably due to unbalanced efforts of oculorotary muscles.[4] Also, a sensory evoked pressure response has been found in the rabbit eye.[5] Mild sensory stimulation produces a transient rise in intraocular pressure amounting to 10 mm Hg in some instances. The potential clinical significance of these observations has not yet been fully explored. However, hope for clinical exploitation of such phenomena is offered through the analysis of long-term continuous records of telemetrically derived physiological data.

Chronically implanted passive transensors require no tubes of wires to pierce the organ being monitored. Hence, normal intracranial or intraocular pressure integrity is maintained. Also, no tracts for bacterial invasion exist. Of over one hundred implantations, none have shown signs of visible irritation related to the implant. Recent histological studies confirm this observation.

Transensor biotelemetry has demonstrated utility in following sensory and other neurogenically induced pressure phenomena; assessing drug effects in conscious versus anesthetized animals; and monitoring intraocular, intracranial and blood pressures under normal physiological conditions. Wherever there is a need to measure pressure close to the body surface, the passive spiral transensor offers a sensitive, wireless method in a small package.

Hard wire telemetry was used in crash protection studies made a decade ago in the Mercury space vehicle program. We found, as you would expect, that acceleration injury could be minimized by a molded total body support or couch. With this equipment, I was able to sustain 25 g acceleration maintained over a 1-minute orbital reentry acceleration pattern associated with emergency conditions in a manned space capsule.[6]

Dr. Pudenz makes a good argument for the services of a qualified design engineer. It is certainly true that new departures in biomedical instrumentation can best be met by a graduate engineer. However, telemetry equipment is becoming available to the extent that many medical instrumentation needs can be met by a competent technician if a design engineer is not available. Installation and operation of existing commercial units can often answer research questions without designing new apparatus.

Since Dr. Pudenz' excellent review, a valuable and interesting new volume of biomedical telemetry by Mackay[7] has been added to those of Caceres and Slater.

References

1. COLLINS, C.C.: Microminiature endoradiosonde for intraocular implantation. *Proc Ann Conf Engin Med Biol*, 8:171, 1966.
2. COLLINS, C.C.: Miniature passive pressure transensor for implanting in the eye. *IEEE Trans Biomed Engin*, BME-14(2):74–83, 1967.
3. OLSEN, E.R.; COLLINS, C.C.; LOUGHBOROUGH, W.B.; RICHARDS, V.; ADAMS, J.E., and PINTO, D.W.: Intracranial pressure measurement with a miniature passive implanted pressure transensor. *Amer J Surg*, 113:727–729, 1967.
4. COLLINS, C.C.; BACH-Y-RITA, P., and LOEB, D.R.: Intraocular pressure variation with oculorotary muscle tension. *Amer J Physiol*, 213:1039–1043, 1967.
5. COLLINS, C.C.: Evoked pressure responses in the rabbit eye. *Science*, 155:106–108, 1967.
6. COLLINS, C.C., and GRAY, R.F.: Pilot performance and tolerance studies of orbital reentry acceleration. *NADC report MA 1.1-7390*, Johnsville, Pa., Sept. 16, 1959.
7. MACKAY, R.S.: *Bio-Medical Telemetry*. New York, Wiley, 1968.

Chapter VIII

FINE STRUCTURE OF CEREBRAL DAMAGE:
Toxic and Mechanical

Anthony J. Raimondi, Fred Beckman, and Joseph P. Evans

In determining the effects of mechanical damage to the grey and white matter of the hemispheres, and brain stem structures, it is desirable to learn whether the observed changes may be considered reversible. It is also of the utmost importance to obtain information concerning the morphological alterations which damaged cerebral cells undergo. Reports in the literature have stressed changes in the extracellular compartment, the intracellular compartment, the basement membrane, and the endothelial cells. These have been part of extensive studies on cerebral edema caused by tin, by freezing lesions, by expanding balloons in the extradural space, etc. The observations have ranged from a simple increase in size of the extracellular space, through changes in form and location of mitochondria, to very characteristic splitting of the myelin lamellae at the intraperiod line with resultant formation of large vacuoles. There have been suggestions that all of the structural changes reported in cases of cerebral edema are secondary to hypoxia.

It would appear, therefore, that a comparison of the morphological characteristics of cerebral edema, secondary to a toxic clinical entity such as lead encephalopathy, could profitably be compared to those in a purely mechanical entity, such as cerebral edema secondary to epidural hematoma in the human being, and the inflation of a balloon in the epidural space of an experimental animal. This presentation consists of just such a comparison. In it, an effort will be made to describe the fine structural characteristics of lead encephalopathy in grey matter, white matter, and the capillaries of both. In addition to this, already published material on the fine structure of mechanical damage will be reviewed for comparison purposes.

The lead encephalopathy tissue which was studied was removed by biopsy from twelve children with proven lead poisoning. All of these children had developed clinical evidence of encephalopathy: focal convulsions and severe papilledema. The biopsy was taken under local anesthesia, and the material fixed in Osmic acid, then processed for electron microscopy in accordance with standard technique. The electron micrographs were taken on an RCA EMU 3G electron microscope at electronic enlargements ranging from 5000 X through 35,000 X, and photographic enlargements obtained as desired.

It is impossible to distinguish morphologically between a capillary in the grey matter and one in the white matter. The basic capillary structure of one or two endothelial cells surrounded by a triple density basement membrane applies to both. Pericytes, completely surrounded by the basement membrane, are often present. In addition to this, perivascular glial cells abut upon the basement membrane. In the grey matter, a process of a neuron may, on occasion, rest in direct contact with the basement membrane of the capillary. In Figure 8–1, it will be noted that the capillary consists of two endothelial cells. Since this tissue was removed by biopsy and, consequently, not fixed by perfusion technique, it will be noted that the capillary lumen has collapsed and that the endothelial cell is distended. The basement membrane is uniform in thickness and has the usual triple

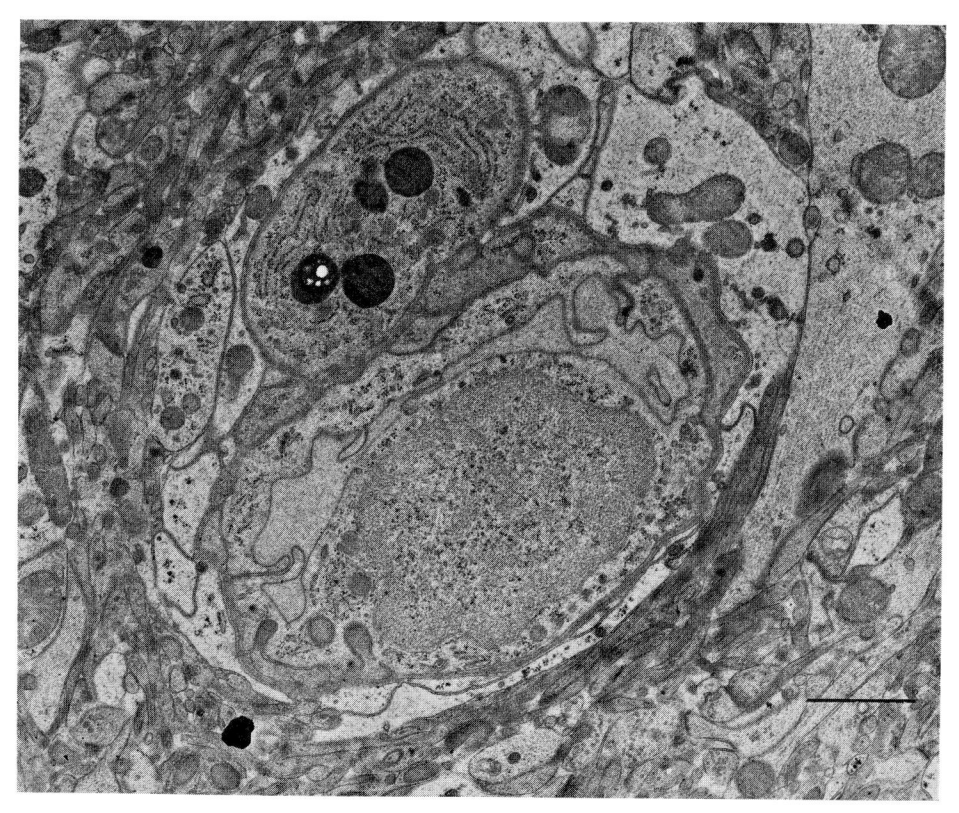

FIGURE 8–1.

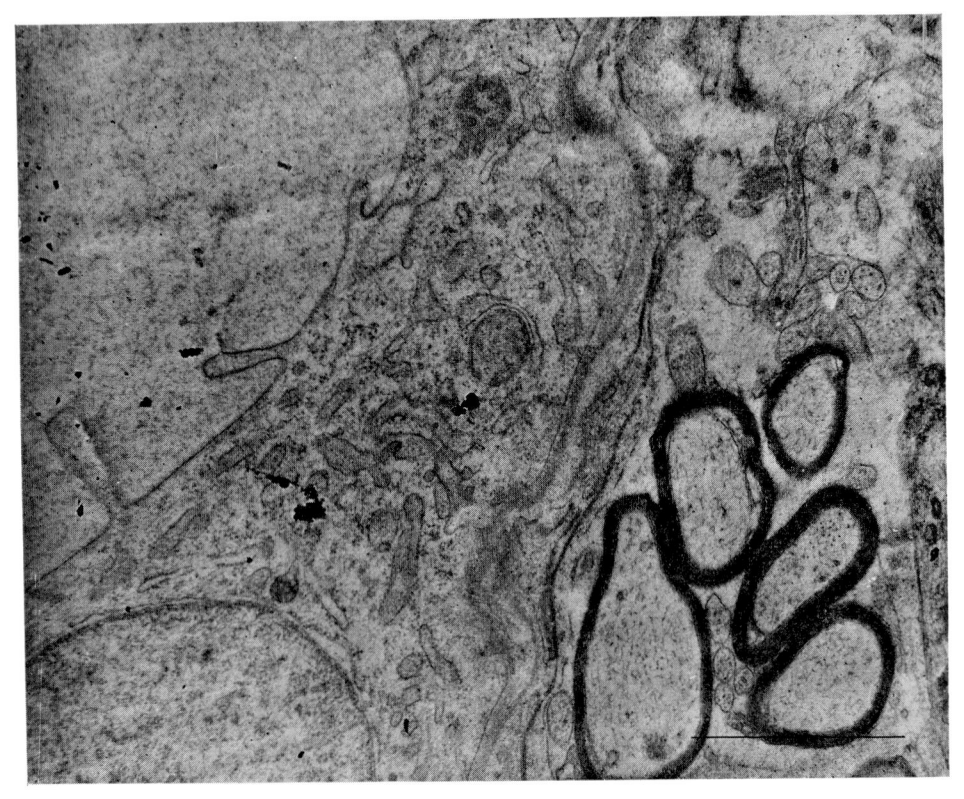

FIGURE 8-2.

density appearance. The pericyte is located at the upper portion of this electron micrograph. It contains four very dense globoid bodies and an abundance of granular ergastoplasm. The perivascular glial cells contain a normal distribution of intracytoplasmic organelles in addition to a flocculent appearing, moderately dense, material. There is a large nonmyelinated axon to the right of the capillary. The remainder of the periglial portion of this electron micrograph is occupied by the neuropil.

In an advanced stage of lead encephalopathy, with severe increase in intracranial pressure, the most obvious morphological changes are quite different in the white matter from what they are in the grey matter. Specifically, in the white matter, the capillary endothelium maintains its normal appearance, though the pericapillary structures are severely altered. In the grey matter, the glial structures maintain a normal appearance, whereas the neuronal structures show signs of distention of the endoplasmic reticulum. On the other hand, in the white matter, the astroglia is maximally damaged whereas the oligodendroglia is moderately well preserved. Again, in the white matter, there are severe changes in the myelin sheaths and ultimately total cellular disintegration. The increase

Fine Structure of Cerebral Damage

in the extracellular space of the white matter, though present in reversible stages of lead encephalopathy, is not nearly as obvious nor as extensive as it is in the irreversible cases.

The endothelial and perivascular changes, as seen in a severe irreversible case of lead encephalopathy, are illustrated in Figure 8–2. The intracytoplasmic compartment of the endothelial cell is well preserved. Mitochondria, ribosomes, and granular ergastoplasm, are all intact. There appears to be an increase in the number of pinocytotic vesicles, but this is moderate. The basement membrane is intact. The perivascular glial cells have disintegrated. There is an extensive extracellular space and the myelinated axons appear to be floating freely within it. The myelin tongues are readily identifiable as are cell processes and patches of glial fibers. This relative preservation of endothelial morphology immediately surrounded by almost total cellular destruction is characteristic of white matter changes in lead encephalopathy.

The changes within the astroglia consist of a progressive distention of the granular ergastoplasm in addition to similar increase in space between the two nuclear membranes, and, lastly, the lamellae of the Golgi appa-

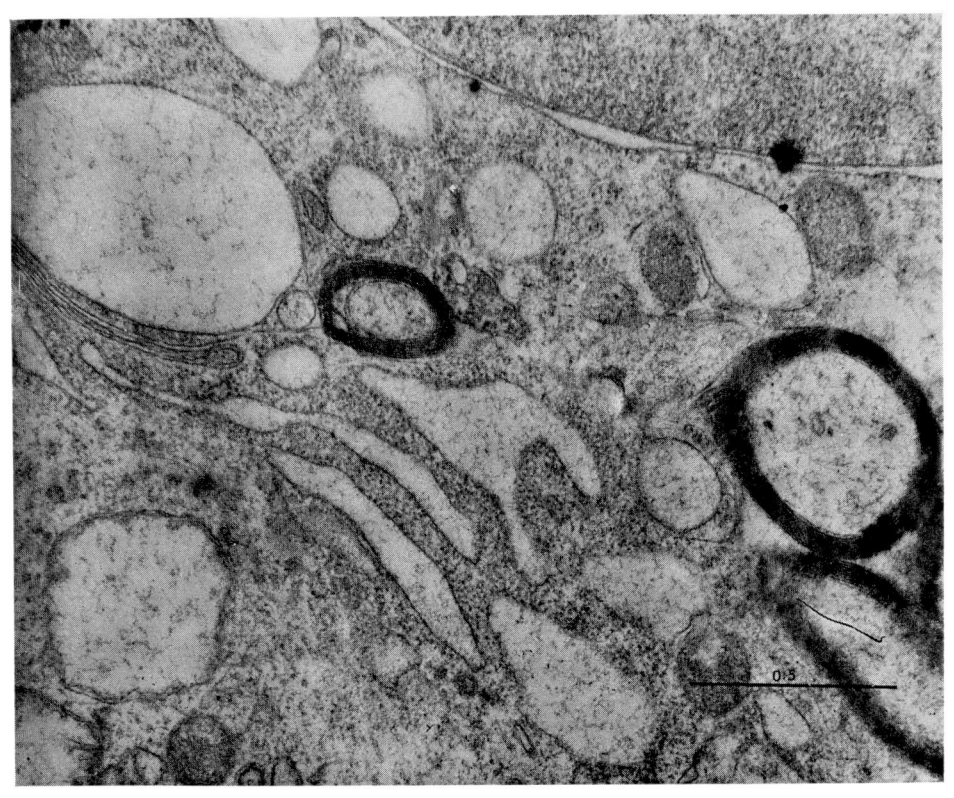

FIGURE 8–3.

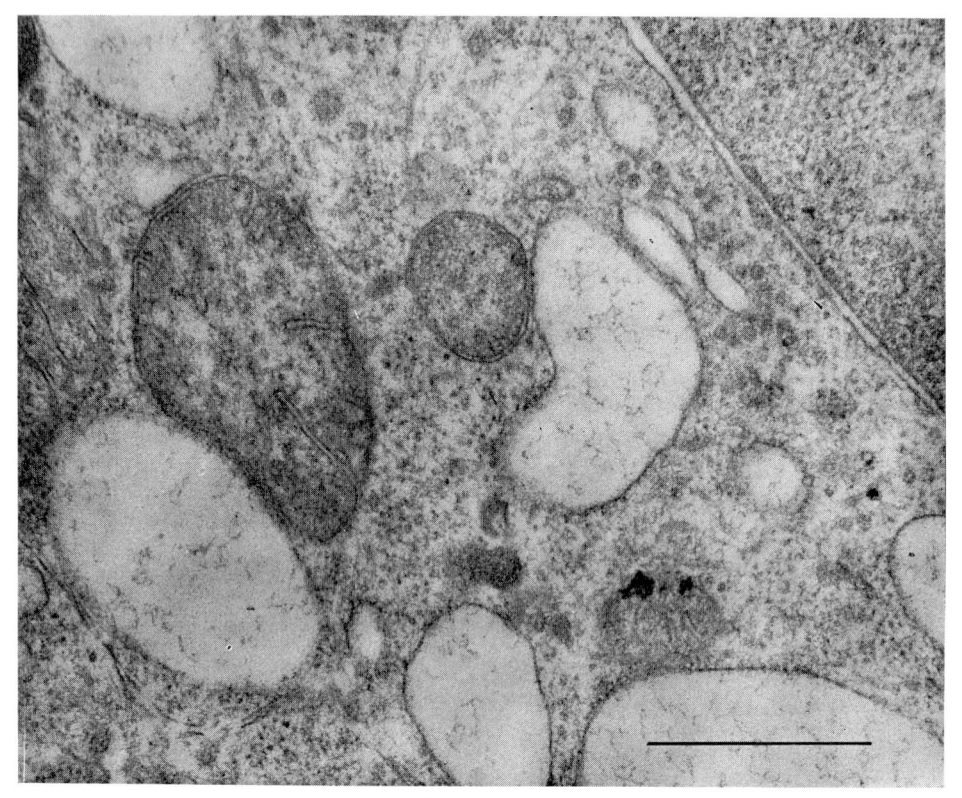

FIGURE 8-4.

ratus. The changes in the granular ergastoplasm are well demonstrated in Figure 8-3. The nucleus is at the upper portion of the electron micrograph. The increase in space between the two nuclear membranes is quite evident as is the distention of the granular ergastoplasm. Notice that at the center of the electronmicrograph, this organelle has so opened as to take the appearance of fissures, whereas there is a vacuolation of the membranous system of the granular ergastoplasm at the upper left of the photograph. Well-preserved myelinated axons are seen. The changes in the appearance and location of the mitochondria are best demonstrated in Figure 8-4. The nucleus is at the upper right of the electronmicrograph, and the two mitochondria are at the center. Each of these microorganelles has come to rest upon the granular surface of the distended granular ergastoplasm. A disintegrating mitochondrion is present at the lower right. Early distention of the Golgi apparatus is well demonstrated in this electronmicrograph. This microorganelle, located in the juxta nuclear position in most cells, consists of a system of vesicles, vacuoles and lamellae. It is the vesicular and vacuolar components, which initially increase in size, and lastly the lamellar component. A comparison of the size of the space

Fine Structure of Cerebral Damage 165

between the two nuclear membranes in Figure 8–4 should be made with that in Figure 8–5. The nucleus in Figure 8–5 is located at the extreme left of the electronmicrograph. The large vacuole containing amorphous flocculent electron dense material is, in essence, the distended space between these two nuclear envelopes. Clusters of ribosomes are accumulated into irregular patches along the outer nuclear envelope. Mitochondria adhere closely to this outer surface. The Golgi apparatus is distended as are the individual components of the granular ergastoplasm. There is evidence of myelin disintegration in the myelinated axon at the extreme right. The axon within this myelin sheath is completely destroyed, and the myelin lamellae are partially destroyed.

The changes within the oligodendroglial elements are not visibly as prominent as those within the astroglia. Figure 8–6 illustrates this point. The nucleus occupies the entire superior portion of the electronmicrograph. The nucleolus is well preserved, and the space between the two nuclear membranes is normal. Kinetosomes are multiple and intact. Within the ectoplasm, the clusters of ribosomes have a normal appearance as do the mitochondria. There is not an increase in size or number of pinocytotic

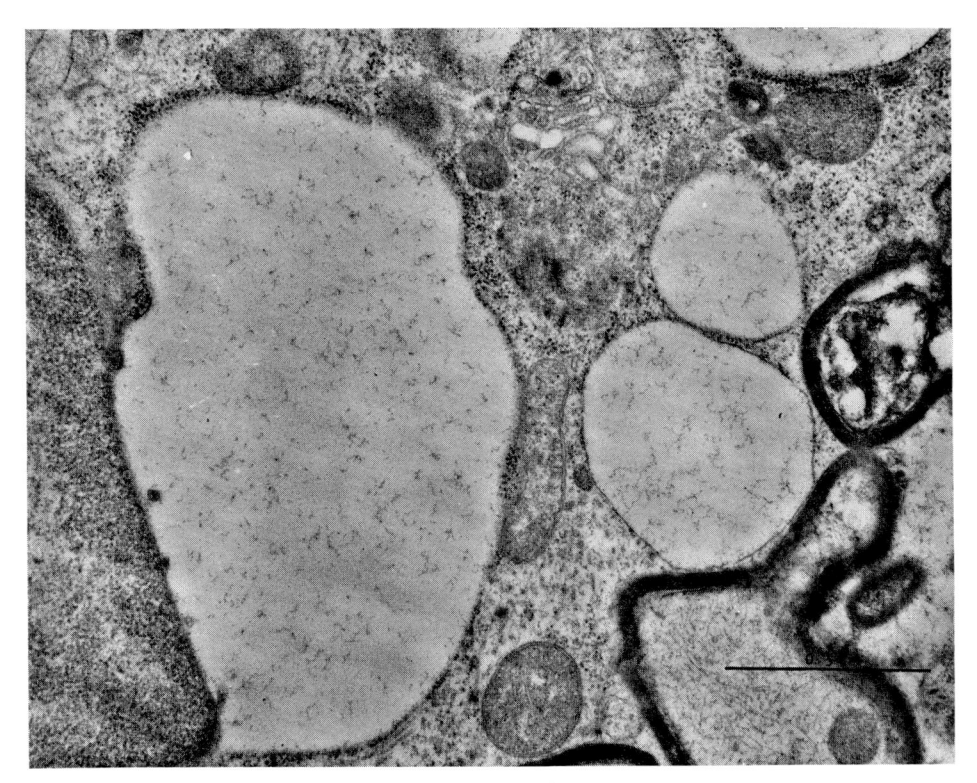

FIGURE 8–5.

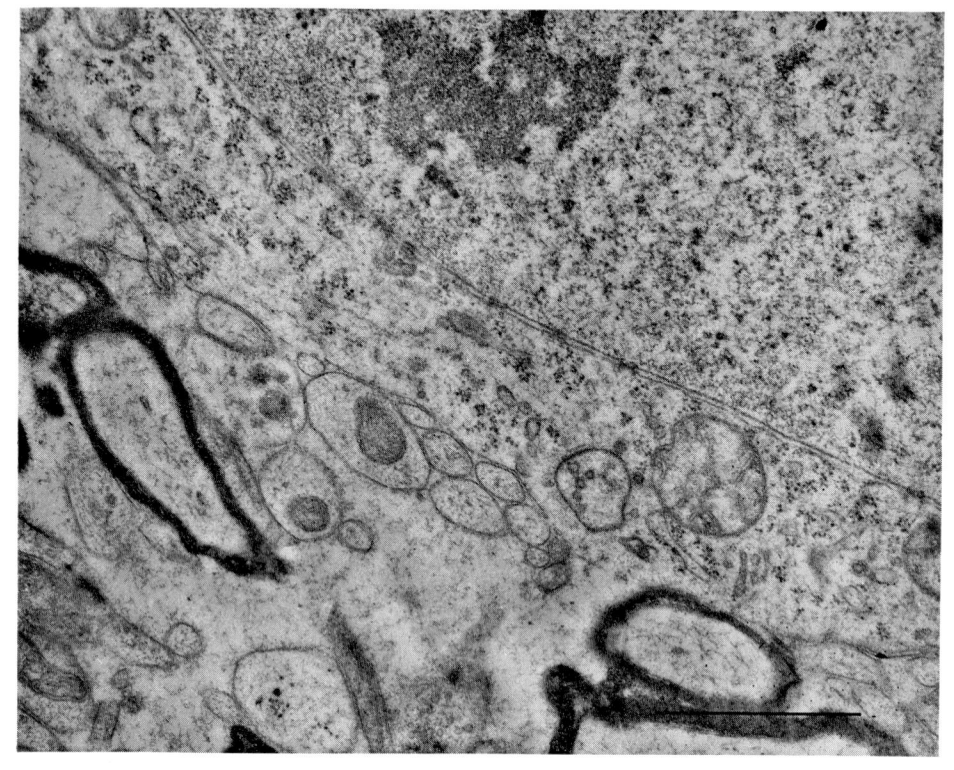

FIGURE 8-6.

vesicles. However, notice that the extracellular space is extensive. Myelinated and unmyelinated axons appear to be floating within this extensive extracellular space. Figure 8–7 is an electronmicrograph of an almost totally destroyed fibrous astrocyte. The nucleus is at the lower right of the photograph. A patch of intracytoplasmic protoglial fibrils is located above the nucleus, and distended granular ergastoplasm to the left of the nucleus. The splitting of the myelin lamellae at the intraperiod line is clearly shown in the myelinated axon located above and to the left of the distended granular ergastoplasm. Less obvious splitting at the intraperiod line is seen in the myelinated axon immediately superior to the nucleus.

As the destruction of astroglial elements continues, the increase in the extracellular compartment proceeds pari passu. It is, of course, not possible to conclude that this severe increase in size of the extracellular space is solely and directly the result of astroglial disintegration. This latter is simply the most obvious morphological change which accompanies the increased volume of the extracellular compartment. Figure 8–8 illustrates a disintegrated astrocyte, at the lower left, and the extensive accumulation of fluid in the extracellular compartment. Well preserved myelinated axons are floating freely within this compartment as are fragments of ectoplasmic microorganelles, and cell processes. At this stage, it is impossible to distinguish between the cerebral edema which is secondary to toxic encephalopathy, and that which results from the presence of an expansile mass over the surface of the brain. It is therefore best to consider this "end stage" cerebral edema from a morphological point of view.

Extremely high resolution electronmicrographs of the myelinated axons permit one to identify the nature and location of changes in the myelin sheaths. Figure 8–9 illustrates myelinated axons and some of the early changes in the myelin sheath. At the lower left, the splitting of the myelin lamellae at the intraperiod line is clearly shown. In the sheaths at the upper left and lower right, the lamellae are fractured and replaced by the patches of electron dense granules. In this same Figure 8–9, a well preserved mesaxon is visualized in the myelinated axon at the center of the electronmicrograph. Figure 8–10 illustrates progressive changes in the myelin sheaths. There is a large cleft which has formed between two myelin lamellae at the intraperiod line. Similarly, there is fracturing of

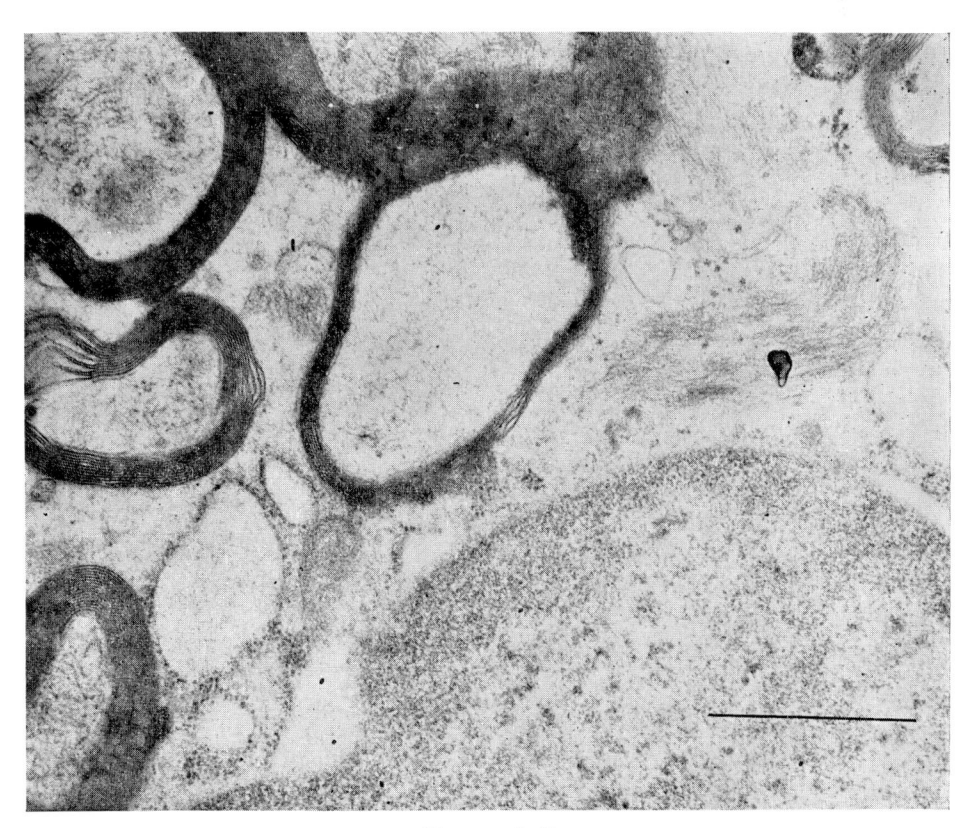

FIGURE 8–7.

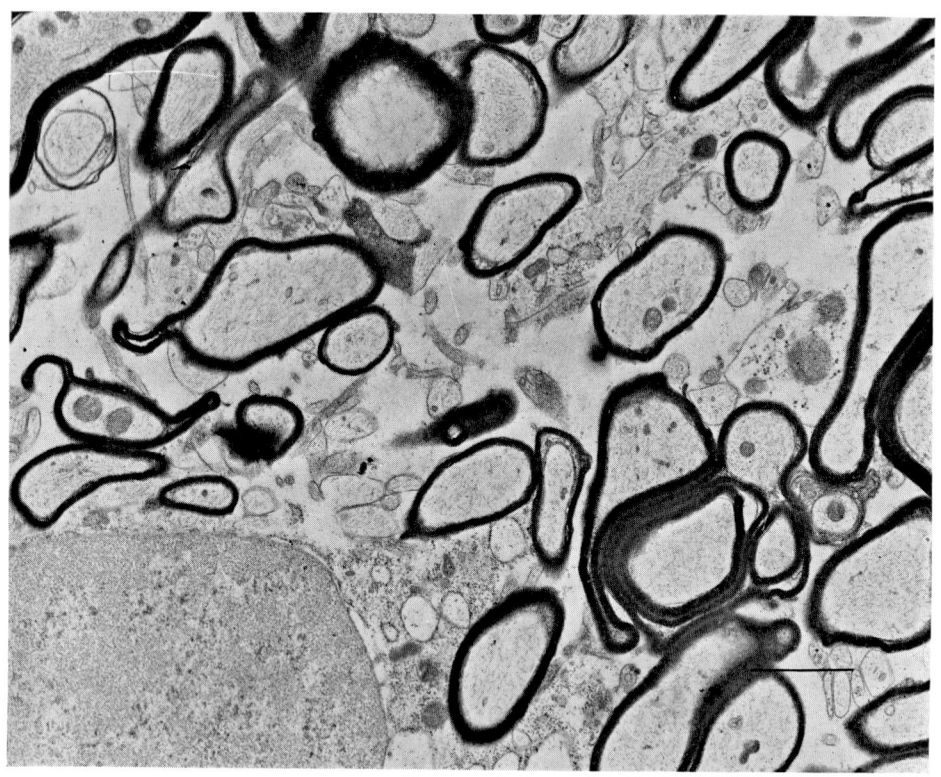

FIGURE 8–8.

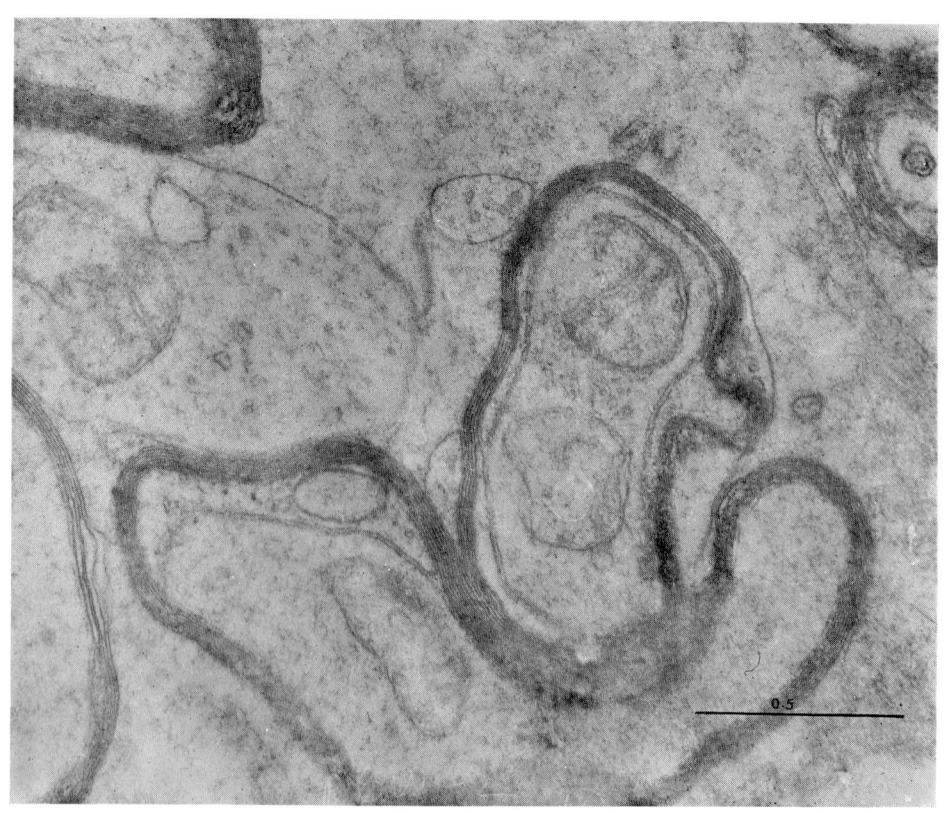

FIGURE 8–9.

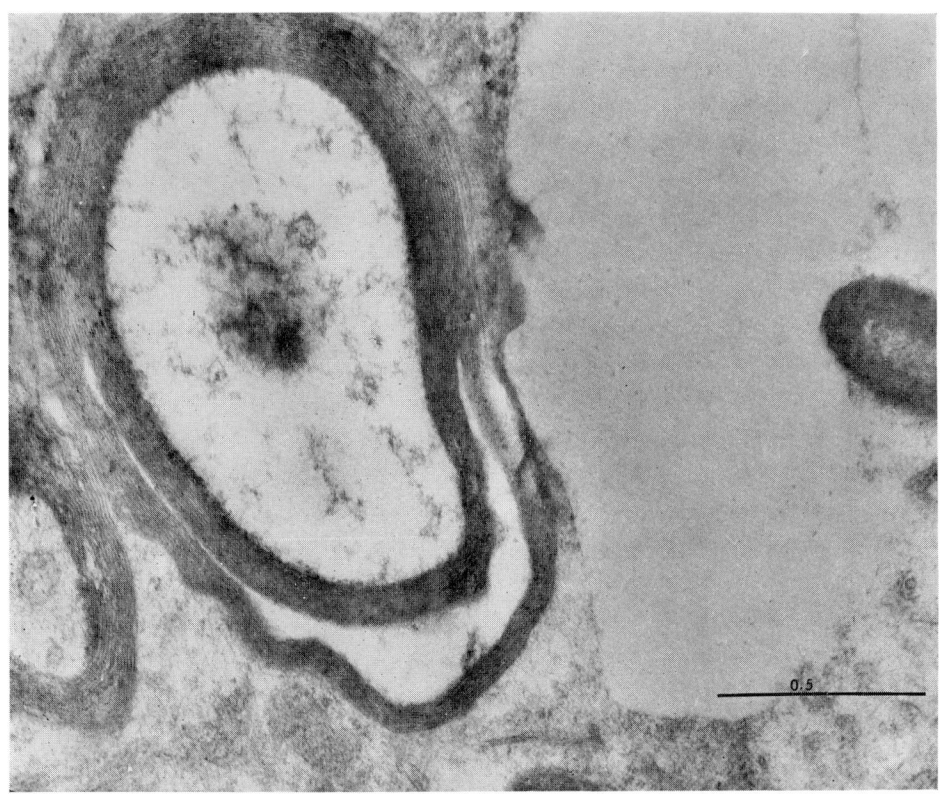

FIGURE 8–10.

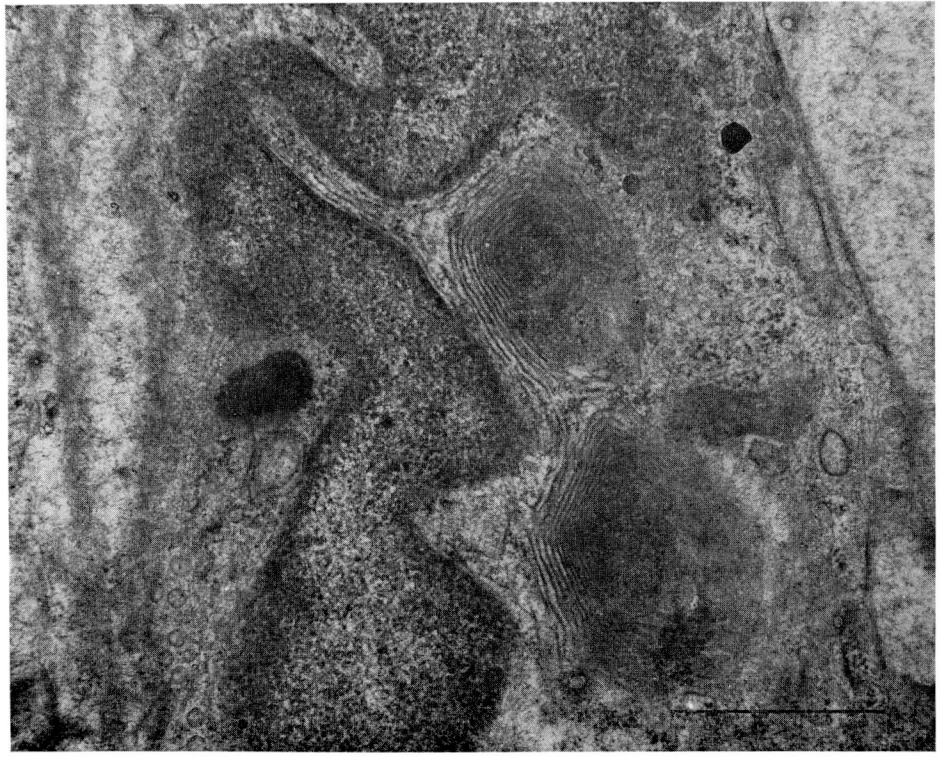

FIGURE 8–11.

170   *Impact Injury and Crash Protection*

the myelin lamellae and the accumulation of electron-dense granules. The axon is completely destroyed.

The changes in the grey matter are much less prominent than those already described in the white matter. This is in keeping with observations on cerebral edema caused by tin intoxication or mechanical damage. Similarly, it has long been known that the most severe morphological alterations which accompany an increase in cerebral volume are within the white matter. Primarily, the grey matter changes are located within the cytoplasm of the endothelial cells of the capillaries and within the granular ergastoplasm of the ganglion cells.

The single most characteristic observation, in the capillary endothelial cytoplasm of the grey matter, has been the formation of lamellar bodies. Figure 8–11 illustrates two of these structures located within the juxta nuclear position. They have a rather dense center which is surrounded by an eccentric array of lamellae. In addition to this, there is a marked increase in the number, size and variability of the pinocytotic vesicles. The changes in the basement membrane are also quite remarkable. Contrasting these endothelial alterations with the paucity of such alterations

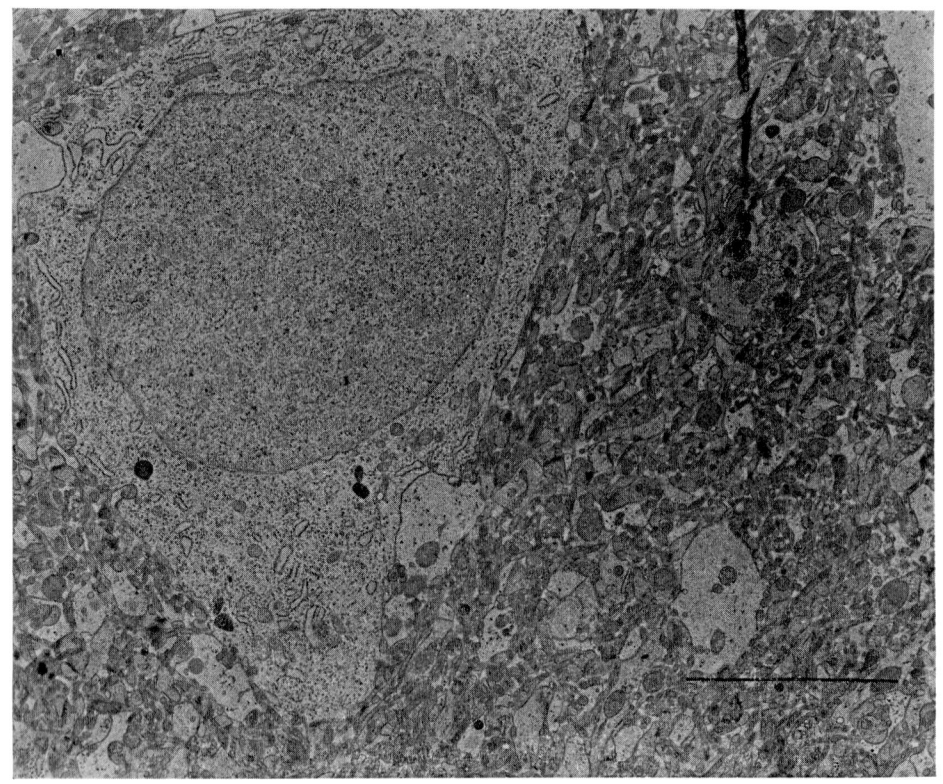

FIGURE 8–12.

in the capillaries of white matter provides one of the remarkable features of the fine structure of lead encephalopathy.

As has already been stated, the glial elements of the gray matter are quite normal in appearance in all stages of lead encephalopathy. Figure 8–12 illustrates an oligodendrocyte and the neuropil of a child with severe increase in intracranial pressure, bilateral papilledema and in deep coma. The oligodendrocyte is entirely normal in appearance, as is the neuropil. In Figure 8–13, which is a higher resolution electronmicrograph, portions of the nucleus and of the intracellular compartment of an oligodendrocyte are well visualized. The mitochondria are intact as are the ribosomes. There is no alteration in the continuity of the cell membrane, nor is there any evidence of intracellular swelling. The extracellular compartment shows only minimal increase in size. In Figure 8–14, which is an electronmicrograph taken at an even higher resolution (108,000 X), a very small portion of the oligodendrocyte and of the neuropil are reproduced. The Golgi apparatus is normal in appearance as are the ribosomes and granular ergastoplasm. The integrity of the plasma membrane is well demonstrated. It should be noted that there is only a minimal increase in size of the extracellular compartment.

The normal appearance of a satellite oligodendrocyte adjacent to a ganglion cell with distended granular ergastoplasm is illustrated in Figure 8–15. The oligodendrocyte is at the right of this electronmicrograph, its nucleus at the far right. The two nuclear membranes show no evidence of swelling nor does the granular ergastoplasm. However, the granular ergastoplasm in the ganglion cell is distended. There is also an increase in size of the extracellular space. Figure 8–16 demonstrates the extensive increase in the space between the lamellae of the granular ergastoplasm of a ganglion cell.

In cerebral edema produced in the experimental animal by the inflation of a balloon in the epidural space, the primary changes are at the expense of the white matter. Specifically, there is an increase in pinocytotic activity at the level of the capillary endothelium with secondary alterations in the appearance of the basement membrane and the perivascular glial cells. Initially, the extracellular space increases in size, and then the perivascular glial cells lose their normal appearance. The glial cells become distended and the cell membrane ruptures. This results in an outpouring of intracytoplasmic contents into the extracellular compartment with further increase in volume of this latter space.

Though there is a distention of the granular ergastoplasm, it is not as obvious nor as consistent as in lead encephalopathy. Lastly, the changes in the glial cells are much more obvious in the astrocytic than in the oligodendrocytic series.

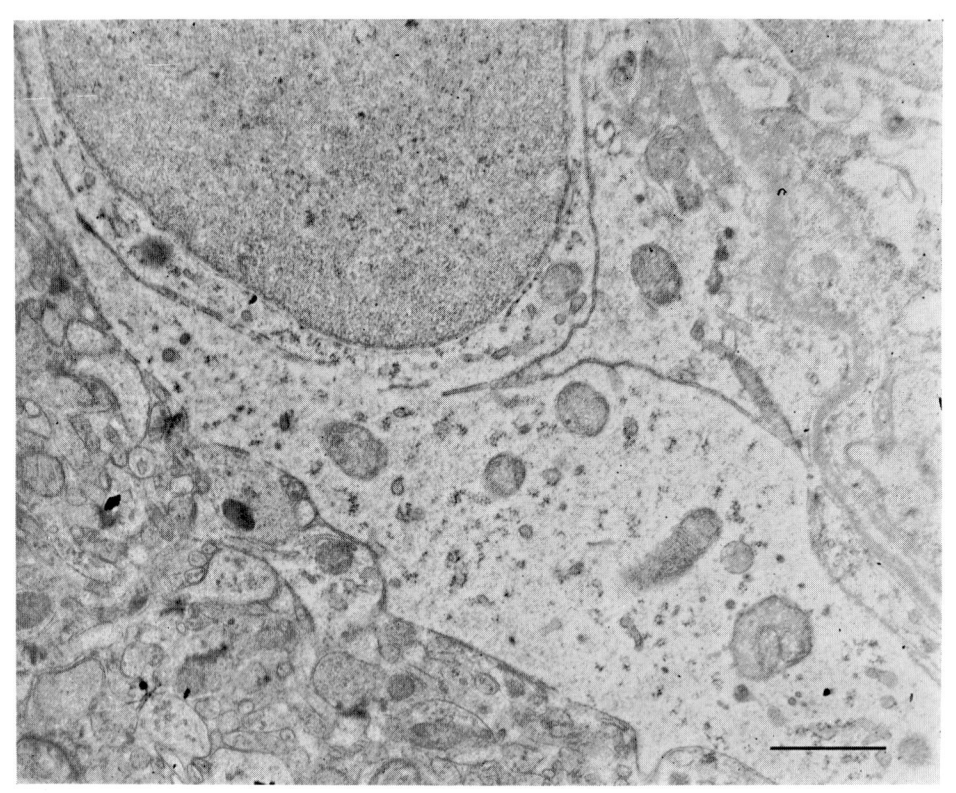

FIGURE 8-13.

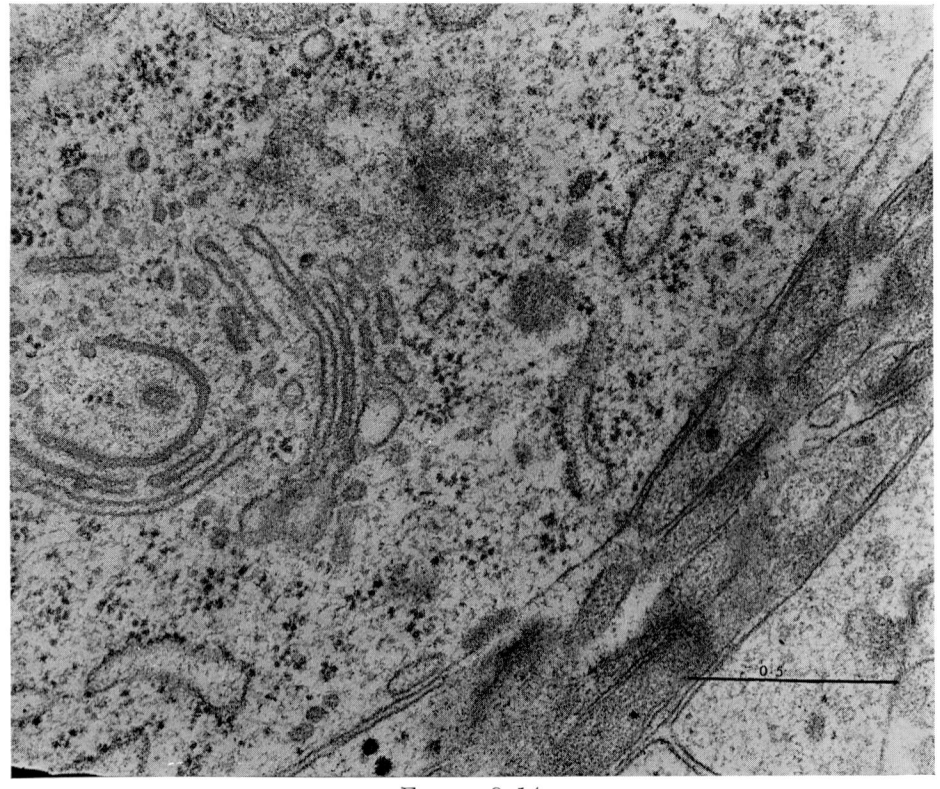

FIGURE 8-14.

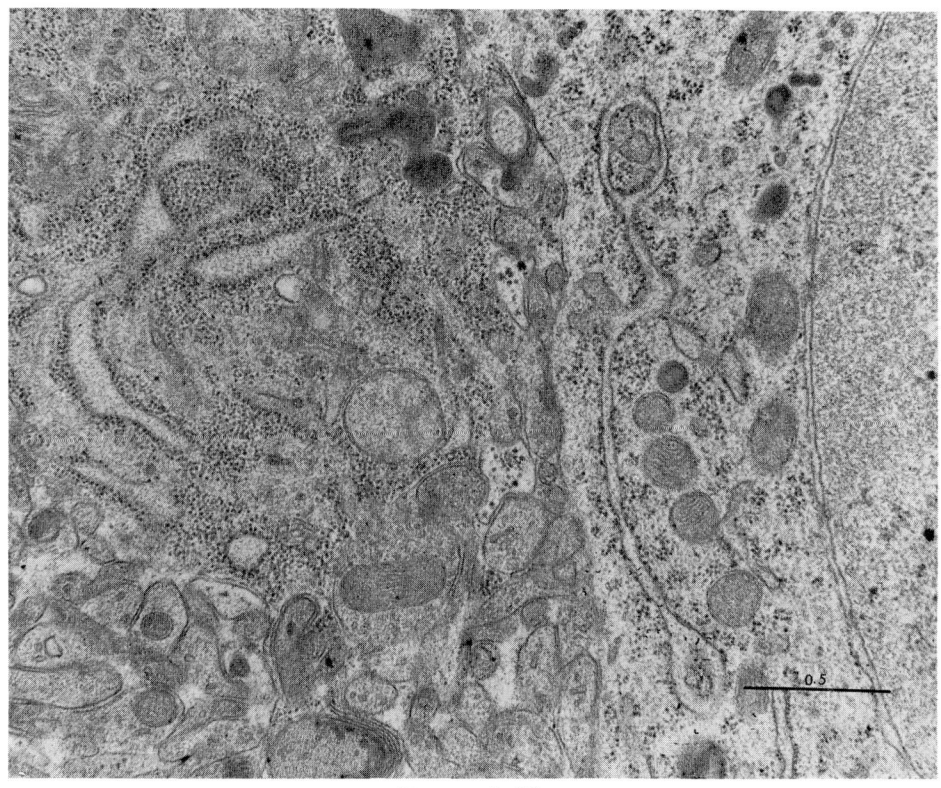

FIGURE 8-15.

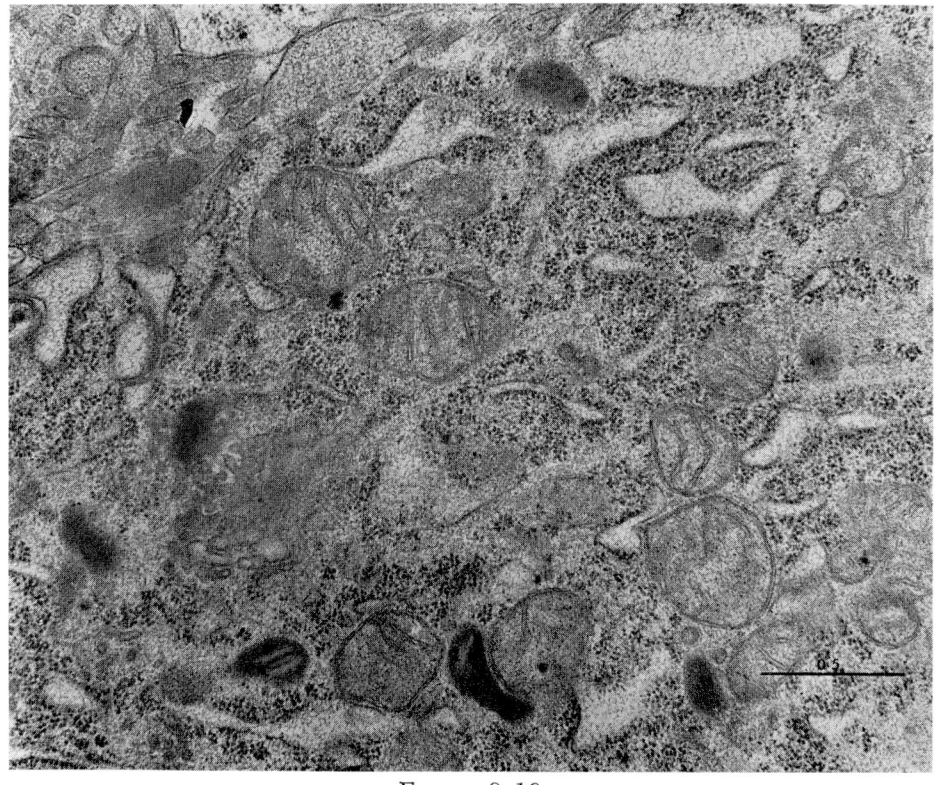

FIGURE 8-16.

174   *Impact Injury and Crash Protection*

Figure 8–17 demonstrates a capillary from an experimental animal following the inflation of a balloon in the epidural space. The material was fixed by the perfusion technique. It will be noted that the capillary is crescent shaped. This is the result of the expansile mass located over the surface of the brain. The endothelial cell appears intact and the basement membrane only minimally altered. However, there is an extensive extracellular space and total disruption of the perivascular glial cells. In Figure 8–18, one notices that the interfascicular oligodendrocyte of the experimental animal has a relatively normal nucleus, but that the ectoplasm is almost completely destroyed. Elements of granular ergastoplasm and one mitochondrion remain. The plasma membrane of this cell is still intact. In Figure 8–19, the pathogenesis of cerebral edema, as caused by

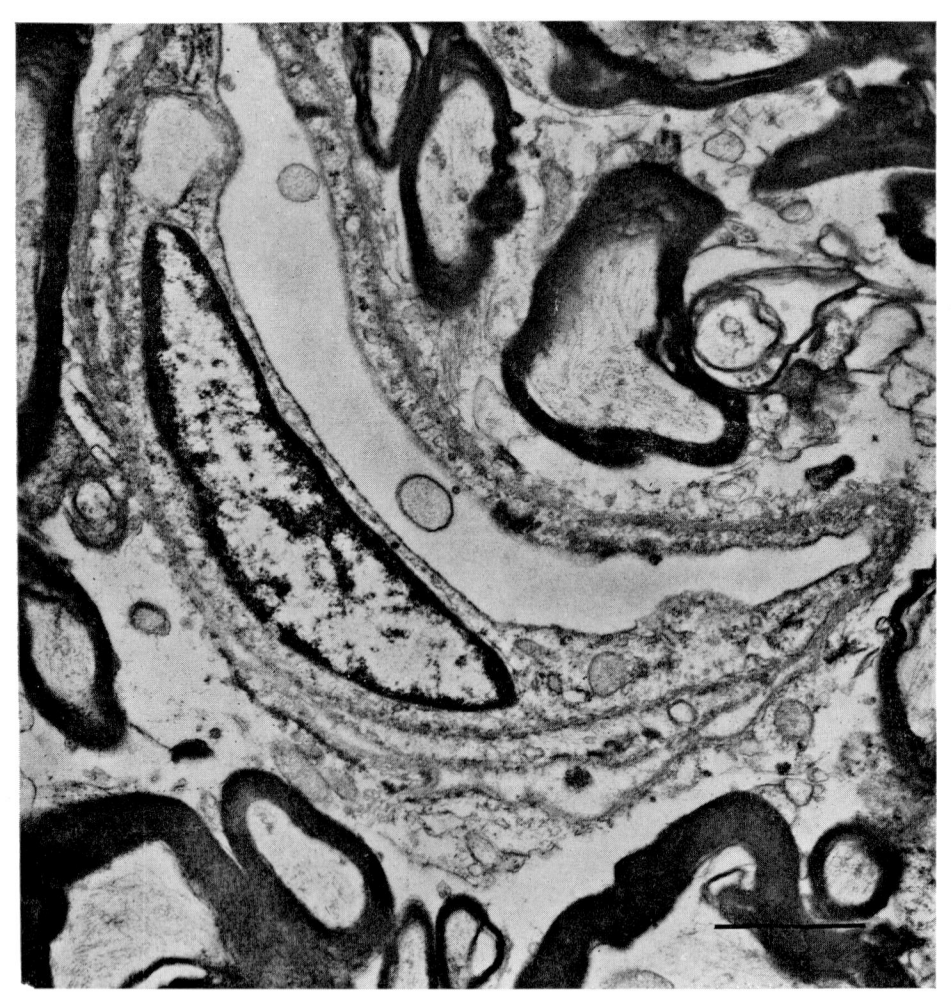

FIGURE 8–17.

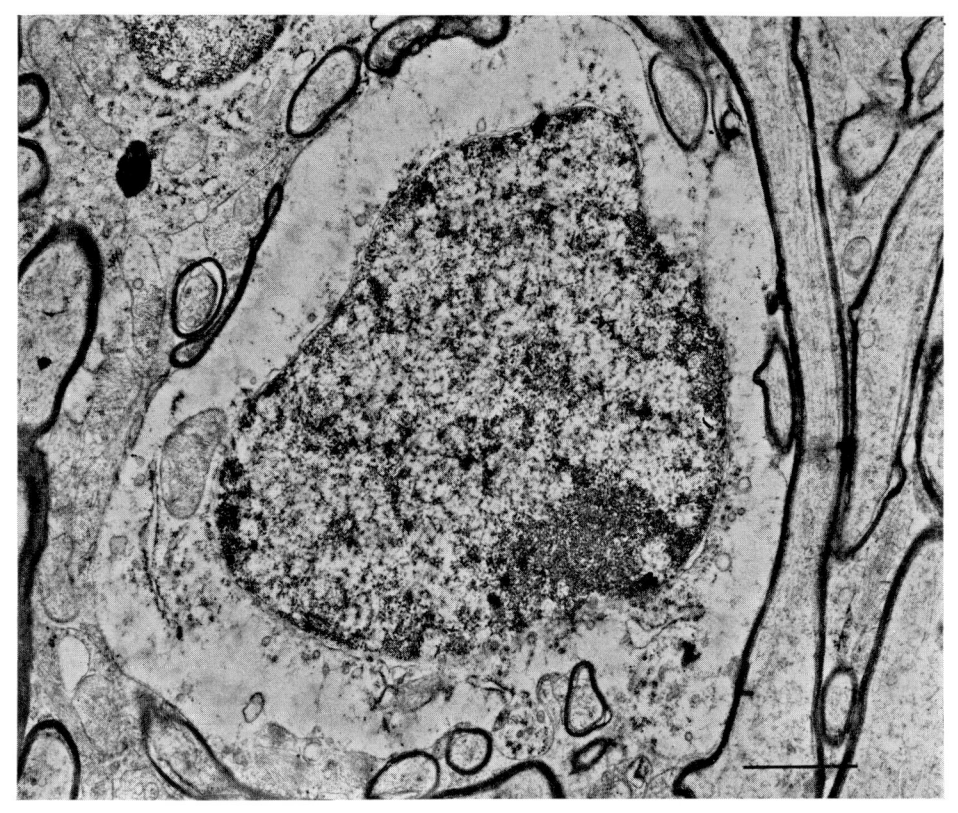

FIGURE 8–18.

an epidural balloon, is visibly demonstrated. At the upper right hand corner, both the capillary endothelium and the basement membrane are visualized. The extracellular space is quite large but the perivascular glial cells are still intact. Cell processes contain an increased number of pinocytotic vesicles which, in turn, contain Ferritin®—a visible tracer which had been used in order to identify the pinocytotic vesicles and determine the direction of flow.

From these observations on the fine structural changes in human lead encephalopathy and in experimental and human cerebral edema, it becomes clear that one may not outline a common sequence of morphological changes for these diverse clinical entities. To be sure, the morphological picture of "endstage" cerebral edema is the same in lead encephalopathy as it is in epidural hematoma. However, if one observes the fine structural changes as they develop, it becomes clear that there is no structural similarity between the various types of cerebral edema. Of course, this does not mean that hypoxia is not a common cause, but it does mean that there is a particular response of white and grey matter to varying toxic and mechanical noxae. One may speculate that a toxic agent, such as lead, interferes with the metabolism of a specific microorganelle, whereas a mechanical agent, such as an epidural hematoma, disturbs the function of all cells and organelles equally. This, however, is pure speculation, and therefore not a matter for the present.

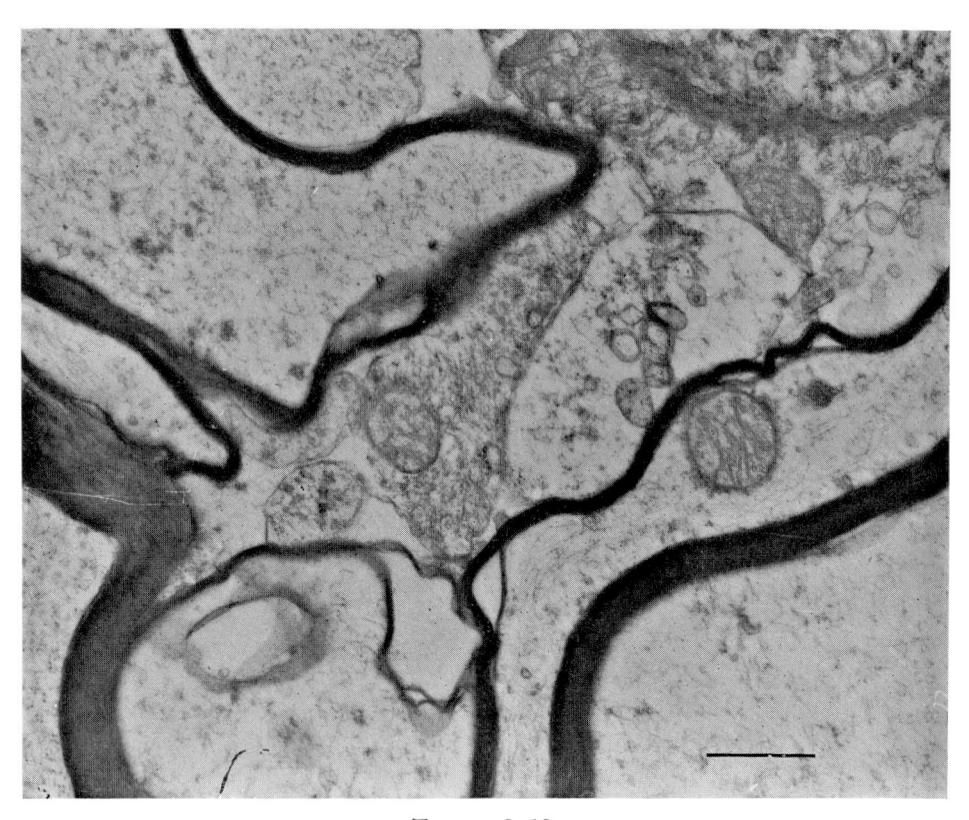

FIGURE 8–19.

DISCUSSION

Joseph P. Evans

Quite properly, in the motor city of Detroit, primary emphasis is being laid on mechanical considerations. All of us familiar with the perduring interest of Dr. Gurdjian over more than three decades are grateful to him and to his associates for their correlation of mechanical and clinical events. We are all greatly indebted to these men, including the late Dr. Lissner.

The approach which my own associates and I have employed over a somewhat similar period of time has laid more emphasis on the purely biological side. Our first interest lay in learning more of the nature and course of intracranial pressure alterations—not the acute impact alterations so effectively studied by Gurdjian and his colleagues, by Walker and his associates, and more recently by Ommaya and his group, but rather the long-term alterations, over hours and days, resulting from compression, both experimental and clinical. The longterm pressure recordings, initiated by Ryder of our then Cincinnati group, gave the first clear indication of the amazing readjustments possible within a physiologic range of the equation:

$$V_{Ic} = V_{Br} + V_{Bl} + V_{Csf} + V_L$$

Where V_{Ic} = volume of intracranial contents
V_{Br} = volume of gray and white matter
V_{Bl} = volume of circulating blood at any particular moment
V_{Csf} = volume of cerebrospinal fluid at any particular moment.
and
V_L = volume of any particular lesion, if one be present.

In utilizing this equation, it is important to bear in mind the different time parameters involved in the several volumes under consideration. Thus neurosurgeons recognize, for example, the early onset of brain swelling which may develop before edema of the brain (V_{Br}) has had time to develop. The rapid development of a lesion, such as an epidural hematoma, (V_L) plays a role, but there is good evidence that distension of the vascular bed of the brain (V_{Bl}) may be a very significant factor.[4]

It was out of these studies that Ishii's balloon experiments grew in the effort to simulate the lesion and the volume changes of an epidural hematoma and its subsequent secondary effects.[2] It was obvious that if we were to understand the full implications of the equation, we had to develop a reliable experimental model. Thus, by the simple expedient of inserting a small balloon into the epidural space, by distending it with known increments of fluid, and by monitoring the physiologic state of the animal by EEG, we were able to mimic one form of head injury, epidural hematoma.

It is *this* model that Dr. Raimondi has employed so effectively in studying the fine structure changes associated with epidural compression, thereby adding greatly to our better understanding of the dynamic changes occurring in the experimental lesion.

The evidence he has presented represents the late changes observed and as he, himself, has been careful to note, it is difficult in the late stages to identify specifically the causative agent and mechanisms responsible for the observed alterations. Elsewhere, he has amplified his observations on pathogenesis.[3]

I am happy to acknowledge here the contribution to our program Dr. Raimondi has made through his energy, skill, and perception—qualities which led before the development of his own independent program to the establishment of the electromicroscopic laboratory in our neurosurgical unit at the University of Chicago.

But structural alterations imply disruptions of physiologic activities, and physiologic changes imply disturbed biochemical reactions. Can we not then look beyond the electronmicroscopic picture?

Utilizing the same experimental model of epidural compression, Ishii has recently been exploring this possibility. Central nervous system tissues differ from those of other body systems in their high lipid content. It is now recognized that cerebral lipids are intimately related to cellular activity. Furthermore, the unit membrane, of which all cell membranes and membranous organelles are constructed, consists of a bimolecular leaflet of lipid bounded by protein molecules. Since it is known that important phases of cellular metabolism are linked to cell membrane integrity, it is not unreasonable to postulate that alteration in the lipid metabolism may affect fundamental cellular processes, e.g., alterations in the plasma membrane may result in abnormalities of membrane transport, those in the mitochondria may be associated with defective ATP synthesis and disruption of energy mechanisms, and those in endoplasmic reticulum with defective protein synthesis. Ishii and his co-workers have, in fact, demonstrated that some cerebral lipids, notably lecithin and ganglioside, do undergo a reversible breakdown following cerebral compression and the animal's cerebral activity corresponds roughly to these metabolic changes in lipids. Please note that I said "a reversible breakdown," for it is always the clinician's hope to reverse the effects of the adverse mechanical processes with which many of the investigators here are primarily concerned.

This is not the place to detail Ishii's extensive studies on lipid metabolism,[4] but it is possible to report that the administration of cytidine nucleotides, important cofactors in the biosynthesis of lecithin—whose content in the white matter is significantly reduced in experimental compression—has reversed strikingly the animal's condition and has improved the EEG pattern.

Observations of this sort, though undocumented in my brief comments, give promise—when coupled with increasing knowledge of membrane biology and of untrastructural alterations—of a more effective therapy directed at altering favorably fundamental biological dysfunction.

Such a promise lessens in no way the imperative need of a better understanding of the mechanical factors involved in injury, but does give hope of improved after-the-fact management of the head-injured patient.

References

1. RYDER, H.W.; ESPEY, F.F.; KIMBALL, F.D.; PENKA, E.J.; ROSENAUER, A.; PODOLSKY, B., and EVANS, J.P.: The mechanism of the change in cerebrospinal fluid pressure following an induced change in the volume of the fluid space. *J Lab Clin Med*, 41:428–435, 1953.
2. ISHII, I.: Brain swelling. Studies of structural, physiologic, and biochemical alterations. In Caveness, W.F., and Walker, A.E. (Eds.): *Head Injury: Conference Proceedings*. Philadelphia, Lippincott, 1966, pp. 276–300.
3. RAIMONDI, A.J.: Experimental cerebral edema: fine structure and pathogenesis. In Caveness, W.F., and Walker, A.E. (Eds.): *Head Injury: Conference Proceedings*. Philadelphia, Lippincott, 1966, pp. 300–321.
4. LANGFITT, T.W.; WEINSTEIN, J.D., and KASSEL, N.F.: Vascular factors in head injury: contribution to brain swelling and intracranial hypertension. In Caveness, W.F., and Walker, A.E. (Eds.): *Head Injury: Conference Proceedings*. Philadelphia, Lippincott, 1966, pp. 172–195.

Chapter IX

IMPLANTED MONITORS

John E. Adams and Carter C. Collins

In our chapter, we shall confine our remarks primarily to monitors implanted for the purpose of recording intracranial pressure continuously or intermittently over a long period of time. Other aspects of telemetry and devices for measuring acceleration and deceleration are covered elsewhere in the program.

The yield from implanted monitors recording intracranial pressure acutely and chronically in experimental situations, as well as in patients with head injuries, has been disappointingly barren. It has not initiated any new concepts or provided knowledge which was not available beforehand or which could be inferred from our previous clinical and pathological observations. Furthermore, the data which have been obtained have not led to any practical gains in the treatment of acutely head-injured patients.

However, with the more refined techniques now available in the form of passive transensors which allow implantation over long periods of time, and which provide increased sensitivity, new information of both theoretical and practical importance may become available.

Prior attempts at measuring the intracranial pressure periodically or continuously may be listed as follows:

Group I. Lumbar puncture
  A. Single
  B. Multiple
  C. Continuous recording
  by the following:
    1) Manometric measurement
    2) Strain gauge

Group II. Ventricular puncture
  A. Single or repeated manometric measurements—using manometers and strain gauges
    1) Recorded
    2) Graphically represented[1]

Group III. Subdural or subarachnoid implanted monitors
A. Subdural balloon[2]
B. Various subdural transducers

Group IV. Radiotelemetry[3,4]

All of the pressure measuring devices which involve connecting the ventricle or the subarachnoid space to the device are short of ideal due to the following (1) Fluid must be removed in making the measurements; (2) The system was frequently blocked by choroid plexus, arachnoid or other anatomical structures; (3) Depending upon the type of linkage, the measurements usually demonstrated considerable lag, lack of sensitivity or effective amplification; (4) Long-term measurements were usually rendered inaccurate by virtue of artifacts such as movement, or change in barometric pressure; (5) There was great difficulty in devising a reliable drift-free automatic device to record continuous long-term measurement without constant surveillance; and (6) Danger of infection was ever-present.

Many of these undesirable features, however, were minimized and excellent long-term recordings of intraventricular pressure were obtained by Lundberg.[5] The use of a subdural balloon by Rothballer obviated the problems of blockage of cerebrospinal fluid in the linkage system. Other pressure transducers have been employed in the subdural space, culminating in a small miniaturized silastic-coated transducer described by Jacobson and Rothballer[6] which allowed continuous recording of subdural pressure. This transducer provided excellent recording of intracranial pressure artifact-free over a long period of time. However the risk of infection remained and the mobility of the patient or experimental animal was limited.

The application of radiotelemetry techniques for the measurement of intracranial pressure was first suggested by Mackay.[3] The first passive transmitter, energized from an external radiofrequency source for the measurement of intraocular pressure, was devised by Collins,[4] and successfully implanted in monkeys for long-term measurement of intracranial pressure by Olsen et al.[7] This passive pressure-sensitive transensor contains no power source and therefore can be very small. It transmits a frequency modulated signal to a location external to the body by virtue of the absorption of a pressure-sensitive resonant circuit contained within the capsule. The original "miniature passive pressure transensor" developed by Collins consists of a short piece of polyethylene-covered glass tubing with mylar diaphragms attached to each end in drum-like fashion. Within the capsule, there is a pair of parallel coaxial spiral copper coils attached to the inner surface of the diaphragms. The pair of coils constitutes a resonant circuit

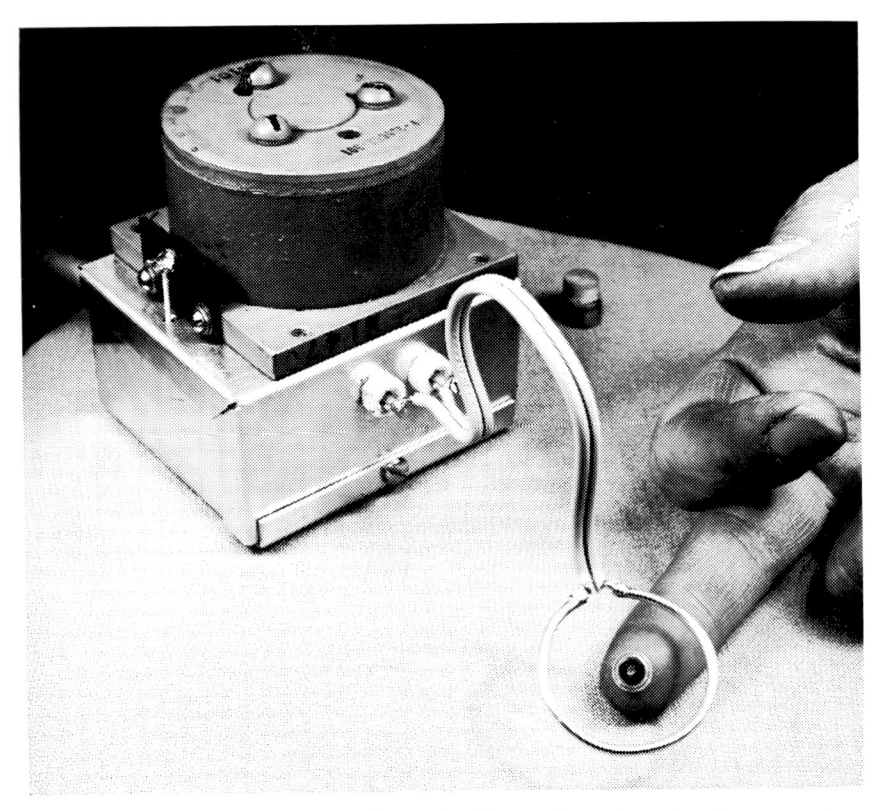

FIGURE 9–1. Transensor resting on fingertip. External sensing circuit is superimposed over transensor.

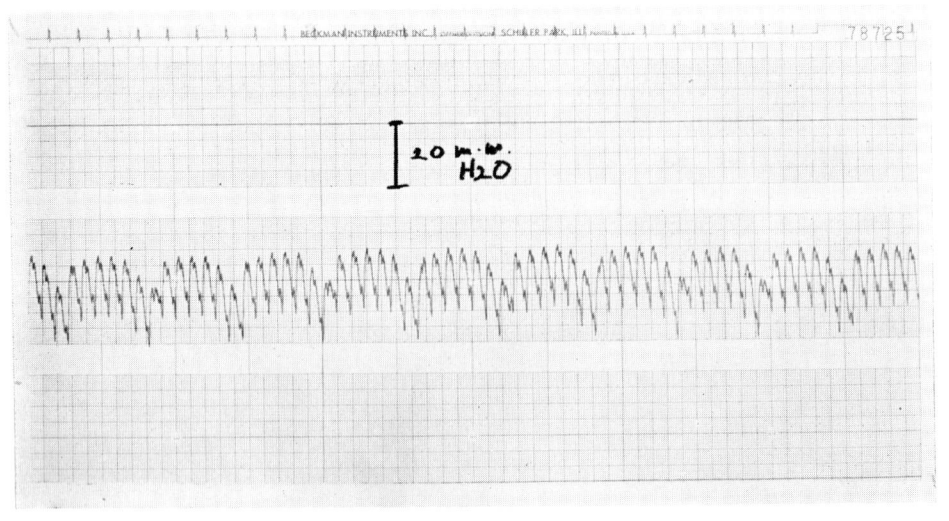

FIGURE 9–2. Time scale—1 second intervals shown in first channel.

in which the frequency is a function of the spacing between the coils which in turn is a function of the pressure on the diaphragm. The transensor, following implantation in the subdural space, is sensed externally by a sweeping grid-dip circuit. The output of the sensing circuit is fed through a low pass filter and the output of the filter is then fed to a penwriter as a continuous record of intracranial pressure.

This original transensor suffered a major disadvantage for long-term intracranial measurement because of the semipermeability and creep of the plastic diaphragms. The resulting drift to lower frequencies caused a shift of the baseline toward higher pressure recordings. A second anticipated disadvantage was biological unsafety resulting from the possible

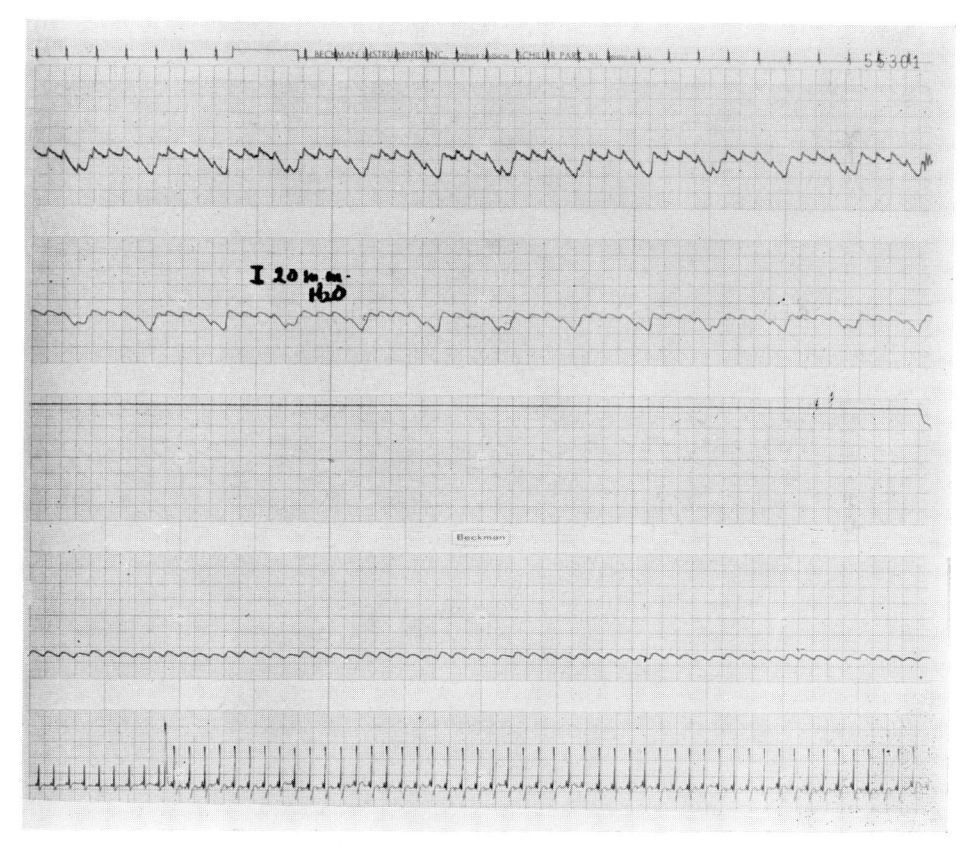

FIGURE 9–3. Recording channels are as follows:
Channel 1—Time scale (1 second intervals)
Channel 2—Internal jugular pressure
Channel 3—Subdural pressure
Channel 5—Carotid artery pressure
Channel 6—EKG

deposition of copper salts in the tissues or in the cerebrospinal fluid if the diaphragms leaked or ruptured.

More recently, Collins[8] has developed a glass transensor (Fig. 9–1) which has functioned successfully and appears to provide an absolutely stable zero baseline and pressure sensitivity indefinitely. Glass would seem to be an ideal material since it is relatively free of elastic anomalies and exhibits no creep or changes of spring constant. It possesses dimensional stability, has a low coefficient of thermal expansion, low loss insulating properties, a high viscosity at ordinary temperatures, and is nonirritating to animal tissues.

In our laboratories, Dr. Earl Olsen[9] has implanted this device in the subdural space of monkeys where they have been maintained over several months in a completely functional state. To date, there has been no evidence of a damping effect by the formation of scar tissue around the

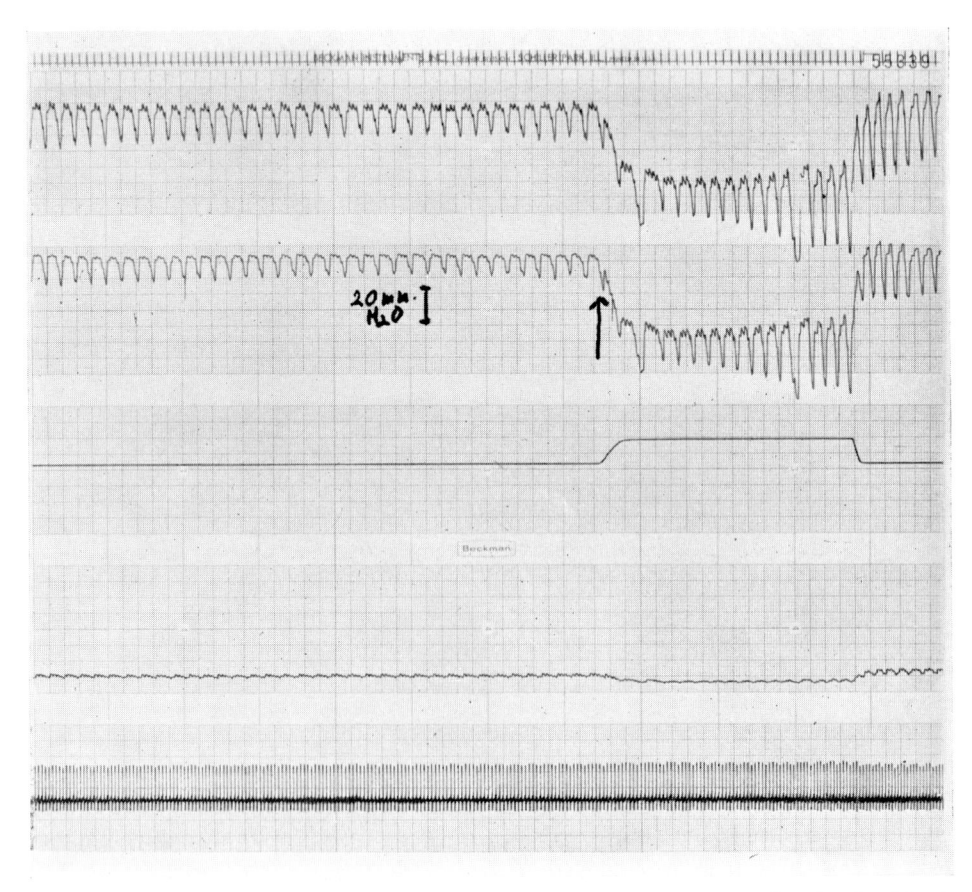

FIGURE 9–4. Same channel assignments as Figure 9–3. At arrow, head of table is elevated, resulting in a lowering of intracranial pressure.

transensor, and the reaction of the meninges and underlying cortex has been minimal.

The graphic display of the intracranial pressure recorded from the subdural space by the original transensor is shown in Figure 9-2. The fluctuation of pressure with respiration, and the arterial and venous dicrotic notches are clearly evident. In Figure 9-3, comparison of the internal jugular, intracranial and carotid artery pressures recorded by the glass transensor are shown. Finally, in Figure 9-4 the effect of change in posture upon jugular, subdural and carotid pressures recorded by the glass transensor may be seen.

REFERENCES

1. GUILLAUME, J., and JANNY, P.: Manométrie intracranienne continue. Intérêt de la méthode et premiers résultats. *Rev Neurol, 84*:131–142, 1951.
2. ROTHBALLER, A.B.: Continuous recording of intracranial pressure in man and animals. Presented at a meeting of the Harvey Cushing Society, Philadelphia, Penn., April 1963.
3. MACKAY, R.S.: Telemetering from within the body of animals and man; endoradiosondes. Caceros, C.A. (Ed.): *Biomedical Telemetry*. New York, Academic, 1965.
4. COLLINS, C.C.: A miniature passive pressure transensor for implanting in the eye. *IEEE Trans Biomed Elect, BME-14*:74–83, 1967.
5. LUNDBERG, N.: Continuous recording and control of ventricular fluid pressure in neurosurgical practice. *Acta Psychiat Neurol Scand* (Suppl. 149), *36*:7–193, 1960.
6. JACOBSON, S.A., and ROTHBALLER, A.B.: Prolonged measurement of experimental intracranial pressure using a subminiature absolute pressure transducer. *J Neurosurg, 26*:603–608, 1967.
7. OLSEN, E.R., et al.: Intracranial pressure measurement with a miniature passive implanted pressure transensor. *Amer J Surg, 113*:721–729, 1967.
8. COLLINS, C.C.: Passive telemetry with glass transensors. *Proc Nat Telemetering Conf*, 1967, pp. 146–151.
9. OLSEN, E.R., et al.: Intracranial tissue studies relating to glass transensors. *Amer J Surg 116*:3–7, 1968.

DISCUSSION

Eldon L. Foltz

The application of this radiosonde to the measurement of intracranial pressure may hold great promise in the future of neurosurgery. Whereas Dr. Adams and Dr. Collins have measured subdural pressure in the monkey by this method, Dr. James Atkinson (of the Barrow Neurological Institute in Phoenix) and I have been working for some time on a transensor to measure the ventricular waveform in humans, particularly in reference to infants with hydrocephalus. We have been fortunate indeed to have had the full cooperation of Dr. Carter Collins, Dr. Adams' confrere, who has contributed very significantly to our efforts. We are now in the third phase of our project to develop a satisfactory radiosonde or transensor for measurement of intracranial pressure in humans. I should like to briefly describe these three phases and point out some of the differences in our efforts as compared to Dr. Adams and Dr. Collins.

Physiological parameters have been demonstrated that were measured in an infant in the operating room under general anesthesia with strictly controlled respiratory pressures and respiratory CO_2 (Fig. 9–5). Carotid blood flow, CSF pressure, ventricular waveform and sagittal sinus pressures were recorded simultaneously. The pressures are recorded by Statham gauges via small catheters and the ventricular waveform is the parameter in which we are particularly interested. This is essentially an isovolumetric measurement demonstrating the water hammer effect within the ventricles of the pulse pressure wave generated by the choroid plexus. You can note the basic respiratory artifact with the superimposed pulse pressure artifact even with a dicrotic notch on the descending face of the pressure wave. This can be correlated easily with the dicrotic notch in the carotid blood flow pattern seen in the first channel. We have done many of these recordings in hydrocephalic infants and now recognize that this ventricular waveform is strikingly augmented whenever the mean pressure is elevated and in its augmented form is apparently characteristic of progressing hydrocephalus. It has, therefore, been our intent to develop a transensor which will measure this ventricular waveform, irrespective of the mean pressure, by means of implanting a radiosonde device.

The first phase of our effort has been described in the November, 1967 Journal of Neurosurgery. We selected a configuration of a transensor which could be easily managed surgically, would fix the geometry of the transensor coil in an advantageous position for detection, and would provide free access to ventricular pressure. Acrylic was selected for the case, and was coated with Insul-X,® a synthetic polymer. The diaphragm material selected was type 302 stainless steel. Electrically, the transensor consists of a parallel tuned circuit containing a capacitance and an inductance. The capacitor has one fixed plate and one plate which is a flexible stainless steel diaphragm. The diaphragm is separated from the fixed plate by an air space of 0.5 mm. The effective diameter of the diaphragm is 8 mm. These stainless steel plates are resistance-welded to a coil of the same material to complete the tuned circuit. The typical working frequency of this unit is 70 MHz. Through a small nylon tubular connection, a silicone rubber ventricular catheter connects the transensor to the ventricular system.

The transensor has been inserted into the skull of infants with the catheter going down a needle tract into the ventricle and the transensor case fitting into an 8 mm burr hole in the skull (Figs. 9–6 through 9–10).

The transensor is fitted securely in the burr hole with the scalp about to be closed over the transensor to hold it securely in place.

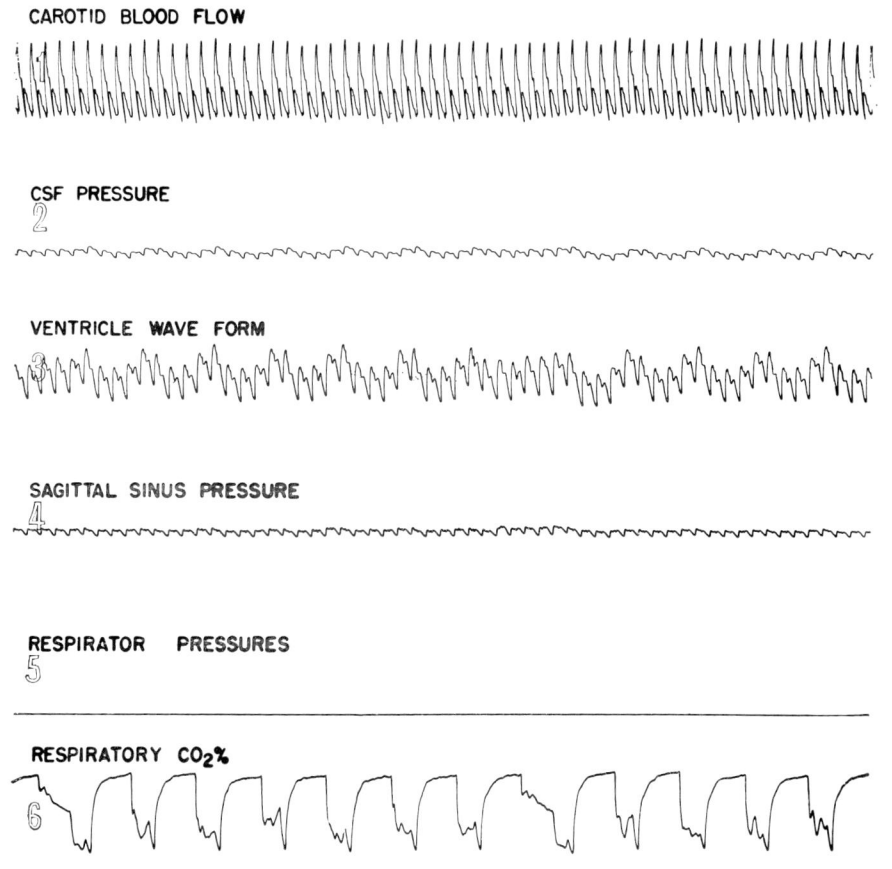

FIGURE 9–5. Measurements of pressures and carotid blood flow in a hydrocephalic infant.

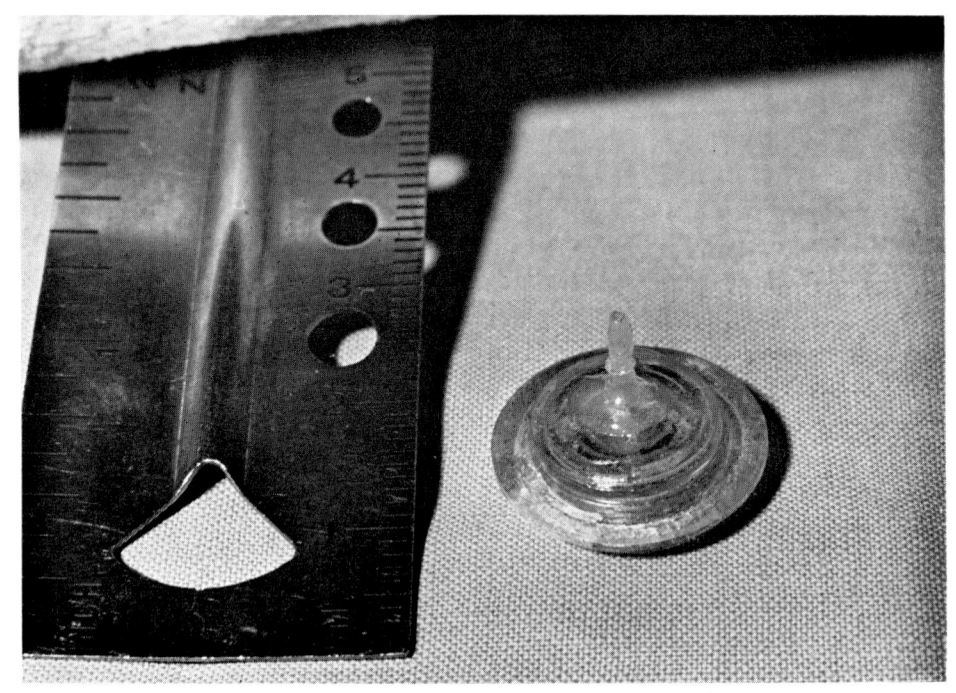

FIGURE 9–6. Transensor capsule to measure ventricular wave form; for implantation in skull with catheter in ventricle.

This transensor is shown in place, diagramatically, with the sensing device. A variation of Collins and Loughborough's panoramic absorption analyzer, incorporating operational amplifiers, was used for detection. The coil of the detecting unit, an inductor of a Nuvistor sweeping grid-dip circuit, can be placed over the implanted transensor and the output fed to a Grass polygraph.

A telemetry readout from this transensor in an infant can be taken. The ventricular pressure recorded by the transensor demonstrated large pressure changes synchronous with respiration. Under the circumstances, neither the transensor nor the strain gauge resolved the reflection of arterial pulse pressure in the ventricular system, which we are so interested in recording. The strain gauge was recorded through an Ommaya reservoir with a 23 gauge needle inserted. The time constant for the telemetry readout in this instance was 2 seconds. As a consequence of this choice, the slow 10-second transient recorded by the external strain gauge system was not recorded by the telemetry system. The noise level of the telemetry system in this application was equivalent to about 5 mm of water.

We found two major disadvantages to this particular system:

1. The transensor case was in actual fact permeable to water over a period of two weeks and therefore shorted out the transensor circuitry;

2. Type 302 stainless steel diaphragms were too insensitive to pick up the rapid transients. A major effort for continuing development was obviously necessary.

In phase 2 of our effort, five of the glass diaphragm transensors described by Dr. Adams and Dr. Collins were given to us by Dr. Collins for trial in humans. These were encased in similar acrylic capsules for both subdural and intraventricular pressure recordings. The subdural capsules were made with open face for direct application on the surface of the brain, again inserted in an 8 mm burr hole and secured only by means of the overlying scalp. Our efforts at using these capsules in the human being have been classified by us as "disastrous." The first such transensor was sterilized by gas sterilization at 14.5 pounds per square inch, and the glass diaphragms were found to be broken and displaced, presumably by this sterilization. The other four, therefore, were not gas sterilized but were wet-sterilized externally, taking the risk that a fracture of the glass diaphragms might produce bacterial and chemical (copper) contamination of the intracranial spaces. These were implanted in pairs, one in the ventricular system and one in the subdural space. Successful subdural pressure telemetry was obtained in two infants, but no successful telemetry from the ventricular transensors was achieved.

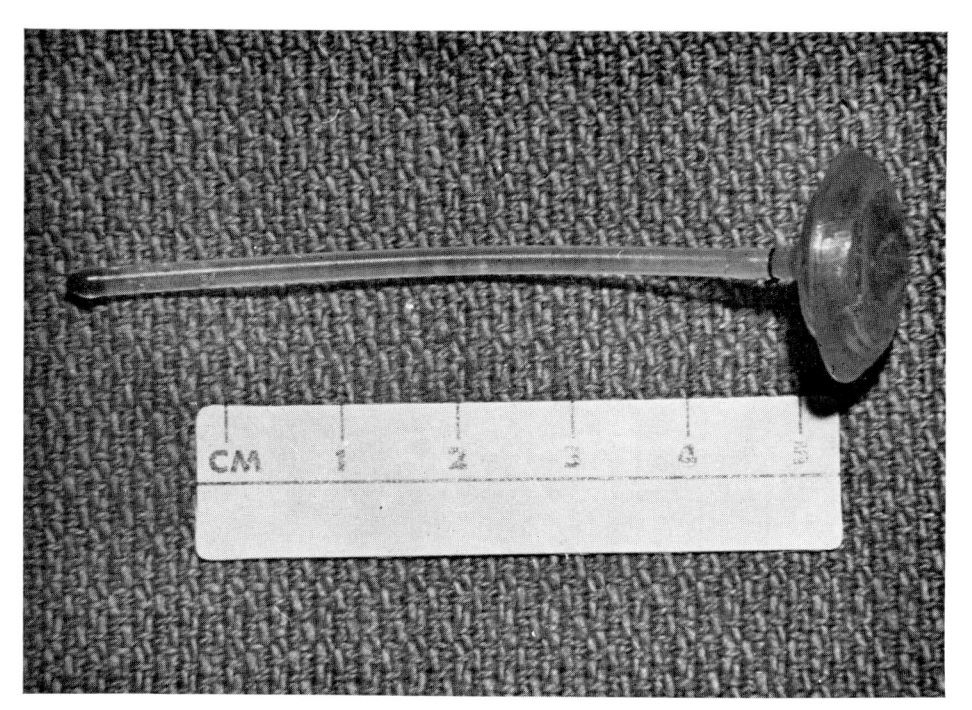

FIGURE 9–7. Transensor with ventricular catheter attached.

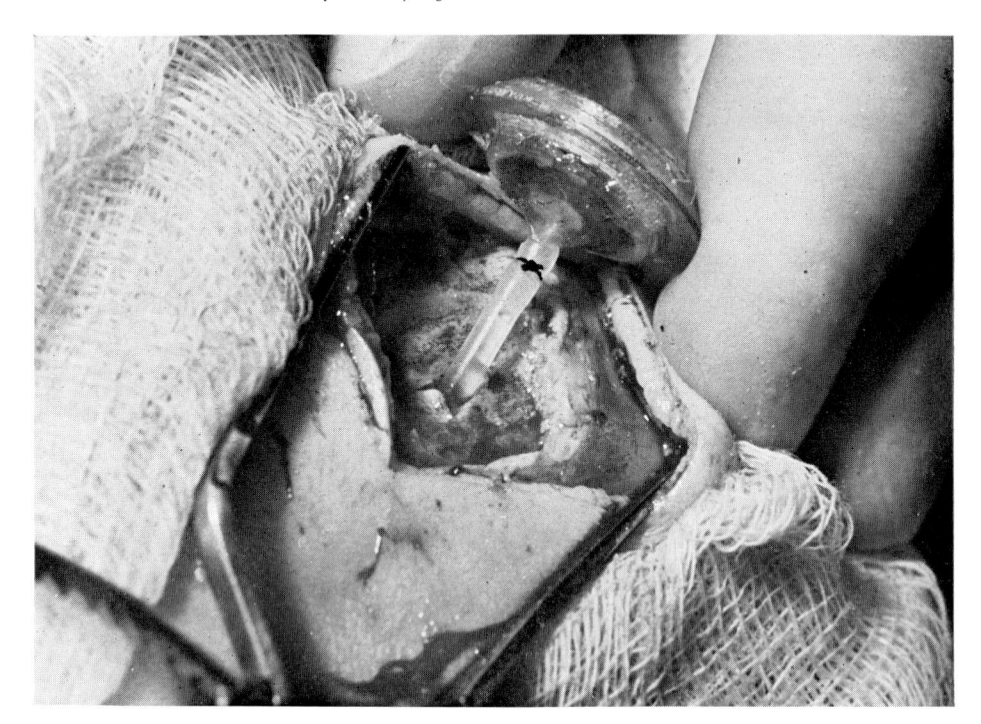

FIGURE 9-8. Implantation of transensor (with ventricular catheter) via burr hole in skull of an infant; scalp incised and open.

In Figure 9-12, the subdural transensor responds to increased pressure from breath-holding and crying, (channel 1) and the same transensor rapidly responds to fontanel compression in Figure 9-13. The effect of compressing a myelomeningocele sac on subdural pressure has been demonstrated in Figure 9-14, wherein the first artifact is increased respirations secondary to pain, followed by 30 percent augmentation of the pulse pressure wave, and at pressure release again deep breathing is secondary to pain input.

The transensors had a life span of only 3 days for the subdural transensors, and we had no viable recording from the intraventricular transensors. These were removed and all four were found to have fractured glass diaphragms without displacement, centered around the center post, and were all highly suggestive of fatigue effect of the glass. It is our presumption that this is secondary to the intense hammering effect of the pulse pressure wave in these infants, considerably greater in magnitude than that experienced by Dr. Adams and Dr. Collins with the monkeys in subdural space. Contamination of the CSF spaces did occur in both instances and infection resulted in one.

In phase 3 of our effort, we have returned to stainless steel as the diaphragm material of choice, and Dr. Atkinson has collaborated closely

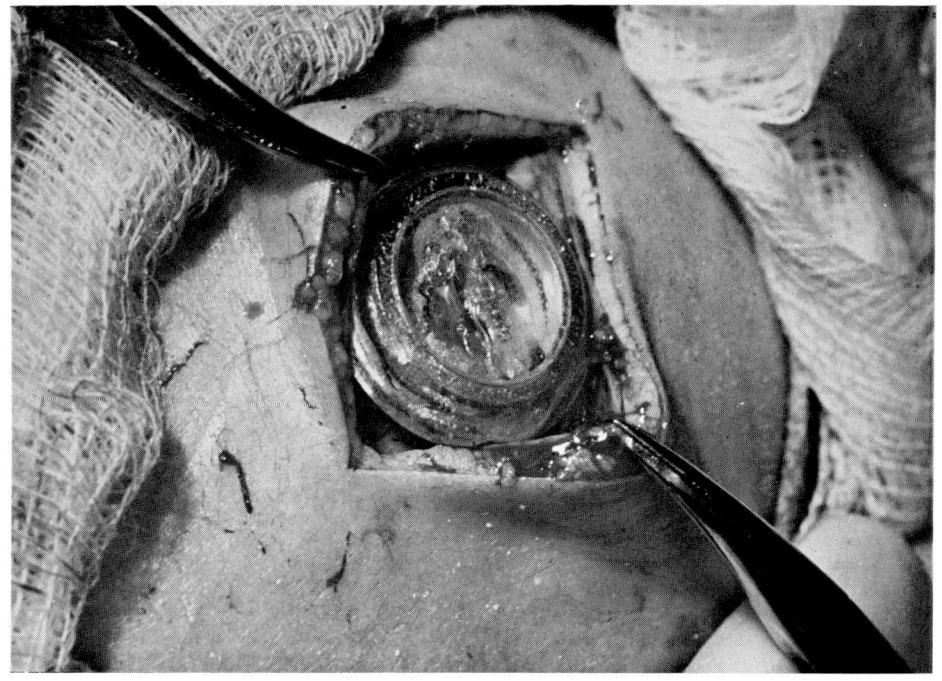

FIGURE 9–9. Transensor in place in burr hole, scalp about to be sutured closed.

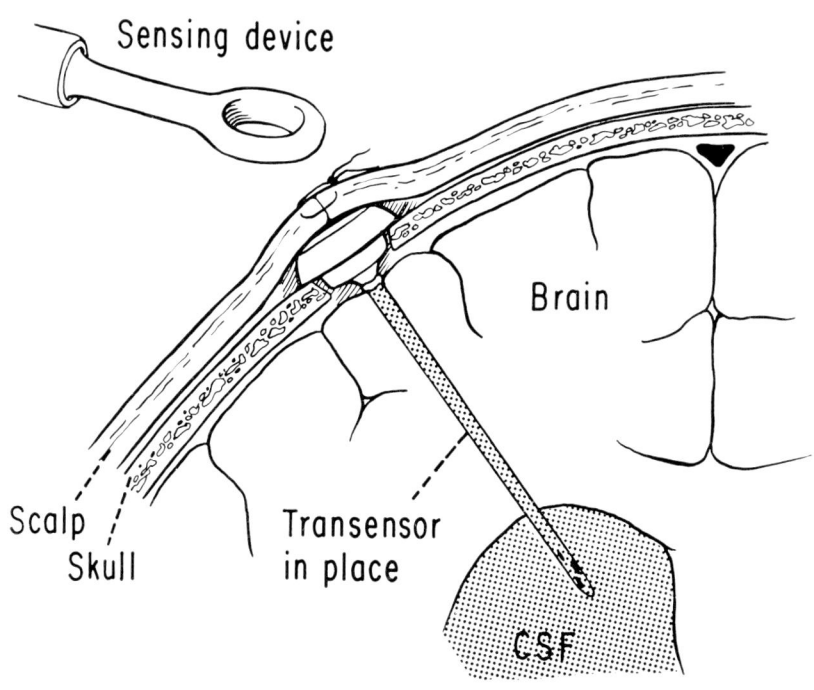

FIGURE 9–10. Diagram of transensor in place in skull burr hole, catheter in ventricle of brain, and sensing device in position externally.

192   *Impact Injury and Crash Protection*

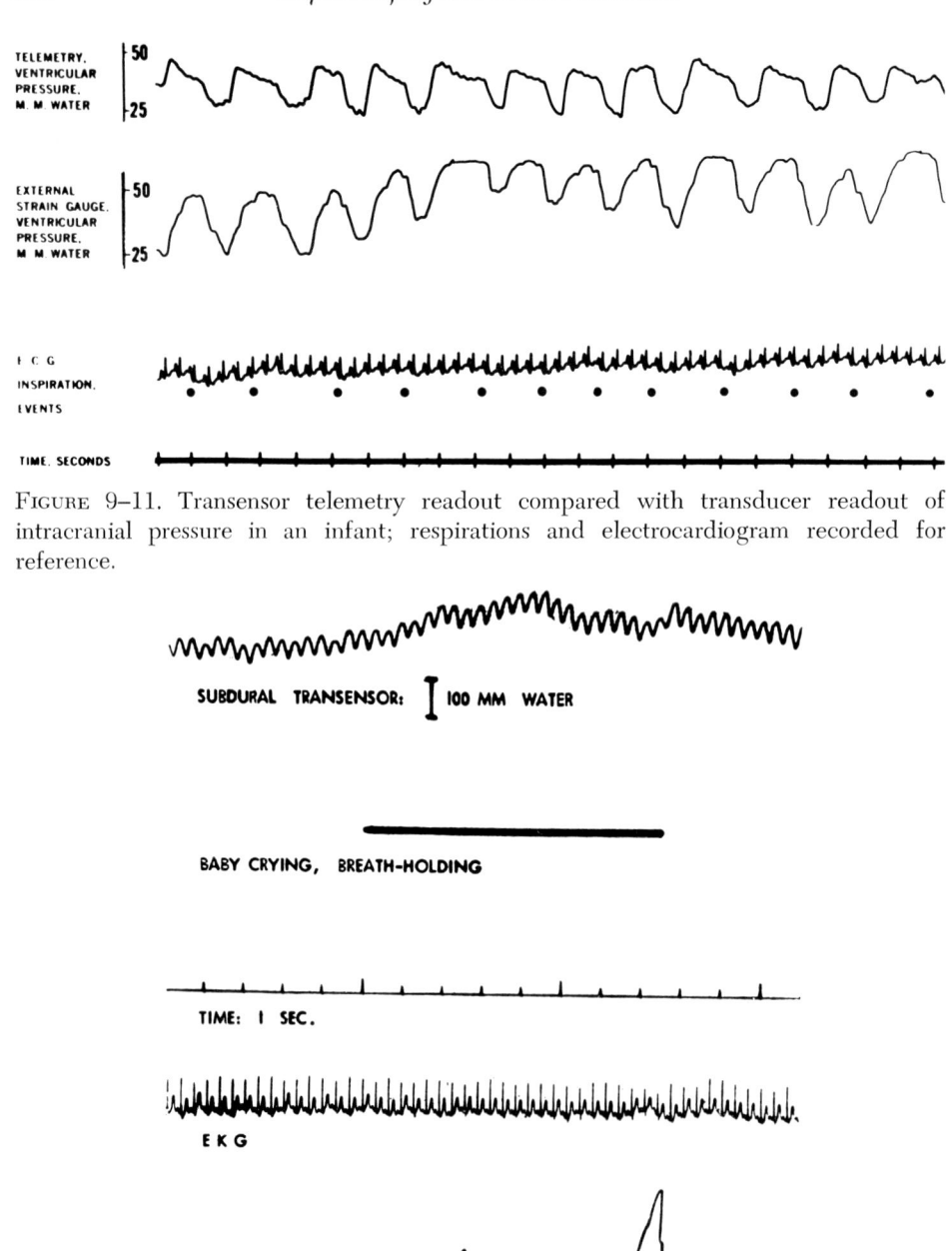

FIGURE 9-11. Transensor telemetry readout compared with transducer readout of intracranial pressure in an infant; respirations and electrocardiogram recorded for reference.

FIGURE 9-12. Subdural transensor readout of intracranial pressure with respiration, EKG, and time references; hydrocephalic baby.

with Motorola in the development of an impermeable case for the transensor. This case is made of a combination plastic material which is extremely hard and appears completely impermeable to water, thus satisfying the need for absolute water impermeability. The stainless steel diaphragms are made of stainless steel 316 with a sensitivity much better than the previous stainless steel diaphragms. This particular transensor, the first of this model, has a sensitivity of 94 MHz when dry (8.3 Kc/mm Hg). This model is currently under continuing development with tissue tolerance studies for the case and further modifications of the diaphragm design in an effort to further improve the sensitivity (Fig. 9–15).

This method of passive telemetry for measurement of CFS pressure appears to have promise, both to measure ventricular as well as subdural pressures. Whether this method or a modification of this will have appli-

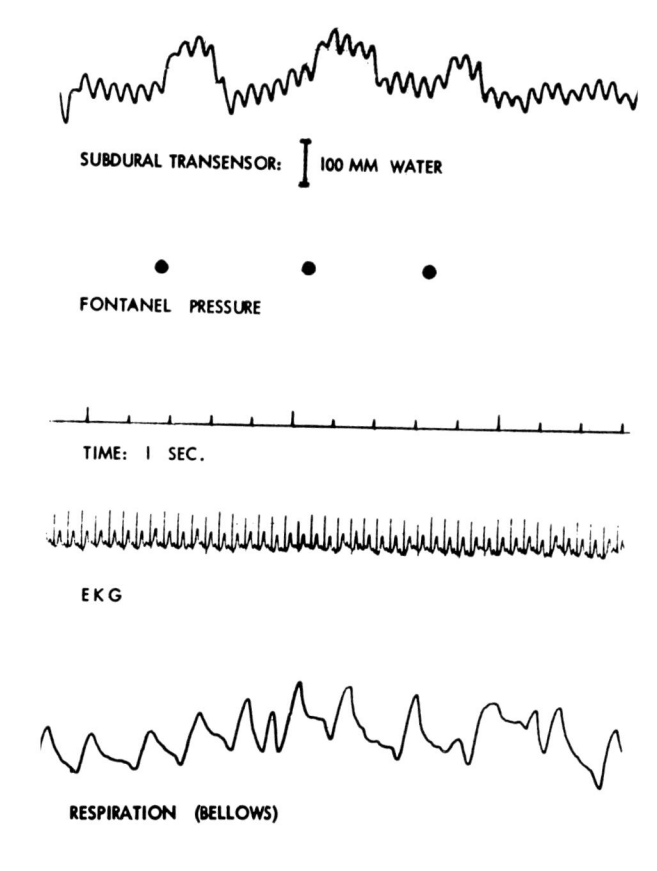

FIGURE 9–13. Subdural transensor response to increasing intracranial pressure by finger compression of open fontanel; hydrocephalic infant.

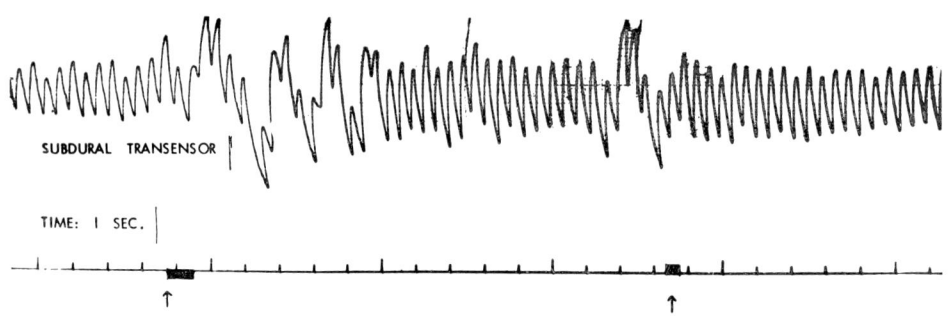

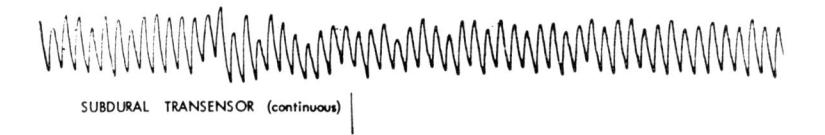

FIGURE 9–14. Subdural transensor response to increasing intracranial pressure by digital compression of myelomeningocele sac; infant with hydrocephalus and myelomeningocele (spina bifida).

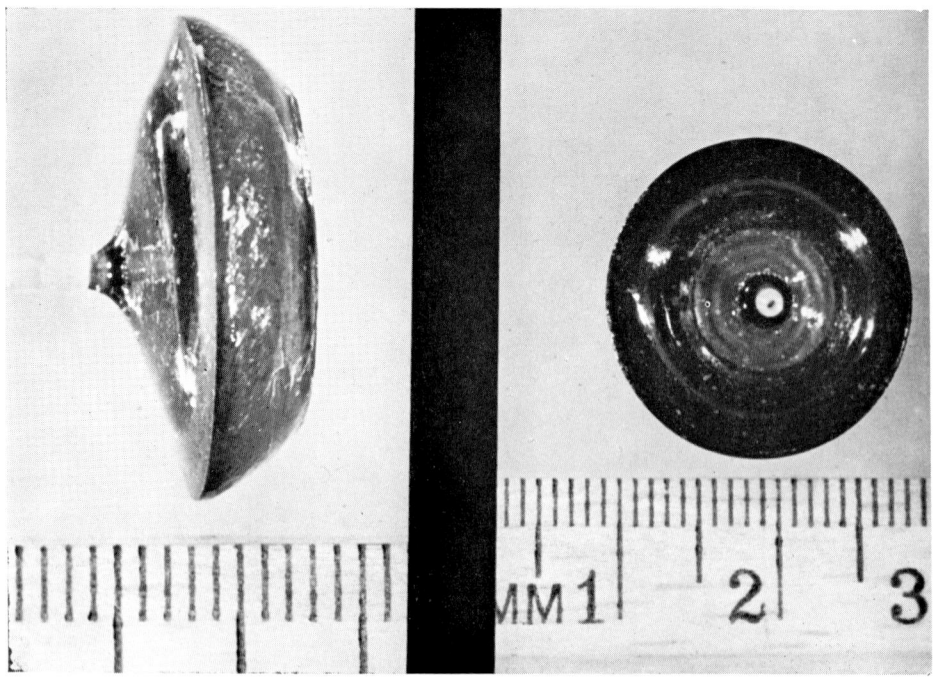

FIGURE 9–15. Latest transensor model using stainless steel diaphragms and new, impermeable casing.

cation in the field of brain trauma remains to be seen. To date, it should seem quite apparent that developmental problems far outweigh the results demonstrated.

Dr. Collins and Dr. Adams are to be congratulated for introducing this pressure telemetry method to neurosurgery.

Chapter X

HIGH SPEED FLASH X-RAY AND CINEMATOGRAPHY IN INJURY RESEARCH

John L. Martinez

The application of systems for the permanent recording of dynamic events for later detailed study has been an inherent part of the growth of injury research. The period between World War II and the present has seen the development of the high level of interest in the mechanics of the human body, its systems and the sensitivity of those systems to trauma. This period has coincided with, partly coincidentally but certainly strongly abetted by, a technological revolution started by the research efforts of World War II and accelerated by the space age endeavors. Hence, it is difficult to determine to what extent the devices and procedures related here spurred biomechanics and injury research or to what degree they evolved as their need became apparent with the development of interest in dynamic phenomena.

One of the surprises experienced in studying high speed motion pictures of an impact phenomenon for the first time is the amount of detail available. Even, perhaps particularly, the most experienced researcher will replay the action sequences, noting one element at a time, making notes, moving on to another segment of action. Sometimes it is useful to alternate between macro- and microscopic points of view—to note detail, but always in the framework of the total action.

As the high speed recording equipment began to be used in situations which had been studied previously by deduction or by interview with injured subjects, it became apparent that the human subject is a most unreliable reporter of short term dynamic phenomena in which he is either a participant or observer. It is interesting to read some of the papers of 20 years ago which attempted to relate injuries produced to an assumed set of body actions which, it is now known, do not occur. The term "whiplash," for example, was first applied to a supposed head-neck action which high-speed photography later indicated was incorrect.

When volunteers are used in tests of moderate violence and the actions recorded with high-speed equipment, the subjects are usually surprised at the extent of the deformations and displacements which they have endured. The subject tends to underestimate the degree of distortion which his body has experienced. Another variable often reported has to do with the state of readiness of the subject. Provided the accelerations and related forces are within the strength capabilities of the subject, his "bracing" for the impact profoundly affects the resulting body actions.

In enumerating the problems of studying body actions prior to the use of high speed equipment—the short time interval which makes human observation unfeasible, the unreliability of the subject himself as a reporter, the change of pattern as a function of subject preparedness—it is suggested that much of the early work which has not been repeated probably should be with the modern aids for recording and displaying the details of impact phenomena.

The equipment used in recording the mechanics of the body include displacement, velocity and acceleration and force transducers, camera oscilloscopes, recording oscillographs, "flash" x-ray systems, x-ray cinematography, and video output systems. This paper will describe the last three systems listed and some of their features and limitations used jointly or singly. X-ray cinematography consists of the cinematographic recording of radiologic images such that the number of exposures per unit time is consistent with the usual standards of cinematography. The techniques of serial fluorography and serial radiography usually do not meet this criterion as they employ a substantially lower frequency rate. X-ray cinematography includes two basic approaches: (1) the direct exposure of a sensitive emulsion to x-rays and, (2) the cinematographic recording of a fluoroscopic image. These methods are referred to as direct and indirect cinematography.

DIRECT X-RAY CINEMATOGRAPHY

Figure 10–1 illustrates direct x-ray cinematography. In the direct method, the x-rays penetrate the subject and expose the film. The recorded image is full size or slightly enlarged depending on the tube-to-subject and subject-to-film distance. The film can be in roll form, running at constant speed if the x-ray pulses are of short enough duration to stop action, but usually the film is advanced serially and keyed to a pulsing system of the x-ray tube so that the subject is exposed to radiation only during film exposure periods, not during advance and indexing time. Cut film, rather than roll film, may also be used, but the handling system is more complex and limits exposure rates to 12 per second in most installations. However, large sizes up to 14 × 14 inches may be handled in direct systems.

X-rays penetrate film very easily and only a very small amount of the

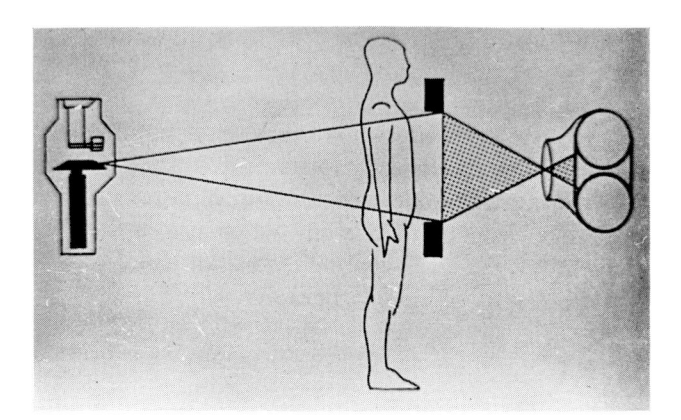

FIGURE 10–1. Direct x-ray cinematography.

available energy goes into exposing the film. To increase the effect, luminescent screens are usually used in intimate contact with one or both sides of the photographic film. The screens are coated with certain inorganic crystalline phosphors chosen for their high absorption coefficients for x-rays and their efficiency in converting some of this energy into light in the wave lengths to which the film is particularly sensitive. Hence, when the x-rays reach the film, there is some direct exposure of the film but the impingment of the rays upon the phosphor coatings produces visible light at the surface of the films with a powerful multiplying exposure effect. Films may be double-coated and used with screens on both sides and, in this arrangement, may show an effective sensitivity an order of magnitude greater than that for the film alone. When dealing with experimental animals, the radiation dose might or might not be of importance, but, in the case of human subjects or where radiation damage could be a complicating factor in an animal study, the usefulness of screens in reducing the dose experienced by the subject is apparent.

In the case of fluoroscopy, the light emitted by the phosphors must be in the visible range, particularly for the dark-adapted retina of the observer. If the fluoroscope screen is to be photographed, serially or cinematographically, then a match between the phosphor characteristics and camera film sensitivity is important.

All fluorescent materials have a time factor for reaching maximum emission and for decaying of the image when excitation ceases. A long decay period is acceptable for much radiographic work but, if the decay period is too long, it can interfere with the generation of the next image in situations where rapid serial exposures are desired or in the case of the use of cinematography of the fluorescent screen.

In the selection of screens, the two performance characteristics sought are the screen speed, which measures the intensity of the usable light given off for a given input radiation energy and the resolution characteristics of the screen. There is some lateral diffusion in the crystalline structure of the phosphors, some self-excitation, and, therefore, the final image is not as valid as it would be with film without screens. A number of screens are available with relative speeds of approximately 1, 3, 5 but with corresponding decrease in resolution of 15, 10, 6 lines per millimeter. Hence in selection of screens, the factors involved are the following: (1) limiting the dose received by the subject, when that is a factor, by choice of screen-film combinations, (2) securing maximum detail consistent with meeting the speed limitations imposed in (1), (3) choosing a phosphor with a decay constant consistent with the frames per second, which are to be recorded in those cases where the same fluorescent area is photographed repeatedly.

This digression on screens was necessary before continuing the description of film-handling systems which impose one limitation on exposure rates in x-ray cinematography. In the case of the cut film systems, each film is mounted together with two screens and the device is loaded with up to thirty-four such films. Continuous-roll film systems, on the other hand, must advance film between a set of intensifying screens, stop, allow pressure to be applied for good contact, release, and advance again. In both systems, there are mechanical limitations which restrict frame speeds to 6 to 12 per second. In another system, the loaded cassettes are mounted on the periphery of a drum and rotate into position, but the system is limited to the number of cassettes which will fit on the drum—usually ten.

In describing the "direct" systems which yield full size or slightly enlarged x-ray pictures, the concept of using the title "cinematography" might seem strained, but the system qualifies if the exposure rates are in the usual motion picture category. When the size of the subject or of the detail studies is sufficiently small, 70 mm films may be used for direct x-ray studies and projected directly since such projection equipment does exist. For larger sizes, photo-copying on standard size movie film will allow projection and study although in most large film systems the total number of frames involved is quite small, usually less than thirty-four.

INDIRECT X-RAY CINEMATOGRAPHY

Indirect x-ray cinematography is much more widely used because it lends itself to recording on standard sized movie film—usually 16 mm. If a television chain is included in the system for direct viewing or tape recording, the term kinefluorography is used. This latter system has advantages of requiring much lower dosages than for camera systems and a large screen output for easy viewing during a procedure as well as the easy recording and replay capability, but is limited to speed ranges at the lower end of the cinematographic scale. The use of an image-intensification system makes the lower dosage possible with a video system.

Indirect x-ray cinematography consists of photographically recording the image on a fluorescent screen (Fig. 10–2) or on the small tube (Fig. 10–3). Since the levels of illumination normally used for fluoroscopic examination of human subjects is too low for practical photographic recording, that system is not used. But with animal subjects and where radiation damage is not of concern, the x-ray intensity can be raised sufficiently high for recording at moderate speeds.

The cinefluorographic system, particularly when used with a video system, permits cinematography at reasonable dosage levels. The image intensification system permits much higher brightness levels at the output screen than in fluoroscopic work, permitting direct viewing or television monitoring. If a recurrent phenomenon is being studied, it can be observed at low radiation levels with the television and direct viewing systems and, after adjustments or injection of opaque materials, switched to camera recording which necessitates much higher dosage levels for a brief period.

In order to limit the dosage received by the subject, the output of the x-ray tube is pulsed in synchronization with the camera. This can be done by energizing the x-ray only while the camera shutter is open or by pulsing the x-ray a given number of times while the shutter is open on each frame. Various control devices are used to coordinate the camera and x-ray actions.

One of the limitations of the cinefluoroscopic arrangement is the size of the area covered, many of the units using a 6-inch diameter field. Some

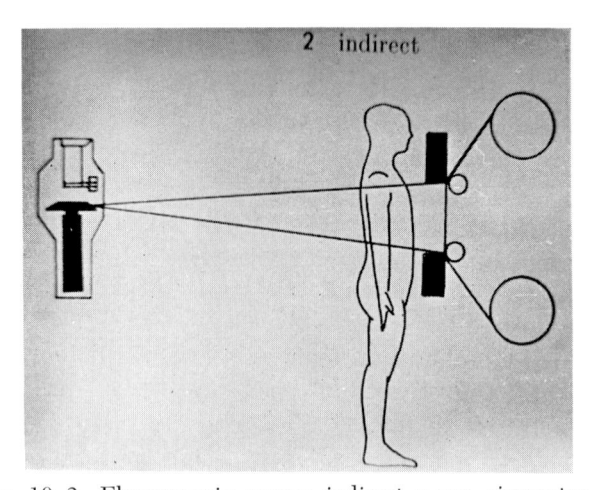

FIGURE 10–2. Fluoroscopic screen indirect x-ray cinematography.

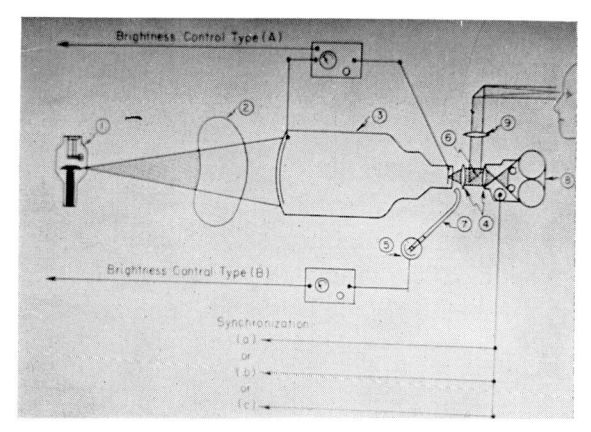

FIGURE 10-3. Schematic diagram of a typical cinefluorographic system. (*From* Michael M. Ter-Pogossian, Washington University.)
1. X-ray tube
2. Part examined
3. X-ray intensifier tube
4. Lenses
5. Photomultiplier tube
6. Partially reflecting mirror used to monitor the image during recording
7. Light pipe
8. Cinematographic camera
9. Field lens

newer equipment provides moderately larger areas. Speeds are still rather low, most units recording at 10 to 60 frames per second, although a newly-developed camera operating at 300 frames per second has been announced.

The television monitoring systems offer several advantages over optical monitoring, including the possibility of using several larger screen monitors, and can be done at the same low radiation levels as the visual monitoring as compared with the increased radiation levels for camera recording. The frames per second limit is controlled by the phosphor decay characteristics and the sweep method used in the television scanning system. Practically speaking, the system will record phenomena of moderate speed—a beating heart, for example—but will "smear" with very rapid motions.

FLASH X-RAY SYSTEMS

Flash x-ray systems are electronic instruments in which energy is stored in capacitors and then discharged quickly through a field emission vacuum tube. They provide an intense burst of x-rays for a short period of time and are quiescent between such discharges. The Field Emission Corporation of McMinnville, Oregon, produces a line of flash x-ray tubes and associated equipment under the name of Fexitron.®

The chief characteristic of these x-ray systems is an extraordinarily high dosage rate for very brief pulse durations so that the dosage per firing is moderate. One model (No. 2350) features a dose rate of 10^8 roentgens second at the tube face but a pulse width or duration of approximately 70 nanoseconds (70×10^{-9} seconds or .07 microseconds).

The power supplies for these systems are usually flexible and the capitance units or pulsers can be arranged to fire after any desired delay from 1 microsecond to 100 milliseconds and through the same x-ray tube or tubes in parallel. When fired through the same tube, frame rates up to 2×10^4 are possible in some models. If the pulsers are arranged to fire through separate tubes, these tubes can be so positioned as to x-ray the subject at various positions along its path—remote from the power supply. Because of the short exposure time required, the flash x-ray system will "stop" most motions and give clear x-ray pictures of dynamic phenomena.

Figure 10–4 shows a typical arrangement of a multiple-tube experimental arrangement. The guinea pig is to be accelerated by (1) the crossbow (2) past x-ray film in a long cassette (3) or series of cassettes, passing between the cassettes and the gun-like tubes. Lead separators are arranged between the tubes to control the overlapping of exposure fields which might otherwise occur. The control panel contains the pulsers and the trigger amplifiers. While the triggers could be set for programmed delays for the firing of the four tubes, it would probably be more appropriate to have the carriage carrying the animal trip microswitches controlling each tube circuit at the correct subject position. Figure 10–5 A and (B) show the detail possible in the study of the dynamic response of organs at the high accelerations and velocities reached. Figure 10–6 is of a monkey in a test vehicle undergoing acceleration.

In the illustration used, the "frame rate," if that term applies, is a matter of the x-ray pulsing only and the problem of getting new film into position

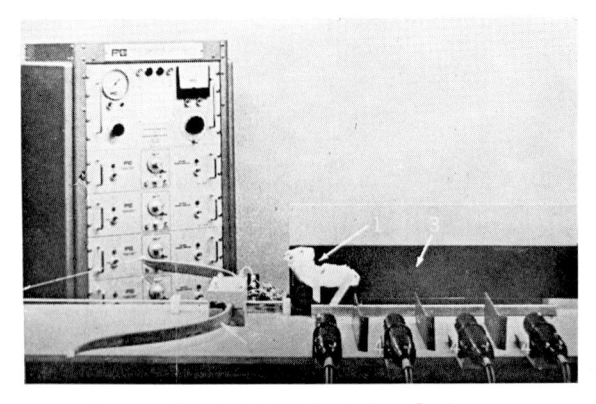

FIGURE 10–4. Multiple tube flash x-ray.

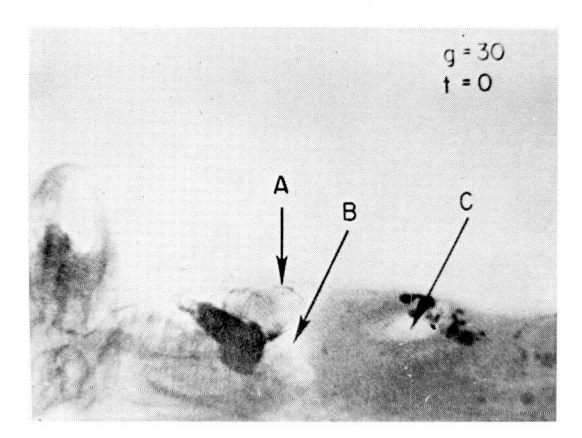

FIGURE 10-5A.

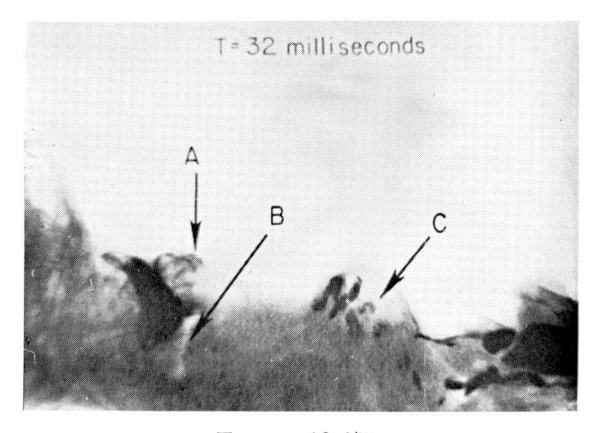

FIGURE 10-5B.
Flash x-rays of mouse under acceleration. (*From* Field Emission Corporation.)
A. Heart, showing compression
B. Diaphragm, showing motion
C. Motion of gas bubble and intestine

is avoided because of the displacements involved. Hence, in using the term frame rate for multiple-gun systems, the potential rate is that of each tube multiplied by the number of tubes in the system and rates of 10^6/second may be approached with four tubes in some systems.

When the subject does not move so conveniently, or does not move at all, the frame rates are likely to be a function of the film handling system. Most systems are limited to 10 to 12 frames per second, and a maximum 34 frames serially, but special arrangements allow higher frame rates. Figure 10-7 shows an arrangement used with four tubes to x-ray an exploding wire. The lead collimators control the portion of the single piece of x-ray film used and would permit four sequential shots at the frame

204 *Impact Injury and Crash Protection*

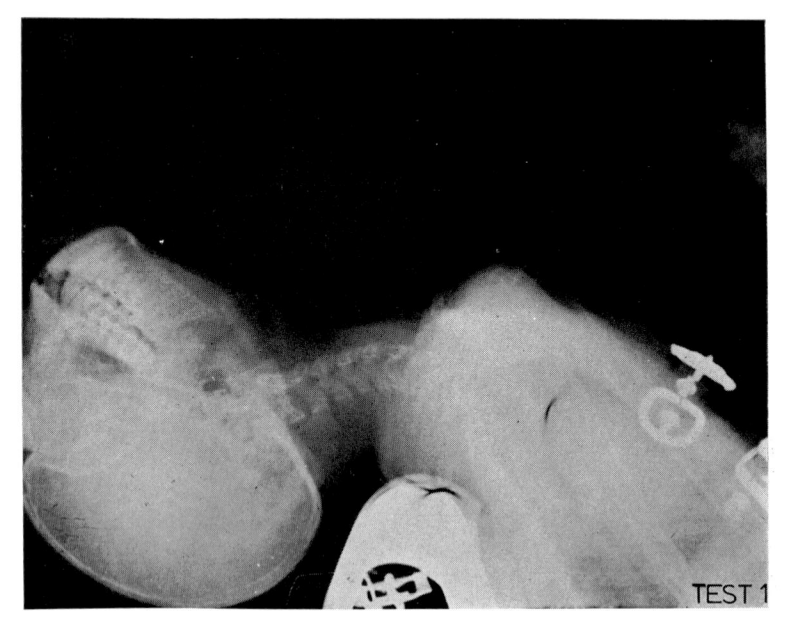

FIGURE 10-6. Flash x-ray film of monkey undergoing acceleration.

rate of the x-ray system. The change in orientation must be evaluated for its effect but is simple geometrically.

A unit designed by the author in conjunction with Dr. Hirsch and Dr. Ommaya, features a large rotating disc containing four cassettes and rotating at 3600 rpm and used with one x-ray tube. A smooth front plate permits placing the disc in almost rubbing contact with the animal—the proximity limiting magnification and penumbra effects. Driven by a synchronous motor, the device can be timed by the trigger delay circuits

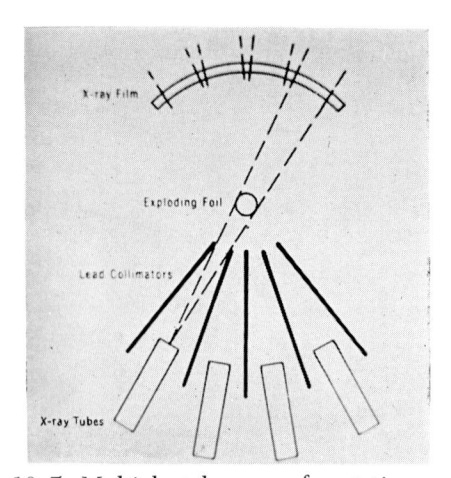

FIGURE 10-7. Multiple tube x-ray for stationary object.

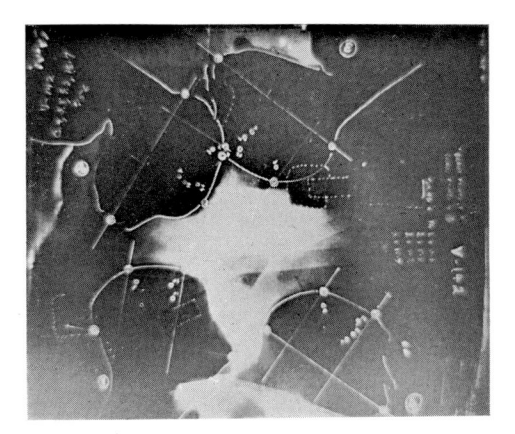

FIGURE 10-8. Multiple x-rays using one tube and 4 rotating cassettes.

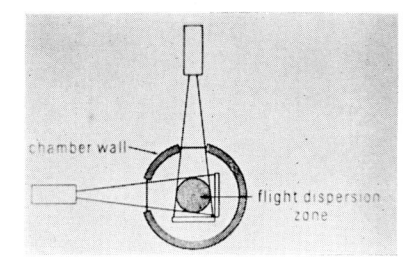

FIGURE 10-9. Orthogonal views obtained with 2 tubes and 2 cassettes.

or by microswitches to fire when each cassette has reached a predetermined position. This arrangement yields a frame rate of 240 frames per second with no overlapping of shots or change of orientation. A set of x-rays taken with the device during impact of a monkey's head is shown as Figure 10-8. Figure 10-9 shows an arrangement using two tubes to obtain a set of orthogonal views.

As spectacular as some of these short duration capabilities are, the flash x-ray systems have not been widely used in diagnostic radiology because of two limitations: (1) The focal spot size in currently-available field emission tubes is of the order of 2 to 5 mm, larger than in conventional x-ray tubes (.3 to 2 mm) which results in less accurate detail and, (2), The tubes are operated at relatively high voltages resulting in the emission of high energy radiation not particularly suited for radiologic examinations.

HIGH SPEED MOTION PICTURES

Most recording of dynamic actions with human and animal subjects is done with high speed motion pictures. Other systems are also used to document movements: the displacement, velocity and acceleration devices mentioned previously. High speed cinematography lends itself to a wide range of uses, alone and in conjunction with other instrumentation. Accelerometers, for example, give excellent information as to the magnitude of acceleration existing *along the axis* of the accelerometer at a given instant. High speed motion pictures could show the orientation of the accelerometer at any moment, allowing correction of the signal. Much of the work with high-speed motion pictures is done by analyzing the pictures for time and displacement data by photographing the subject in front of a grid. Velocity and acceleration data can be obtained by graphical or mathematical analysis of the same data.

With the advent of fine high speed films, including color films, camera speeds have increased rapidly in the last 10 years. While 500 to 1000 frames per second is sufficiently fast for many biomechanics studies, many modern cameras have capacities to 9000 frames per second and speeds as high as 44,000 are readily available. In spite of the high film speeds available, higher speeds require intense lighting and wider apertures—the latter resulting in loss of clarity and depth of field. Hence, the ordinary practice is to use as low a speed as will stop action, as small an aperture as possible consistent with lighting availability or heating restrictions imposed by the subject.

One difficulty with high speed cameras is that the speed is variable during the start-up period. The camera must be started early enough so that it is essentially up to speed before recording the test action. Several devices can be used to validate the test time at a given frame. (1) Many cameras have electronic speed controls, sometimes as an accessory, which will regulate the speed within 1 per cent of a constant value after once reaching test speed. (2) Timing light generators are available which will trigger neon glow lamps and thereby put timing marks on the camera film on a 10, 100 or 1000 cycle per second basis. Thus data can be taken and accurately evaluated even in the case of a camera which is running at other than indicated speed or in a nonregulated system. (3) A timing device—a synchronous motor driving a disc, a circuit pulsing a timing light—can be included in the framing of the test subject and become a part of the data display.

COMBINATION OF SYSTEMS

The systems discussed and other nonphotographic instrumentation are frequently used together for correlation purposes and for the unique information yielded by each device. For example, accelerometers, velocimeters and high-speed photography with a grid background give a great deal of information although with substantial overlapping. The grid background often used in photographic systems, incidentally, is not actually needed as a grid can be introduced at the time of projection for data-taking purposes.

Other combinations of instrumentation are appropriate. The "flash" x-ray system, when used with high speed cinematography, will give internal and external views of the same phenomenon. If the triggering system for the x-ray unit is arranged to cause a light to flash and a timing mark signal is sent to a recording oscillograph where acceleration or velocity data is being taken, the resulting x-rays can be classified as to time, acceleration, and velocity at that moment and, if the photography was from the proper perspective, the external view can be correlated with the x-rays.

An interesting development is the radiation system where both electronic and x-ray radiation are emitted from a single source. The "betagraphs" produced are high contrast electron shadographs, capable of defining small objects or even vapors. The x-rays produced are capable of deep penetration. If a single cassette is appropriately loaded with electron sensitive and x-ray sensitive films, simultaneous exposure can be obtained with this dual radiation. While clinical applications of this kind of radiation are unlikely because of extremely high radiation levels, the dual output with films which can be superimposed yielding detail not possible with either system alone seems of great significance. The name Febetron® is used by Field Emission for these systems.

In summary, the rapid development of instrumentation capable of recording events occurring at high speeds and of extremely short duration has given experimenters in biomechanics tools of great capability. Experimental techniques for the evaluation of the physical properties of the various tissues of the human body under dynamic loadings are being developed, largely based on such instrumentation.

The dynamic as well as the static properties of the body and its tissues must be better defined for the current research in biomechanics to have the maximum eventual clinical use.

DISCUSSION

Voigt R. Hodgson

This chapter contains interesting detail about which many of us using the equipment are often unaware. The rotating disc devised by Mr. Martinez and his colleagues to move x-ray film under a subject at rates up to 240 frames per second, to allow four sequential exposures using a single tube, is an advancement in the science of cineradiography. This will provide resolution sufficient to observe internal body displacements under many dynamic situations, but is still about one order of magnitude too slow for recording a sequence of exposures during short term events, i.e. less than 0.004 of a second. A specific example will show the advantages pointed out by Mr. Martinez in the use of flash x-ray equipment to observe the behavior of biological tissues under dynamic loading.

Consider the two flash x-rays of a monkey head, shown in Figure 10–10. The head is shown on the left before impact, and the exposure on the right was delayed 0.0005 of a second after striker contact with the head. This event produced a peak force of 1260 pounds during a pulse lasting 0.0015 of a second. The head of the animal was free to move and the result-

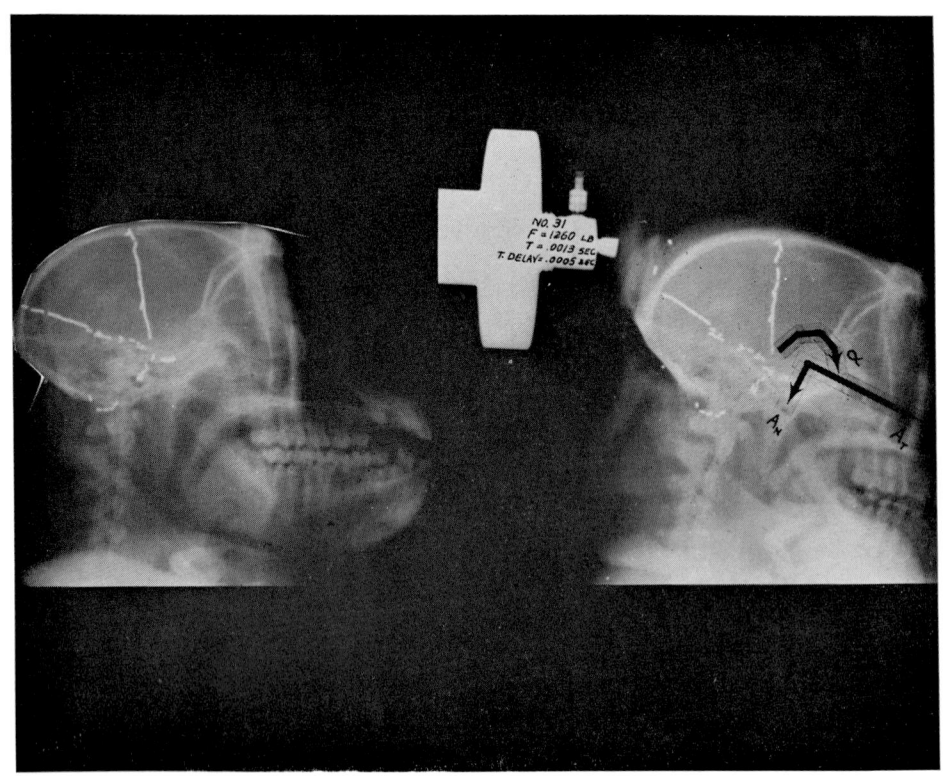

Figure 10–10. Flash x-ray before (left) and during impact to the occiput of a stumptail monkey.

ing motion from this impetus was a combination of translation and rotation. Three lines of lead tags were impregnated in the brain from the top to the base, from the occipital to the base, and across the foramen magnum as shown, to interpret relative displacements in the brain tissue. It has been charged that the displacement experienced by these tags does not represent true brain movement because of the high density of lead compared to brain tissue. This appears to be valid criticism, but a more detailed look at the experiment will show that it does not invalidate the results.

The tags were cut from resin core solder 0.027 of an inch in diameter, 0.125 of an inch long, each weighing approximately 6.6 mg. Specific gravity is therefore about 5.6 instead of 11.34 for pure lead. The limiting maximum stress condition for tissue loading against the end of a tag axially aligned with the direction of accelerated motion of 1000 g, would therefore be only about 25 psi.

The motion of the head during this blow to the occiput, as indicated by the x-rays and high speed photographs, is forward and down, therefore, the inertia forces should be rearward and up. There is no gross observable strain indicated by the lines of tags near the top of the head where inertia forces should be maximum (See overlay of these x-rays in Dr. Thomas' paper). However, two to three millimeters of downward displacement is indicated at the foramen magnum where the inertia forces should have an upward component.

Either of two things could be happening to explain this apparent displacement: (1) Inertia forces are acting on the head to cause the vertebral column to stretch more than the spinal cord, thereby tending to pull the skull off the brain, which seems unlikely; (2) Due to inertia of the contents inside the accelerated skull, pressure gradients arise which act to deform the brain at the foramen magnum. Displacement of the tags represents deformation rather than flow. Evidence from this monkey experiment and from other flash x-ray experiments in the dog indicates that the brain moves grossly in proportion to and in phase with applied force, and returns to its original shape after the force application like an elastic body.[1]

In summary, it appears that rather than invalidating the information gained from this experiment, the use of lead tags (resin core solder) enhances the evidence from this experiment. The tags do not indicate gross movement in areas of highest acceleration where the largest inertia forces act but they do move down at the foramen magnum where the inertia forces are lower and caudal cephalid.

Reference

1. HODGSON, V.R.; GURDJIAN, E.S., and THOMAS, L.M.: Experimental skull deformation and brain displacement demonstrated by flash x-ray technique. *J Neurosurg*, XXV(5):549–552, 1966.

DISCUSSION

Simple Radiographic Techniques for Recording Brain Motion During Acceleration

Donald J. Sass

The purpose of this discussion is to describe a simple radiographic technique, which has been found useful for recording relative motion of visceral organs in cats during whole body vibration. Preliminary results indicate that the technique will provide information concerning brain motion in cats and monkeys during whole body vibration. Similar radiographic methods are suggested in this discussion for future investigations with other acceleration stresses.

The chapter by Hirsch, Ommaya, and Mahone which appears in this book discusses two methods which they used for estimating the natural frequency of rotation of the monkey brain. One method used clinical cineradiography equipment to record the motion of radiopaque markers* implanted in the brain when the monkey's head was shaken by hand. The other method used ultra-high speed motion picture photography to record the motion of brain sulci during impact to the skull. A transparent Lexan calvarium had been chronically implanted in these monkeys using a technique similar to that of Pudenz and Shelden. From their experiments, Hirsch et al. estimate the rotational frequency of the brain to be between 5 and 10 Hz.

The frequency measurements of Hirsch et al. have two possible sources of error. In the Lexan dome experiments, the natural frequency of the brain depends upon how closely the artificial dome replaces the resected calvarium. A larger dome will lower the natural frequency and vice versa. The second source of error is in frame rate. Clinical cineradiography equipment does not place timing marks on the film and frame rates may vary by as much as 25 per cent from their nominal value.

The relative displacements measured with either method did not exceed 2 mm. Resolution is therefore a limiting factor when radiographic methods are used in this application. This is particularly true with high speed flash or pulsed x-ray equipment because the total radiation during each film exposure is small with current equipment. The technique to be described employs high radiation output, relatively inexpensive x-ray equipment.

Editors Note: *From* The Bureau of Medicine and Surgery, Navy Department, Research Task No. MR005.04–0037. (Supported in part by NASA contract R-10.)

* Silicone rubber impregnated with tantalum. Specific weight equivalent to that of brain tissue.

Resolution is better than when low level cineradiography equipment is used, and the sources of error mentioned are eliminated.

The technique is as follows. Cats or small monkeys are immersed in a lucite tank as illustrated in Figure 10–11. Water immersion is used as a restraint to prevent relative motion between the animal and table during vibration. An x-ray cassette is mounted vertically on the table adjacent to the immersion tank and x-rays are directed through the head onto the film. If the film exposure is sufficiently long, then relative motion between radiopaque markers in the brain and film during vibration will produce a blur in the marker image, and the size of this blur will vary with the degree of relative motion.

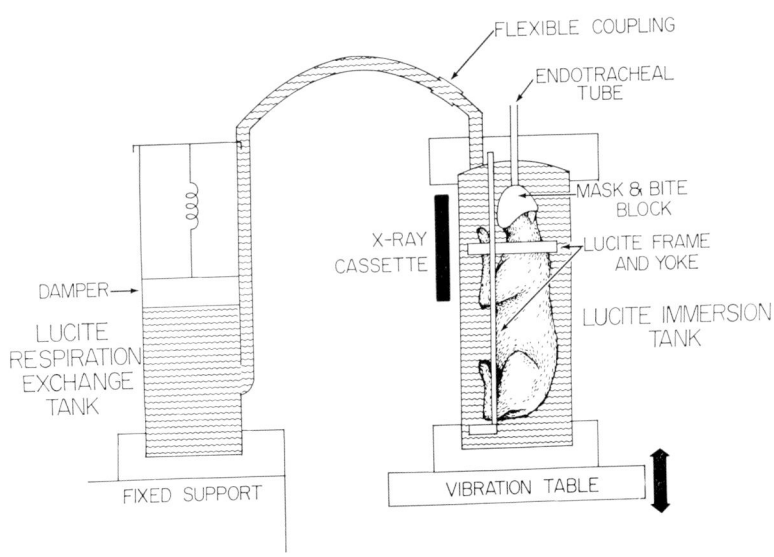

FIGURE 10–11. Water immersion scheme for investigating visceral motion during vibration.

Figure 10–12 is a roentgenogram of a cat made during sinusoidal vibration at 8 Hz 0.4 inch D.A. Film exposure time was 0.8 seconds. The ventricles were opacified with Pantopaque® in this film which is presented to illustrate the technique. Relative motion between different parts of the brain can be demonstrated in a single film using markers placed in the areas of interest. The natural frequency will be measured with this technique by vibrating monkeys with markers at several discrete frequencies over the frequency range of 2 to 20 Hz.

The technique can be further developed as follows. An x-ray cassette is mounted flat on a circular table which can be made to rotate as a roulette wheel or oscillate with harmonic motion about its center of rotation.

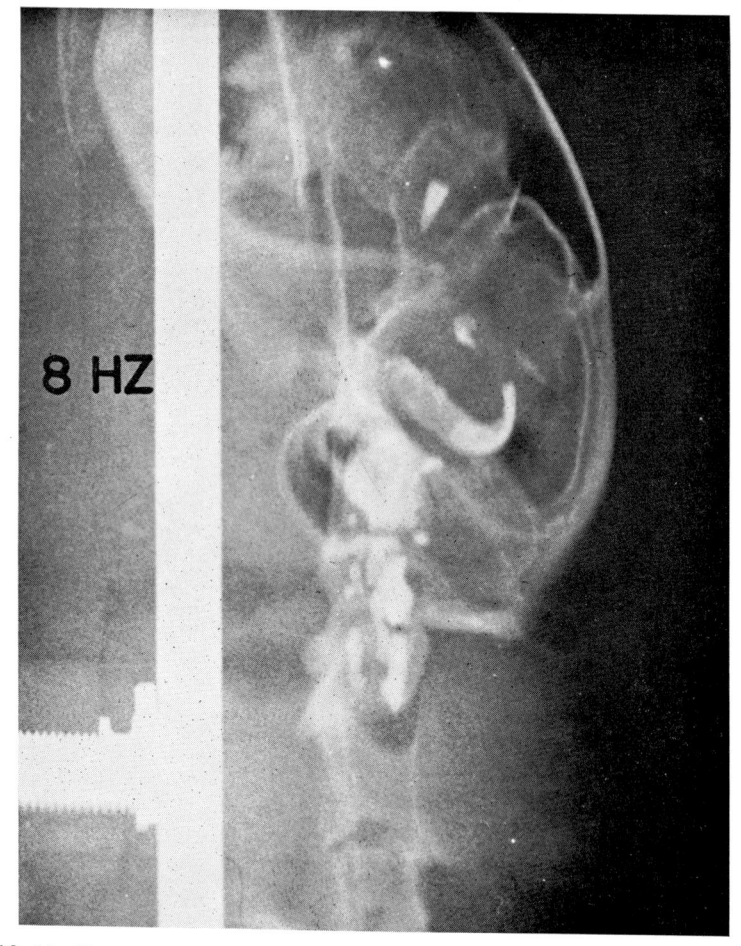

FIGURE 10–12. Roentgenogram made during whole body vibration. 8 Hz 0.4" D.A. ±1.5 g. Exposure time 0.8 seconds. Ventricles opacified with Pantopaque.

Figure 10–13 illustrates the method. The immersion tank is placed over the film with the center of rotation passing through the animal's head, e.g., at the temporomandibular joint. X-rays are directed through the tank onto the film. Relative brain motion can be recorded during abrupt deceleration of the spinning table or during harmonic rotation, similar to the method of Martinez which used gelatin models of the brain. Water immersion is used to minimize acceleration of the test animal. The effects of pure angular acceleration can be studied in the living animal without skull impact or flexion in the cervical region and without linear acceleration. This relatively simple and inexpensive technique may prove to be a satisfactory model for testing the effects of pure angular acceleration on brain motion and concussion.

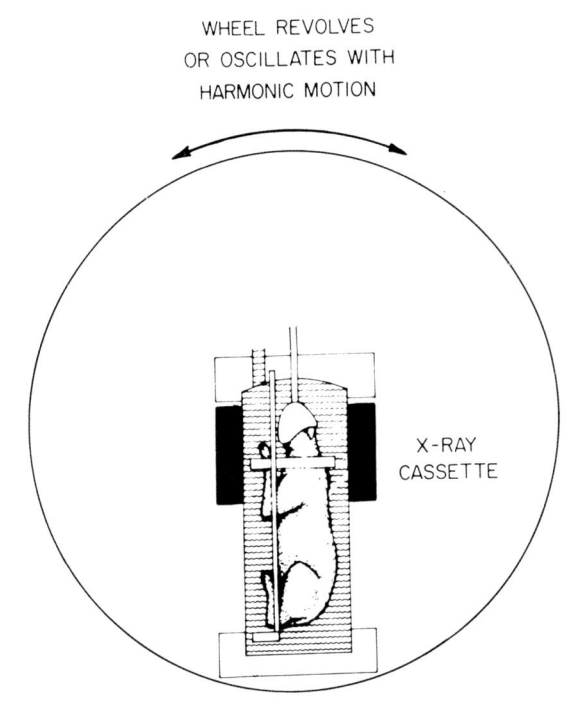

FIGURE 10–13. X-ray technique for investigating rotational motion of the brain during angular acceleration or abrupt deceleration. Also proposed as a model for experimental concussion.

Chapter XI

MATHEMATICAL MODELS FOR INJURY PREDICTION

RAYMOND R. MCHENRY

INTRODUCTION

Mathematical modeling is a technique of physical research in which simplified idealizations are substituted for actual objects, or systems, to make them more amenable to analysis and to aid understanding. Most forms of engineering analysis may be viewed as applications of this technique, in the sense that they involve thinking about physical systems in terms of corresponding mathematical systems that exhibit conditionally equivalent behavior. For example, in engineering analyses of mechanical systems, mathematical abstractions such as point masses, rigid bodies, massless elastic springs, homogeneous and isotropic materials, point forces, rigid frames, etc., are routinely used to form idealizations which embody the essential features of the actual systems, while permitting analytical simplifications. Applications of the modeling technique to several aspects of biomechanics research have received increasing attention in recent years.

The current widespread availability of large-capacity computer facilities has greatly extended the scope of mathematical modeling. Whereas, past analyses of complicated physical systems have required great ingenuity in the selection of extensive simplifying assumptions and in the approximate solution of equations, it is now technically feasible to obtain exact solutions for virtually any equations that can be derived. As a result of this fact, the emphasis in mathematical modeling has shifted from the techniques of simplification and solution of approximate (e.g., linearized) equations to those of derivation of more accurate and detailed equations and logic for "equivalent" mathematical systems.

EDITORS NOTE: This paper is based on research that has been supported by the U.S. Public Health Service, Injury Control Program, National Center for Urban and Industrial Health, Cincinnati, Ohio, Contracts No. PH 108–65–174 and PH 86–68–23, and by the Automobile Manufacturers Association, Contract No. CC-137.

Raymond R. McHenry is the Head of the Engineering Mechanics Section, Transportation Research Department, Cornell Aeronautical Laboratory, Inc.

The adequacy of a selected mathematical model is dependent, of course, on the nature and objectives of the particular analysis. The desired degree of solution detail determines the extent of coarseness of definition that is allowable in the modeling process. In general, the development of an appropriate model is achieved most efficiently by starting with simple analytical representations and adding complexity only to the extent found necessary. The general procedure of development of a mathematical model is outlined in Figure 11–1.

OBJECTIVES OF MATHEMATICAL MODELING IN BIOMECHANICS RESEARCH

In biomechanics, as in all branches of physical research, the primary objective of mathematical modeling is to achieve an understanding of relationships that govern the behavior of physical objects, or systems, and an ability to predict how they will behave under given circumstances. A predictive capability is an essential part of scientific knowledge of any subject, and it generally cannot be acquired from experiments alone. As a minimum, there must be a theoretical framework within which the experimental data can be interpreted. A conditionally validated mathematical model can be applied, within the limitations of its simplifying assumptions, to organize and interpret observational material and also to determine approximate values of parameters that are not directly measurable.

In the following paragraphs, some representative mathematical models of different aspects of acceleration responses of the human body are briefly described, with particular emphasis given to the prediction of injury. The specific objectives and the limitations of each model are indicated. A comprehensive review is not attempted, in view of the existence of other recent and excellent reviews of the general subject matter.[1,2]

REPRESENTATIVE MODELS

Existing mathematical models that are relevant to the present review may be categorized as attempts at either (1) direct or (2) indirect predictions of injuries in given acceleration exposures. Within the context of the present discussion, "direct" prediction of injury is taken to mean that the actual injury mechanism is modeled (e.g., tissue strain). "Indirect" prediction is taken to mean that the acceleration or the dynamic loading is predicted for one or more portions of the body and that the injury potential of these items is evaluated in terms of separately determined tolerance information.

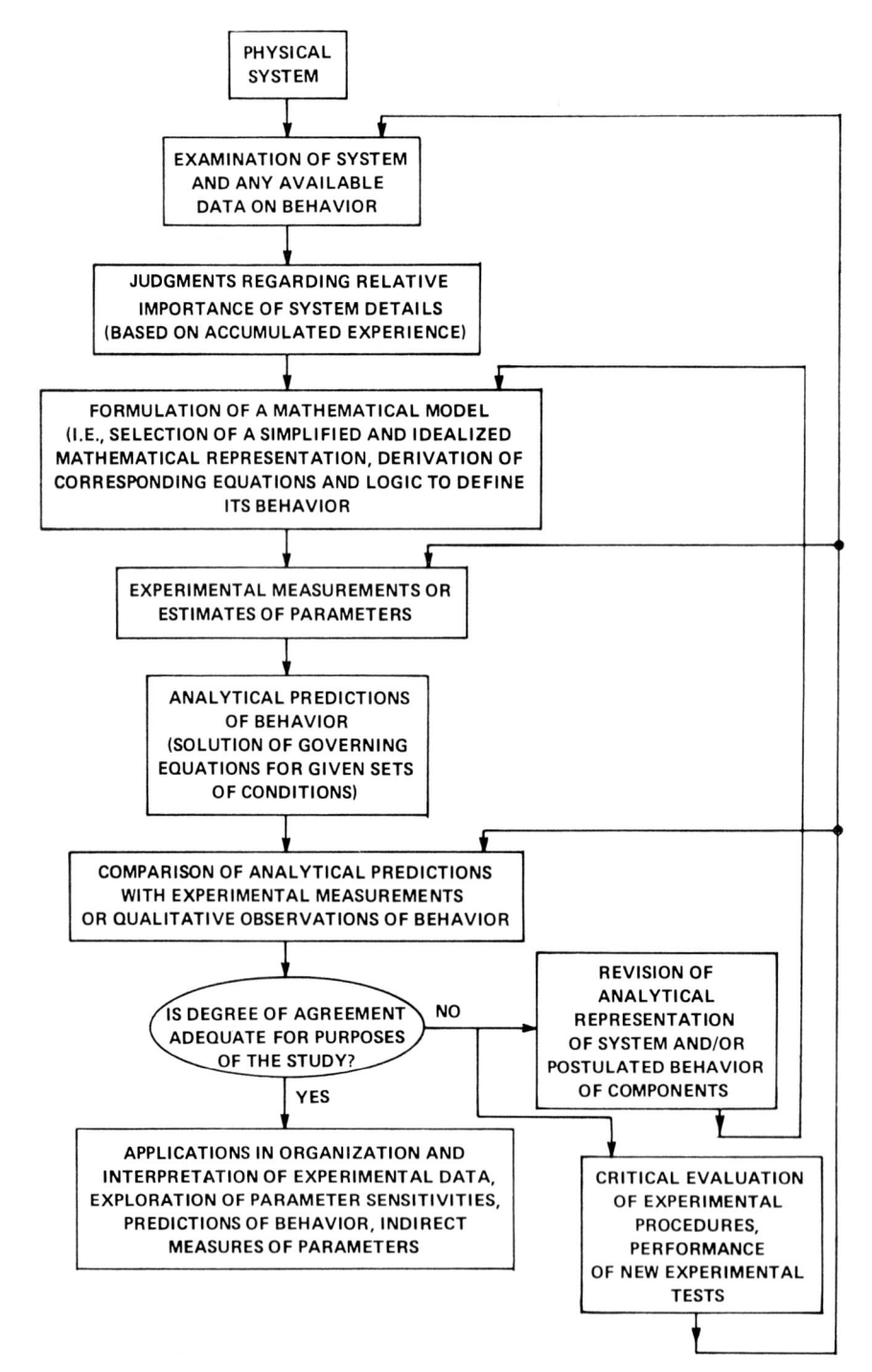

FIGURE 11-1. Procedure of model development.

It should be noted that a similar categorization can be made of physical simulations in the sense that most anthropometric dummies are designed to withstand extreme exposures without damage, while producing acceleration and force measurements that are interpreted in terms of separately determined tolerance levels. Recent developments in dummies, such as the frangible "Sophisticated Sam"[3] and the UCLA-Sierra "trauma-indicating" dummy[4] are aimed at achieving direct indications of injury as, of course, are cadaver and animal test specimens.

Direct Injury Prediction

Lumped-Parameter Models

Several simple, lumped-parameter models (e.g., see Fig. 11–2) are described by Payne[5] with which measurements of whole body human tolerance in the positive spinal and transverse directions and of head tolerance have been extrapolated. The "spinal" models depicted in Figure 11–2 assume a properly supported erect posture. The limiting item of

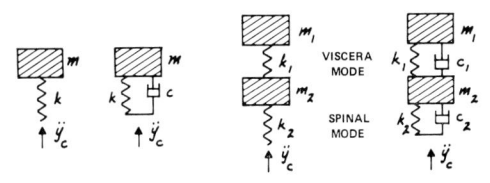

FIGURE 11–2. Models for spinal compression (Payne,[5]).

response (i.e. the injury predictor) is taken to be the peak spring strain in the spinal mode. Tolerance plots are generated for given waveforms of acceleration time-histories, corresponding to predictions of compression fracture thresholds. The several indicated directions of exposure are treated in a similar manner. However, each direction is treated separately. In each case, full restraint is assumed (i.e. effects of posture changes are not included).

A more elaborate model of the human body, for exposure to spineward-accelerations and to external pressure loads, is described by von Gierke[2] (see Figure 11–3). The described model is treated, for simplicity, as a passive linear system. The assumption is made that injury is produced by relative displacements within the system, and curves of constant critical tissue strain (i.e. injury thresholds) are calculated and plotted for the various subsystems. With the availability of more extensive applicable biological data, the model can, of course, be extended to include non-linear effects and time-varying constraints (e.g., muscular actions). The major limitation, therefore, is seen to be the restriction to purely spineward acceleration vectors and to the condition of erect posture.

218   *Impact Injury and Crash Protection*

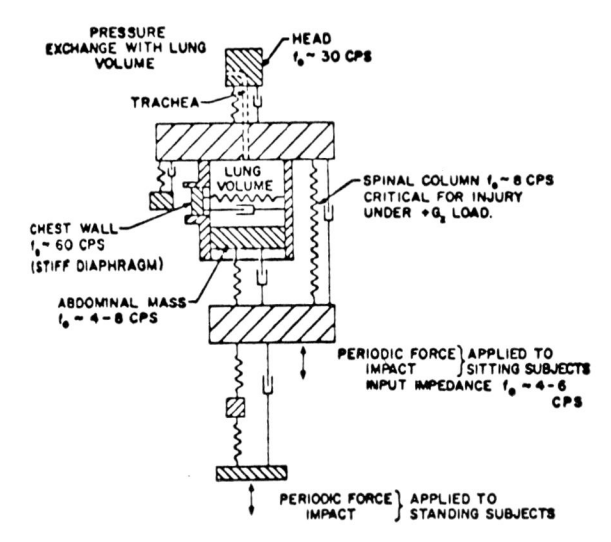

FIGURE 11-3. Mechanical model of the human body exposed to g_z vibration or impact and to external pressure loads (acoustic, blast, decompression loads) (Von Gierke[2]).

The mathematical model of the head and neck that is described by Martinez, et al.,[7] (see Fig. 11-4) can be viewed as a development aimed ultimately at direct prediction of injury, in the sense that it simulates the body mechanism (i.e. the head-neck action) associated with the specific injury of interest, "whiplash." As more definitive injury criteria are developed for the "whiplash" type of injury (e.g., maximum deflection of the neck, rotational acceleration of the head), the analytically predicted actions can be compared with injury thresholds. The model, as described, is limited to planar motions in rear collisions and to linear system char-

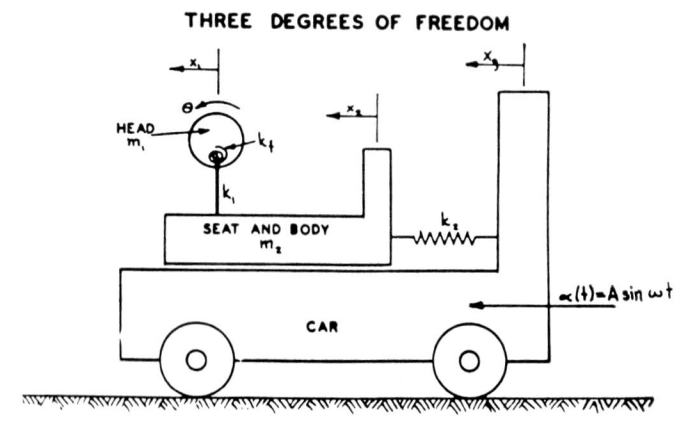

FIGURE 11-4. Head-neck model (Martinez, et al.,[7]).

acteristics. However, reference 7 indicates that continued development, to include damping and friction, is in progress.

A Proposed Distributed-Parameter Head Model

A long-range program of research that includes the development of a mathematical model to predict head injury has been proposed by Goldsmith.[6] For the theoretical part of the program, he proposes starting with a dynamic analysis of the responses to point impact of an elastic spherical shell filled with an ideal compressible fluid (Fig. 11-5). The proposed analytical development would proceed with variations of the shape and/or thickness of the shell and the viscous properties of the fluid until an experimentally validated model of the human head has been achieved. Goldsmith suggests that the applicability of the method of finite elements should be explored in relation to the proposed shell analysis.

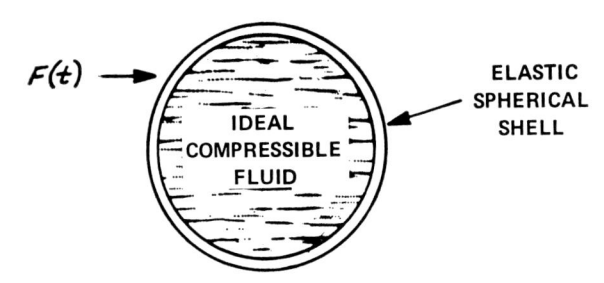

FIGURE 11-5. Schematic of a proposed head model (Goldsmith[6]).

The task of interpreting analytical results from the proposed head model in terms of trauma would require the combined efforts of physicians and scientists. Such efforts would include, for example, consideration of the shearing effects in the brain produced by skull distortion and head rotation, further study of the mechanism of cavitation and determination of the elastic limit and fracture strength of the skull.

It would appear to be desirable to also include early consideration of an appropriate simulation of the inertial loading and constraints imposed by the neck.

Indirect Injury Prediction

In the case of automobile collisions, large and highly variable changes can occur in the position and orientation of the occupant, even with the use of existing restraints. The automobile case is further complicated by the wide ranges of occupant size and weight that must be taken into consideration in safety improvements. In view of the complicating factors, several highly simplified mathematical models have been developed to explore fundamental relationships within the occupant-restraint-compartment system. Gross interpretations of injury potential, either absolute or relative, have been based on separately determined tolerance information or on selected measures of severity. These models may, therefore, be viewed as indirect predictors of injury.

Point-Mass Models

A highly simplified, point-mass representation of an unrestrained occupant (Fig. 11-6) has been applied by Martin and Kroell[8] to study the gross effects of initial occupant spacing on the interior crush depth in frontal automobile collisions. Evaluations of the relative injury potential

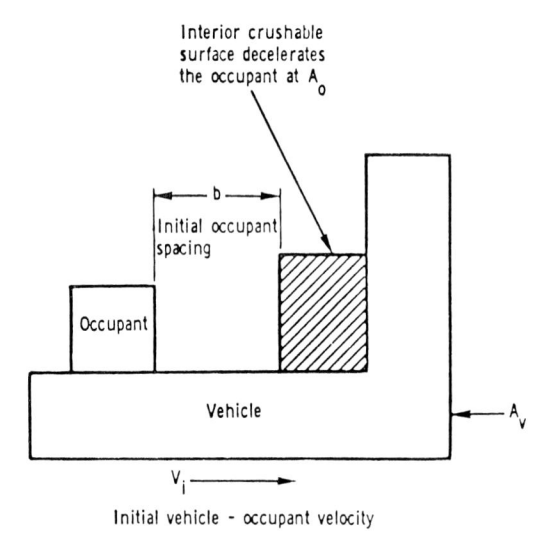

FIGURE 11-6. Single mass occupant model (Martin and Kroell,[8]).

were based on the predicted interior crush depth (i.e. a gross indication of the severity of the "second collision").

Point-mass models have also been used by Egli[9] and Grime[10] in fundamental studies of the behavior of a restrained occupant in a frontal automobile collision (e.g. see Fig. 11-7). Egli's evaluations of injury potential were based entirely on consideration of the occupant (i.e. the point-mass) deceleration. Grime's evaluations of relative injury hazards were based on predictions of the velocity with which the simulated occupant would strike the vehicle interior, with consideration also given to the level of occupant deceleration produced by the restraints.

The limitations of the described point-mass models were, of course, both fully recognized and clearly stated by the cited investigators. The models were aimed only at investigations of fundamental relationships in purely frontal collisions.

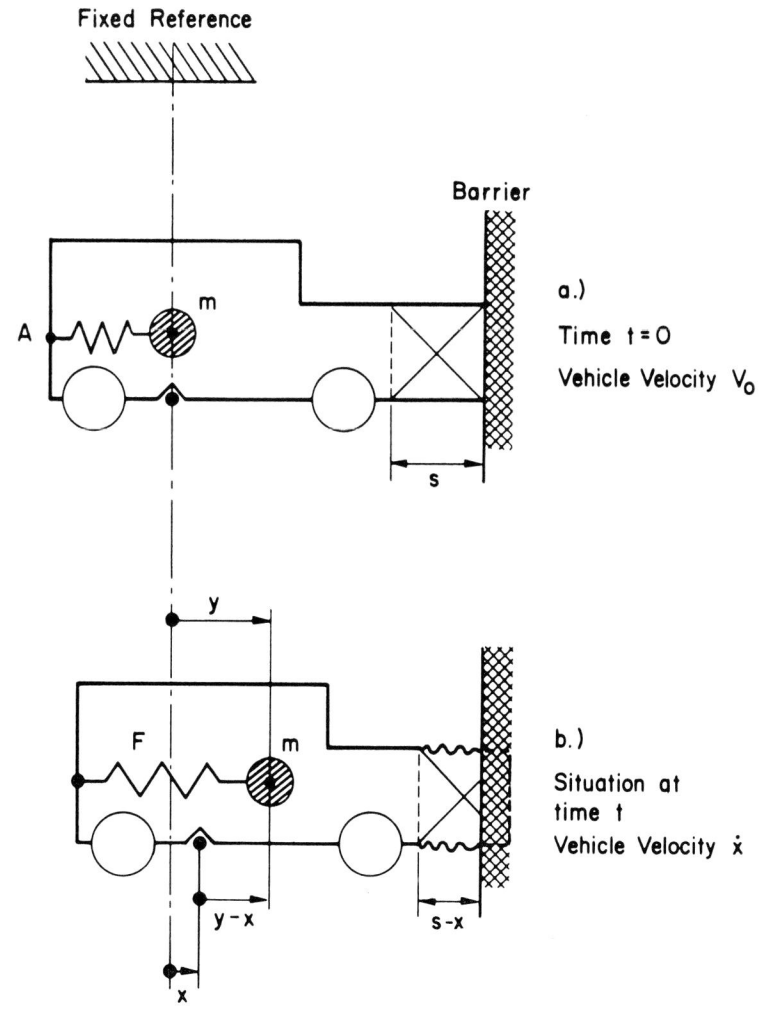

FIGURE 11-7. The crash system (Egli,[9]).

Two-Mass Models

Somewhat more complicated, two-mass models of restrained occupants in frontal automobile collisions have been developed and applied by Ryan and BeVier[11] and Renneker.[12] Ryan's study (Fig. 11-8) was limited to an approximate representation of a lap belt restraint. Renneker's study (Fig. 11-9) included the cases of lap belt and lap belt plus upper torso restraint. In the Ryan study, interpretations of injury potential were based on the magnitude of the predicted hip acceleration. Renneker's interpretations were based on the magnitudes of the predicted belt loads.

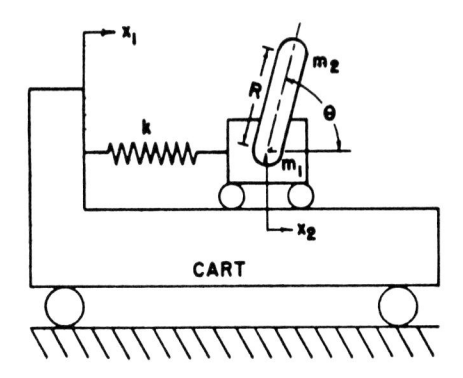

NOTATIONS:
m_1 - mass of body excluding upper part of body
m_2 - mass of upper part of body.
k - stiffness of belt.
x_2 - displacement of hip.
θ - angular displacement of upper part of body
x_1 - displacement of cart.

FIGURE 11–8. Two-mass model (Ryan and Bevier,[11]).

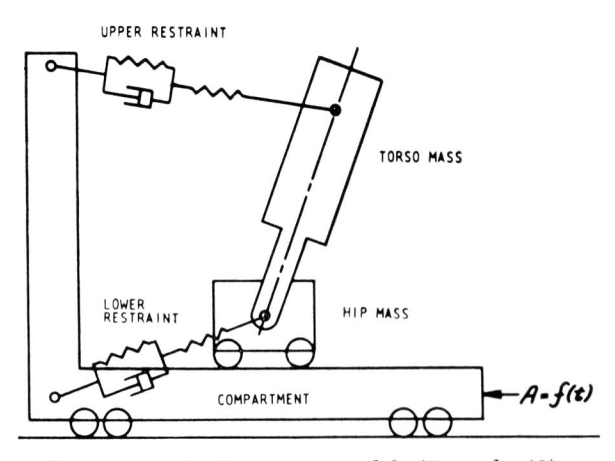

FIGURE 11–9. Two-mass model (Renneker[12]).

The CAL 11-Degree of Freedom Model

A relatively elaborate mathematical model of the automobile crash victim in longitudinal (i.e. fore and aft) collisions has been developed by the Cornell Aeronautical Laboratory, Inc. (CAL).[13,14] In the development of the more recent refinements and modifications,[14] CAL has worked with the Analytical Model Simulation Committee of the Automobile Manufacturers Association, Inc. This model (Fig. 11–10) will be described in greater detail in view of both its complexity and the author's detailed

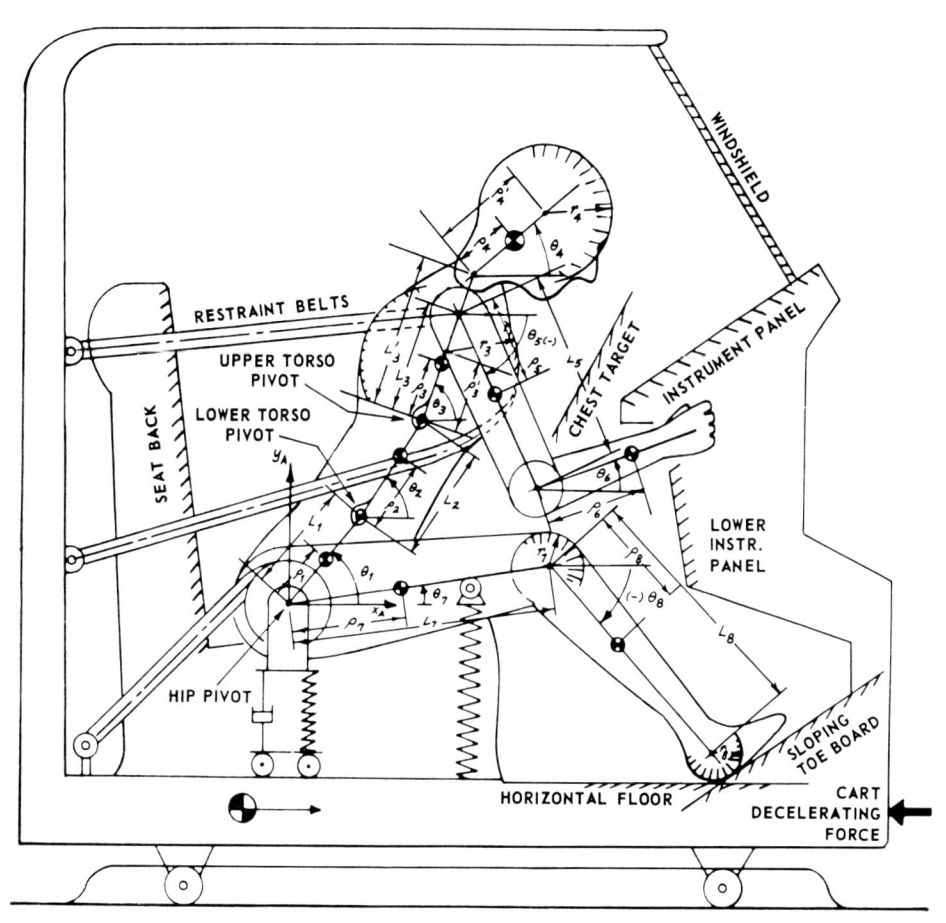

FIGURE 11-10. Mathematical model of human body and restraint system on test cart (11 degrees of freedom).

familiarity through direct involvement with this research. Injury hazard assessments in the case of the CAL model have been based primarily on evaluations of the accelerations and forces predicted for several components of the body (i.e. head, chest and pelvis), in terms of separately determined tolerance information. However, in one application,[15] a gross measure of the relative hazards associated with spinal bending, on the basis of the predicted energy absorption in torso bending, was developed and applied.

The CAL research program has been aimed at a simulation of whole body kinematics and of the inertial loading of restraint belts and body areas that impact the vehicle interior, rather than at a detailed treatment of biomechanical characteristics. The human body has, therefore, been approximated by an articulated assembly of rigid mass segments, with dimensions and inertial properties that are sufficiently representative to provide characteristic motions of the torso and extremities.

Solution Forms

The digital computer calculations have been programmed for two forms of time-history solutions.

In the first form, where occupant-to-vehicle interactions are simulated, the free response of the complete 11-degree-of-freedom system depicted in Figure 11–10 is determined. A general form of vehicle-stopping mechanism, that responds to the velocity and displacement of the vehicle, decelerates the system from an initial velocity. With this form of solution, the adequacy of a test sled and its stopping mechanism for a physical simulation of actual vehicle collisions can be evaluated (i.e. the effects of interaction on the resulting deceleration time-history of the sled can be determined).

In the second form of solution, the forced response of the 10-degree-of-freedom articulated body is determined with an experimental or idealized time-history of vehicle deceleration serving as the forcing function.

Simulation of Belt and Impact Forces

The belt, contact (i.e. corresponding to impact against interior surfaces of the vehicle), and seat forces on the occupant are calculated from the relative displacements and velocities within the system during a stepwise numerical integration of the equations of motion. A nonlinear load-deflection subroutine is applied to each of the force-generating components in turn, for which the analytic geometry of the simulation indicates the possible existence of a force. The resulting forces are applied in the equations of motion during the particular increment of time.

The load-deflection relationship in each of the force-generating components is treated in the manner depicted in Figure 11–11. A general poly-

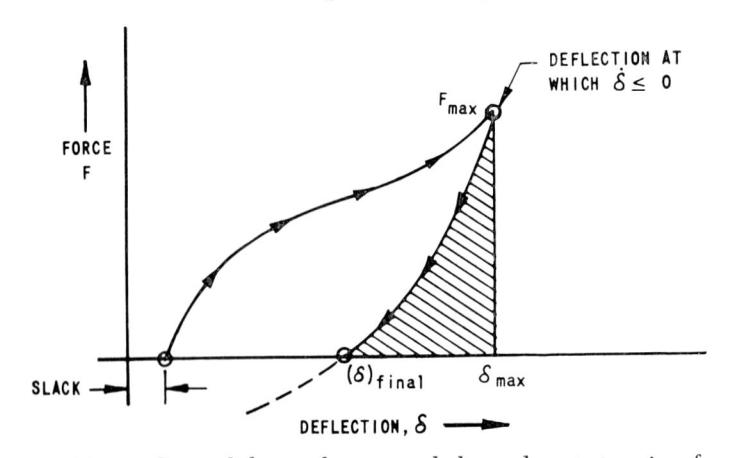

FIGURE 11–11. General form of contact, belt, and cart-stopping forces.

nomial function of deflection and the velocity of deflection, representing the composite load-deformation properties of the force-generating component and the corresponding portion of the occupant, is used to generate increasing loads. For decreasing loads, the load-deflection relationship is represented by a parabolic function of deflection that is determined from specified (input data) ratios of (1) conserved energy to total absorbed energy, and (2) residual deflection to maximum deflection.

Joint Representation

Each of the joints in the simulated body includes adjustable friction. Some of the joints also include adjustable motion-limiting stops and adjustable elasticity.

In the earlier version of the computer program,[13] exploratory developmental changes resulted in a nonuniform analytical treatment of the various joints in the simulated occupant. Also, certain deficiencies in the simulated, joint stops were indicated in the initial validation study reported in reference 13. The large magnitude, high frequency spikes that occurred in the calculated head and chest accelerations, and the insufficient joint recovery after the engagement of stops were found to have been caused, in large part, by the use of completely nonconservative analytical treatments of the joint stops. The earlier forms of treatment of the joint stops were based on the results of static measurements of the Alderson F-50 AU dummy; however, the dynamic behavior of that dummy as observed in films of the test series reported in reference 13 and in the corresponding acceleration traces, indicated that a portion of the joint-stop energy was conserved and returned to the adjacent body segments.

Changes were, therefore, incorporated,[14] aimed at the achievement of an improved and uniform analytical treatment of the occupant joints. The changes include the incorporation of two similar third-order polynomial stops (for positive and negative relative motion) in each joint, with a capability for unsymmetrical placement in relation to initial joint angularity and with independently adjustable linear elasticity about the initial position, in addition to the existing adjustable coulomb friction. Each joint stop also has the capability for a variable amount of energy dissipation. The mechanism for energy dissipation in the joint stops is a hysteresis loop formed by unloading along a curve similar to the loading curve but shifted toward larger angular displacements. The general form of the present joint-stop representation is depicted in Figure 11–12.

Since no data are known to be available on the actual dynamic characteristics of dummy or human joint stops, the parameters indicated in Figure 11–12 have been adjusted to limit the relative angularity between adjacent body segments to the maximum values observed in the more severe tests of the initial validation series.[13] The amount of energy dissi-

FOR LOADING $(SGN\ \theta_r = SGN\ \dot{\theta}_r)$,

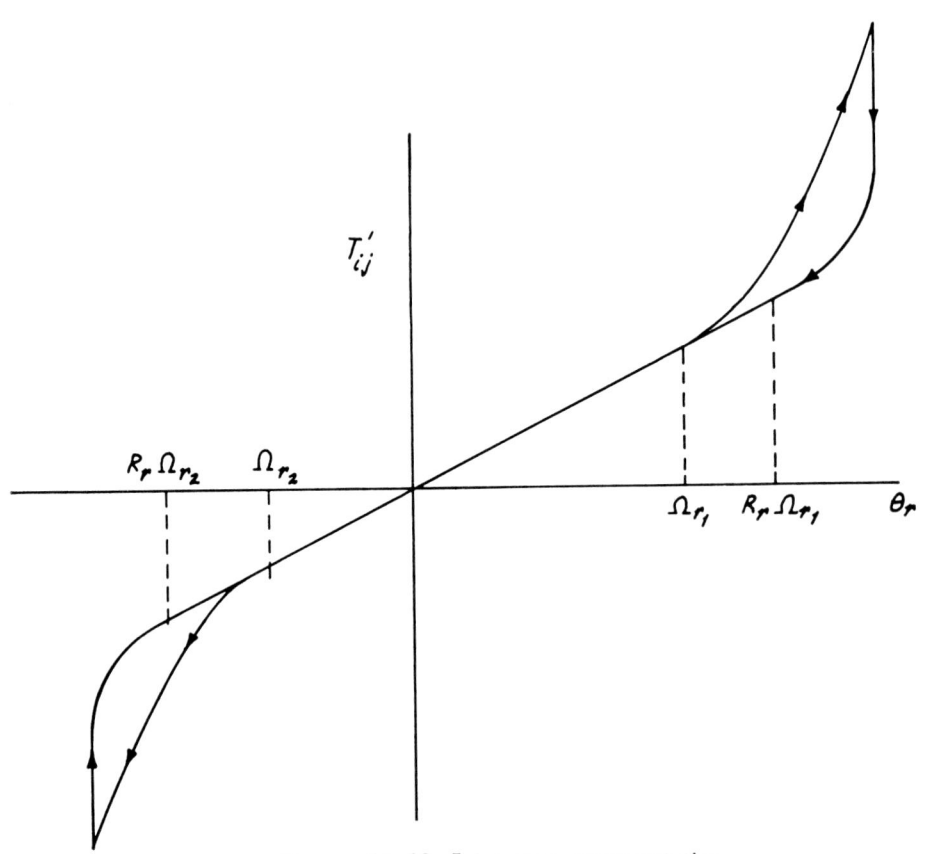

$$T'_{ij} = \begin{cases} K_r(\theta_r), & \text{FOR } \Omega_{r_2} \leq \theta_r \leq \Omega_{r_1} \\ K_r(\theta_r) + K_{r_1}(\theta_r - \Omega_{r_1})^2 + K_{r_2}(\theta_r - \Omega_{r_1})^3, & \text{FOR } \theta_r > \Omega_{r_1} \\ K_r(\theta_r) - K_{r_1}(\theta_r - \Omega_{r_2})^2 + K_{r_2}(\theta_r - \Omega_{r_2})^3, & \text{FOR } \theta_r < \Omega_{r_2} \end{cases}$$

FOR UNLOADING $(SGN\ \theta_r \neq SGN\ \dot{\theta}_r)$

$$T'_{ij} = \begin{cases} K_r(\theta_r), & \text{FOR } R_r\Omega_{r_2} \leq \theta_r \leq R_r\Omega_{r_1} \\ K_r(\theta_r) + K_{r_1}(\theta_r - R_r\Omega_{r_1})^2 + K_{r_2}(\theta_r - R_r\Omega_{r_1})^3, & \text{FOR } \theta_r > R_r\Omega_{r_1} \\ K_r(\theta_r) - K_{r_1}(\theta_r - R_r\Omega_{r_2})^2 + K_{r_2}(\theta_r - R_r\Omega_{r_2})^3, & \text{FOR } \theta_r < R_r\Omega_{r_2} \end{cases}$$

FIGURE 11-12. Joint stop representation.

pation in the joint stops (i.e. the extent of the energy dissipation beyond that produced by the measured values of friction) has been estimated on the basis of the observed recovery after engagement of the stops.

Acceleration Filter

In the present form of the CAL simulation, the articulated, rigid-body representation of the occupant, in combination with simulated step discontinuities (e.g. coulomb friction) and the discontinuities inherent in a digital form of solution, tends to generate response frequencies that are higher than those of an actual physical system (i.e. an anthropometric dummy, a cadaver or a living subject). Also, the data gathering equipment used in accelerator sled and full-scale crash experiments has inherent low-pass filtering characteristics which are frequently extended by means of auxiliary low-pass filters, to eliminate unwanted high frequencies. For these reasons, the unfiltered acceleration outputs of the computer simulation tend to include response frequencies that are substantially higher than those in related experimental data.

The function of any filter is, of course, to remove unwanted frequency ranges from a time-history, and its use ultimately rests on the assumption that data outside the selected frequency range are of no significance in the phenomenon under investigation. In much of the available data on human tolerances, the effects of both unintentional and intentional filtering are present. As a result, the rates-of-onset and peak values of acceleration that are associated with experimental injury thresholds generally reflect the effects of low-pass filtering. The recent incorporation in the CAL simulation of an adjustable digital filter[14] with completely defined performance characteristics, permits direct comparisons between calculated and measured acceleration responses with similar frequency contents.

Computer Graphics Display

To ease the task of interpretation of the rather extensive output information, a computer graphics display of the simulated occupant kinematics has been developed (see Figures 11–13 and 11–14). The display is produced either on an XY plotter or on a cathode ray tube.

The top rows of Figures 11–13 and 11–14 show frames from motion pictures of sled tests that physically simulated frontal collisions at 10 mph. The anthropometric dummy in the sled tests was restrained by a lap belt in Figure 11–13 and by a lap and torso restraint in Figure 11–14. The bottom rows of the two figures show corresponding frames from a computer-generated display based on the mathematical model of occupant response.

Computer-generated motion pictures have also been produced by means of a flying spot scanner which traces the occupant, in its computed position and orientation, with a dot of light on a cathode ray tube. A new position for the dummy is computed for each frame. A camera, with its shutter open, exposes a single frame for each display. In this way, a motion picture is made frame by frame.

Current Status

The general agreement between responses measured in sled tests (with anthropometric dummies) and predictions of the mathematical model has

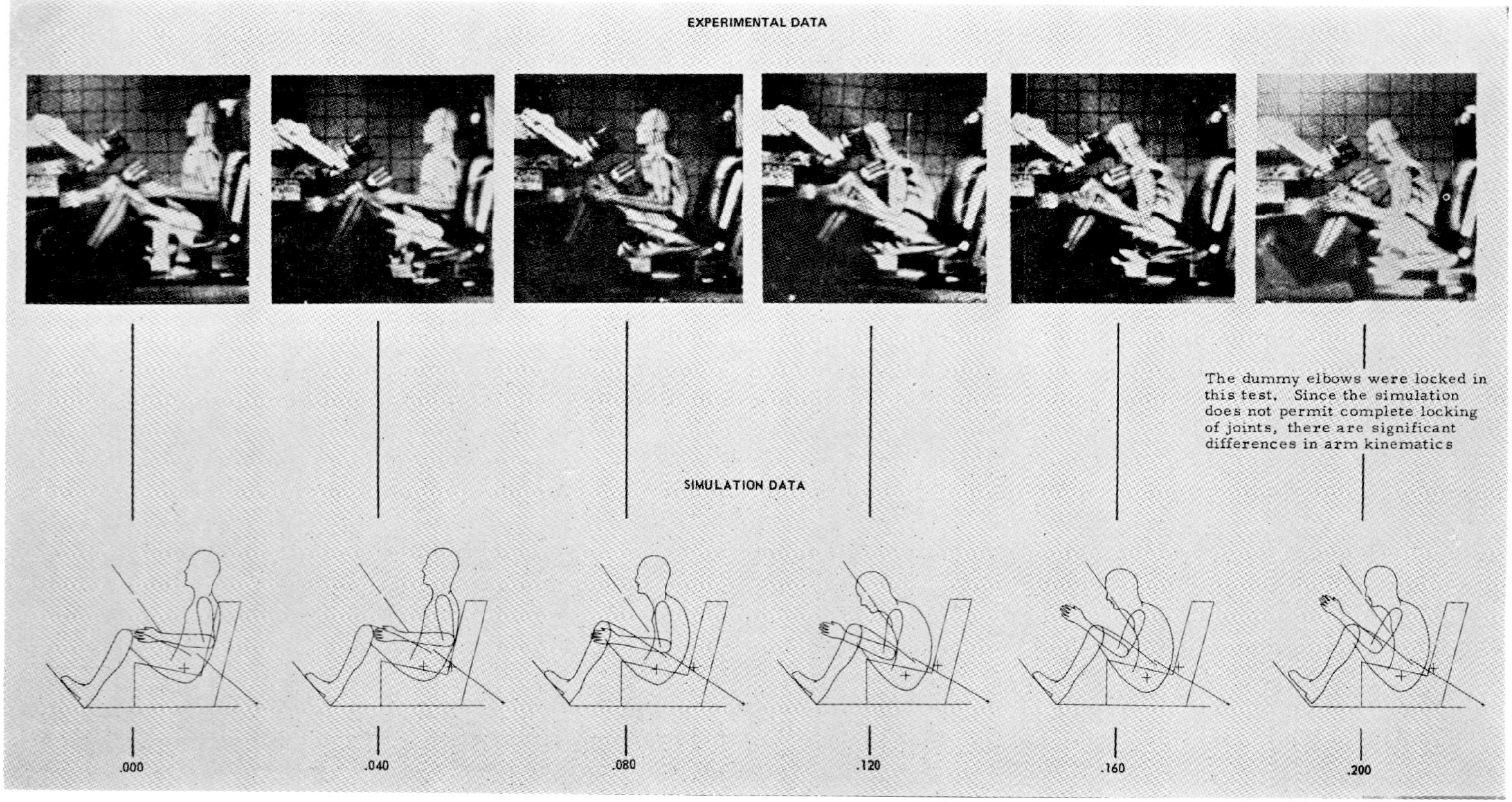

FIGURE 11–13. Dummy kinematic comparison lap belt restraint–cart velocity 10 mph.

FIGURE 11–14. Dummy kinematic comparison lap and torso restraint—cart velocity 10 mph.

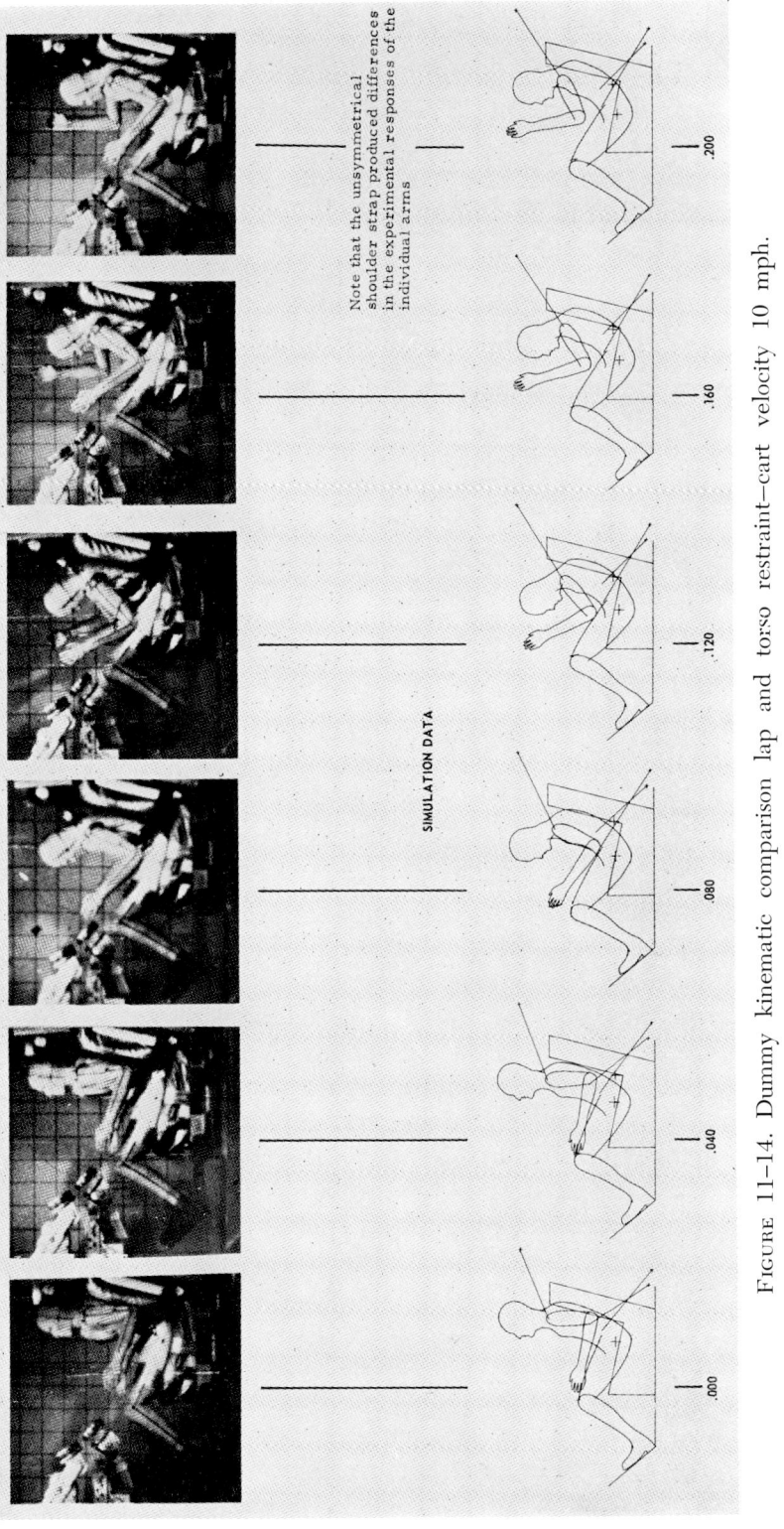

been found to be quite good, particularly following the recent incorporation of several refinements.[14] Comparisons have been made in occupant kinematics, the timing of events, the general levels of peak values and in waveforms of time-histories. A continuing program of development is in progress, aimed at further improving the detailed correlation with experiments and at extending the generality of the mathematical model.

LIMITATIONS OF MATHEMATICAL MODELING

While mathematical models for injury prediction have not yet progressed to the point where admonitions concerning excessive confidence are necessary, consideration of limitations is appropriate in relation to expectations for future developments.

In reference 16, Golomb lists pitfalls inherent in mathematical modeling. He refers, of course, to models in more highly developed fields than injury prediction. However, some of his admonitions that are pertinent to anticipated future developments related to the present topic, are repeated here:

1. "No model is ever a perfect fit to reality. Deductions based on the model must be regarded with appropriate suspicion."
2. "Don't apply any model until you understand the simplifying assumptions on which it is based and can test their applicability."
3. "Don't limit yourself to a single model. More than one model may be useful for understanding different aspects of the same phenomenon."

Mathematical models can never replace experiments, but they can constitute a valuable supplement to experiments as means of interpretation and extrapolation of results. A capability of extrapolation is particularly important in the case of automobile collisions, where the wide distributions of occupant sizes and weights, conditions of restraint and accident speeds and types make a purely experimental approach unfeasible. A definitive program of experiments with a proposed safety improvement would require a large number of sizes of test specimens, and the cost of the required number of experiments would tend to be prohibitive. Also, it is difficult to repeat experimental test conditions. The cumulative effects of variations in the occupant position, slack in restraints, muscle tone in the test subject, the detailed waveform of the vehicle deceleration time-history, etc., tend to produce a poor repeatability. Since the occupant-restraint-vehicle collision system in the so-called "second collision" is highly nonlinear, it is not possible to directly extrapolate experimental results.

Thus, while caution must be exercised in the application of mathematical models, they are seen as an essential part of future biomechanics research, particularly in relation to automobile collisions.

PROBABLE FUTURE DEVELOPMENTS

Biomechanics research is predominantly experimental at the present time. However, as it attracts more extensive study by dynamicists and as more quantitative data are generated, it appears likely that computer-based (i.e. highly detailed, nonlinear) mathematical models will play an increasingly important role. The following sequence of developments is foreseen for such mathematical models.

Extension of Planar Whole Body Models

The incorporation of generalized, lumped-parameter representations of individual organs and subsystems of the body (i.e. for multidirectional excitation) into a whole-body, articulated and deformable model of the skeletal structure is the next logical step in the extension of planar models. Such an extension will be aimed at the provision of direct indications of injury for arbitrary planar acceleration vectors and for a variety of conditions of restraint. It should also be noted that the effects of time-varying muscular restraints can be quite readily explored in such a mathematical model by means of tabular inputs for joint restraints and for the bending stiffness of the spinal structure.

Initial exploratory research directed toward this ultimate goal is currently in progress at CAL.

A Three-Dimensional Whole Body Model

For the case of the automobile crash victim, whose exposure includes oblique vehicle collisions with substantial angular accelerations, a three-dimensional mathematical model appears to be an essential supplement to experiments. Such a model could be applied in studies of kinematics, inertial loading and regions of contact with the vehicle interior for different occupant sizes and weights, conditions of restraint and ranges of exposure severity.

In view of the obvious analytical complexities, the initial version of a three-dimensional model will probably be an articulated rigid-body representation similar to the existing CAL planar model of the automobile crash victim.[14] It will, therefore, be an indirect predictor of injury.

A computer graphics display of an articulated three-dimensional human figure, such as that described by Fetter[17] (see Fig. 11–15), would appear to be most helpful in the development, validation and application of a three-dimensional simulation. The display described by Fetter is currently being used by Boeing to animate personnel subsystems studies (e.g., extreme reach capabilities).

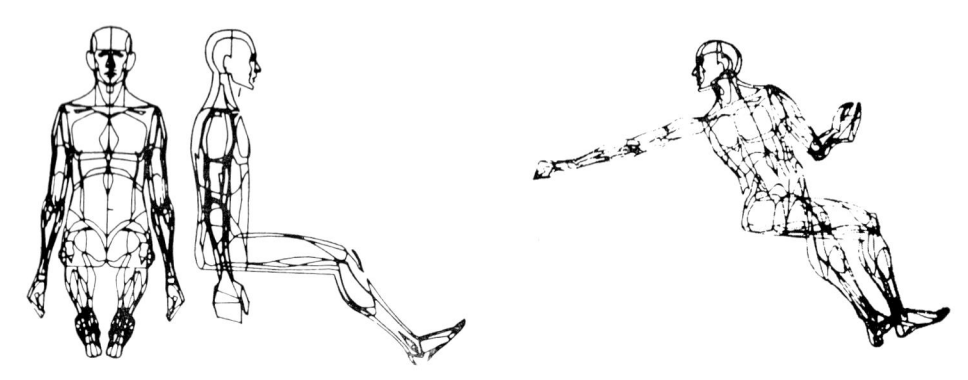

FIGURE 11–15. Computer graphics display of 3-dimensional human figure (*from* Fetter).

Detailed Models of Body Components

Detailed models of body components, such as that proposed by Goldsmith[6] for the head, are expected to be developed in programs of research that will be concurrent with those of the whole body models described in items 1 and 2. The extent to which such detailed submodels need be integrated into the whole body models will be determined by the degree of interaction that is found to exist. Where interaction effects are not significant, the whole body models can provide loading conditions for auxiliary injury predicting submodels.

CONCLUSIONS

The simplified nature of the models that have been discussed reflects the present early stage of development of analytical techniques for the biomechanics of injuries in acceleration exposures. The human body is a highly complicated nonlinear mechanism which has been modeled only in a gross manner for limited forms of acceleration exposure. However, the vast existing technology of engineering mechanics has not yet been fully brought to bear on the problem.

The growing interest among dynamicists and engineers in this area of research, particularly in relation to automobile safety, is expected to produce a greater future emphasis on mathematical models. Also, the rapidly developing technology of computers and computer applications is expected to play a major role in making acceleration responses and injury predictions amenable to analytical study.

Mathematical models are seen as an essential part of future biomechanics research, particularly in relation to automobile collisions.

REFERENCES

1. ROBERTS, V.O.; STECH, E.L., and TERRY, C.T.: Review of mathematical models which describe human response to acceleration. *ASME Paper No. 66–WA/BHF–13*, Nov. 27-Dec. 1, 1966.
2. VON GIERKE, H.E.: Biodynamic response of the human body. *Appl Mechanics Rev*, Dec. 1964, pp. 951–958.
3. BLOOM, A.; CICHOWSKI, W.G., and ROBERTS, V.L.: Sophisticated Sam–a new concept in dummies. *SAE Paper No. 680031*, Detroit, Jan. 8–12, 1968.
4. SEVERY, D.M.: Human simulations for automotive research. *SAE SP–266*, Jan. 1965.
5. PAYNE, P.R.: The dynamics of human restraint systems. Impact acceleration stress. National Academy of Sciences, National Research Council, *Publication 977*, 1962, pp. 195–257.
6. GOLDSMITH, W.: The physical processes producing head injuries. *Proceedings of the Head Injury Conference.* Philadelphia, Lippincott, 1966, pp. 350–382.
7. MARTINEZ, J.L.; WICKSTROM, J.K., and BARCELO, B.T.: The whiplash injury–a study of head-neck action and injuries in animals. *ASME Paper No. 65–WA/HUF–6*, Nov. 7–11, 1965.
8. MARTIN, D.E., and KROELL, C.K.: Vehicle crush and occupant behavior. *SAE Paper No. 670034*, Detroit, Jan. 9–13, 1967.
9. EGLI, A.: Stopping the occupant of a crashing vehicle–a fundamental study. *SAE Paper No. 670038*, Detroit, Jan. 9–13, 1967.
10. GRIME, G.: Safety cars. *Road Research Laboratory, Report No. 8*, Harmondsworth, 1966.
11. RYAN, J.J., and BEVIER, W.: *Safety Devices for Ground Vehicles.* Mechanical Engineering Dept., University of Minnesota, Minneapolis, Sept. 1, 1960.
12. RENNEKER, D.N.: A basic study of "energy-absorbing" vehicle structure and occupant restraints by mathematical model. *Proceedings of SAE Automotive Safety Dynamic Modeling Symposium*, Anaheim, California, Oct. 12, 1967.
13. McHENRY, R.R., and NAAB, K.N.: Computer simulation of the crash victim–a validation study. *Proceedings of the Tenth Stapp Car Crash Conference, SAE Paper No. 660792*, Nov. 8–9, 1966.
14. SEGAL, D.J., and McHENRY, R.R.: Computer simulation of the automobile crash victim–revision No. 1. *CAL Report No. VJ-2492-V-1*, Dec. 1967.
15. McHENRY, R.R., and NAAB, K.N.: An analytical investigation of the causes of "submarining" responses of anthropometric dummies in tests of automobile restraint harnesses. *CAL Report No. YM-2250-V-1*, Dec. 1966.
16. GOLOMB, S.W.: Mathematical models–uses and limitations. *Astronautics and Aeronautics*, Jan. 1968, pp. 57–59.
17. FETTER, W.A.: Computer Graphics. A Presentation to the American Society for Engineering Educators Annual Meeting, Pullman, Washington, June 20–24, 1966.

Chapter XII

COMPARISONS OF RESEARCH IN INANIMATE AND BIOLOGIC MATERIAL:
Artifacts and Pitfalls

Elisha S. Gurdjian, M.D., D. Gonzales, M.D., Voigt R. Hodgson, M.S., L. Murray Thomas, M.D., and S. W. Greenberg, B.S.

The application of information obtained from animal experimentation to problems of human physiology and pathophysiology has been criticized occasionally because certain functional responses in the lower forms and humans are not exactly similar. Excision of the motor cortex in the dog and the cat causes but slight disability. This disability is worse in the monkey and is very marked in the human when the cortical areas are destroyed by injury, tumor or failure of the blood supply to the motor area. On the other hand, many physiological responses in the monkey compare favorably with those in the human. It is the prerogative of the scientist to make use of dependable experimental information, recognition being given to its limitations. He should know the differences in response, and how findings in the lower forms may not apply to certain human organs and functional patterns.

The utilization of inanimate tissues for study immediately after death points to several limitations. After death, there is termination of physiologic processes, chemical alteration of tissues and loss of certain physical properties such as elasticity, strength, stiffness, etc. Physical properties may be altered in different degrees in different tissues. But in spite of the death of the animal, tissues may be responsive for a short period of time. The brain may be shown to have the ability to absorb O_2 and eliminate CO_2; the heart may be capable of rhythmic contraction; blood vessels and involuntary muscles may respond to certain chemical and electrical stimuli. Certain inanimate tissues are particularly valuable for study of their mechanical behavior, their strength characteristics and patterns of deformation.

Editors Note: This research has been supported by U.S. Army Medical Research and Development Command, Grant # DA 49-193-MD-2603 (Mechanism of Head and Neck Injury).

RESEARCH ON THE MECHANICAL PROPERTIES OF SKULL AND OTHER SKELETAL STRUCTURES

The comparison of results of living and dead specimens has been important in our laboratory since we have utilized human cadaver material for the study of certain mechanical properties of the skull and other bones of the body. The deformation patterns of the skull in the living monkey under anesthesia, the same monkey dead with skull contents intact, and the dried (but kept moist) skull of the same animal, have been studied in our laboratory by the utilization of the Stresscoat* technique. The same was done with the dog. The patterns were similar in the live, the dead with contents intact, and the dry skull of the same animal. (Fig. 12–1) The

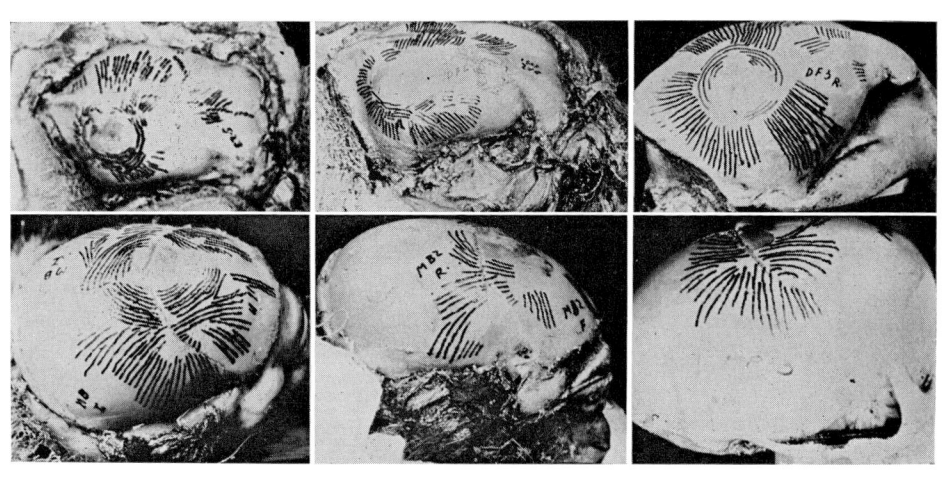

FIGURE 12–1. Stresscoat pattern of deformation of the skull in the dog, above, and monkey, below. From left to right, live specimen under anesthesia, dead animal with skull contents intact, and dry skull of animal, respectively.

deformation of the human skull with scalp removed but facial and basal soft tissues intact was compared with patterns of deformation of dry skulls (kept moist). The findings were similar (Fig. 12–2). A paper written by the senior author with the late Prof. Lissner in December, 1945,[4] discusses these findings.

Certain quantitative determinations with the stresscoat were reported in 1946.[5] It was discovered that blows in various areas of the skull required different levels of energy for threshold deformation patterns. A midoccipital blow caused cracks in the lacquer with 8 inch-pounds of energy, whereas

---

* Stresscoat is a brittle lacquer. It is applied on the material for study of its deformations. Cracks appear in the lacquer due to bending and tensile stresses. The tensile stresses on the exterior of the skull result in cracks in the lacquer on the external surface. The tensile stresses on the internal surface of the skull result in cracks of the lacquer applied on the internal surface of the skull. Thus the deformation patterns of the skull following an impact may be studied by this technique.

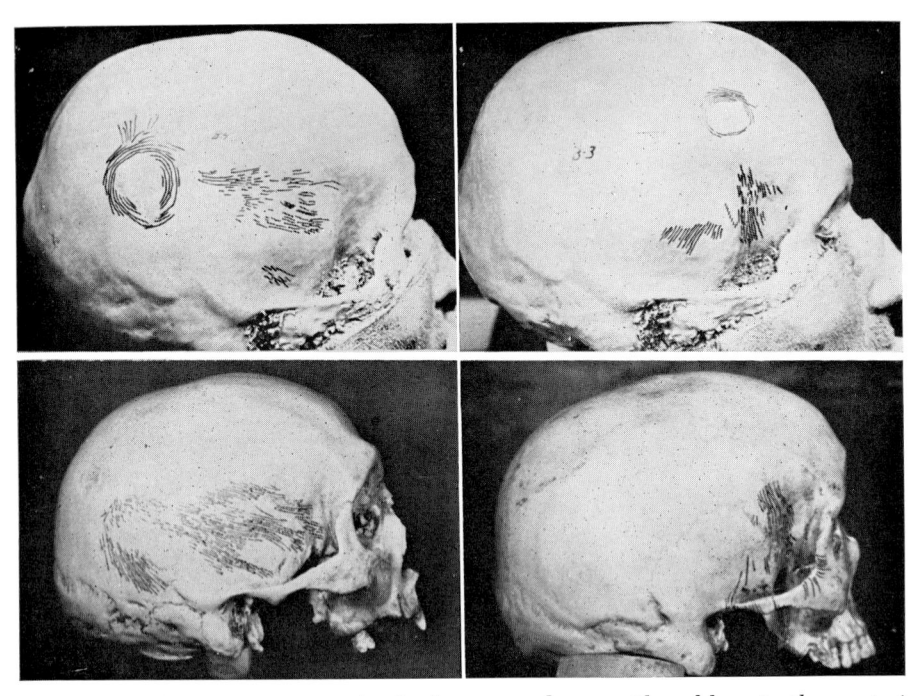

FIGURE 12-2. Stresscoat pattern in the human cadaver with a blow in the posterior parietal and lateral frontal areas. Above, with soft tissues of base and face intact; below, dry skulls. Note similarity of pattern in the two groups of specimens.

in the parietal area, the energy requirement for beginning cracks was 12 inch-pounds. In later work, the threshold deformations due to impacts of twelve areas of the skull were studied. It was found that with midoccipital impacts, the weakest point in 38 per cent of the specimens was lateral to the foramen magnum in the occipital squama, while in 29 per cent, the midline occipital bone extending to the middle of the foramen magnum was the site of threshold deformations. In 15 per cent, following a midoccipital impact, there were inferior parietal deformations; in 5 per cent, deformations of the lambdoid area; and in 4 per cent, midline vertex threshold deformation patterns. "The proof of the pudding is in the eating" is a reasonable statement and may be applied to the question of linear skull fracture and its predictability on the basis of the Stresscoat work.

About 70 per cent of skull fractures seen clinically are linear. Unlike in the laboratory, many accidents involve more than one impact during the few milliseconds of the accidental injury. However, in many clinical cases, a single impact in a given area may be assumed by the presence of a contusion or laceration. There is good agreement of prediction of linear fracture site between the experimental work done on cadaver skulls and the human experience in accidental impact injuries. Midoccipital impacts have a high incidence of agreement, second only to anterior parietal impacts with an incidence of 83 per cent temporal fracture predictions.

Linear fractures result from elastic deformation of the skull. The area of impact is inbended; distal to the area of inbending, the skull undergoes outbending. A linear fracture is initiated in the outbended portion of the skull, extending toward the point of impact and in the opposite direction. In Figure 12–3 the Stresscoat pattern following a midoccipital blow shows the primary stress level to be about the foramen magnum.[6,7] In Figure

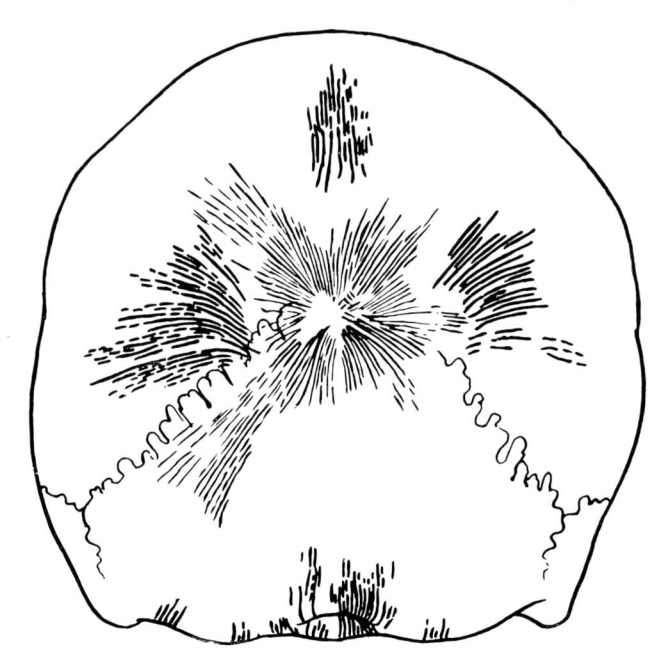

FIGURE 12–3. Stresscoat deformation pattern with a midoccipital blow in the human skull (kept moist). Area of primary stress level is about the foramen magnum. The four groups of cracks in the lacquer are on the external surface of the skull surrounding the central lozenge-shaped cracks which were on the internal surface of the skull.

12–4, a midoccipital blow on a cadaver skull has resulted in a linear fracture extending from the center of the foramen magnum to the area of impact. In this specimen, there are also laterally placed fractures about the foramen magnum. In Figure 12–5 are two clinical cases in which the areas of impact were contused and are shown by the wires. The fractures of the occipital squama are comparable to the cadaver fracture and predictable by the stresscoat pattern.

Another example is the analysis of the formation of a linear fracture in the parietotemporal area, seen experimentally in the cadaver and shown in Figure 12–6. The site of impact has been marked by the black circle.

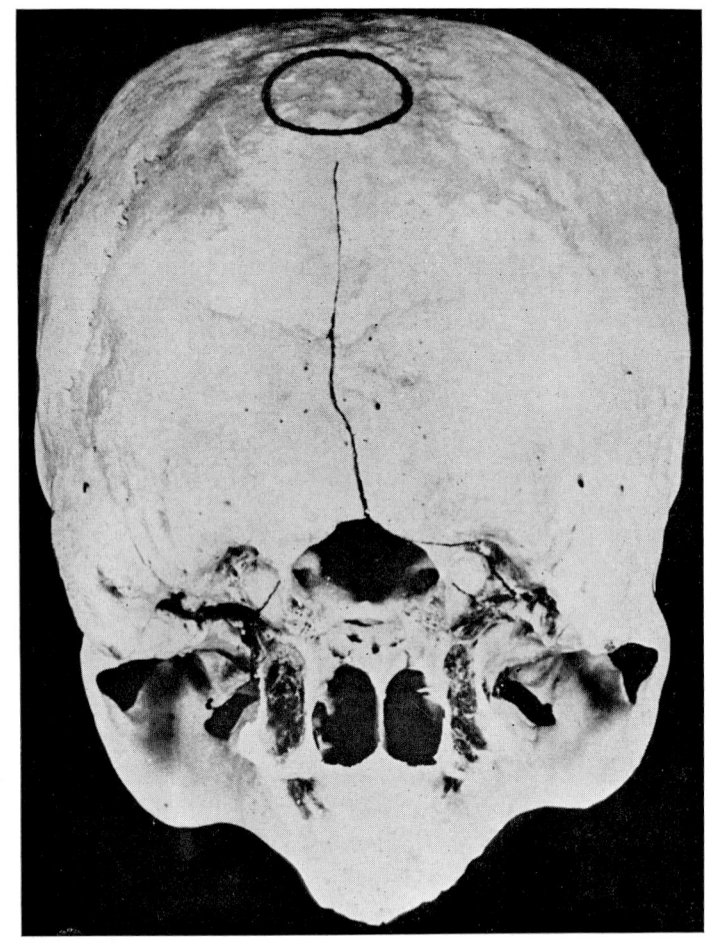

FIGURE 12–4. Experimental skull fracture due to a midoccipital impact in the human cadaver. Note that the fracture is wider apart at the foramen than at the point of impact.

This fracture resulted from elastic deformation of the skull. The area of impact was inbended and distal to the area of inbending in the temporal area; there was outbending of the skull. In this outbended region, a fracture in the skull was initiated as a result of tensile forces. The crack then extended toward the point of impact and toward the base of the skull. The outbended portion also caused outbending of the zygomatic arch with a fracture. The fracture line proceeded toward the point of impact because following the initial inbending, the area became outbended; hence the fracture line was drawn to its center because in an outbended state, the impact area was a region of stress concentration. This explanation is borne out by the Stresscoat pattern following an anteroparietal impact. The area of primary stress level is in the temporoparietal junction (Fig. 12–7). In

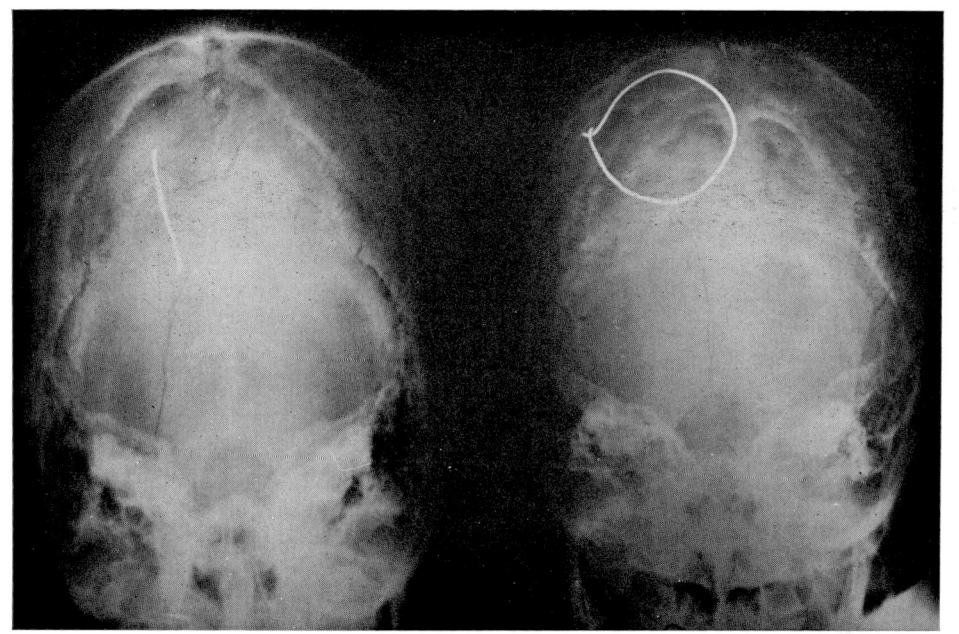

FIGURE 12-5. Wires show the site of impacts which were contused in two patients. The associated skull fracture is near the midline to the right and lateral to the foramen magnum to the left.

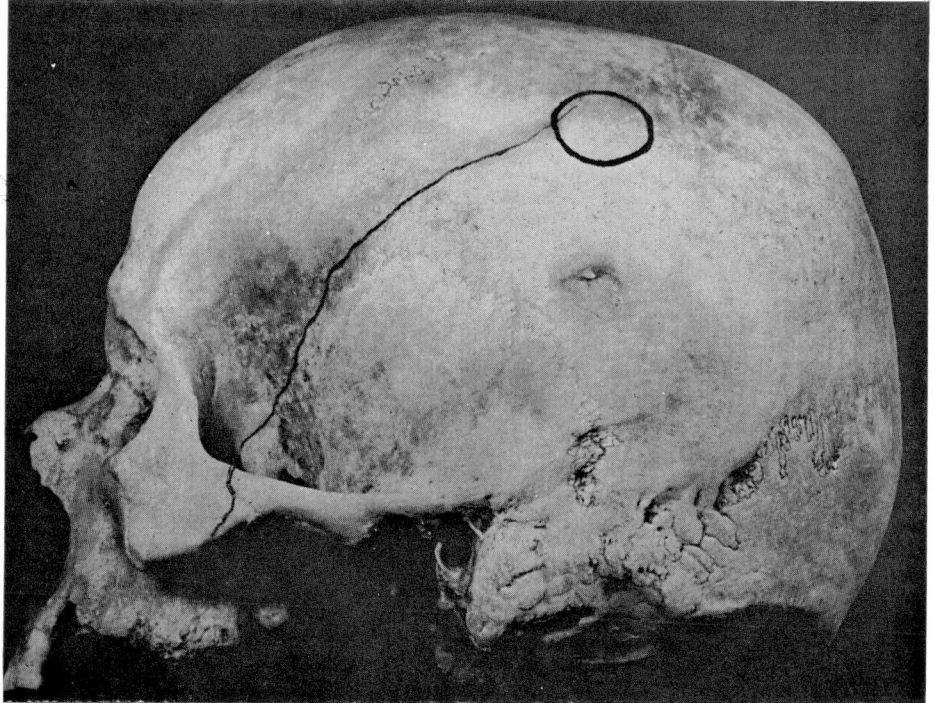

FIGURE 12-6. Experimental skull fracture in the human cadaver following a parietal impact. Note that the temporal portion of the fracture is wider than at the point of impact. The outbending of the temporal area where the fracture was initiated also resulted in outbending of the zygomatic arch with fracture.

240   *Impact Injury and Crash Protection*

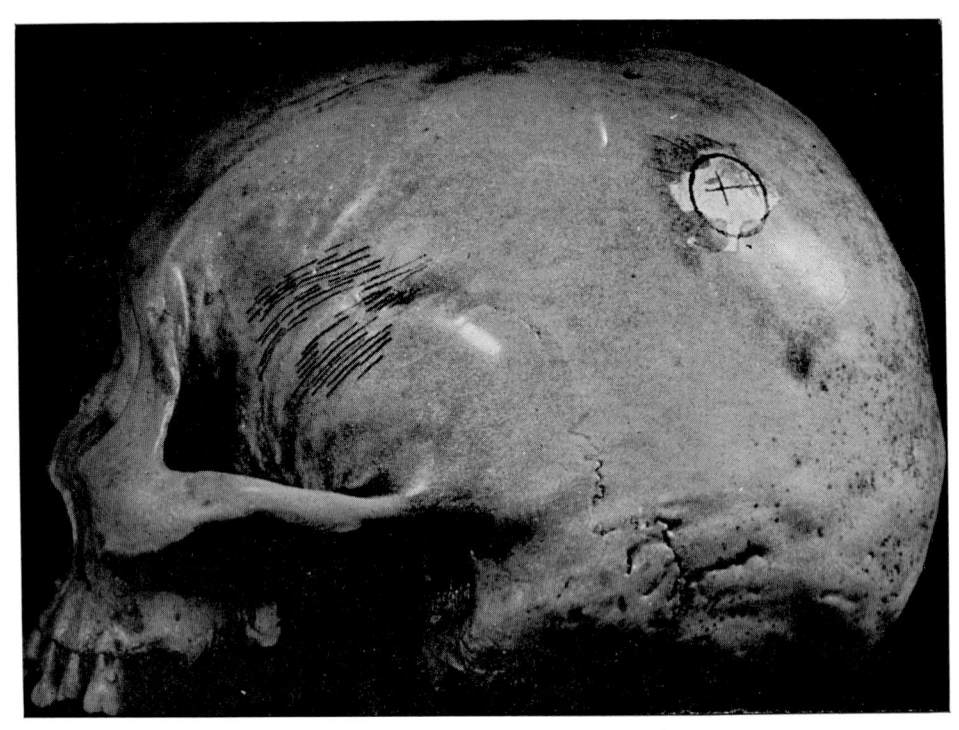

FIGURE 12-7. Stresscoat pattern following a parietal blow. Area of primary stress level in the temporal region.

Figure 12-8 is shown a diagram of the deformation pattern. It is in the outbended portion of the skull where the fracture is initiated. In Figure 12-9 is shown a clinically observed skull fracture. The area of impact was contused and is marked with a radiopaque wire. It should be noted that the fracture is more separated in the temporal region rather than in the area of impact. In fact, it was initiated at a distance from the point of impact and then proceeded toward the point of impact as well as toward the base of the skull.

The problem of depressed and perforated fractures need not concern us in this discussion, since the production of depression and perforation is due to the application of high velocity energy with a blunt or pointed object. There is failure of the skull in the area where the energy is applied.

The cranial deformations with low velocity impacts are dependent upon the shape and configuration of the skull and to a lesser extent its composition. Buttresses influence the deformation patterns; chance thin and thick areas influence it; the presence of previously inflicted defects in the skull alter its pattern. Some persons have narrow (scaphocephalic) shaped heads; others have more spherical heads; still others have a head shape

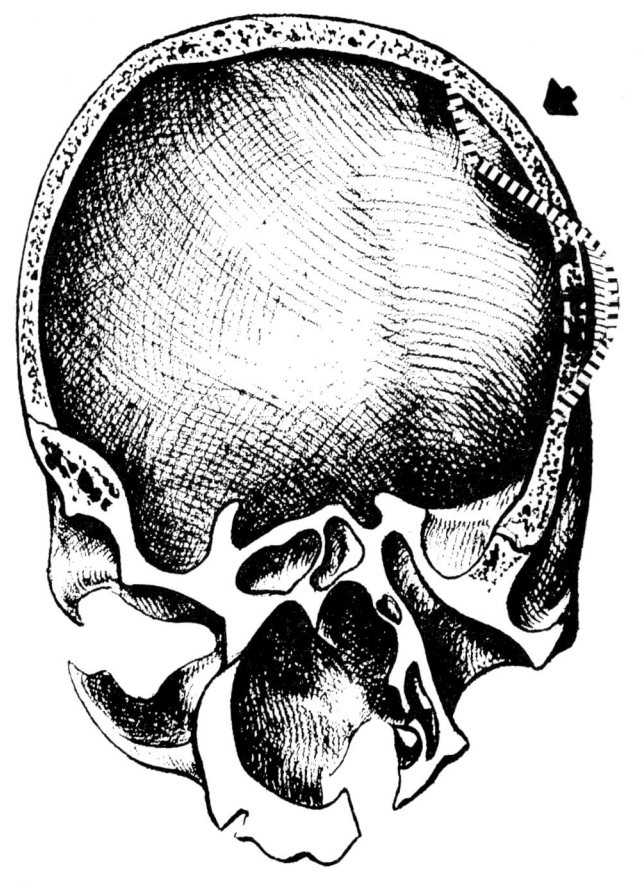

FIGURE 12–8. The artist's view of the deformation pattern. Area of impact is inbended and the temporal region surrounding the area of impact is outbended. Fracture is initiated in the temporal region and extends toward the point of impact and toward the base.

narrow from the back to the front (anteroposterior) and long from the top to the bottom (superoinferior) (brachycephalic, oxycephalic). The stress patterns in an unusually shaped skull are understandably different One can predict the deformation patterns in a perfect sphere with the deformations being equidistant from the point of impact. The skull is not a true sphere; hence its patterns of deformations will vary depending upon its shape and configuration. However, skull shape and configuration generally are similar; hence the deformation patterns in different specimens are comparable.

The deformation patterns in the dog and the monkey are not similar to those in the human cadaver because of differences of shape and configuration. However, the studies in the lower forms showed a consistent

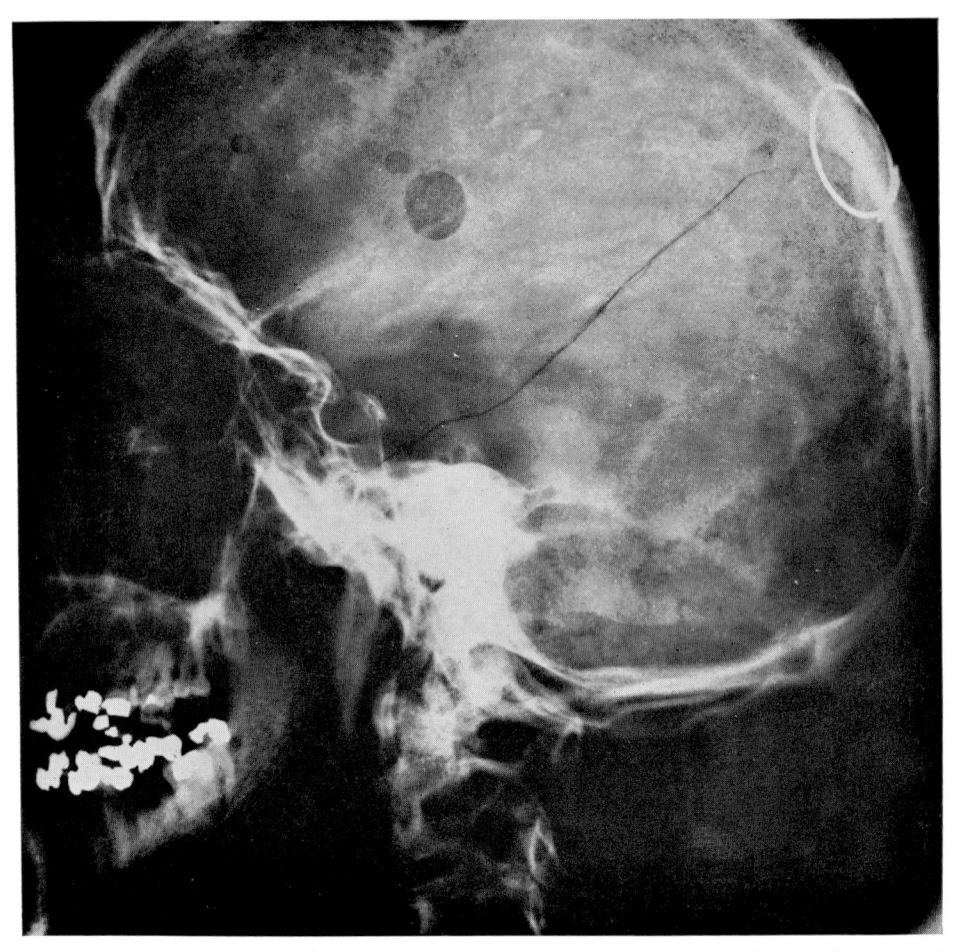

FIGURE 12-9. Linear skull fracture in a patient, the area of impact being shown with a circular wire. Note again that the fracture is wider away from the point of impact than at the point of impact.

similarity of pattern in the live, dead, and dry skulls. Obviously such correlation could not be studied in the human. The fact that the deformation patterns in the skulls of the live and dead monkey and dog are similar makes the experimental use of the human cadaver material more tenable.

Aside from deformation patterns studied with Stresscoat, an investigation of strength of material is necessary to help complete the study of the mechanical properties of cranial and other bones. Experimental studies of the strength of various skeletal structures have been conducted in our laboratories. Roberts and Lissner[10] studied the effects of constant acceleration and varying levels of jerk (g/sec) on embalmed cadavers and living systems in the dog. There was good correlation in the dynamic responses of the vertebrae in the living and dead animal. In the transition region between a dynamic load factor of one and the terminal maximum plateau (the overshoot), the living vertebra in the animal under anesthesia was 20 per cent more sensitive. Evans and King[3] studied the physical properties of cancellous bone. The compressive strength was different depending upon whether a cubic (.79 cm^2) or a rectangular piece was used (2.2 cm x .79 cm). The strength was higher for the cubic shaped specimen.

This paper reports on preliminary load-deflection test results on the skull and tibia of the dog. The tests have been conducted in the dog under anesthesia, in the freshly sacrificed animal, in the embalmed state, with bones tested kept moist, and in the dry specimens of the same animal. In a few, the dry specimen has been immersed in 10 per cent formalin solution for several days and retested in the remoistened state.

Methods and Material

Mongrel dogs weighing 15 to 28 kg were anesthetized with sodium pentothal (50 mg/cc/kg). Through a median incision of the head extending from the middle of the forehead-nose junction to the middle of the neck, the skull was exposed (Fig. 12–10). The temporal muscles were reflected and excised. Electrocoagulation was used to control bleeding. The tibia-fibula complex was prepared as shown in Figure 12–11. The tibia was exposed equidistant from the steel pins supporting the bones (Fig. 12–12). Because of variation among animals, the experiment is designed to test each animal against itself in the several conditions.

Skull Tests

Testing the skull *in vivo* presents the most difficult control problems. After exposure, the skull is fitted into the loading fixture as shown in Figure 12–10. Since the dimensional features of the skull are never parallel on the two sides, toggle pads are used on the loading heads on either side of the skull. Small nipples in the pads fit into one sixteenth diameter holes drilled into the skull for locating purposes. The skull is loaded at a rate of approximately 0.17 inch per minute to a maximum load of 250 pounds and then unloaded to zero at the same rate. The load is applied by a hydraulic cylinder through a BLH load cell while simultaneously recording the deflection of the skull by means of a linear displacement transducer. The output of the transducers is fed into an XY plotter for automatic recording of the load deflection and hysteresis characteristics of the specimen. The animal is then sacrificed by intravenous injection of KCl without altering the loading setup and then retested in the fresh condition.

To obtain better mechanical control, tests to determine changes in

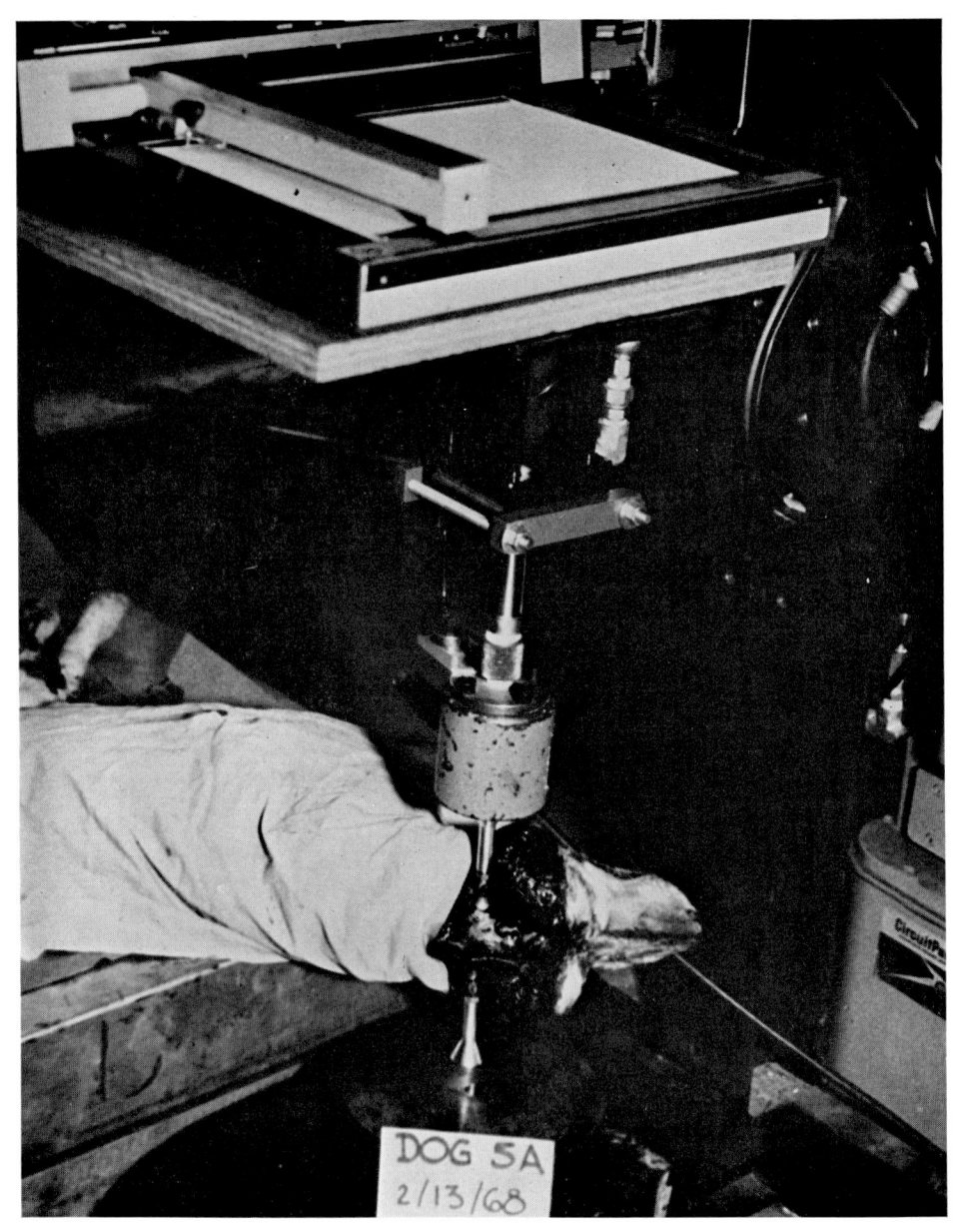

FIGURE 12–10. Load deflection technique being used to study the deflection of dog skull in the anesthetized animal.

physical characteristics of the skull in the several states of preservation were conducted in the fixture shown in Figure 12–13. This mechanism has a pin (0.375 of an inch in diameter) to prevent rotation by holding the skull through the maxilla bones approximately at the infraorbital foramen. The load is applied around a guide pin (0.250 of an inch in diameter)

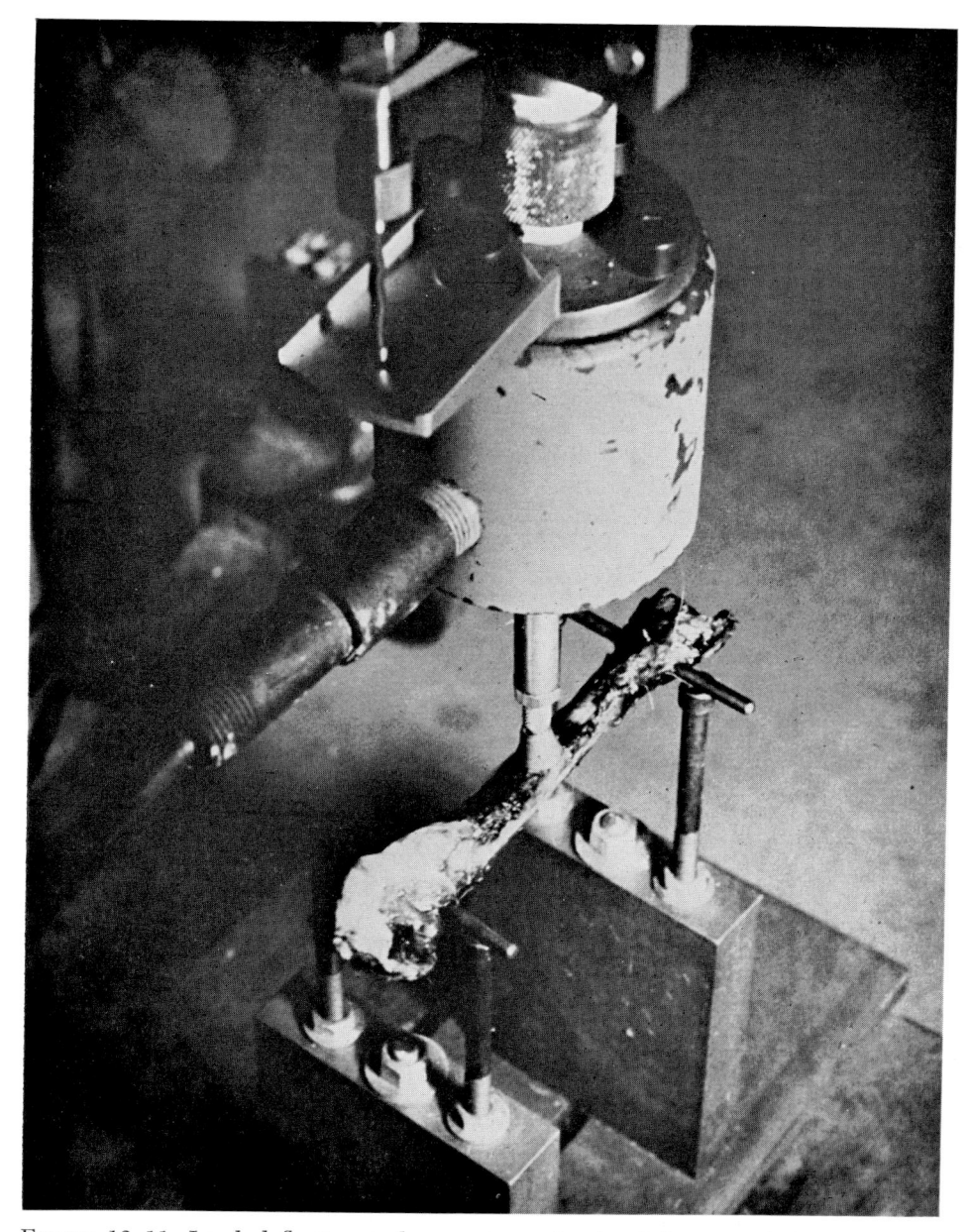

FIGURE 12-11. Load deflection technique to study the deflection of the freshly removed tibia of the dog.

through the parietal bones at the most prominent aspect above the zygomatic arch. The compressive force is distributed to the skull on both sides through a low melting (117°F) metal alloy pad. The metal was cast on the skull and around the load guide pin to provide a form-fitting pad with 0.250 of an inch inside diameter, 0.750 of an inch outside diameter, and

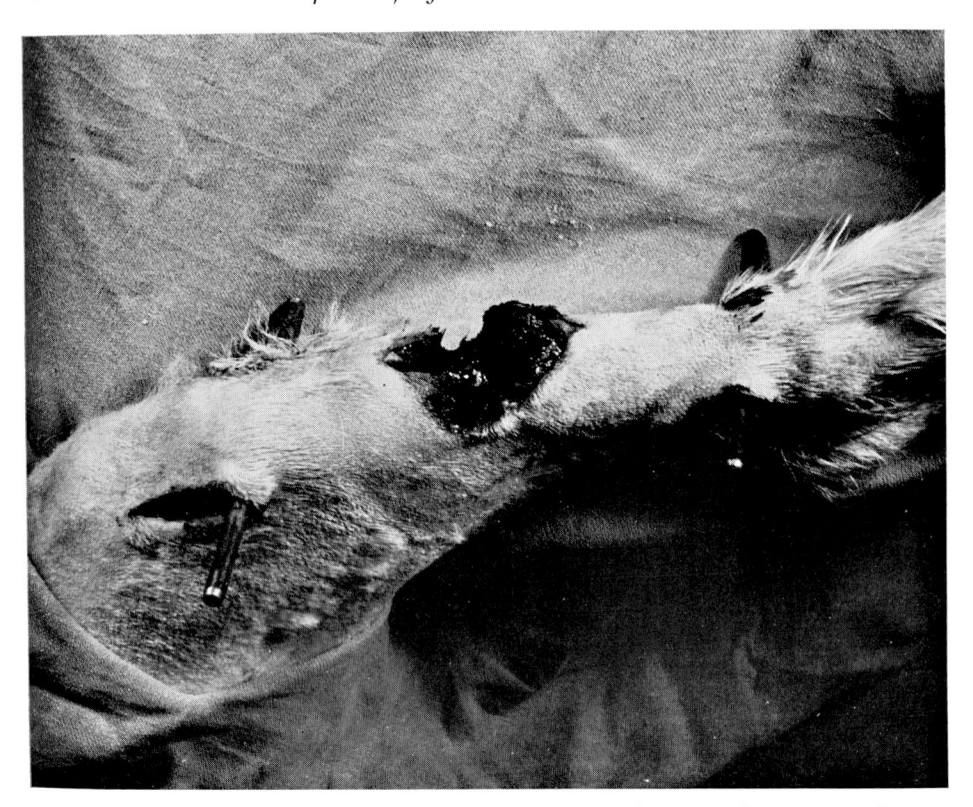

FIGURE 12–12. Preparation of the tibia in the dog. The bone has been exposed equidistant from the supporting pins in preparation for the deflection test.

varying thickness (maximum 0.188 of an inch). Under load the pads displayed negligible deflection compared to that of the skull. The same pair of pads were used with each skull throughout the series of tests.

Each skull was loaded in the fresh condition (1 hour after death) to 200 pounds (approximately ½ ultimate strength) at a slow rate of about 0.001 inch per second. The load was released at about the same rate. Similar tests were repeated after the following: (1) soaking 1 week in a 10% formalin solution; (2) a second week of soaking in saline; (3) a third week of drying to a constant weight over $CaCl_2$ in a vacuum dessicator; (4) a fourth week of remoistening the skull in saline. In each condition the skull was loaded to 200 pounds to stabilize the system. The test was repeated three times and the data was recorded as the average of the last three tests.

Tibia-fibula Tests

Each tibia-fibula is perforated transversely near its epiphyses and hardened steel pins are inserted as shown in Figure 12–12. The shaft of the

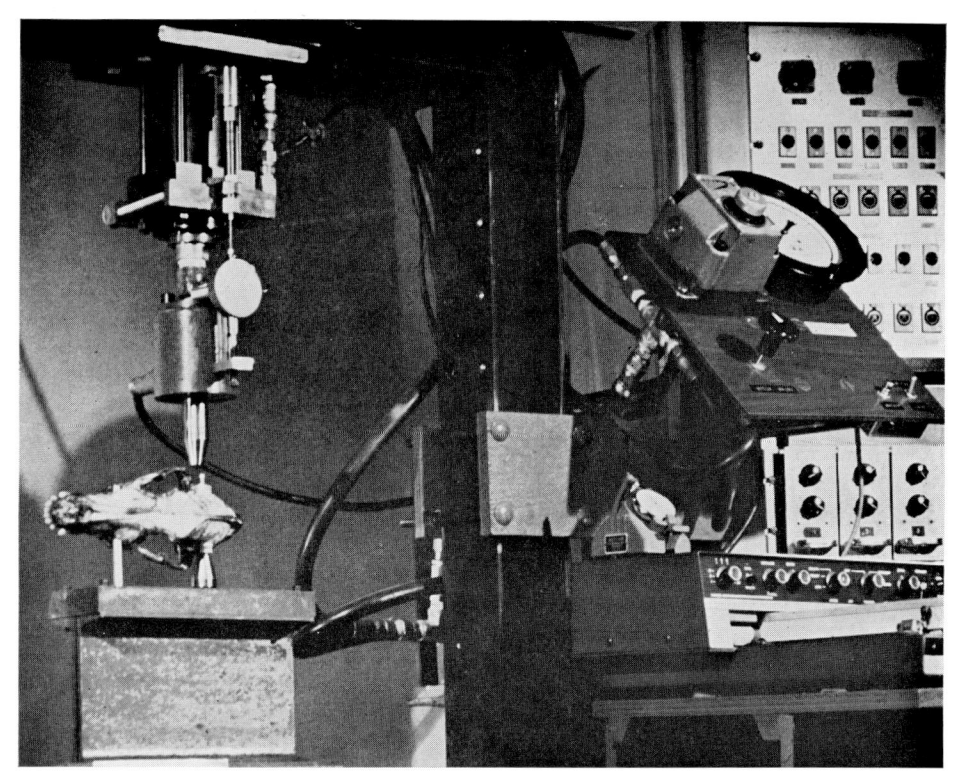

FIGURE 12–13. Test setup to determine the load-deflection characteristics of the dog skull in the fresh condition and several states of preservation.

tibia is then exposed midway between the pins. A one-sixteenth of an inch in diameter hole is drilled into the bone for the purpose of locating the pad nipple, thus giving a reference for successive retesting at weekly intervals. The right hand tibia-fibula complex is then placed in the loading fixture as shown in Figure 12–12 and loaded *in vivo* to complete failure. The left tibia-fibula complex is then tested *in vivo* to 50 per cent of the fracture load which occurred on the right side. The bone specimen is then allowed to unload itself at the same rate as loaded. Load-deflection and hysteresis characteristics are recorded as before. The load is applied to the shaft in the anteroposterior direction in a parasagittal plane and is performed three times in succession for comparative elimination of artifacts. The animal is then sacrificed and the same specimen is retested shortly after death (fresh condition). After excision the bone is preserved by immersion in 10% formalin for 1 week. The specimen is retested at 1 week intervals for 3 weeks in the wet condition for comparison of results under prior conditions (Table 12–III).

Results

Since the *in vivo* skull tests are difficult and very time consuming, the *in vivo* to fresh *in situ* experiments were devised to eliminate the living tests if results were similar. Table 12–I indicates that the changes in stiffness which occurred among a group of five animals fell within ± 5 per cent; therefore the *in vivo* skull tests have been eliminated (See also Fig. 12–15.)

Shown in Table 12–II are the load-deflection characteristics, at 200 pounds of force of ten skulls in several states of preservation compared to their characteristics in the fresh (dead 1 hour) condition. The mean changes, standard deviation and 95 per cent confidence limits, all given in terms of percentages, are listed below in Table 12–II.

Table 12–III was constructed to statistically quantify the changes be-

TABLE 12-I
LATERAL LOAD SPRING RATES FOR THE SKULL OF THE DOG *IN VIVO* AND *FRESH-IN SITU*

Sample	Dog	Spring Rate lb./in. In Vivo	Fresh In Situ	% Change
1	1X	3740	3580	−4.3
2	2X	3030	2987	−1.4
3	13A	3766	3944	+4.7
4	14A	5750	5900	+2.6
5	15A	10000	10500	+5.0
Average............		5257	5382	+2.4
Standard deviation = 4.6%				

tween *in vivo*-fresh and fresh-wet embalmed for the tibia-fibula of the dog. Mean increase in stiffness of 3.3 per cent, standard deviation of 12.2 per cent and −6.9 to 13.5 mean per cent change in stiffness expected for 95 per cent of the population, were calculated using the changes from *in vivo* to the fresh condition. For the fresh to wet embalmed condition the mean change was 8.4 per cent increase in stiffness, standard deviation 15.5 per cent and expected mean of −4.6 to 21.2 per cent change in stiffness.

In Figure 12–14 ultimate strength of the *in vivo* tibia-fibula complex compared with the embalmed counterpart are shown. This embalmed specimen was dessicated for 1 week until it manifested a constant weight. It was then remoistened for 1 week in a 10% formalin solution. Figure 12–14 shows that the embalmed specimen is slightly stiffer, and that it fractured at a higher load than the live bone. In Table 12–IV are shown ultimate strength characteristics of tibia-fibula complex *in vivo* and after embalming, drying and remoistening.

TABLE 12-II
STATISTICAL ANALYSIS OF CHANGES IN SPRING RATE OF DOG SKULLS DUE TO SEVERAL STATES OF PRESERVATION

Sample No.	Dog No.	S.R.* lb./in. Fresh	S.R. lb./in. EMB.	% Change P	P²	S.R. lb./in. Moist	% Change P	P²	S.R. lb./in. Dry	% Change P	P²	Remois- tened	% Change P	P²
1	2	8000	8333	4.16	17.3	7410	−7.38	54.4	9080	13.6	185	7690	−3.8	14.4
2	3	8333	9080	8.97	80.4	8690	4.3	18.5	9530	14.3	205	8690	4.3	18.5
3	4	9530	13320	39.8	1584	10520	11.1	123	10520	11.1	123	11750	23.3	543
4	5	3775	3845	1.85	3.42	3775	0	0	4260	12.7	161	3775	0	0
5	6	9080	8700	−4.18	17.5	9530	4.8	23.1	9530	4.8	23	9530	4.8	23.1
6	7	7410	7690	3.80	14.3	8000	8.0	64.0	9530	28.6	818	7690	3.8	14.4
7	8	9080	10000	10.1	102	10520	15.8	250	11750	29.3	858	10000	10.1	102
8	9	12500	15380	23.1	533	12500	0	0	16670	33.2	1103	10520	−15.7	247
9	10	10000	9080	−9.2	84.6	10520	5.2	27.0	12500	25.0	625	10000	0	0
10	11	9530	11100	16.5	272	11100	16.5	272	11100	16.5	272	10000	5	25
TOTAL				94.9	2739		58	832		176	4373		31.8	987

Fresh-embalmed
$D = 9.5\%**$
$S = 14.3\%$
$\mu = -0.3, 19.3***\%$

Fresh-moist embalmed
$D = 5.8\%**$
$S = 5.5\%$
$\mu = 2.0, 9.6***\%$

Fresh-embalmed dry
$D = 17.6\%**$
$S = 11.9\%$
$\mu = 9.5, 25.7***\%$

Fresh-embalmed remoistened
$D = 3.2\%**$
$S = 9.9\%$
$\mu = -3.6, 10***\%$

KEY.
* Spring Rate
** All changes referred to fresh condition 1 hour after death
*** 95% confidence limits
D = mean change
S = standard deviation
All values corrected for small sample size.

TABLE 12-III
STATISTICAL ANALYSIS OF CHANGES IN SIMPLY SUPPORTED CENTER LOAD SPRING RATES FOR THE TIBIA-FIBULA COMPLEX OF THE DOG IN VIVO-FRESH-WET EMBALMED

Sample No.	Dog No.	Spring Rate* In Vivo	Spring Rate* Fresh	% Change (P)	P^2	Spring Rate* Fresh	Spring Rate* Wet Embalmed	% Change (P)	P^2
1	3	2240	2500	11.6	135	2500	2310	− 7.6	58
2	4	940	790	−16	256	790	940	19	361
3	5	3950	3570	− 9.6	92	3570	2780	−22.1	488
4	6	2210	2500	13	169	2500	2940	17.6	310
5	7	2150	2420	12.6	159	2420	2940	21.5	463
6	8	2460	2880	17.1	292	2880	3060	6.2	38
7	9	1810	1830	1.1	1.2	1830	2130	16.4	269
8	10	2360	2270	− 3.8	14.4	2270	2630	15.8	250
Total				26	1119			67.4	2237
Average				3.3				8.4	

In Vivo—Fresh:
Standard Deviation = 12.2%.
Expected Mean Percentage Change in Population = −6.9%, 13.5% (95% confidence limits).
Fresh—Wet Embalmed:
Standard Deviation = 15.5%.
Expected Mean Percentage Change in Population = −4.6%, 21.2%.
* lb./in.

TABLE 12-IV
ULTIMATE STRENGTH OF TIBIA-FIBULA COMPLEX IN VIVO AND EMBALMED*

Sample	Dog	Specimen	Load—lbs. In Vivo	Embalmed*	% Change
1	5A	RH	357		
		LH		375	+ 5.0
2	6A	RH	350		
		LH		318	− 9.1
3	7A	LH	333		
		RH		220	−34.0
4	8A	RH	290		
		LH		378	+30.3
5	9A	RH	320		
		LH		380	+18.8
6	10A	RH	305		
		LH		393	+28.8
7	12A	RH	378		
		LH		352	− 6.9
8	14A	RH	268		
		LH		360	+34.3
9	15A	RH	395		
		LH		425	+ 7.6

* Fracture test performed after embalming, successive deflection testing, drying and remoistening.

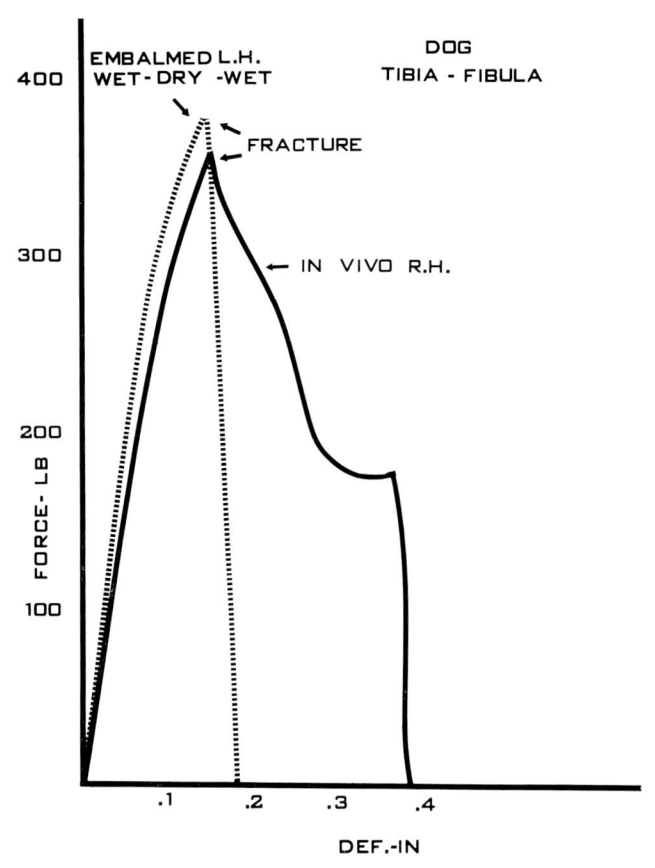

FIGURE 12–14. Fracture of the live and embalmed tibia. The embalmed specimen appears to be somewhat stiffer.

Conclusions

The deformation patterns of the skull in the monkey and the dog compare favorably with those in the live animal under anesthesia, dead animal with contents intact and the dry skull of the same animal (kept moist). These are qualitative comparisons. Human dry skull patterns are similar to those of the cadaver with the vertex bones exposed. Studies in the human cadaver have given us valuable information on the mechanism of linear fracture in the living human. These correlations indicate the value of cadaver material in biological research.

Recent studies among 10 dogs in our laboratory show that the static deflection characteristics are about the same in the living dog skull and the freshly sacrificed specimen. After one week in a 10% formalin solution the skull exhibits an increased stiffness of 9.5 per cent with standard de-

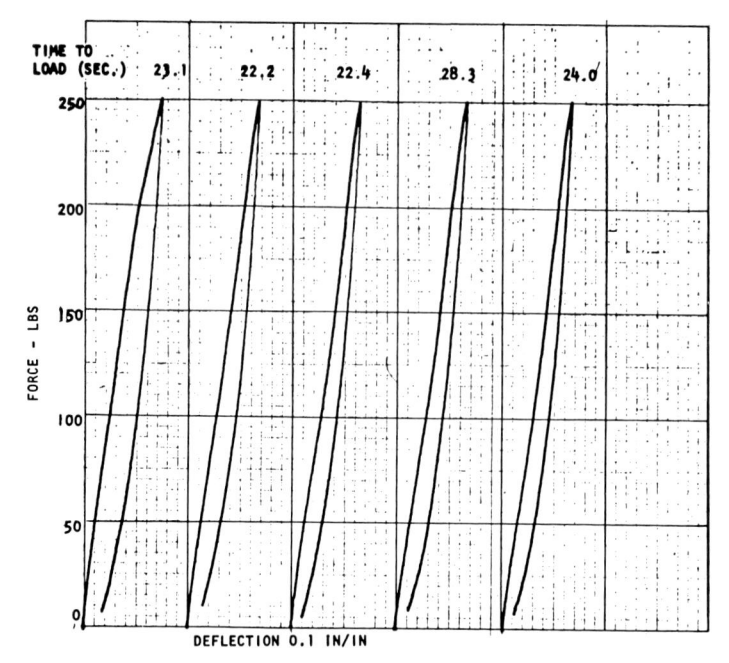

FIGURE 12–15-A. Repetitive loading of the in vivo skull of the dog. Average load rate—0.17 in/min.

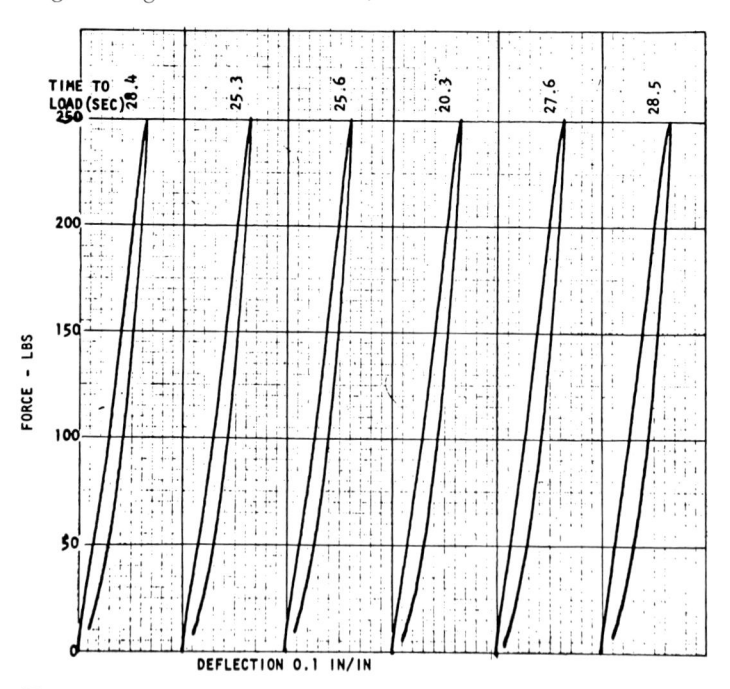

FIGURE 12–15-B. Repetitive loading of dog skull within 15 minutes after death. Average load rate—0.17 in/min.

In vivo and fresh *in situ* comparisons of skull deformation in Dog 13A. In this case there was an increase in the spring rate of 4.5 percent from *in vivo* to fresh, 15 minutes after death.

viation of 14.3 per cent, from the fresh condition. When the embalmed skull is soaked in a saline solution for one more week the spring rate is only 5.8 per cent stiffer than that of the fresh skull with standard deviation of 5.5 per cent. Drying the skull for 1 week to a constant weight causes the bone to become stiffer by 17.6 per cent on the average, with a standard deviation of 11.9 per cent. When remoistened, the bone returned closer to its fresh condition spring rate, showing a mean increased stiffness of only 3.2 per cent, standard deviation of 19.9 per cent. Results in the tibia-fibula complex were similar to those obtained for the skull.

REFERENCES

1. EVANS, F.G., and LEBOW, M.: Regional Differences in some of the physical properties of the human femur. *Appl Physiol*, 3 (10), April 1951.
2. EVANS, F. GAYNOR: Significant differences in the tensile strength of adult human compact bone. *Proceedings of the First European Bone and Tooth Symposium*. New York, Pergamon, 1964, pp. 319–331.
3. EVANS, F. GAYNOR, and KING, ALBERT I.: Regional differences in some physical properties of human spongy bone. Evans, F. Gaynor (Ed.): *Biomechanical Studies of the Musculo-Skeletal System*. Springfield, Thomas, 1961, pp. 49–67.
4. GURDJIAN, E.S., and LISSNER, H.R.: Deformation of the skull in head injury (a study with the stresscoat technique). *Surg Gynec Obstet*, 81:679–687, 1945.
5. GURDJIAN, E.S., and LISSNER, H.R.: Deformations of the skull in head injury studied by the "stresscoat" technique. Quantitative determinations. *Surg Gynec Obstet*, 83:219–233, 1946.
6. GURDJIAN, E.S.; WEBSTER, J.E., and LISSNER, H.R.: The mechanism of skull fracture. *Neurosurg*, VII(2):106–114, 1950.
7. GURDJIAN, E.S.; WEBSTER, J.E., and LISSNER, H.R.: The mechanism of skull fracture. *Radiology*, 54(3):313–339, March 1950.
8. MCELHANEY, J.H.: Dynamic response of bone and muscle tissue. *J Appl Physiol*, 21(4), 1966.
9. MCELHANEY, J.; FOGLE, J.; BYARS, E., and WEAVER, G.: Effect of Embalming on the mechanical properties of beef bone. *Appl Physiol*, 19(6), 1964.
10. ROBERTS, V.L., and LISSNER, H.R.: A correlation between cadaver and *in vivo* results. Patrick, Lawrence M. (Ed.): *Proceedings of the Eighth Car Crash and Field Demonstration Conference*, Detroit, Wayne, 1966.
11. SEDLIN, E.S.: A rheologic model for cortical bone—a study of the physical properties of human femoral samples. *Acta Orthopaed Scand* (Suppl. 83), 1965.
12. YAMADA, M.D.: *Human Biomechanics*. Kyoto Prefectural University of Medicine, Kyoto, Japan, 1963.

DISCUSSION

A. EARL WALKER

The basic research of Dr. Gurdjian and his team over the years has clarified many of the mechanisms of head and neck injury. Obviously, although their studies were finally to be applied to man, it was impossible to utilize the human subject for such studies. Consequently, Dr. Gurdjian has now inquired into the validity of transferring the findings in lower animals and in cadavers to the clinical problems of the human being. This is certainly a pertinent question and one which is worthy of considerable attention at this time. Dr. Gurdjian has noted the changes which might occur in the physical properties of bone after death and after their removal from their normal physical-chemical environment. He finds that the forces applied to a cadaver produce approximately the same degree and same kind of osseous disturbances as similar forces applied to the living individual. Consequently, the findings obtained in the cadaver would seem to be applicable to man.

One might inquire into the physical changes which occur as the living becomes the dead skull, and which modifies the pattern of deformation. Unquestionably there is a change in the water content of the bone after death and changes in the colloidal constituents of various tissues of the skull. These alterations may well modify the degree of absorption of forces applied to the bone. However, insofar as the lines of stress are concerned, Dr. Gurdjian has shown that the dissemination of the applied force is similar. Even the presence of the supporting structures of the skull and the enclosed brain, subarachnoid space and its fluid do not greatly modify the deformation pattern of the skull.

I am somewhat surprised at this finding for I should have thought that the presence of a semifluid substance within the skull case would dampen the stresses. However, I suppose the techniques are measuring phenomena too rapid to be modified by a fluid media with a low periodicity. This factor plays a role in the closed head injuries of infants in whom the relationship between fracture and brain damage is unpredictable.

Dr. Gurdjian and his associates have critically examined the deflections and deformities of the skull showing that the differences in the living and dead tissue are negligible. Certainly the differences introduced by using cadaver skull are less than the variability resulting from the use of varying types or vectors of force. Furthermore, the stress patterns point out that the site is more important than the violence of the applied force in determining a fracture. From the clinical standpoint, we note that in closed head injuries, frontal and occipital traumas are much more common than violence to the side of the head. Consequently, if a fracture occurs, it is likely to radiate into the frontal sinus or to the occipital foramen. On the other hand, blows or missiles lacerating the scalp are more common in the central regions and cause fractures radiating into the temporal bone and crossing the grooves of the middle meningeal arteries producing an extradural hematoma. A knowledge of the propagation of the stress is then of value in assessing the probable site of injury to intracranial structures.

Dr. Gurdjian mentioned that morphological skeletal variations between individuals might be an important factor in determining the presence and direction of fractures. In other words, the dissipation of a force applied to a dolichocephalic skull would probably produce stress patterns quite dissimilar to those induced in a brachycephalic skull. Not much attention has been paid to the influence of the cephalic morphology on the pattern of stress. This would seem to be a subject for scientific inquiry since the buttressing of the dolichocephalic and brachycephalic skull with quite different patterns of stress might require special designs for helmets and safety gear.

PART III

TOLERANCE TO IMPACT

Chapter XIII

METHODS OF ESTABLISHING HUMAN TOLERANCE LEVELS:
Cadaver and Animal Research and Clinical Observations

LAWRENCE M. PATRICK and TAKASHI B. SATO

NEED FOR HUMAN TOLERANCE LEVELS

With over 100,000 accidental deaths in this country each year, mostly from violent impacts, it is essential that improvements in the conditions providing these injuries and fatalities be made. To do this, it is necessary to provide design data on what the human body can stand which can be used to eliminate the injury conditions. An illustration for the requirements for optimum design is readily available from the automobile accident conditions in which approximately half of the fatalities occur. To illustrate the difficulty of the problem, it should be pointed out that a whole body tolerance level of 40 g requires a minimum stopping distance of 36 inches from a velocity of 60 mph. This is the ideal situation with uniform or constant deceleration while from a practical standpoint much greater distances are required. As shown in Table 13-I, about 57 inches is required with the more common half sine pulse from 60 mph.

If optimum safety designs are to be achieved, it is essential that the basic design data—namely, the human tolerance to impact—be obtained with as great an accuracy as possible, and that the values be established

TABLE 13-I
STOPPING DISTANCE FOR CONSTANT AND HALF SINE ACCELERATION PULSES FOR MAXIMUM ACCELERATIONS OF 40 AND 80 G UNITS

Velocity		*Stopping Distance in Inches*			
		40 g Max		*80 g Max*	
mph	ft./sec.	Constant Accel.	Half Sine	Constant Accel.	Half Sine
10	14.7	1.0	1.6	0.5	0.9
20	29.3	4.0	6.3	2.0	3.1
30	44.0	9.0	14.2	4.5	7.1
40	58.6	16.0	25.2	8.0	12.6
50	73.4	25.0	39.3	12.5	19.7
60	88.0	36.0	56.6	18.0	28.3

at as high a level as possible so the necessary stopping distance from a given velocity will be minimum. Or conversely, protection can be provided from the greatest velocity for the available stopping distance.

Fortunately, most automobile accidents are either the forward force or rear force type which provides maximum stopping distance, and most of the data available on human impact tolerance is for impact in the fore and aft direction. There is less distance on the sides of automobiles for protecting the occupant with the present geometrical shape of the vehicle in which it is not practical to put more than three people in a single file position. If the same decelerating distance is to be provided for side impact as for front impact, it will be necessary to eliminate the current three abreast seating arrangement or make the cars wider since even with two abreast the necessary stopping distance cannot be achieved for protection from side impact. Fortunately, velocity change is less in side impact. Thus, in an intersection type accident (side impact), the struck car generally has a change in velocity of about half the initial velocity of the striking car while in a frontal force accident in a barrier situation the change in velocity is the full impact velocity. The side of the vehicle as currently designed does not have the resistance to penetration or intrusion into the passenger compartment that is available from the front impact where the engine and vehicle structure are more rigid and provide additional protection.

If maximum benefit is to be achieved from human tolerance data, it is necessary to consider new concepts without being restricted to the present configurations. However, if the new concepts are to be successful, they must stay within the framework of fundamental physical laws. Some of the advanced designs under consideration include a seat with the restraint systems fastened to it rather than to the structural frame members in the vehicle, and airbags to provide passive protection without the need for the occupants to don a restraint system. Other innovations that might be considered include repositioning the occupant at the time of impact to provide the maximum impact resistance or to reposition the environment to remove the impact injury-producing components. In side impacts, the sides or doors must be provided with energy-absorbing structures that will permit the change in relative velocity without injury and without compromising the integrity of the passenger compartment. Perhaps the best way to accomplish this is to design the front end of vehicles so that when they strike the side of another car, it is forced over the rigid front end frame and engine structure to minimize the intrusion of the striking car into the passenger compartment. This can be accomplished with the side impact where the striking vehicle can always be made to go under the struck vehicle, while it is not feasible for front impact where it would be impossible to determine which of the vehicles in a head-on accident is going to go over the other.

Another place where human tolerance is required, if advances in safety are to be made, is in the pedestrian impact which accounts for about 20 per cent of the automobile fatalities in this country. It is obvious that the pedestrian is at a distinct disadvantage when a 4,000 pound vehicle impacts an individual that weighs from 40 or 50 pounds (child) up to perhaps 250 pounds. There are two major types of injury: (1) the injury from forces applied during the collision or when striking the roadway, and (2) the crushing injuries received in the run-over condition. Pedestrian protection can be achieved by deflecting him out of the path of the car without producing forces high enough to cause injury or by absorbing the impact energy by deforming the vehicle exterior. This latter approach is obviously only satisfactory at very low velocities. The deflection is also a difficult problem with which to cope, since if the pedestrian is deflected over the car, there is a probability of severe injuries from hitting the roadway. Thus, the deflection problem requires a method of establishing ways of preventing impact to the roadway or at least insuring that when the pedestrian strikes the roadway he will do so in a manner that will not produce major injury. As the foregoing paragraphs point out, there is little question about the need for human tolerance data to minimize injury. The problem is how to establish human tolerance to impact levels which is the subject of this paper and is discussed in subsequent sections.

TOLERANCE LEVELS

Before getting into details of human tolerance levels, it should be pointed out that there is a rather large range of physiological variations in tolerance level so that it is not possible to establish a single tolerance level that will be safe for all individuals. A range or level suitable for the "average" individual is meant when a tolerance level is referred to in this paper. Thus, an injury tolerance level that would produce a moderate injury in the majority of the population will probably produce serious or fatal injuries for a few and no injuries for others.

Human tolerance can be based on the following: (1) voluntary, (2) injury threshold, (3) moderate or (4) severe injury levels. The voluntary injury level is that level which volunteers are willing to be subjected to and is usually well below the injury level. Injury threshold refers to impact conditions which are just below those that will result in injury. The moderate injury level is that level where some injury occurs, but complete recovery is expected with no permanent deformities. The severe injury level is any level up to fatality. Obviously, the severe injury level is not a satisfactory design level. With requirements for protection from higher and higher impact velocities it is probably advisable to use the moderate injury level for designing safety devices instead of one of the subinjury categories. If a lower level is used, then it is impossible to provide protection from the high velocities encountered in automobile collisions. With a properly established moderate injury tolerance level, there will be a certain segment of the population consisting of those least able to withstand impacts that will receive serious injuries. The major part of the population will receive only reversible moderate injuries, while those able to withstand the greatest impacts will receive no injury whatsoever. It is important to understand that the best design criteria are those which will provide the maximum protection for the maximum number of people at the maximum impact velocity for any given condition.

Tolerance levels must be established for each type of impact exposure and each type of injury ranging through soft tissue damage, bone damage, internal organ injury and other types of trauma. Included in the parameters that affect impact tolerance, and consequently must be recognized in the tolerance level, are the following: impact site, area, direction, velocity, mass, surface hardness, surface roughness, age, sex, physical condition and size.

It should be emphasized that lesions from previous trauma, congenital defects and other abnormalities will affect the results of injuries from the impact environment. Thus, an individual with an aortic aneurysm which might rupture spontaneously at any time can probably withstand only a very mild chest impact. Thus, he would fall well out of the protection level for designs based on moderate injury tolerance levels.

The most commonly used methods of establishing human tolerance levels are listed below:

1. Controlled tests with human volunteers
2. Human cadaver research
3. Animal research
4. Research with anthropomorphic dummies
5. Clinical observations
6. Mathematical models

All of these methods contribute to the overall knowledge, and all of them have shortcomings that should be recognized. The object of this chapter is to discuss the various methods of establishing human tolerance to impact and to point out some of the pitfalls associated with each. Finally, a table of human tolerance levels will be presented.

Voluntary Limits

Col. John Paul Stapp[1] is the pioneer in voluntary impact studies. He used his own body as the experimental subject for many of the early research programs at military bases. He used high speed sleds for determining the maximum force levels a human can stand when restrained with lap and shoulder harness. His early runs at Holloman Air Force Base on the rocket sled, Sonic Wind, are outstanding examples of human exposure to voluntary acceleration conditions. He experienced a change of velocity of over 600 mph with accelerations in excess of 40 g.

Others who have contributed to voluntary tolerance limits include various military researchers associated with Col. Stapp and Prof. James Ryan at the University of Minnesota,[2] Lombard,[3] Armstrong,[4] Patrick,[5] Mertz[6] and Zaborowski.[7] There are many others, and no attempt will be made here to list them all.

Voluntary whole body tolerance is based on the results of human experiments on centrifuges, sleds and a few deliberate automobile crashes. The aforementioned Sonic Wind ride by Colonel Stapp is the outstanding example of human sled research, but other investigators are contributing to the store of voluntary human tolerance with sled tests with the occupant in forward-facing, rear-facing and side-facing positions to represent forward-force, rear-force and side-force collisions. With a lap belt and upper torso restraint it appears that a 40 g deceleration[8] for a change in velocity up to the 70 or 80 mph encountered in an automobile is a survivable limit.

The whiplash environment has been studied on a sled at simulated impact speeds up to 44 mph by Mertz.[6] This mode of impact apparently is one of the few in which the proper design of the environment can eliminate the injury, with the design criterion being the voluntary limit rather than some injury limit. At the 44 mph simulated rear-end collision, the volunteer felt no apprehension over the possibility of head or neck injury. It is expected that with adequate design of the seat and head support to prevent hyperextension that rear-end collisions up to 60 mph can be withstood with no injury whatsoever. This is the one exception to the design requirement for a moderate injury tolerance level. It also illustrates the advantage of having the forces distributed over a large part of the body.

In addition to the whole body experiments conducted on the sled and centrifuge, impact to individual body components is one of the essential needs for design criteria. Kroell[9] and Patrick[10] have studied the individual body impacts to the head, chest, knee and combinations thereof. Gurdjian,[11] Lissner,[12] Patrick[13] and others, have established a head tolerance curve which is a function of acceleration magnitude and time. Other investigators have also found that the duration of impact is an important parameter in tolerance. Gadd[14] has devised a method that is widely used for evaluating the time-magnitude acceleration pulse to eliminate mathematically the human error that was involved in previous evaluation of the pulse. Most of the head impact data is for forehead impact, so considerable research is required to provide additional tolerance data on impact to other parts of the head.

Linear acceleration is the most common parameter used to indicate the injury potential of head impact. Other parameters that have been considered include force, angular acceleration, pressure and displacement. The acceleration criterion has the advantage that it can be measured during the impact by attaching accelerometers to the head opposite the point of impact. The other parameters are more difficult to measure and interpret, and require that the impacting surface be instrumented which is often difficult and not accurate.

Voluntary tolerance limits are indicative of the maximum that a volunteer will withstand, but are generally well below the injury level. Human tests have the advantage of providing realistic data and are important as an end point in establishing other types of tolerance levels. The response of human volunteers can be used to validate other types of experiments including those with human cadavers and anthropomorphic dummies. This is accomplished by comparing the response data from volunteer, cadaver and anthropomorphic dummy tests at the same level of impact. Good correspondence at the voluntary levels provides confidence in the results at higher levels.

Human Cadaver Experiments

Human cadavers are advantageous in human tolerance experiments, since the mass distribution and structure is identical to the living human. Also, the cadaver with proper preparation has the same degrees of mobility as the living human. Obviously, the physiological responses are not present, and the muscular reactions cannot be duplicated exactly. However, there are ways in which the effect of the muscles can be simulated such as adding external, flexible braces, which provide increased stiffness to the joints. This latter technique has been used to a limited degree with only mediocre results.

At Wayne State University, the use of cadavers has been an important tool in establishing human tolerance levels for approximately 30 years. These experiments run the gamut from individual body components to whole body acceleration. Generally, the approach is to provide a response to a particular environment from a human volunteer. The identical environment is used for the cadaver experiments with a comparison of the human volunteer and the cadaver results made at a subinjury level. After the correlation with the volunteer at low impact levels, the cadaver is subjected to progressively higher impact levels until structural damage (bone fracture) occurs.

Gurdjian and Lissner were early advocates of this type of biomechanics research.[11,12] Their work was instrumental in establishing the tolerance of the human head to impact. They combined human cadaver research with animal research and clinical observations to provide a comprehensive picture of injury to the head.

The use of cadavers is illustrated in papers by Evans,[15,16] Kroell,[9] Mertz,[6] Patrick,[10] Hodgson,[17,18] Gurdjian,[11] Huelke[21] and others.

Animal Research

Physiological responses are used to measure the effect of impacts to animals including brain and organ reactions which are not available in cadavers. Ommaya,[19] Gurdjian,[20] Hodgson,[22] Martinez,[23] Wickstrom,[24] Snyder,[25] Higgins[26] and many others have reported on animal research. The advantage, of course, is the physiological response and the injuries that can be observed by clinicians similar to those observed in accident cases with humans. The disadvantage is that all animal responses are not similar to those of humans, particularly since the experiments are conducted with the animal anesthetized.

The species difference is the major drawback of the use of animals. The animals used in animal research include the dog, cat, goat, sheep, cattle, primates and several species of rodents. The primates appear to have the greatest importance, and many people feel that this type of research is the best way to establish the human tolerance to impact.

Correlation between the animal and the human is the major problem involved. Ommaya[19] has suggested concussion correlation between the monkey and the human to be based on angular acceleration. He derives a relationship between primate and man in which the angular acceleration to produce concussion in man varies inversely as the ⅔ power of the mass of the brain on the assumption that the brains have similar properties and shapes. While there is some question whether the extension of this ⅔ power ratio is valid for the human because of variation in shape and possibly material properties, and possibly because concussion is a function of some parameter other than angular acceleration, there does appear to be some correlation that will ultimately be determined. Verification may eventually be obtained by a comparison with known injuries and the physical parameters such as angular acceleration to produce the injuries. However, the present state of the art does not permit an accurate extrapolation of injury parameters from animals to humans.

While the exact correlation between human and animal research is not yet available, the mechanism of injuries to various organs can be studied quite accurately with animals. If the mechanism of the injury is known, the methods of combatting the injury can be established with better accuracy than would be the case if the injury mechanism is unknown. Roberts[27] has studied the aortic injuries in animals and found them to be quite similar in appearance to those observed in accident victims.

Clinical Observations

The use of clinical observations for establishing human tolerance levels to impact has been underway for many years. Huelke and Gikas,[28] Nahum and Siegel,[29] States[30] and others have reported on clinical observations relating to injuries and in some instances an estimate of the conditions producing the injuries have been made. An extension of this technique is expected to produce the most reliable human tolerance data.

In order for this data to be of importance it is essential that a quantitative physical measure of the conditions producing the injury be obtained. This approach is being undertaken at Wayne State University through a contract with GSA[31] in which clinical injuries from accident cases are being studied and compared with experimental results. Cadavers are used in these experiments and the exact conditions producing the injuries are studied in the laboratory with the same type of vehicle. The victims' injuries are reported on an appropriate form by the emergency room physician. A team of doctors and engineers then classifies the injuries according to a scale developed for this purpose. The deformation of the interior of the vehicle is carefully measured and is used as a method of obtaining the exact environmental conditions. For example, when a given head impact produces a certain deformation in the instrument panel and a corresponding injury to the victim, the conditions are reproduced in the laboratory by varying the impact conditions until the same deformation is produced with the same type of vehicle and a cadaver as the occupant. Forces or accelerations are measured on the cadaver in the laboratory crashes so when the same deformation is obtained in the laboratory as was present in the accident, the forces or acceleration to produce the injury are known. By using a large number of impacts of this type, it is expected that a degree of injury as a function of head acceleration will result. Similar studies are being conducted on steering wheel impact. An extension of this principle to other injury conditions will provide a measure of human tolerance to impact based on actual injury conditions. Again, it should be pointed out that for this information to be valid, it is necessary to have a quantitative measure of the forces or accelerations and times to produce the injury.

Investigations with Anthropomorphic Dummies

The automotive companies,[32,33] Severy,[34,35] and others, are conducting research in simulated impact environments using anthropomorphic dummies as the subjects. Sophisticated instrumentation permits the acceleration and forces associated with the impact to be recorded accurately. Unfortunately, the anthropomorphic dummies currently available do not simulate the human body and the reactions of the body to the impact satisfactorily. However, with continued improvement in the dummies, this technique should be valuable in predicting injuries from any impact environment that can be described and reproduced experimentally

The manufacturers of anthropomorphic dummies are continually revising the dummies to incorporate the latest information available on the dynamics required to simulate humans. As more data become available, the dummies will become more sophisticated and ultimately will provide a means of studying injury potential of all types including internal injuries. Dummies with frangible components and simulated organs which will show "bone" fracture and "organ" injury similar to that of humans under the same impact conditions are being developed. Unfortunately, these sophisticated dummies cannot be completed until physical measurements corresponding to the injuries are available. When the many variables are considered, it appears that years of research will be required before a true trauma-indicating dummy becomes available.

Mathematical Models

The role of the mathematical model must be mentioned. Just as the sophisticated dummy could replace all other subjects in crash research, the mathematical model can theoretically replace the dummy when enough data and large enough computers become available. McHenry[36] and Austin[37] are proponents of mathematical models for the occupant and the vehicle. Eventually, it might be possible to design a vehicle and evaluate its safety characteristics without going farther than the computer. When that day arrives, optimization techniques will result in the safest car possible.

At the present time, McHenry's 11 degree of freedom model is pushing the capabilities of the computer, and it does not approach the number of variables required for complete human simulation. Similarly, even the most advanced mathematical model of the automobile does not approach the complexity required if all types of collisions (external and internal) are to be considered. Nevertheless, the mathematical model will undoubtedly play an increasingly important role in automobile and other types of safety.

HUMAN TOLERANCE LEVELS

Finally, a summary of human tolerance to impact is an essential part of this paper. Table 13–II is a compilation of tolerance levels considered useful in automotive safety. The source and method of obtaining the levels are included. A cursory examination of the table shows it to be woefully incomplete. This, then, is the challenge to those engaged in safety research —COMPLETE THE TABLE.

REFERENCES

1. STAPP, J.P.: Human exposure to linear deceleration. The forward-facing position and the development of a crash harness. *AF Technical Report No. 5915*, Dec. 1951, Pt. 2.
2. RYAN, J.J.: Reduction in crash forces. *Proceedings of the Fifth Stapp Conference.* 1962, pp. 48–89.
3. LOMBARD, C.F.; AMES, S.W.; ROTH, H.P., and ROSENFELD, S.: Voluntary tolerance of the human to impact accelerations of the head. *J Aviation Med*, April 1951, vol. 22.
4. ARMSTRONG, R.W.: First summary report of the national bureau of standards tests at Holloman Air Force Base. Verbally presented at National Bureau of Standards, Oct. 1967.
5. PATRICK, L.M.: Human tolerance to impact—basis for safety design. *SAE Transactions*, 1966.
6. MERTZ, H.J., JR., and PATRICK, L.M.: Investigation of the kinematics and kinetics of whiplash. *Proceedings of the Eleventh Stapp Conference.* 1967, pp. 175–206.
7. ZABOROWSKI, A.B.: Human tolerance to lateral impact with lap belt only. *Proceedings of the Eighth Stapp Conference.* 1966, pp. 34–69.
8. STAPP, J.P.: The problem: biomechanics of injury. *The Prevention of Highway Injury.* Ann Arbor, U. of Mich., 1967.
9. KROELL, C.K., and PATRICK, L.M.: A new crash simulator and biomechanics research program. *Proceedings of the Eighth Stapp Car Crash Conference.* 1966, pp. 185–228.
10. PATRICK, L.M.; KROELL, C.K., and MERTZ, H.J., JR.: Forces on the human body in simulated crashes. *Proceedings of the Ninth Stapp Conference.* 1966, pp. 237–259.
11. GURDJIAN, E.S.; WEBSTER, J.E., and LISSNER, H.R.: Observations on the mechanism of brain concussion, contusion, and laceration. *Surg Gynec Obstet, 101:* 680–690, Dec. 1955.

12. LISSNER, H.R., and GURDJIAN, E.S.: Experimental cerebral concussion. *ASME Paper No. 60–WA–273*, 1960.
13. PATRICK, L.M.; LISSNER, H.R., and GURDJIAN, E.S.: Survival by design—head protection. *Proceedings of the Seventh Stapp Conference.* 1965, pp. 483–499.
14. GADD, C.W.: Use of a weighted-impulse criterion for estimating injury hazard. *Proceedings of the Tenth Stapp Conference.* 1967, pp. 164–174.
15. EVANS, F.G., and LISSNER, H.R.: Studies on pelvic deformations and fractures. *Anat Rec, 121:*141–166, Feb. 1955.
16. EVANS, F.G.; LISSNER, H.R., and LEBOW, M.: The relation of energy, velocity, and acceleration to skull deformation and fracture. *Surg Gynec Obstet*, Nov. 1958, vol. 107.
17. HODGSON, V.R.; LANGE, W.A., and TALWALKER, R.K.: Injury to the facial bones. *Proceedings of the Ninth Stapp Conference,* 1966, pp. 144–163.
18. HODGSON, V.R.; LISSNER, H.R., and PATRICK, L.M.: The effect of jerk on the human spine. *ASME Paper No. 63–WA–316*, Nov. 1963.
19. OMMAYA, A.K.; YARNELL, P.; HIRSCH, A.E., and HARRIS, E.H.: Scaling of experimental data on cerebral concussion in sub-human primates to concussion threshold for man. *Proceedings of the Eleventh Stapp Conference.* 1967, pp. 47–52.
20. GURDJIAN, E.S.; LISSNER, H.R., and PATRICK, L.M.: Concussion—mechanism and pathology. *Proceedings of the Seventh Stapp Conference.* 1965, pp. 470–482.
21. HUELKE, D.F., and BURDI, A.R.: Location of mandibular fractures related to teeth and edentulous regions. *J Oral Surg*, Sept. 1964, vol. 22.
22. HODGSON, V.R.; GURDJIAN, E.S., and THOMAS, L.M.: Experimental skull deformation and brain displacement demonstrated by flash x-ray technique. *J Neurosurg*, XXV:549–552, 1966.
23. MARTINEZ, J.L.: Study of whiplash injuries in animals. *ASME Paper No. 63–WA–281*, Nov. 1963.
24. WICKSTROM, J.; MARTINEZ, J.L.; JOHNSTON, D., and TAPPEN, N.C.: Acceleration-deceleration injuries of the cervical spine in animals. *Proceedings of the Seventh Stapp Conference,* 1965, pp. 284–301.
25. SNYDER, R.G.; YOUNG, J.W., and SNOW, C.C.: Experimental impact protection with advanced automotive restraint systems: preliminary primate tests with air bag and inertia reel/inverted-Y yoke torso harness. *Proceedings of the Eleventh Stapp Conference,* 1967, pp. 271–285.
26. HIGGINS, L.S., and SCHMALL, R.A.: A device for the investigation of head injury effected by non-deforming head accelerations. *Proceedings of the Eleventh Stapp Conference,* 1967, pp. 35–46.
27. ROBERTS, V.L.: Experimental studies on thoracic and abdominal injuries. *The Prevention of Highway Injury.* Ann Arbor, U. of Mich., 1967.
28. HUELKE, D.F.; GIKAS, P.W., and HENDRIX, R.C.: Patterns of injury in fatal automobile accidents. *Proceedings of the Sixth Stapp Conference*, Nov. 1962.
29. NAHUM, A.M.; SEVERY, D.M., and SIEGEL, A.W.: Automobile accidents correlated with collision experiments: head-on collisions. *Proceedings of the Ninth Stapp Conference.* 1966, pp. 303–316.
30. STATES, J.D.: Case studies of racing accidents. *Proceedings of the Eighth Stapp Conference.* 1966, pp. 251–257.

TABLE 13-II
HUMAN TOLERANCE TO IMPACT

Body Area	Loading Direction or Position	Description	Subject	Trauma	Vel. ft./sec.	Accel. g units	Time msec	Force lbs	Source (See References)
Total	Supine	Fall on packed garden earth	Human	No injury	54	140 ave.			38
Total	Supine	Fall on crusted snow—3½ foot deep crater	Human	No injury	178	141 ave.			39
Total	Seated	Eyeballs out—military vol. Torso, lap belt	Human vol.	No injury	226–50	45 peak	230		40
Total	Seated	Eyeballs in—military vol. Head, torso and lap belt support	Human vol.	No injury	208–112	35 peak	160		40
Total	Seated	Eyeballs down—military vol. Optimum restraint system	Human vol.	No injury		35 peak			40
Total	Seated	Eyeballs down—some fract. during ejection	Human	Occasional vertebral fract.		20 peak			41
Forehead	A-P*	Cadaver, animal and clinical analysis	Cadavers	Mild concussion deduced	60	80	30		42
Forehead	A-P	Severity Index $\int a^{2.5} dt = 1000$ max.	Hypothet.						43
Forehead	A-P	6 inch diam. × ½ inch thick metal target, unpadded	Human vol.	No injury			5	peak 400	44
Forehead	A-P	6 inch diam. × ½ inch thick metal target, padded	Human vol.	No injury			32	peak 285	44
Forehead	A-P	2.5 inch diam. flat padded impactor	Cadaver	Skull fract. (threshold)			4	2000	45
Full face (inc. forehead)	A-P	Padded, deformable metal instr. panel	Cadaver	No fract. Probable brain damage to humans	60	165 peak			46
Cheek (zygoma)	Arch	2.5 inch diam., flat padded impactor	Cadaver	Fract. threshold			9	480	45
Cheek (zygoma)	Arch	2.5 inch diam., flat padded impactor	Cadaver	Fract. threshold			19	360	45
Cheek (zygoma)	Arch	1.1 inch diam., flat padded impactor	Cadaver	Fract. threshold			7	250	45
Upper jaw	A-P	1.1 inch diam., flat padded impactor	Cadaver	Fract. threshold			22	160	47

Body region	Direction/Restraint	Test condition	Subject	Result	(col)	(col)	Ref
Jaw (mandible)	A-P	2.5 inch diam., flat padded impactor	Cadaver	Fracture (threshold)		6	45
Jaw (mandible)	A-P	1.1 inch diam., flat padded impactor	Cadaver	Fracture (threshold)	17	600	47
Neck (larynx)	A-P	Excised larynx	Hog	Fracture		275	48
Shoulder	A-P	Steering wheel rim (each shoulder)	Cadaver	No fracture	36	65	49
Upper torso (thorax)	A-P	Total load—steering wheel impact—collapsible column	Cadaver	No fracture	36	500	49
Shoulder	Shoulder belt	Load on shoulder belt	Human vol.	No injury		1800	50
Chest	Midsternum	Impact to 6 inch diam. padded target	Cadaver	Rib fracture	25	770	51
Pelvis	Lap belt	Impact sled with lap belt	Human vol.	No injury		1200	52
Pelvis	Lap belt	Force calculated from peak accel. on buckle and total subj. weight	Human	No injury		2800	53
Knee, thigh, hip	Seated	Dynamic knee impact to 6 inch diam. padded target with force along femoral axis	Human vol.	No injury		5000	51
Knee, thigh, hip	Seated	Dynamic knee impact to 6 inch diam. padded target with force along femoral axis	Cadaver	Femur fracture		1050	51
Knee, thigh, hip	Seated	Dynamic knee impact to 6 inch diam. unpadded target with force along femoral axis	Cadaver	Patella fracture		1500	51
Lower leg	Transverse	Concentrated impact load at distal third of lower leg	Cadaver			1500	51
Neck	Hyper-extension (whiplash)	Seated position—rear-end collision	Human vol.			1000–	54, 55
Neck	No head support	Simulated 15 mph rear-end collision	Human vol.	None			56
Neck	Rigid head support	Simulated 44 mph rear-end collision	Human vol.	None		340	56

* A-P—Anterior to posterior.

31. General Services Administration Contract No. GS-00S-56359 entitled Establishing Human Tolerance to Automobile Steering Wheel and Instrument Panel Impact. With Wayne State University granted July 1, 1965.
32. LUNDSTROM, L.C.; KELLY, A.H., JR., and LaBELLE, D.J.: Crash research for vehicle safety. *SAE Paper 831A*, April 1964.
33. FREDERICKS, R.H.: Automobile crash research. Presented at SAE Detroit Section Meeting, Nov. 1962.
34. SEVERY, D.M., and MATHEWSON, J.H.: Automobile barrier and rear-end collision performance. Presented at SAE Summer Meeting, June 1958.
35. SEVERY, D.M.; MATHEWSON, J.H., and SIEGEL, A.W.: Automobile side-impact collisions, series II. *SAE Paper 491A*, March 1962.
36. McHENRY, R.R; SEGAL, D.J., and DELEYS, N.J.: Computer simulation of single vehicle accidents. *Proceedings of the Eleventh Stapp Conference*. 1967, pp. 1–34.
37. AUSTIN, C.E.; BRAUBURGER, R.A., and KANSAL, S.C.: Computed implemented design of automobile interiors. *Proceedings of the Tenth Stapp Conference*. 1967, pp. 116–125.

Sources (Table 13-II)

38. DeHAVEN, H.: Mechanical analysis of survival in falls from heights of fifty to one hundred and fifty feet. *War Med*, 2:586–596, July 1942.
39. KIEL, F.W.: Hazards of military parachuting. *Milit Med*, 130:512–521, 1965.
40. STAPP, J.P.: The problem: biomechanics of injury. *The Prevention of Highway Injury*, 1967, pp. 159–164.
41. Personal communication with Cdr. C.L. Ewing, MC, USN, who found occasional vertebral fractures in aircraft ejections at 20 to 24 g.
42. STAPP, J.P.: Review of air force research on biodynamics of collision injury. *Proceedings of the Tenth Stapp Car Crash Conference*, 1966, pp. 325–342.
43. GADD, C.W.: Use of weighted impulse criterion for estimating injury hazard. *Proceedings of the Tenth Stapp Car Crash Conference*, 1966, pp. 164–174.
44. PATRICK, L.M.: Voluntary male subject, no injury. (unpublished).
45. HODGSON, V.R.: Tolerance to facial bones in impact. *Amer J Anat*, Jan. 1967.
46. DANIEL, R.P., and PATRICK, L.M.: Instrument panel impact study. *Proceedings of the Ninth Stapp Car Crash Conference*. 1966, pp. 165–179.
47. HODGSON, V.R.; NAKAMURA, G.S., and TALWALKER, R.K.: Response of the facial structure to impact. *Proceedings of the Eighth Stapp Car Crash Conference*. 1966.
48. GADD, C.W.: Rupture threshold, bare larynx of hog. 1965 (unpublished).
49. GADD, C.W., and PATRICK, L.M.: System versus laboratory impact tests for estimating injury hazard. SAE Engineering Congress and Exposition, Detroit, Jan. 1968.
50. ARMSTRONG, R.W.: First summary report of the national bureau of standards tests at Holloman Air Force Base. Verbally presented at National Bureau of Standards, Oct. 1967.
51. PATRICK, L.M.; KROELL, C.K., and MERTZ, H.J.: Forces on the human body in simulated crashes. *Proceedings of the Ninth Stapp Car Crash Conference*, 1965.
52. RYAN, J.J.: Human crash deceleration tests on seat belts. *Aerospace Med*, 33: 167–174, 1962.

53. Stapp, J.P., and Enfield, D.L.: Evaluation of the lap-type automobile safety belt with reference to human tolerance. *SAE Paper 62A*, June 1958. [(5000#) calculated from accelerometer reading on buckle]
54. Young, J.W.: Threshold value for tibia fracture, male cadavers (aged 29–57). 1967 (unpublished).
55. Young, J.W.: Mean value for 12 male cadaver legs, tibial fracture. 1967 (unpublished).
56. Mertz, H.J., and Patrick, L.M.: Investigation of the kinematics and kinetics of whiplash. *Proceedings of the Eleventh Stapp Car Crash Conference*. 1967, pp. 175–206.

DISCUSSION

L. Murray Thomas

The various efforts to determine, to the best degree possible, the tolerances that humans can stand in various forms of impact injury have been presented.

One of the difficulties that we have been faced with all along, in this particular work, is the problem of trying to determine how you can protect against one kind of injury, without adding substantially to the danger from some other form of injury. Although the seat belt may have helped in many situations, there are more intra-abdominal injuries related to seat belts, improperly used to be sure, but at least related to one form of protection. Any effort which can be made to find the tolerances that people can stand, without life-endangering or disabling injury, is important.

It is important to continually go back to the human, continually go back to the cadaver, continually go back to the animal experiments, and work the three in conjunction with each other. If the anthropomorphic dummies are being used, put this in the group too. Do not spend all of your time working on animal experiments, or on cadavers, without going to the human. It is very difficult to do what I have said, except in a few institutions. We have been very fortunate here at Wayne. Our Anatomy Department has been able to provide us with cadavers for experimentation, and we have been able to correlate these with animal and dummy work. And we have been very fortunate to have a supply of at least body parts to do the same kind of correlative study.

Chapter XIV

PHYSICAL FACTORS RELATED TO EXPERIMENTAL CONCUSSION

Voigt R. Hodgson

INTRODUCTION

This chapter is an attempt to enumerate and define the roles of the most important physical factors related to concussion in the experimental animal from blunt impacts to the head. It is based upon a series of head injury experiments utilizing thirty-seven monkeys, ten dogs and ten cats. The results and conclusions of other researchers are liberally included to point up areas of unanimity or disagreement or inadequacies in this writer's experience.

Physical agents, related to head injury by investigators, have been head accelerations (from a direct blow),[1,2,4,6,19] including translational,[1,2,4,6,19,23,25] and rotational,[7,12,21] as a peak value,[1,2,4] average value,[19] or mean value, associated with pulse duration[6] impulse[19] energy[19] velocity.[1,19] Others have associated angular acceleration[20,22] produced on a small primate whiplash sled, with concussion. Still others have related concussion to neck stretch,[14] mentioning but without giving any values for, amount of force and rate of application or time duration.

Many have concluded that as far as injury to the brain or brain stem is concerned, the ultimate physical cause is shear stress. Holbourne[12] pointed out that the bulk modulus (resistance to volume change) of brain tissue is large compared to its modulus of rigidity (resistance to change in shape). Therefore, he concluded that if brain tissue is considered to react to stress like other materials, brain injury is most likely produced when shear stresses arise as a result of angular acceleration of the head. He reasoned that linear accelerations tend to produce compression and rarifaction strains which because of the high bulk modulus of brain matter have no injurious effects. Shear strains produced by linear acceleration, according to Holbourne, are produced mainly in the neighborhood of foramena, where tissue has a tendency to be extruded or sucked in and in the neighborhood of ventricles owing to the slight difference in density between CSF and brain tissue. He concluded that these shear strains produced by linear acceleration could be neglected compared to those produced by rotational acceleration. He cited Grundfest's experiment in which an isolated nerve continues to conduct when subjected to 10,000 psi pure hydrostatic pressure.

Gurdjian and Lissner[5] reasoned that pressure gradients observed in their experiments arising out of acceleration or deformation of the skull would produce shear stress particularly in the brain stem area. However, Gurdjian, et al.,[6] have also emphasized that in general, a head impact produces both translational and rotational motion as well as deformation of the skull with resultant brain injury from relative motion in the brain and between brain and skull. Gurdjian and Lissner[5] used a two dimensional photoelastic model to show that the region of the craniocervical junction is a region of high shear stress concentration. Ommaya, et al.,[22] support Holbourne's[12] angular acceleration-shear stress theory.

Unterharnscheidt and Sellier[23,25] have emphasized that head accelerations and skull deformations produce intracranial pressure changes which result in cavitation at the antipole and at points of skull outbending. They suggested that the term "cortical foci of cavitation" be used to describe brain lesion and hemorrhage due to this low pressure phenomenon. Gross[3] has produced experimental cavitation by impact to water filled flasks.

Shock waves have been discounted as a source of injury to brain tissue by Unterharnscheidt[23] because even the shortest impact duration caused by a blow to the human head (.002 of a second) is one order of magnitude longer than the transit time of pressure waves across the brain (0.00013 of a second).

These investigations were carried out under varying conditions of species and injury production and the possibility exists as shown by Thomas[24] that they may not all have been investigating the same phenomena. Therefore, it is understandable that although some injury factors are agreed upon there are many areas of disagreement. It is the purpose of this paper to present some recent results which may help to improve the understanding of experimental concussion.

METHODS

Data similar to that shown in Figure 14–1 were obtained after impacts to a group of thirty-seven monkey, ten dogs, and ten cats for the purpose of comparing the physiological response and to determine the physical factors most related to the degree of concussion. The experiment was designed to obtain the velocity, mass, and energy of the striking missile and the force-time history of the impact. All animals were in the lightly anesthetized state, responsive to stimuli affecting the reflexes listed in

PHYSIOLOGICAL MANIFESTATIONS OF CONCUSSION

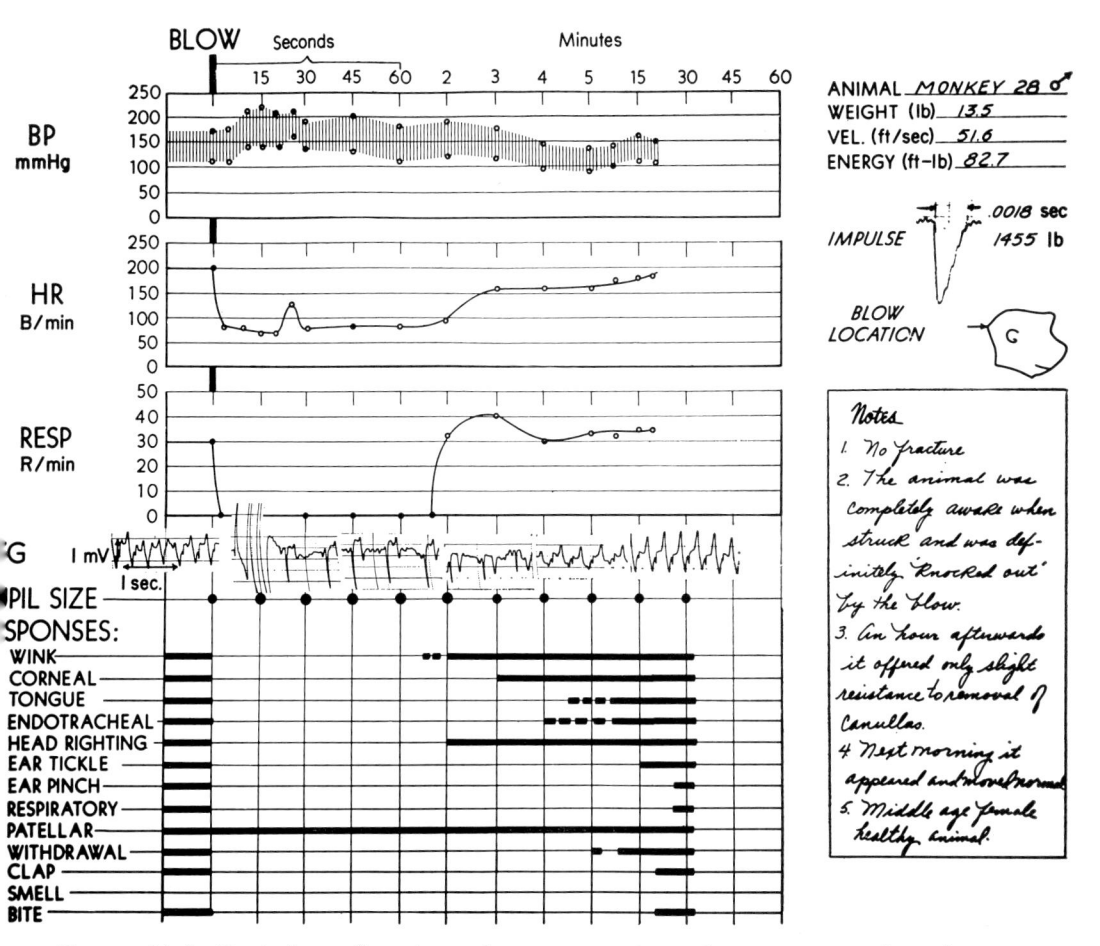

FIGURE 14–1. Typical manifestations of severe experimental concussion without fracture in the stump-tail monkey.

Figure 14–1. Blows were delivered to the occipital ridge in the monkey. The cats and dogs were struck on the sagittal crest or occipital protuberance. The striker was a solid steel cylinder weighing 2 pounds, with a ¼ inch thick hard rubber face, 1 inch squared area. It was accelerated to the desired level and then guided at constant velocity into impact with the head. The dogs and cats were mongrel, of various sizes, age and sex. In the monkey group were animals of several species including rhesus, babboon and stumptail. In the discussion of monkey experimentation to follow, only results on twenty-seven of the stump-tail variety are included. This group contained animals ranging from young mature to old but active, male and female, weighing from 10 to 23 pounds, all in apparently good health. Heads of the animals were removed and weighed after the experiment. The cats and dogs exhibited similar but more sensitive physiological changes in response to a blow compared to those seen in the monkey. However, variations among the cats and dogs may have obscured any relationship between physical factors, and therefore results in these two species will not be discussed in much detail.

RESULTS

Physiological Changes

Typically, an animal (dog, cat, stump-tail monkey) after receiving a blow to the head of sufficient intensity, will exhibit changes similar to those shown in Figure 14–1. There is usually, as shown here, a rise in blood pressure, a slight increase in pulse, bradycardia, a period of apnea for up to 2 minutes. Confused EKG exhibiting such things as inverted T waves, rhythm irregularities, and other evidences of an irritated and ischemic heart, an increase in pupil size (only slight in the monkey) and loss of response to stimuli as listed in the lower left of Figure 14–1. In the case of this animal, (Monkey 28), all of the reflexes and responses were knocked out for at least 2 minutes except the patellar reflex which is controlled in the cord. This blow delivered by a 2 pound striker moving at 51.6 feet per second, energy 82.7 feet per pounds, produced an impulse of 1460 pounds maximum force, duration 0.0018 seconds. The animal was unresponsive to any stimuli for 2 minutes. It did not exhibit a bite or respiratory reflex, or respond to sound for over 20 minutes, and was very weak an hour after the blow. It was judged to have received a severe concussion. The next morning, the animal appeared and moved normally and did not suffer a fracture. It was a middle aged, healthy, female animal weighing 13.5 pounds.

Evaluation of the degree of concussion suffered by an animal was done on a relative basis for each species. An animal which experienced a loss of at least one of the eight or ten responses to mechanical stimuli which were checked, was deemed to have received a minimal concussion. This formed the basis for five degrees as follows: subminimal, minimal, moderate, severe, and lethal. A subminimal effect was manifested by at most a momentary change in the amplitude or rate of EKG, EEG, respiration, heart rate, pulse, or blood pressure, but no response loss. To help establish whether a blow had a minimal, moderate, or severe effect, the amount of change and time duration to return to normal of the above mentioned physiological parameters and response to mechanical stimuli, as well as cardiac ischemia and rhythm irregularities evidence by the EKG records, were utilized. Since each animal displayed a unique response, several difficult decisions arose while grading the effects of a blow. However, a neurosurgical resident conducted an independent evaluation of the degree of concussion, as indicated by EKG changes, and his evaluations agreed closely with those of the author, who used response and physiological changes other than EKG as a criterion. Among thirty monkeys there was agreement in twenty-six experiments, and in the remaining four there were only minor differences.

Physical Factors Related to Injury

Shown in Figure 14-2 is a typical force-time history of an impact to the head of a monkey. With this amount of information, plus the weight and velocity of the striker and the weight of the animal's head, it is possible to compare the physiological effect to at least the following physical factors:

1. Force
2. Impulse
3. Energy

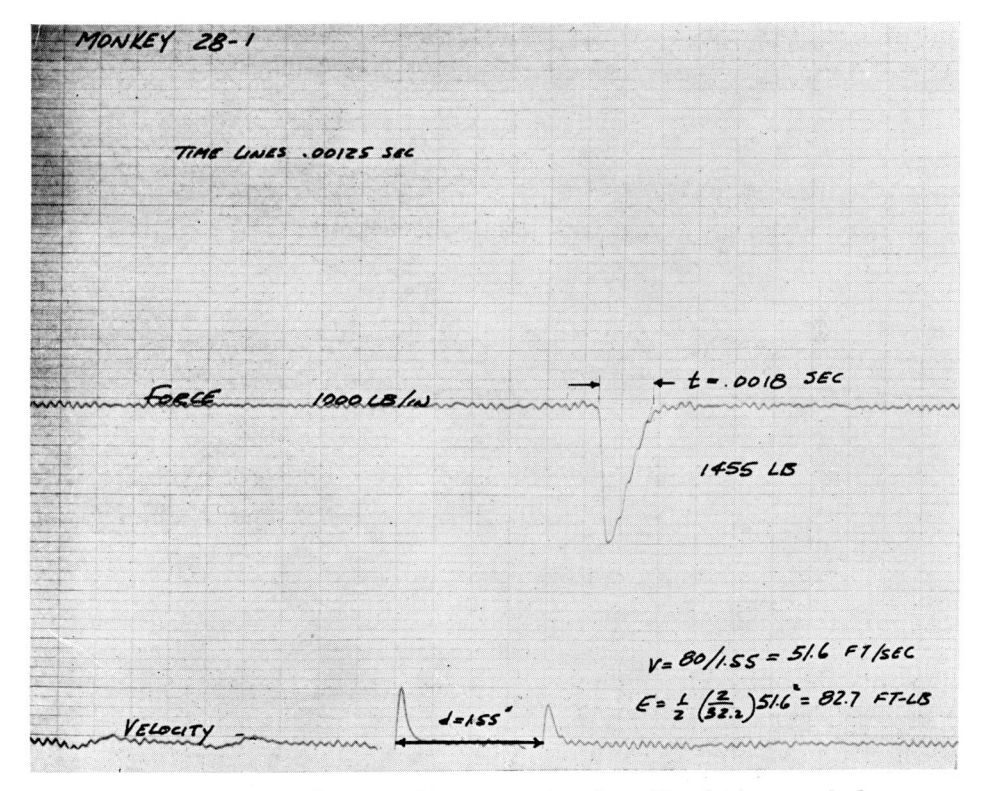

FIGURE 14-2. Force-time history of impact to monkey 28 which caused the severe physiological changes in Figure 14-1.

4. Energy absorbed
5. Power absorbed
6. Apparent head acceleration (force/head mass)
7. Jerk
8. Frequency spectrum

These terms are defined as follows:

Force is taken to mean the peak value.
Impulse is the integral (area) of the force-time curve taken over the time duration (T) of the pulse, i.e. the integral from 0 to T of F(t) where F(t) indicates force as a function of time as illustrated in Figure 14–2.
Energy refers to the kinetic energy of the striker prior to impact ($\frac{1}{2}mv^2$).
Energy absorbed (E_a) is derived as follows:

$$E_a = E_1 - E_2 \tag{1}$$

$$E_1 - E_2 = \tfrac{1}{2}mv^2 - \tfrac{1}{2}m(v - \Delta v)^2 \tag{2}$$

where E_1 and E_2 are the initial and post impact kinetic energy of the striker; m is the mass of the striker; v is the initial velocity of the striker; Δv is velocity change of the striker ($\int_0^T a\,dt$), caused by the impulse, lasting T sec., where a = force per striker mass.
Power absorbed is energy absorbed divided by pulse duration.
Apparent head acceleration is obtained by dividing peak force by the mass of the monkey's head severed from the base of the occipital, across the outer edge of the foramen magnum and including the mandible.
Jerk is the time derivative of acceleration, calculated here however to be peak rigid body head acceleration divided by rise time.
Frequency Spectrum of the pulse describes the continuous distribution of vibrational energy in a pulse from 0 to ∞ Hz.,[16] but for our purpose the frequency is limited to the range 0 to 5000 Hz.

Each of the above parameters was compared to physiological response in a manner illustrated in Figure 14–3. All of the data was plotted in this manner, identifying the monkeys along the bottom, with the nine animals which received fracture shown on the right, and graduation of the physical parameter listed on the ordinant. The physical data was examined for statistical correlation with injury by the analysis of variance method of dividing the data up into three bands of parameter level, each containing nine animals and excluding animals 16 and 29 which received depressed fractures. The method is illustrated in Table 14–I which shows the calculations for predicting the probability of relationship of force/head mass to the degree of head injury. Force/head mass (acceleration) is considered as a dose of a central nervous system trauma producing agent. The dosages

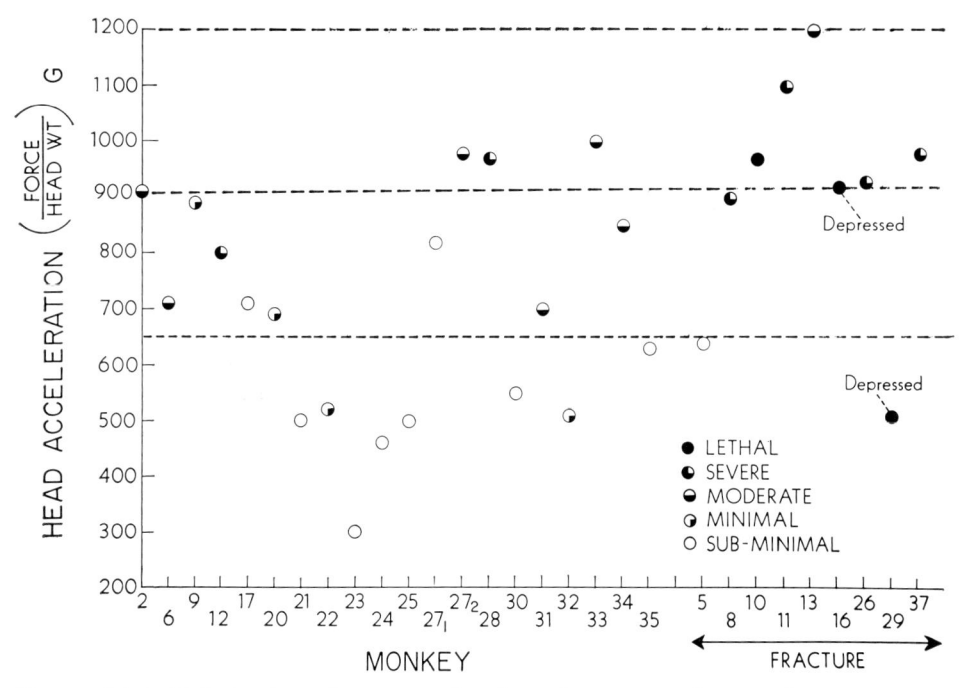

FIGURE 14-3. Relationship of apparent head acceleration to degree of concussion in the stump-tail monkey.

are bands of acceleration, containing nine animals each, in the ranges 300 to 650 g, 650 to 900 g, and 900 to 1200 g (pulse duration 0.0015 to 0.0025 sec.). The degree of injury is broken into five levels: subminimal, minimal, moderate, severe and lethal and these are assigned relative values of 0, 1, 2, 3, 4, for the purpose of quantifying the physiological effect. The average degree of injury in each band are as shown in Table 14-I: 0.22 (between subminimal and minimal) for 300 to 650 g; 1.4 (between minimal and moderate) for 650 to 900 g; and 2.8 (between moderate and severe) for 900 to 1200 g. The rest of the table shows the steps in obtaining Snediker's F factor which for this case was 26.5, giving a probability of much less than 1 per cent that the relationship between apparent head acceleration and the degree of concussion occurred by chance.

Table 14-II shows the probability of relationship to monkey head injury of all physical factors treated in the above manner. Force, impulse, power absorbed and energy absorbed, as such, must be rejected as being related since the probability of chance relationship is 10 per cent or greater. When these factors are put on a specific basis by dividing through by head weight, all appear to be related to experimental concussion, but force/head mass showed the best relationship. (See lower part of Table 14-II. See also the plot of data with line of least squares in Fig. 14-4.)

TABLE 14-I
PROBABILITY OF RELATIONSHIP OF APPARENT HEAD ACCELERATION (FORCE/HEAD WT.) TO DEGREE OF CONCUSSION IN THE STUMP-TAILED MONKEY BY ANALYSIS OF VARIANCE METHOD
(Acceleration considered as a dose of CNS trauma-producing agent)

F/W Band –G– No. in Group	300–650 y	y²	650–900 y	y²	900–1200 y	y²	CODE
1	0	0	0	0	2	4	0—subminimal
2	0	0	0	0	2	4	1—minimal
3	0	0	1	1	2	4	2—moderate
4	0	0	1	1	3	9	3—severe
5	0	0	2	4	3	9	4—lethal
6	0	0	2	4	3	9	
7	0	0	2	4	3	9	
8	1	1	2	4	3	9	
9	1	1	3	9	4	16	
Total	2	2	13	27	25	73	
Av. Deg. of Conc.	0.22		1.4		2.8		
$(\Sigma y)^2$	4		169		625		
$(\Sigma y)^2/9$	0.44		18.8		69.5		
$\Sigma y^2 - (\Sigma y)^2/9$	1.56		8.2		3.5		

$\Sigma[\Sigma y^2 - (\Sigma y)^2/9] = 1.56 + 8.2 + 3.5 = 13.3$

$\Sigma \bar{y} = \frac{2 + 13 + 25}{9} = 4.45; \Sigma \bar{y}^2 = \frac{4 + 169 + 625}{81} = 9.85$

$9[\Sigma \bar{y}^2 - \frac{(\Sigma \bar{y})^2}{3}] = 9[9.85 - \frac{4.45)^2}{3}] = 29.2$

Summary of Results:

Source of Variation	Sum of Squares	Deg. of Freedom	Variance
F/W Level	29.2	2	14.6
Deg. of Conc.	13.3	24	0.55
Total	47.5	26	

$F_{2.24} = 26.5$ (p < 0.01) relationship between F/W and degree of concussion occurred by chance.

TABLE 14-II
STATISTICAL RELATIONSHIP OF PHYSICAL PARAMETERS TO MONKEY HEAD INJURY

Parameter	Snediker's F Factor	Probability of Chance	
Force (F)	2.5	P = 0.1	
Power Absorbed (P.A.)	1.5	P > 0.1	Reject as being
Impulse (1)	0.9	P > 0.1	related to injury
Energy Absorbed (E.A.)	0.3	P > 0.1	

Above parameters put on a specific basis by dividing by head weight (W).

F/W	26.5	P < 0.01
P.A./W	14.5	P < 0.01
1/W	11.6	P < 0.01
(F/W)/R.T.* ("JERK")	11.3	P < 0.01
EA/W	9.0	P < 0.01

* R.T. refers to rise time as shown in Figure 14–5.

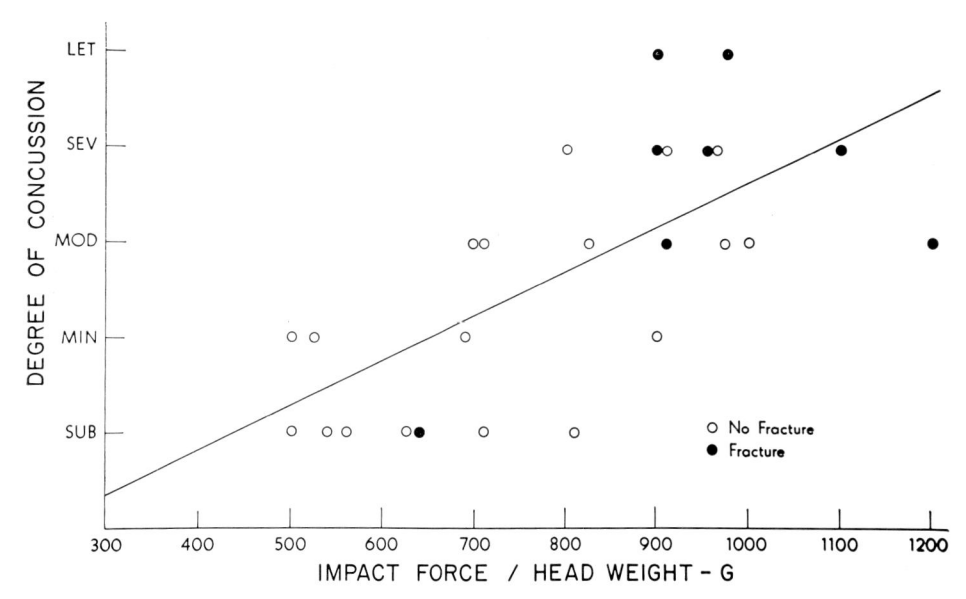

FIGURE 14-4. Degree of concussion versus peak apparent head acceleration (impact force/head weight–g) for the stump-tail monkey occipital blows.

Specific impulse, $1/W = \int_0^T (F/W)\, dt$ is also the velocity change experienced by the head. The pulse time duration varied from 0.0015 to 0.0025 seconds, so velocity change amounts to modifying apparent head acceleration by a time factor. Since apparent head acceleration (peak value) still showed up best in this analysis, the stump-tail monkey brain appears to be sensitive to acceleration rather than velocity change. Equation 3, or the spectrum for any shape pulse, expresses the fact that if a shock pulse is short compared to the natural period of the system on which it acts, the severity of the shock should be determined by area of the pulse (velocity change) alone.[15,16] It follows that the pulses were of the same order of magnitude or longer than the important natural period(s) of the head. These results seem to indicate that for this species, the skull first resonance (near 500 HZ)[10] is more important than the brain resonance (below 20 HZ).

It can be seen in Figure 14-3 that there are several monkeys such as number 9 and 27-1 for example which experienced high acceleration but did not have a proportionally severe effect. Consequently, a frequency spectrum analysis was conducted on the pulses according to a method shown by Karkevich[15] to obtain the normalized modulus of a general shaped pulse according to equation 3.

$$\frac{S}{F_{max}T} = \frac{\frac{\sin(\pi f \Delta t)}{\pi f}\sum_{n=0}^{k-1} F\{(n+\tfrac{1}{2})\Delta t\}e^{-i\omega(n+1/2)\Delta t}}{F_{max} T} \quad (3)$$

Where K is the number of rectangular elements of width Δt the pulse of F_{max} amplitude, T time duration, is broken into; $F\{(n+\tfrac{1}{2})\Delta t\}$ is element amplitude and F is frequency. The spectrum is a useful description of a pulse as an indication of the distribution of vibratory energy and how it can excite resonant systems having any natural frequency from zero to infinity. In general, the shorter the pulse duration, the broader the frequency spectrum, and the more severe the shock to resonant systems.

It was noted that in many of those cases in which monkeys sustained a fracture, the force-time pulse was shaped somewhat like a terminal sawtooth. Therefore the spectrum was plotted for both the rise portion and full pulse, according to equation 3, as shown in Figure 14–5 for monkeys 9, 27-1, 12 and 28. Note that the rise times for monkeys 9 and 27-1 were both near 1 millisecond which is relatively long compared to the rise time of monkeys 12 and 28 pulses. Consequently, the rise-time spectra of 9 and 27-1 are not as broad as the other two, and this is possibly the reason for less damage. In general it was noted that those animals which

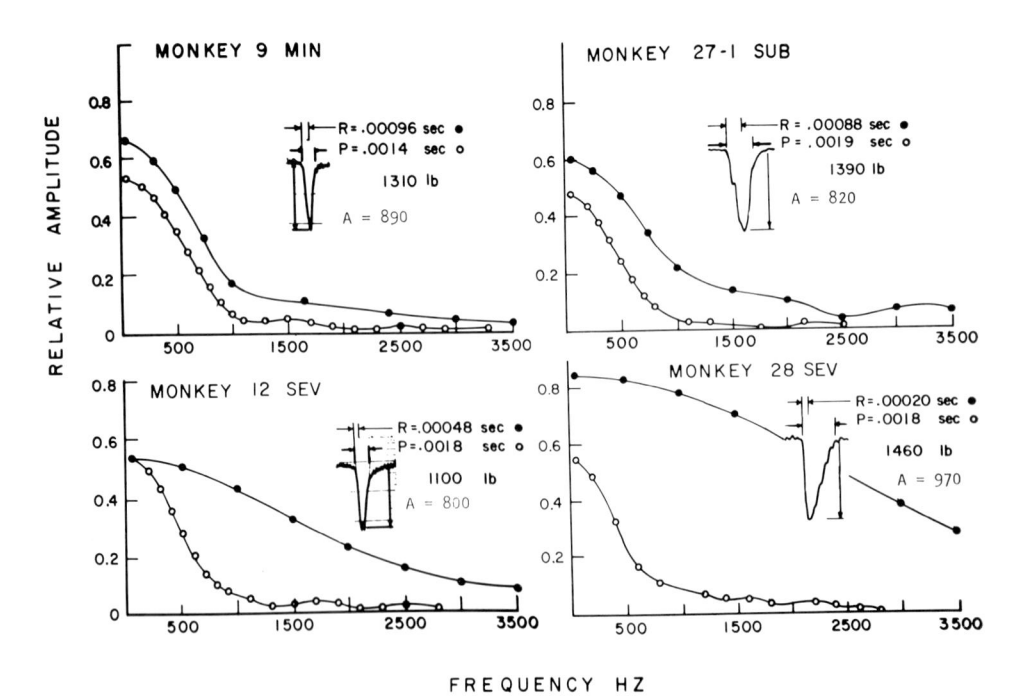

FIGURE 14–5. Plot of normalized modulus of frequency spectrum for rise time portion and full pulse of force-time records for monkeys 9, 27-1, 12 and 28.

suffered the most severe damage experienced both high acceleration and short rise time.

SUMMARY

It has been shown that for these series of experiments, force per head mass, which has units of acceleration (F/W)g is the one physical parameter most related to monkey head injury, including fracture and neural damage leading to loss of response to stimuli and cardiac difficulties. Force alone could not be statistically related to injury. Doubtless, for each individual monkey in this experiment, force level would be related to degree of injury as shown in Figure 14-6 for Monkey 19. This shows the changes in force and acceleration and pulse duration as velocity of impact is increased, for multiple blows to the same anesthetized animal, indicating the level of apparent injury threshold and total response loss. The head weights of the monkey population in this experiment varied from 1.1 to 3.0 pounds, therefore, a given force level accelerated each one differently. By dividing force by head mass, correlation between degree of injury for the population is obtained. For example, Monkey 25 with a head weight of 3.0 pounds displayed no outward effect from a 1500 pound blow, whereas Monkey 28, head weight 1.5 pounds, displayed symptoms of a severe head injury from a 1550 pound blow (duration 0.0016 of a second in both cases). When put on a specific basis, (F/W)g, this means approximately 500 to 1000 g respectively for these two animals, and now it is apparent why the effect of the blow was different.

The relationships of impulse, energy absorbed and power absorbed to monkey head injury were shown to be improved when divided by head weight. The reason for this is similar to the case of force, they are all size dependent in their effect, i.e. small animals cannot absorb as much energy as larger animals. This effect could be overlooked by an experiment using a uniform size group from one species. In a group of similar size animals of one species, struck under similar conditions which produced short* pulse durations, impulse may be a good criterion of head injury, but not in the general case. The same can be said for velocity and kinetic energy as others have pointed out.[25]

It is necessary to look to other measurements and observations to understand why the monkey brain is acceleration sensitive. Consider the measurements made during one impact of a multiple blow experiment to a more deeply anesthetized animal (Monkey 23, Blow 5) as shown in Figure 14-7 (multiple blow experiments are not included among the twenty-seven animals used to compare physiological and physical param-

---

* Short relative to skull first mode of stump-tail (T ≅ 0.002 of a second).

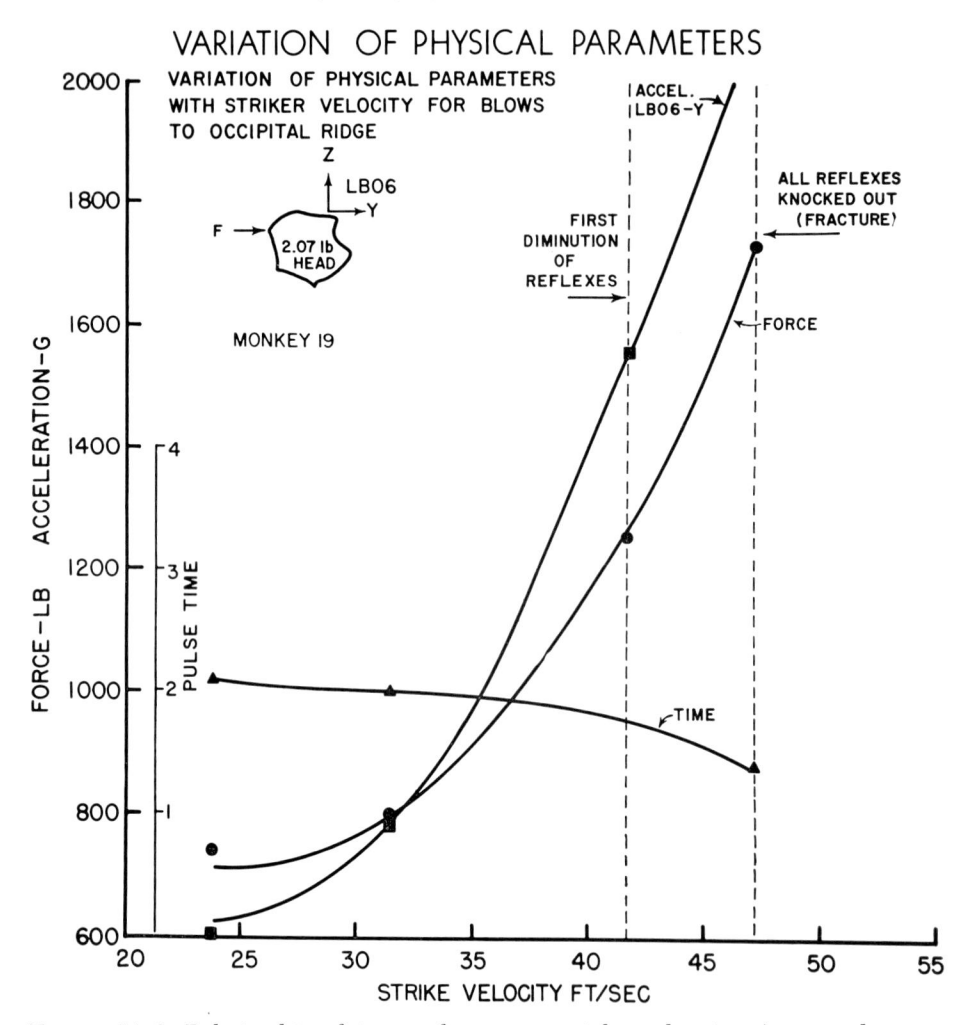

FIGURE 14–6. Relationship of impact force, tangential acceleration (measured on top of head) and pulse duration versus velocity of striker for blunt impact to the occipital ridge of the stump-tail monkey.

eters except for Monkey 27–1,2). These records indicate that initially there is a high pressure on the blow side and near −1 atmosphere pressure opposite the blow. A positive pressure exists initially against the top of the skull above the foramen magnum, and within 0.003 of a second has reversed to a negative value. Despite reversals elsewhere, it is interesting to note that the pressure opposite the blow remains negative throughout the pulse except for a positive spike near the end. The maximum head accelerations measured at the top of the skull parallel to the striker force (see monkey head outline in Fig. 14–7) with an Endevco triaxial accelerometer, Model #2228B, is 800 g, and that normal to the skull relatively

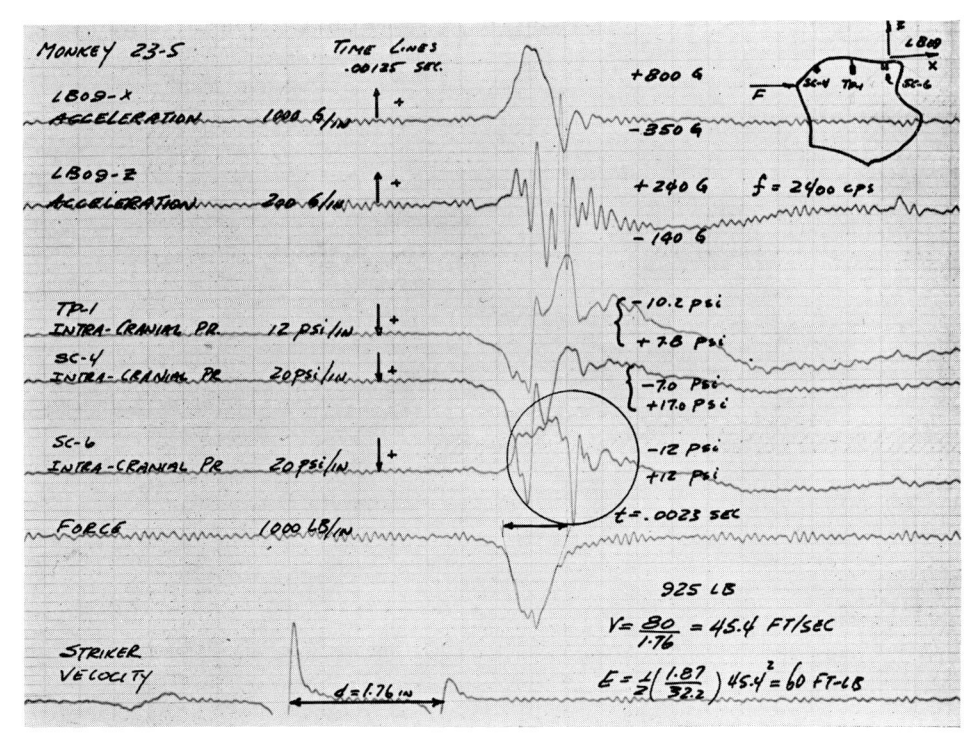

FIGURE 14–7. Impact record of head acceleration, force, velocity and intracranial pressure changes for monkey 23, blow 5. Note especially the positive pressure on the blow side (SC–4) and sustained negative pressure opposite the blow followed by a sharp positive spike (circled record).

small if the vibrations are ignored. The value of force per head mass is 925/2.7 g = 342 g. If this were head center of mass acceleration then it would indicate high angular acceleration was taking place but calculations would be very uncertain since the neck forces are unknown. It is required to measure accelerations at two points on the skull, (assumed to be a rigid body) with biaxial accelerometers, assuming plane motion) to determine angular acceleration. This was attempted in several monkey multiple blow experiments including that to monkey 20, blow 3, the record of which is shown in Figure 14–8. The pickups were oriented as shown in Figure 14–9. For the instants of one-half maximum acceleration on the rise, at maximum, and one half maximum on the fall as measured on LB09-Y, the calculated head CG accelerations and angular accelerations are as shown. The CG acceleration had a predominant P-A component and maximum angular acceleration was 42,000 rads per second squared. Higgins, et al.,[7] have reported lethal effects in the squirrel monkey for rotational accelerations about the head CG as high as 286,000 rads per

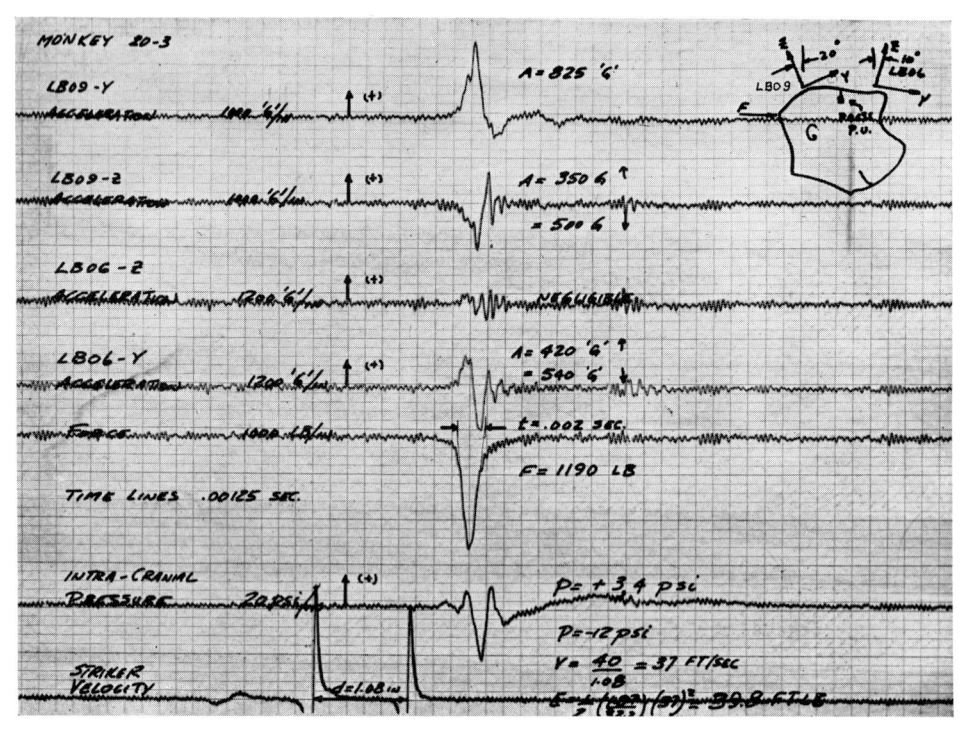

FIGURE 14-8. Typical record of multiple acceleration in recordings on the head of the stump-tail monkey. Measurement of biaxial accelerations at two points on the skull for the purpose of determining angular acceleration and head center of gravity acceleration-components at any instant during impact to monkey 20, blow 3. (See Appendix V).

second squared. Ommaya, et al.,[20] have theorized 40,000 rads per second squared for durations longer than 0.0065 of a second as necessary to cause concussion to 99 per cent of Rhesus monkeys subjected to whiplash, and 7,500 rads per second squared for man. By comparison, Mertz and Patrick,[17] using 2 biaxial accelerometers in whiplash experiments with a volunteer and human cadavers reported maximum angular accelerations of 200 and 500 rads per second squared for the two specimens, respectively, for a 10 mph impact, and 700 rads per second squared for the cadaver only, for the severe 23 mph collision simulation. These values occurred near 150 milliseconds after initial impact.

In a whiplash type injury, angular acceleration may be a good criterion, but because of the small size, skull vibrations, skin movement relative to the skull, and extreme violence it is very difficult to accurately obtain angular head accelerations due to direct impact to the head. Consequently, it is unwise to use angular accelerations as an index of head impact injury. The fact that force per head mass shows the best relation to head injury

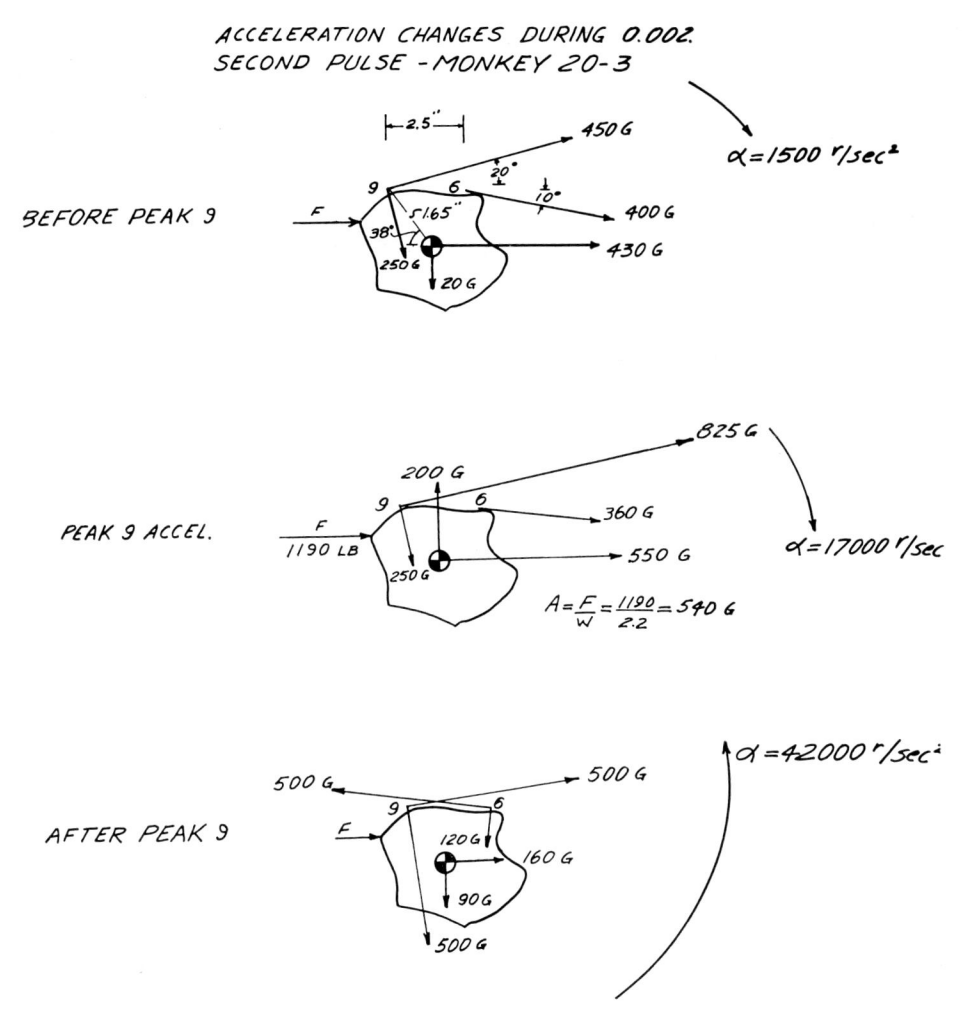

ACCELERATION CHANGES DURING 0.002
SECOND PULSE - MONKEY 20-3

BEFORE PEAK 9

$\alpha = 1500 \text{ r/sec}^2$

PEAK 9 ACCEL.

$A = \dfrac{F}{W} = \dfrac{1190}{2.2} = 540 \text{ G}$

$\alpha = 17000 \text{ r/sec}$

AFTER PEAK 9

$\alpha = 42000 \text{ r/sec}^2$

FIGURE 14–9. Center of gravity acceleration components and angular acceleration for the head of monkey 20, blow 3.

in this species, despite the wide variation in size, sex, age, variation in head motion, rise time, and pulse duration, emphasizes its utility as a head injury parameter in the experimental animal.

The evidence above indicates that in general, a head impact to the monkey is accompanied by rapidly changing stress gradients acting on and throughout the brain. These are caused by interference of parts of the skull due to relative translational and rotational accelerations between skull and brain, and between different parts of the brain, and by fluid pressure of the spinal fluid. The irregular geometry of the skull and brain, the complex dynamics of impact and the difficulties involved in cranial vault measurement, make it obvious that accurate definitions of these stress patterns will not soon be devised. However, some idea of their effect on the brain can be obtained from elementary mechanic considerations as follows. Consider a rigid closed container, symmetric with respect to the x-y plane and subject to acceleration parallel to the x axis according to Figure 14–10A. Consider an element of liquid in the filled container.

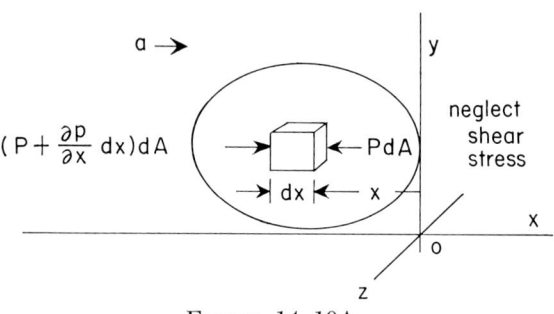

FIGURE 14–10A.

According to Newton, the summation of forces in the x direction will be as follows:

$$\left(P + \frac{\partial p}{\partial x} dx\right) dA - p dA = \rho_f dV a \qquad (4)$$

$$\frac{\partial p}{\partial x} = \rho_f a \qquad (5)$$

where, P = pressure
ρ_f = density of fluid (mass/unit volume)
dx = element of length
dA = element of area
dV = element of volume
a = acceleration

Integrating in the negative direction

$$P = -\rho_f a x + C \qquad (6)$$

Assuming acceleration (a) is sufficient to cause a minimum (gage) pressure (P = −K) boundary condition at x = 0, therefore

$$C = -k \qquad (7)$$

and equation 6 becomes

$$P = -\rho_f a x - k \qquad (8)$$

Where P = pressure, ρ_f = density, a = acceleration, x = distance from the leading edge (x = 0) of the container. This is the equation of the linear pressure gradient which will be set up in the fluid inside the rigid, filled, accelerated container.

Let there be a cube of elastic material immersed in the accelerated container as shown in Figure 14–10B. The cube is assumed to have a different density (ρ_c) than the fluid (ρ_f). (Assume the cube to be tethered with an elestic cord so that it would neither rise or sink in the static condition.)

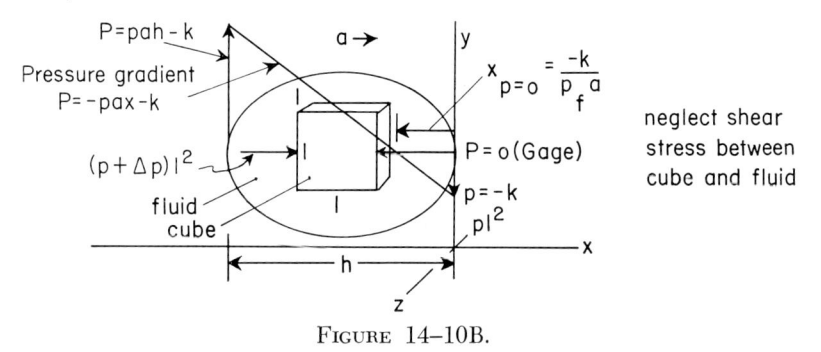

FIGURE 14–10B.

If $\ddot{x}$ is the acceleration of the cube then

$$\Sigma F = m\ddot{x} \tag{9}$$

$$-Pl^2 + (p + \Delta p)l^2 = \rho_c l^3 \ddot{x} \tag{10}$$

$$\Delta p = \rho_c l \ddot{x} \tag{11}$$

$$\ddot{x} = \Delta p / \rho_c l \tag{12}$$

From equation 8

$$dp = -\rho_f a \, dx \tag{13}$$

or in finite terms

$$\Delta p = \rho_f a l \quad (\text{since } x = -l) \tag{14}$$

Therefore (12) becomes

$$\ddot{x} = \frac{\rho_f}{\rho_c} a \tag{15}$$

If

$$\rho_c > \rho_f \tag{16}$$

Then

$$\ddot{x} < a \tag{17}$$

If the liquid is spinal fluid and the cube is brain substance, values for density will be approximately:

$$\rho_f = 1.02 \qquad \rho_c = 1.04$$

Consequently, equation 15 indicates that the brain substance acceleration would be slightly lower than the container. In terms of head displacement, if we assume a half sine acceleration pulse

$$\frac{d}{dt}\left(\frac{dx}{dt}\right) = a_{max} \sin \omega t \qquad (\omega \text{ is circular freq.}) \qquad (18)$$

It follows from double integration, with the conditions that displacement (x), and velocity (v) are zero at T = 0, that

$$x = \frac{a_{max}}{\omega} t - \frac{a_{max}}{\omega^2} \sin \omega t \qquad (19)$$

$$\text{For } t = T \text{ (pulse duration) and } \omega = \pi/T \qquad (20)$$

$$x = \frac{a_{max} T^2}{\pi} \qquad (21)$$

Letting T = 0.002 of a second and a_{max} = 800 g, for example,

$$x = \frac{800 \times 386 \times 4 \times 10^{-6}}{\pi} \cong 0.4 \text{ of an inch}$$

Using relation (15) for the brain acceleration in (21), brain displacement would be

$$x = 0.392 \text{ of an inch} \qquad (23)$$

Consequently the relative displacement interference between skull and brain would be only 0.008 of an inch.

If the energy of impact to such a rigid container is increased from a low level, opposite blow pressure will decrease and the blow side pressure will increase. The near −1 atmosphere pressure is the lowest level that can be sustained in a fluid system at the opposite pole. However, subsequent higher energy blows cause higher pressures on the blow side. Thus, the plane of 0 pressure continues to move toward the opposite pole as demonstrated in Figure 14–10C. Of course if there is an elastic opening such as the foramen magnum condition in the head, this zero point will be influenced by the hole, probably on a time-dependent basis.

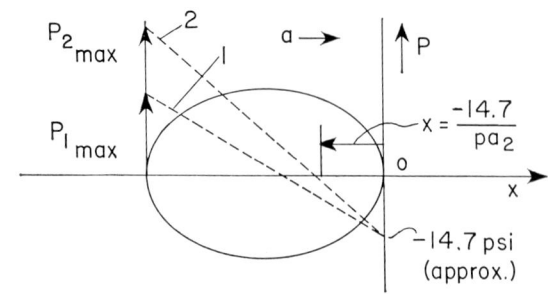

FIGURE 14–10C. Pressure gradients in rigid container. 1 corresponds to acceleration a_1, 2 to a_2, $a_1 < a_2$. Both accelerations sufficient to cause −1 atmospheric pressure @ leading edge.

Physical Factors Related to Experimental Concussion 293

This effect can be seen by the plot of initial maximum values (See record of Fig. 14-7) versus velocity for monkey 34 as shown in Figure 14-11. Once the opposite pole pressure reached the minimum pressure value of near −1 atmosphere around 600 g (measured on the skull) it leveled off, but the impact side pressure continued to increase up to the point of fracture. If the container discussed above is constrained by connection to a heavier mass below and it is struck above its center of gravity, the result will be translational and rotational acceleration which will cause relative acceleration among the brain tissues and will exaggerate the pressure gradient effects.

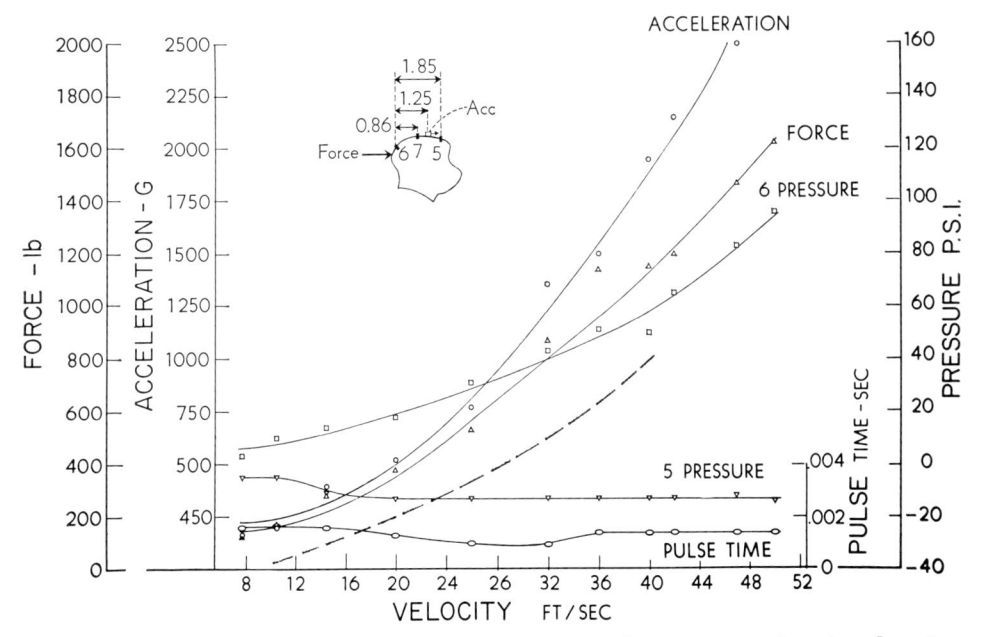

FIGURE 14-11. Plot of force, acceleration, intracranial pressure and pulse duration versus velocity of impact for occipital blows to the stump-tail monkey 34.

From the foregoing simplified models, some concepts of actual intracranial forces and movements can be deduced. Stress measurements have been measured on the skull and pressure changes have been recorded in the CSF during impact, but brain stress and deformation must be inferred at present by other than direct measurement.

If small pieces of lead solder tags are implanted in the brain, there would be a tendency for them to move relative to the tissue when the head is accelerated due to the high specific gravity of the solder (5.6). However, we do not know much about the physical properties of the brain *in vivo*. The brain was considered by Holbourne[12] to be an elastic body. It appears to the touch to be somewhat plastic. Recent tests using

294   *Impact Injury and Crash Protection*

flash x-ray techniques to observe lead tag movement in the brain indicate that in its mileau the brain behaves predominantly as an elastic body.[9]

Consider the monkey skull flash x-rays in Figure 14–11. This shows an x-ray of monkey 31 prior to impact, overlayed with a flash x-ray taken during impact. A string of lead tags across the foramen magnum of this deeply anesthetized animal has been displaced downward 2 to 3 mm, sometime during this 0.002 of a second pulse. The x-rays indicated that the head had gone through both translational and rotational motion during the interval (as illustrated in the sequence of high speed camera film frames in Fig. 14–12). Shortly after the blow the tags were observed in their original positions. Other tests using 0.020 of a second, 20 psi pressure

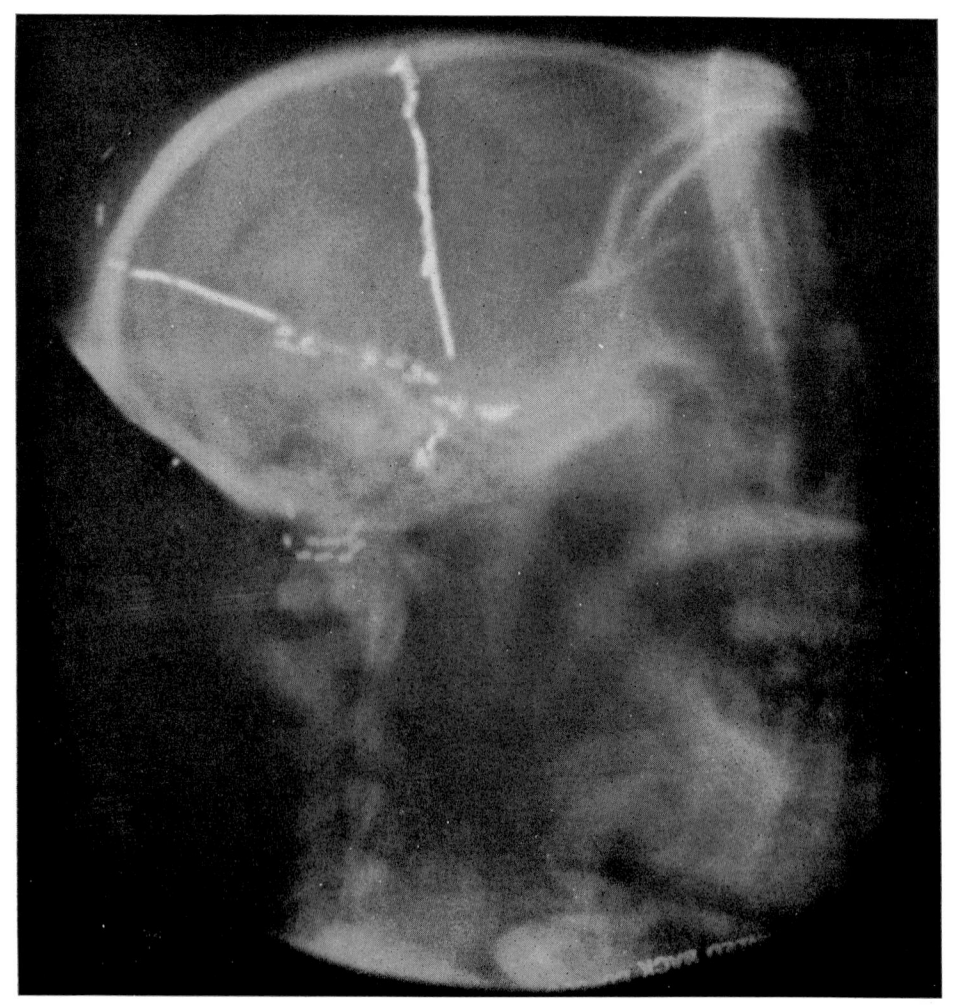

FIGURE 14–12. Flash x-ray of monkey head during impact overlayed on static x-ray before impact to show downward movement of lead tags across the foramen magnum.

pulses transmitted through a trephine against the dura of a stationary animal indicate that the displacement and return occurs in phase with the applied force.[11] It is noted in the figure, that the lines of lead tags running toward the base from the top and rear of the skull show no evidence of gross movement due to shear strain or inertia forces due to either translational or rotational acceleration, while the line of tags across the foramen magnum has changed shape and position. The tags are constrained from observable movement by the neural tissue-blood vessel visco-elastic matrix except at the foramen magnum where they are constrained to move with the tissue. It appears that the sequence of cause and effect is this: The head receives both translational and rotational impetus with a predominant P-A component at the CG, thereby causing inertia forces to arise which set up a complex pressure gradient to act on the brain surface forcing it out of the foramen magnum. Blows of a certain direction such as one delivered P-A with an upward component could initiate an action in which inertia forces would tend to aid the pressure gradients, which they create, to extrude the brain. For example, among the ten dogs used in this experiment, five were struck on the sagittal crest normal to the top of the head and five were struck on the occipital protuberance in the P-A direction approximately 30 degrees to the vertebral axis. Four out of five of the latter were lethal due to respiratory arrest while the blows on the crest only produced from minimal to severe effects. In this dog experiment, it seemed that blow location and line of action were more related to effect than anything else.

The other effect pressure forces can have on the tissue is possibly to cause air bubbles or cavitation in spinal fluid or brain tissue in regions of low pressure as has been pointed out by several workers.[3,23,25] Consider the pressure pulses measured opposite the blow to a human cadaver and a two dimensional plastic model of a sagittal section of the human skull and brain, shown in Figures 14-13 and 14-14, respectively, for comparison with the record for monkey 23-5 shown in Figure 14-7. (pertinent pressure measurements are each circled). All exhibit a similar pattern of being flattened out at a near −1 atmosphere pressure followed by a positive spike near the end of the pulse. The model and cadaver were filled with Dow-Corning sylgard gel using a 10% catalyst to produce a consistency which except for being stickier, felt like live brain to the touch. The initial overshoot on the model and cadaver records is an indication that the gel adhesive properties allow it to support more than −1 atmosphere tension. This effect was not observed in the monkey in which the pickup was mounted flush with the inner table, after piercing the dura to permit spinal fluid to flow around the diaphragm. Minimum pressure at the opposite pole occurred around 170 g for frontal blows to the cadaver and model

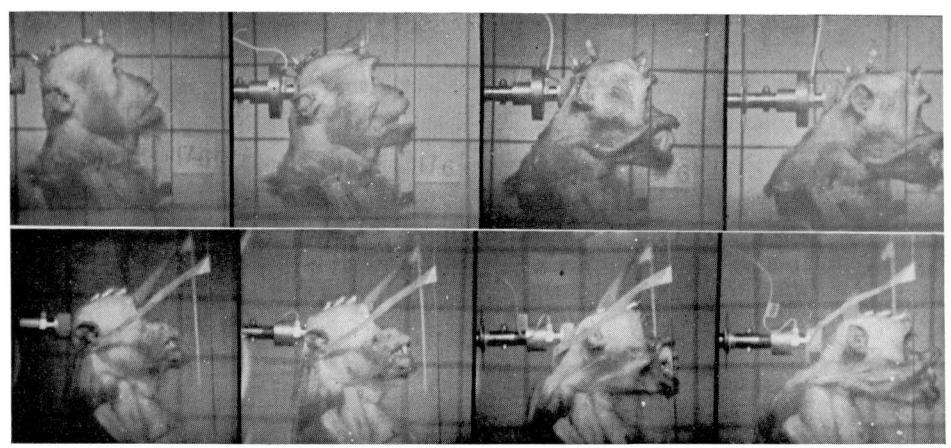

FIGURE 14–13. Typical head movement during and following impact to the occipital bone of the stump-tail monkey. *Top:* animal dead 24 hours (somewhat stiff). *Bottom:* anesthetized animal.

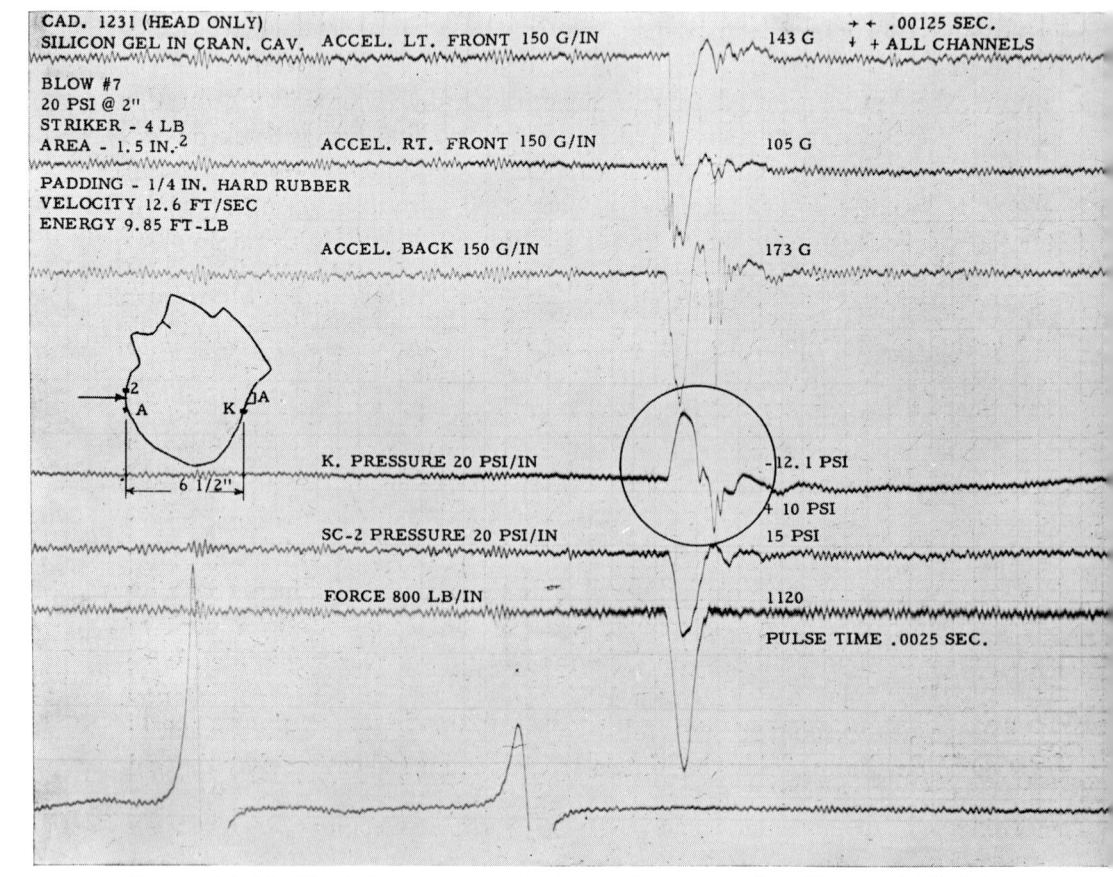

FIGURE 14–14. Physical measurements during impact to the silicon gel filled human cadaver head. Note especially the counter pole negative (gage) pressure followed by a positive spike and its effect on the nearby accelerometer mounted in the skull.

(each measuring 6 inches across the cranial cavity) and 500 to 600 g in the monkey as indicated in Figure 14-15.

These accelerations are approximately proportional to the ratio of major axes lengths measured in this cadaver and monkey: 6 inches per 2 inches. This geometric relation between acceleration necessary to produce this phenomena may provide some assistance in establishing acceleration tolerance limits in man for relatively long duration pulses. It has been observed, however, that bending modes are excited for short duration pulses to the forehead of the human cadaver which produce acceleration amplification on the occiput as high as twice the center of mass acceleration calculated from force per head mass.[8] Figure 14-16 demonstrates this amplification effect for pulses below 0.003 to 0.004 of a second to the forehead of a cadaver. Pulses longer than this produce essentially rigid body motion. Whenever 170 g was experienced on the occiput opposite a frontal impact (in one gel filled and one water filled 6 inch cadaver head, and on 6 inch model) the gage pressure measured on the inner wall of

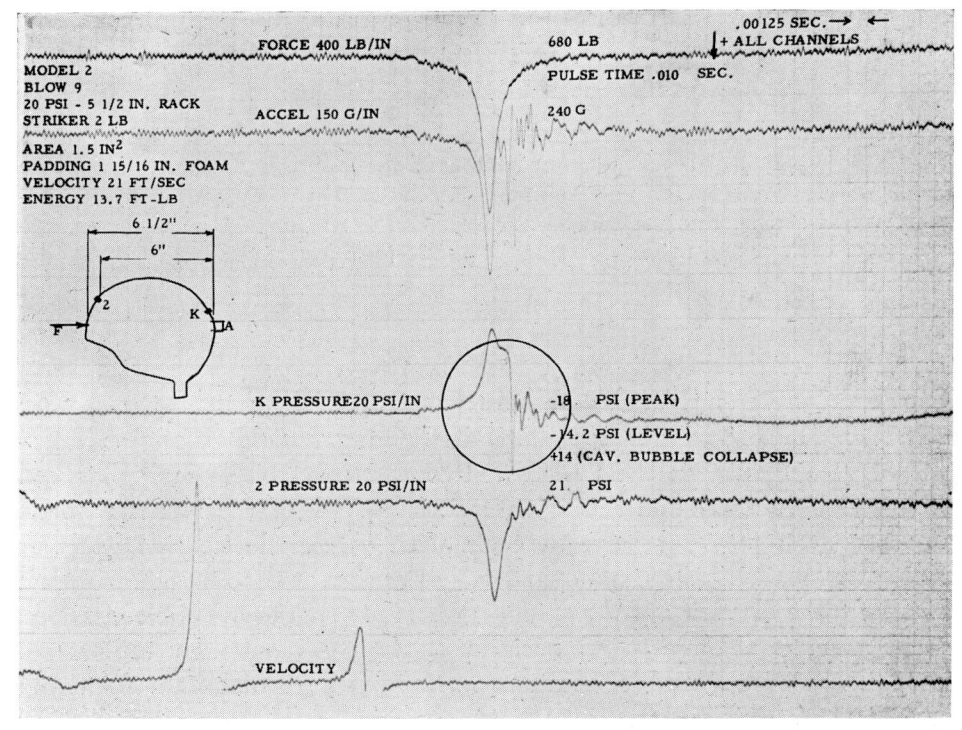

FIGURE 14-15. Physical measurements during impact to the silicon gel filled two dimensional model of the human head. Note the similarity to the cadaver counter pole acceleration and pressure records. The model pressure recording is slightly more developed because the peak acceleration was 240 g whereas the cadaver acceleration was a threshold value of 173 g.

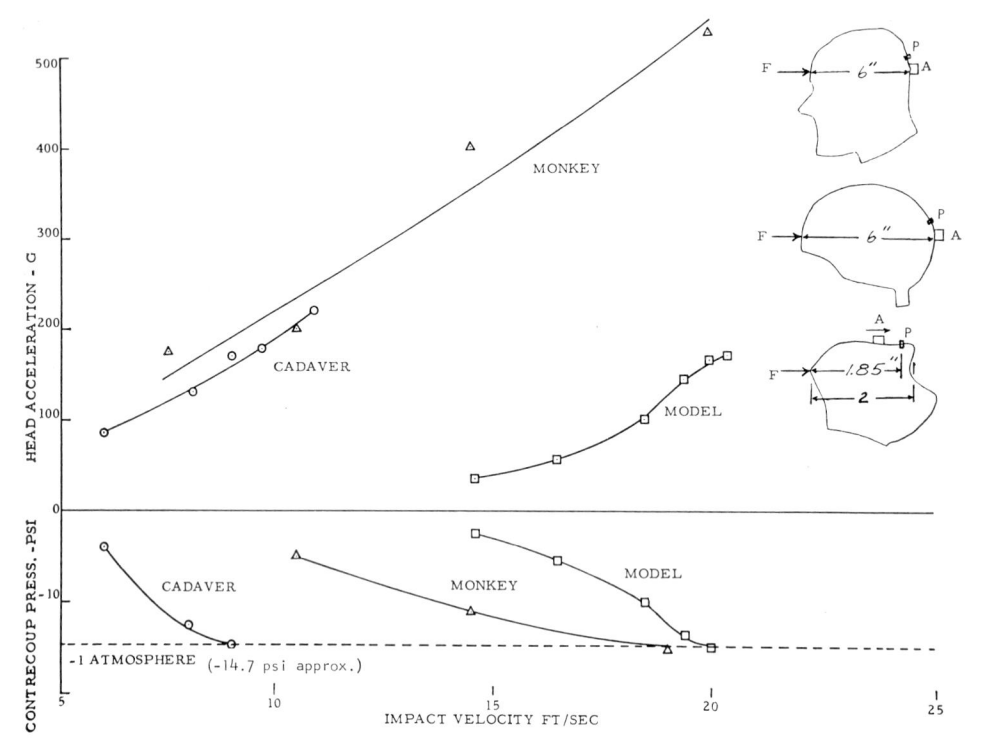

FIGURE 14-16. Plot of acceleration, and intracranial pressure both measured opposite the blow versus velocity for multiple impacts to the human cadaver head, two dimensional model and anesthetized monkey. Acceleration to produce −1 atmosphere opposite blow: cadaver and model—170g; monkey—500 to 600 g.

the occiput began to display the characteristic low pressure phenomena indicated in Figures 14-7, 14-13, 14-14 and 14-17.

Figure 14-17 demonstrates the presence of pressure gradients in a sagittal section model of the human skull. Back lighting filtered through a translucent screen outlines the model in two frames taken from high speed film before (above) and during impact. The shell of the model is made of fiberglass reinforced polyester resin with ¼ inch lucite side walls. A soft spring-loaded piston in a cylindrical extension at the foramen magnum simulates the elasticity of the spinal cord. Many small air bubbles trapped in the silicon gel brain in the occipital area are expanded by the sudden drop in pressure (bubble duration 0.002 second) which is a minimum at the wall. This sudden change in pressure could be responsible for hemorrhage as pointed out by Unterharnscheidt and Sellier.[23] The collapse of bubbles such as these or possibly cavitation in spinal fluid could have produced the positive pressure spikes noted near the end of the pressure records in Figures 14-7, 14-13, 14-14 and 14-18.

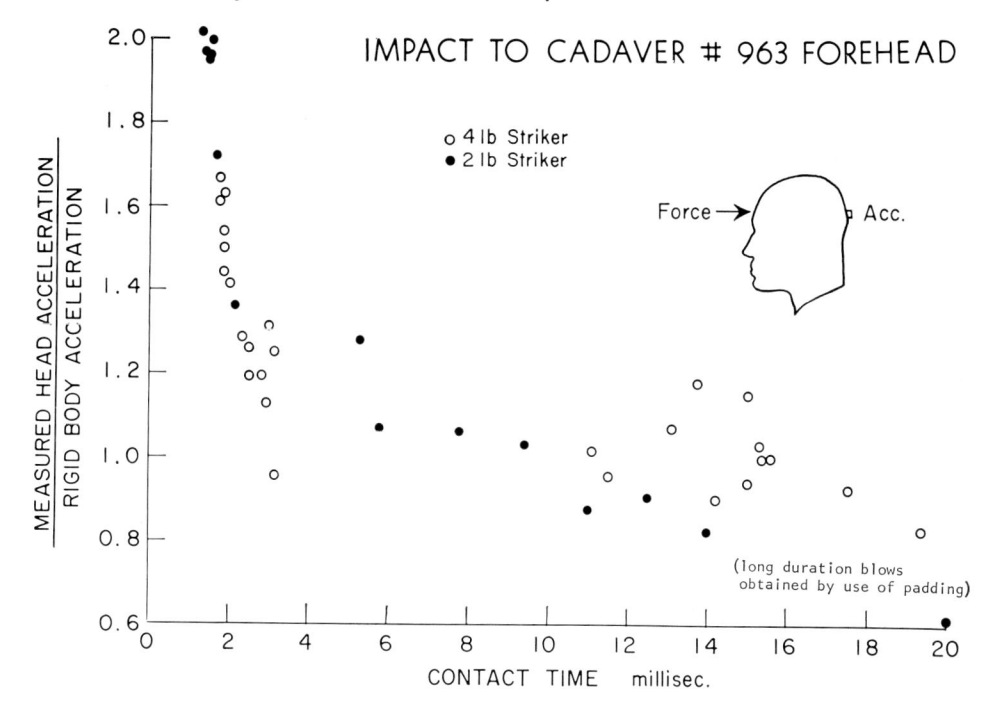

FIGURE 14-17. Acceleration amplification opposite the blow due to bending mode excitation in the human cadaver for short duration impacts (below 0.003 to 0.004 sec.). Intracranial pressure measurements opposite the blow are related to accelerations on this surface.

CONCLUSIONS

1. For this series of experiments in the monkey, force, impulse, energy absorbed, and power absorbed were not related to head injury.

2. All of the factors listed in 1. appeared to be related to injury when put on a specific basis by dividing by head weight (head weight ranged from 1.1 to 3 pounds in this population of twenty-seven stump-tail monkeys of various age and sex).

3. The single parameter most related to experimental concussion in the monkey was apparent head acceleration (peak impact force per head mass).

4. Most severe head injury (concussion with or without fracture) was suffered by those animals which experienced both high acceleration and short rise time.

5. Pressure gradients arising from translational and rotational acceleration of the head are responsible for producing distortion around the brain stem and upper cord.

6. Pressure gradients arising from accelerations and skull deformation can

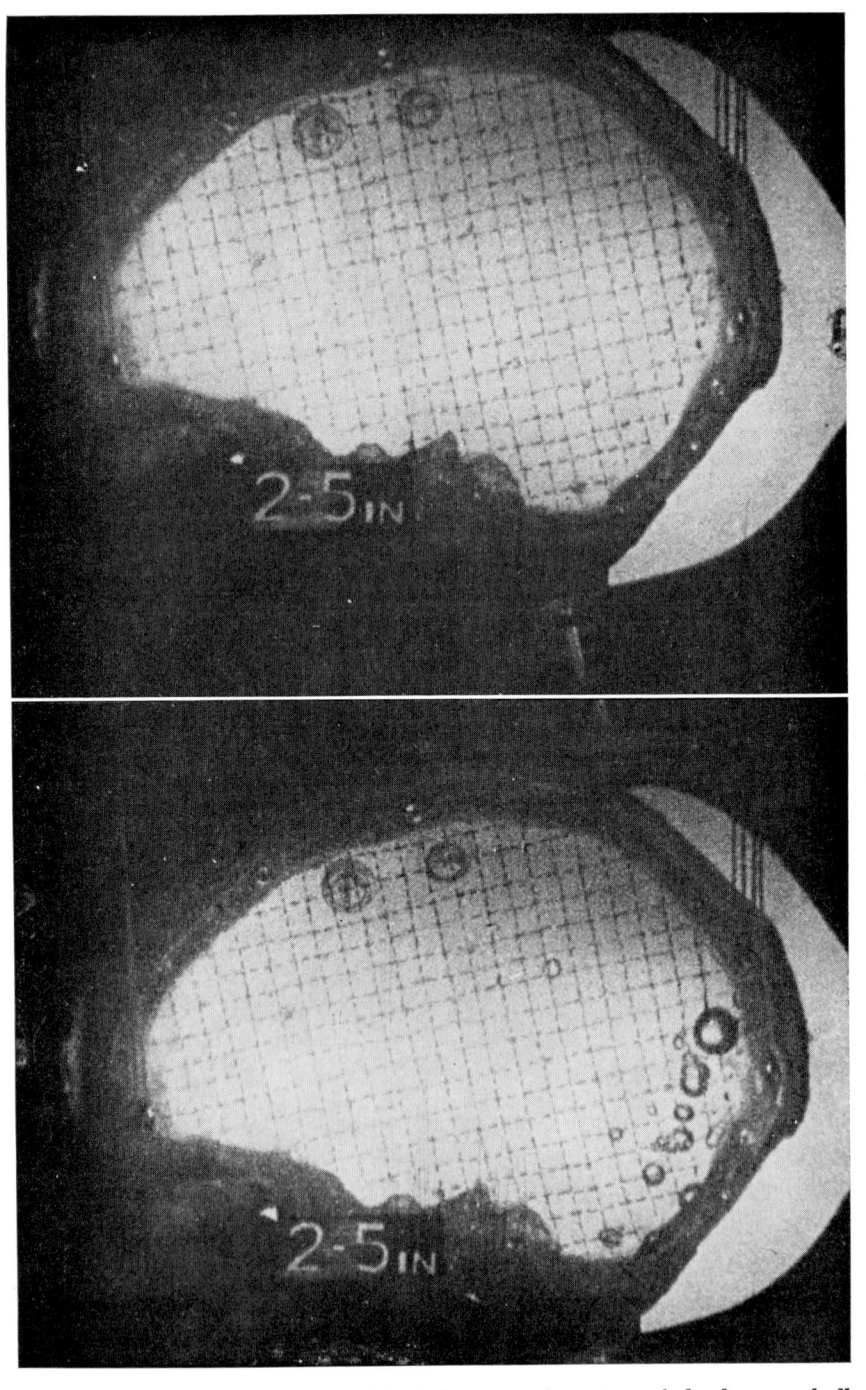

FIGURE 14–18. Two-dimensional model of the sagittal section of the human skull and brain before impact (above) and during impact (0.002 sec.).

cause low pressure particularly on the opposite blow side, such as air bubble formation and possibly cavitation resulting in hemorrhage or brain tissue damage.

REFERENCES

1. DENNY-BROWN, D.E., and RUSSELL, W.R.: Experimental cerebral concussion. *Brain*, 64:93–164, 1941.
2. FRIEDE, R.L.: Experimental acceleration concussion. *Arch Neurol*, 4:449–462, 1961.
3. GROSS, A.G.: A new theory on the dynamics of brain concussion and brain injury. *J Neurosurg*, 15:548–561, 1958.
4. GURDJIAN, E.S.; LISSNER, H.R.; LATIMER, F.R.; HADDAD, B.F., and WEBSTER, J.E.: Quantitative determination of acceleration and intracranial pressure in experimental head injury. *Neurology*, 3(6):417–423, June 1953.
5. GURDJIAN, E.S., and LISSNER, H.R.: Photoelastic confirmation of the presence of shear strain at the craniospinal junction in closed head injury. *J Neurosurg,18*: (1):58–60, 1961.
6. GURDJIAN, E.S.; LISSNER, H.R., and PATRICK, L.M.: Protection of the head and neck in sports. *JAMA*, 182:509–512, Nov. 3, 1962.
7. HIGGINS, L.S., and SCHMALL, R.A.: A device for the investigation of head injury effected by non-deforming head accelerations. *Conference Proceedings Eleventh Stapp Car Crash Conference.* Oct. 1967, pp. 35–46.
8. HODGSON, V.R.; GURDJIAN, E.S., and THOMAS, L.M.: The determination of response characteristics of the head with emphasis on mechanical impedance techniques. *Proceedings of the Eleventh Stapp Car Crash Conference.* SAE, N.Y., N.Y., 1967, pp. 79–85.
9. HODGSON, V.R.; GURDJIAN, E.S., and THOMAS, L.M.: The development of a model for the study of head injury. *Proceedings of the Eleventh Stapp Car Crash Conference.* SAE, N.Y., N.Y., 1967, pp. 286–292.
10. HODGSON, V.R.: Head Impact Response of Several Mammals Including the Human Cadaver. Office for Graduate Studies. Wayne State University, June 1968.
11. HODGSON, V.R.; GURDJIAN, E.S., and THOMAS, L.M.: Experimental skull deformation and brain displacement demonstrated by flash x-ray techniques. *J Neurosurg*, 25(5):549–552, 1966.
12. HOLBOURNE, A.H.S.: Mechanics of head injury. *Lancet*, 11:438–441, 1943.
13. HOLBOURNE, A.H.S.: The mechanics of trauma with special reference to herniation of cerebral tissue. *J Neurol*, 1944, vol. 1.
14. HOLLISTER, N.R.; JOLLEY, W.P., and HORNE, R.G.: Biophysics of concussion. *WADC Technical Report 58–193.* ASTIA Document No. Ad 203385, Sept. 1958, pt. 1
15. KHARKEVICH, A.A.: *Spectra and Analysis.* Consultants Bureau, New York, 1960.
16. KITTELSEN, K.E.: Measurement and Description of Shock. *Bruel and Kjaer Technical Review No. 3*, 1966.
17. MERTZ, H.J., and PATRICK, L.M.: Investigation of the kinematics and kinetics of whiplash. *Conference Proceedings Eleventh Stapp Car Crash Conference.* 1967, pp. 175–206.

18. Morrow, C.T.: Shock spectrum as a criterion of severity of shock impulses. *J Acoustical Soc Amer*, 29(5):596–602, 1956.
19. Ommaya, Ayub K.: Experimental head injury in the monkey. *Head Injury—Conference Proceedings*. 1966, pp. 260–275.
20. Ommaya, A.K.; Yarnell, P.; Hirsch, A.E., and Harris, E.H.: Scaling of experimental data in cerebral concussion in sub-human primates to concussion threshold for man. *Proceedings of Eleventh Stapp Car Crash Conference*. Oct. 1967, pp. 47–52.
21. Ommaya, A.K.; Rockoff, D.; Baldwin, M., and Friauf, W.S.: Experimental concussion a first report. *J Neurosurg*, 1964, vol. 21.
22. Ommaya, A.K.; Hirsch, A.E., and Martinez, J.L.: The role of whiplash in cerebral concussion. *Proceedings of Tenth Stapp Car Crash Conference*. 1966, pp. 314–324.
23. Sellier, K., and Unterharnscheidt, F.: The mechanics of the impact of violence on the skull. Excerpta Medica International Congress series No. 110, *Proceedings of the Third International Congress of Neurological Surgery*. Copenhagen, August 1965, pp. 87–92.
24. Thomas, L.M.: Mechanism of head injury. *Impact Injury and Crash Protection*. Detroit, Wayne, May 1968.
25. Unterharnscheidt, F., and Sellier, K.: Mechanics and pathomorphology of closed brain injuries. *Head Injury—Conference Proceedings*. 1966, pp. 321–341.

DISCUSSION

Ayub K. Ommaya

This chapter analyzes data on twenty-seven stump-tail monkeys to support the contention that force of head impact divided by head weight (expressed as acceleration in g units) displays the "best relation to experimental concussion." The purported acceleration sensitivity is then explained in terms of resultant intracranial pressure gradients which cause high levels of shear stress concentration in the brain stem and upper spinal cord. This is suggested as the prime cause of cerebral concussion, whereas the negative components of the pressure waves induce "cavitation" which is indicated to be the cause of various brain lesions, in particular, contrecoup hemorrhages.

At the very outset, I would like to emphasize that these conclusions cannot be accepted as anything but nonsequiturs if they have been advanced as *true* definitions of the physical factors related to concussion. If, however, they are advanced as hypotheses requiring factual confirmation or refutation by further experiment, I would certainly agree most wholeheartedly. The reasons for this emphasis on the necessity of proof will be discussed in a series of four questions.

I. What is the statistical validity of the five levels of injury response described?

The categories of subminimal and fatal are probably true but there is no proof available for the reality of the three other categories as being indeed separate entities. In order to obtain the category of minimal injury, (onset of concussion) an assumption was made that the loss of any *one* of about ten physiologic responses is equally indicative of the onset of cerebral concussion. Thus, the loss of such low level reflexes as the palpebral, corneal, pinna, head-righting and patellar reflexes were equated with the more highly integrated response of withdrawal to painful stimuli. Even if one were to concede the propriety of this assumption, the investigator proposing such a classification of the response to head impact would still have to show how the five groups numbered 0, 1, 2, 3, and 4 are statistically different from each other in terms of the actual values of the physical factor indicated as causing the injury. This is an essential requirement before one can begin to test for statistical correlation between cerebral concussion and any physical factor. A statistical correlation is strictly the correlation factor "r" which shows the degree of association between two variables x and y. The data presented in this chapter do not show such correlation, because the statistical technique used (analysis of variance) only shows that the three groups of animals receiving the head injury at three dose levels of acceleration are indeed statistically different from each other. These differences cannot however be used to claim a valid relation between the variable of acceleration and that of concussion, because in two of the three groups (Groups 1 and 2 in Table 14–I) both concussed (1, 2, 3 and 4) and nonconcussed (0) animals are mixed to obtain a so-called "average degree of concussion." At best, all that can be said from these data is that for levels of acceleration between 900 and 1200 g, (the animals of group 3 in Table 14–I) every stump-tail monkey out of nine subjected to head impact was either concussed or killed by the blow. For levels of acceleration between 300 and 900 g, the remaining eighteen monkeys displayed concussion in only 50 per cent (nine out of eighteen). If this finding is statistically true, it would confirm our prediction that 100 per cent cerebral concussion in monkeys with a brain weight of about 100 gm should be found if occipital head impacts produce head accelerations exceeding 900 g.[1,2] In our experiments, we used rhesus monkeys (*Macaca mulatta*) in which the brain weight is similar to that of the stump-tail monkey although the skull thickness, muscle mass and body weight are much less. This thinness of the rhesus skull, and its minimal protection by a thin, scantily muscled scalp, may be the explanation why we were unable to demonstrate 100 per cent concussion experimentally without producing skull fracture. Contrary to the data in this chapter, we eliminated animals with skull fracture from our statistical analysis. Our experimental data lay between the 10 per cent and 70 per cent concussive levels with theoretical prediction of the 90 per cent level (Fig. 14–19). However, it is important to point out that the value of such experimental data lies in the adequacy with which they may be extended to predict thresholds of concussion in man. For this reason, it is important to establish the 10 and 50 per cent levels of injury as well as the 100 per cent levels discussed. When we examine the data provided in this chapter, we note that there is considerable scatter of concussed and nonconcussed points between 450 and 900 g with only one datum point (nonconcussed) below 450 g. It is therefore not possible from these data to establish the following: (a) whether the true 50 per cent concussive level lies in the range examined (450 to 900 g) or in the range below 450 g, and (b) where the 10 per cent concussive level would be found.

II. Why is it "unwise to use angular accelerations as an index of head impact injury"?

The difficulty of making a measurement cannot invalidate it and should never be cited as a sufficient reason for not making it or for labeling serious attempts at such measurement as "unwise." Our recent publications have stressed that there are *two* very good reasons why it is extremely important

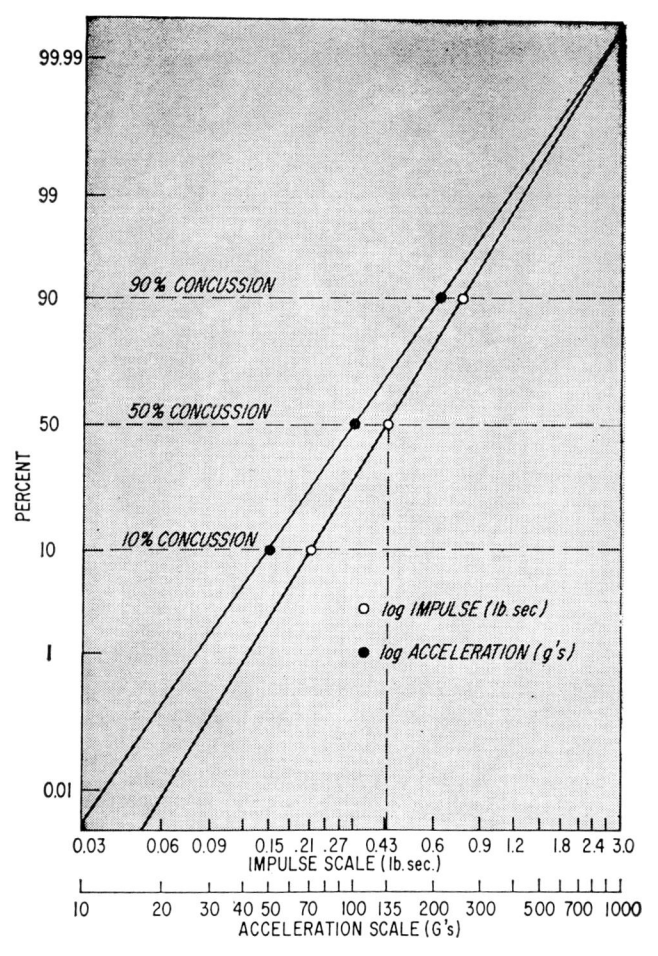

FIGURE 14-19. This is a plot of our data on over one hundred Rhesus monkeys (*Macaca mulata*) subjected to occipital head impacts (short duration blows having duration < 20 msec) measured in terms of the impulse of the blow (unit = lb.sec.) calculated from the area under the recorded force curve, and the resultant head acceleration (unit = g = 32 ft./sec.^{2}) recorded by linear uniaxial miniature accelerometers screwed into the skull. The experimental data were subjected to probit transformation, treating the physical factors of impulse and acceleration as injury dosages. This plot was made on logarithmic probability paper whereon actual data points ranged between the 5 and 75 percent levels. The 10 percent and 50 percent levels for concussion are thus experimentally proven. The 90 percent and higher levels of concussion for any group of subhuman primates with brain weights of about 100 gm were theoretically *predicted*. It should be noted that the data of V. R. Hodgson for the stump-tail monkey (brain weight = 100 gm approx.) would tend to confirm our prediction of the level of head acceleration at which concussion should occur in 100 percent of animals (> 900 g).

to measure the angular acceleration produced by head impact. Firstly, because we showed that a statistically significant correlation between the levels of two physical factors (force of impact to the head—in units of impulse—and the measured peak linear acceleration of the head) and the onset of cerebral concussion in 50 per cent of rhesus monkeys *no longer held* when a neck collar was applied before identical or high levels of impact were given to the head.[3,4] This neck collar was shown not to reduce linear head acceleration or the force input, but significantly lowered the angular acceleration of the head while raising the 50 per cent threshold for cerebral concussion. This observation was crucial for the second reason that is imperative to measure the angular acceleration produced by head impact. This is because it will provide the kind of data required for experimental testing of Holbourn's theory of the mechanics of brain injuries; to date this theory has been the best available approximation of all the known physical, physiological and pathological observations on traumatic injury to the brain and capable of explaining the greatest number of experimental observations including those of Wright, Hollister et al., Friede and of Underharnscheidt and Sellier. Later, we will present our latest data which provides the first comprehensive experimental evaluation of the role of angular acceleration in the genesis of cerebral concussion produced either by direct head impact or indirect "whiplash" injury.

III. What is the evidence that intracranial pressure gradients produced by impact result in "concentrations of shear stress in the brain stem" which constitutes the mechanism of concussion?

The data adduced in this chapter to support this contention consist of a series of animal and artificial model experiments from which no such conclusions can be inevitably drawn without much further proof. The experiment using lead pellets and high speed x-rays which is quoted in this paper can be misleading on two counts; firstly, there is no evidence that the measurement of a maximal 2 to 3 mm pellet displacement was controlled for the radiologic error due to minimal alterations in the relative angles between the x-ray beam and the planes of symmetry of the head. Even if one were to grant this measurement as a real one, there is still no evidence that such pellet displacement bore *any* relationship to actual brain displacements (because of the widely different densities of brain tissue and lead) or to cerebral concussion.

IV. Where is the experimental evidence for "cavitation" as a cause of hemorrhage and other brain lesions after head injury?

To the best of my knowledge, the theoretical statements of Ward, Sjovall, Gross, Underharnscheidt and Sellier are not supported by any evidence stronger than the demonstration of bubble formation in various inanimate fluids such as the silicone gel used by the author of this chapter. The total distribution of lesions, predicted by the cavitation hypothesis, has never been demonstrated in actuality in either animal or man. Invoked as the physical explanation for so-called "contrecoup" brain hemorrhages, the cavitation hypothesis is unable to explain such well documented pathologic observations as the essentially identical brain hemorrhages and contusions of the subfrontal and anterotemporal regions resulting from impact to either the frontal or occipital regions of the head.[5] The slight experimental evidence that *does* exist for cavitation in biologic tissues would suggest that it is difficult to produce for such short durations of negative pressure. Thus Wilson has shown that rapidly produced negative pressures 15 to 30 mm Hg *below* the vapor pressure of water have to be sustained for relatively long durations (minimum of 30 seconds and maximum of 10 minutes in eight exposures) before visible cavitation appears in the tissues of the human head.[6] Cavitation, as a significant injurious mechanism in head injury, remains therefore an interesting hypothesis, and we are currently planning animal experiments to test it as directly as possible.

In conclusion, the only point which I can recognize as being a valid inference from the data given confirms our prediction that subhuman primates having a brain weight of approximately 100 gm will experience cerebral concussion in almost 100 per cent of cases when the freely movable head is subjected to occipital impacts producing linear accelerations exceeding 900 g. The "dosage" of this physical factor exhibits a wide range between the level required for *onset* of concussion in say 10 per cent of animals and that required for concussion in 100 per cent of animals (65 g to >900 g). This wide range was true for our data in the rhesus as it appears to be for the stump-tail monkey. The crucial common factor of course is not the weight of the head but the weight of the brain.

References

1. OMMAYA, A.K.; HIRSCH, A.E.; FLAMM, E.S., and MAHONE, R.H.: Cerebral concussion in the monkey: An experimental model. *Science, 153*:211–212, July 1966.
2. OMMAYA, A.K.; FAAS, F., and YARNELL, P.: Whiplash injury and brain damage. An experimental study. *JAMA, 204*:285–289, April 1968.
3. OMMAYA, A.K.; ROCKOFF, S.D., and BALDWIN, M.: Experimental concussion. A first report. *J Neurosurg, 21*:249–265, April 1964.
4. OMMAYA, A.K.; HIRSCH, A.E., and MARTINEZ, J.: The role of whiplash in cerebral concussion. *Proceedings of the Tenth Stapp Car Crash Conference.* New York, Soc of Automotive Engineers, 1966, pp. 197–203.
5. COURVILLE, C.B.: Coup-contrecoup mechanism of cranio-cerebral injuries. *Arch Surg 45*:19–43, July 1942.
6. WILSON, C.L.: Production of gas in human tissues at low pressures. *Report No. 61–105*, USAF School of Aviation Medicine, Brooks AFB, Texas, August 1961.
7. HOLBOURN, A.H.S.: Mechanics of head injuries. *Lancet, 245*: 438–41, 1943.

Chapter XV

VOLUNTARY HUMAN TOLERANCE LEVELS
John P. Stapp

INTRODUCTION

The primary instrument for measuring the effects of mechanical force on man is man. All other living or dead surrogates or inert simulators of man have real time significance only to the degree with which they can be correlated, calibrated or extrapolated to living human dimensions and reactions. Consistency and repeatability of measurements on living or dead surrogates and inert simulators find practical application in design, performance or compliance testing within ranges of man-rated values. In the case of human response to mechanical force, these values are determined by static and dynamic stress analysis of man. The wide variety of physical properties of component tissues and their complex architecture in the human body make measurements and their interpretation difficult. Variations in psychological and physiological reactions of any one man, and individual differences in response among many men to the same mechanical force test exposure make the results less than exact, by engineering standards for stress analysis. Nevertheless, useful statistical ranges of effects occurring between limits, analagous to the precedent of pharmacological assays, are as acceptable in predicting the inexact behavior between statistical boundaries of biological materials, as exact end points are for predicting consistent and repeatable failure parameters of inert materials. Pharmacological effects of drugs are tested on statistical samples of appropriate animals of a uniform strain to determine the minimum effective dose, the minimum lethal dose, and the dose fatal to half the animal subjects. These values are expressed as quantity of drug per unit weight of animal. The drug is then tested on humans to find the minimum effective dose in drug units per unit weight of human. Correlation with animal results provides a coefficient for extrapolating the minimum lethal and 50 per cent lethal values for man. Further testing with numerous subjects explores the gamut of variables such as age, sex, allergic or freak reactions and cumulative effects before establishing a safe therapeutic dose and frequency of administration for human patients. This is why medicine, unlike engineering, is referred to as a practice. The practice, nevertheless, is valued for its effectiveness, if not its exactness, in terms of health restored and lives saved. The use of human volunteers to determine thresholds and limits of exposure to mechanical force, and in particular, to evaluate whole body response to decelerative force, is limited by experimental hazards. Fortunately, no new designs are in prospect for the two basic models in three colors and many sizes of the human body, so that the growing accumulation of data on human responses to mechanical force should remain current for the foreseeable future.

BACKGROUND

The first clear statement of the problem of dynamic stress analysis of man was by Siegfried Ruff,[53] in relation to the requirements of military aviation. He distinguished between static and dynamic stresses, comparing their effects on elastic deformation and impact tensile strength of tissues. He further compared prolonged acceleration with brief impact acceleration, describing the factors determining tolerance to the latter as follows: (1) peak acceleration, (2) time of exposure, (3) momentum, or time integral of the forces, (4) jolt, or third derivative of distance with respect to time, and (5) the nature of the forces of inertia and the site of application of the body. He devised a pendulum swing with a radius of 15 to 26.5 feet, with a seat snubbed by a shock cord after dropping to the vertical position with a human volunteer seated facing forward with seat belt, or seated facing backward with a high back rest and head cushion. A load cell in the snubbing cable and an accelerometer mounted on the seat provided measurements. In the forward facing position with a 16 inch wide belt, subjects sustained 2,200 pounds loading in .10 second duration with nausea and slowing of the pulse which he related to vagus nerve stimulation, and ultimate loads of 3,300 pounds with no injury at a peak of 18.0 g. He compared this with a crash in which crew men survived uninjured after exposure to 26.0 and 3,740.0 pounds force. He rated the 1941 military aircraft seat belts of the German Air Force at 20.0 for one to several tenths of seconds, tolerated without injury. High speed motion pictures of subjects in swing tests indicated the need for shoulder straps to prevent hyperflexion around the belt and to prevent wedge-shaped vertebral body fractures occasionally observed in pilots crashing with the seat belt alone. He considered the maintenance of upright posture during forward deceleration a more important function for the shoulder straps than that of absorbing decelerative forces.

Simulation of aircraft crash impact with occupants seated facing backward was also accomplished on the swing seat to 4750.0 pounds at 28 to

30 g without injury. No further tests were done because aircraft engineers protested that aft-facing seats and floor attachments in 1942 commercial planes could not be stressed to exceed 4,500 pounds of force.

Ruff also investigated static and dynamic compression loading of the vertebral column in the longitudinal axis. Fresh cadaver vertebral column segments were compressed in a static test machine to find the breaking load on each of the lower five thoracic and all five lumbar vertebrae. He estimated 868 inch pounds compression limit to fracture the first lumbar vertebra when applied to the whole spinal column. A stress strain analysis of the vertebrae in the living spinal column was accomplished by placing a subject supine on an x-ray table with heels, hips and shoulders supported on skate boards, while compression increments of 22 pounds were applied between the head and feet, up to 132 pounds, taking x-rays of the lower eight thoracic and five lumbar vertebrae at each increment. By measuring the compression of intervertebral discs and resultant reduction of space between vertebrae at each increment, strain was determined, and from it the percentage loading of each vertebra by body weight in the upright position. This percentage times gravities to equal the static break load for each vertebra previously determined on fresh cadaver static tests was supposed to equal the dynamic accelerative load range of tolerance for the vertebra. He obtained values of 18.2 to 25.7 g from these calculations. Tests with human subjects in upward ejection seats of a catapult test tower resulted in lumbar spinal fractures for three out of four subjects exposed to 26 gravities for .005 seconds duration, indicating that tolerance for acceleration increases as the time of exposure decreases, if the time of exposure is less than .005 seconds. For corroboration, he exposed himself to deceleration on the swing seat, with the seat suspended in the supine, buttocks forward position up to 20.0 g, sustaining sciatica-like pain of several weeks duration as a consequence. He recommended a 7,700 pound test forward facing crash harness consisting of 4,500 pounds belt, and two shoulder straps of 1,600 pounds test each, converging on an 88 square inch belt plate, with adequate strength seat and attachment points for restraints and seat. He also recommended 4,500 pounds 20 g backward facing seats for air transport passengers.

Interest in impact deceleration survival in the United States began with the analysis of human falls from higher than 50 feet, begun by De Haven[53] at Cornell University. These inadvertent human experiments roughed out the parameters of human impact survival limits, ranging from survival with no injury to survival with severe injuries. From his estimates, De Haven reasoned that a peak of 200 times gravity could be survived during impact under optimum conditions.

The analysis of human falls by Snyder,[64] of parachute accidents by

Kiel,[41] and of professional high divers by Schneider et al.[57] provides data on survival limits for whole body impact acceleration well beyond safe experimentation levels with human volunteers.

Just as in Germany, human experimentation on effects of deceleration impact was undertaken as a military requirement, with the human volunteer subjects covered by the contingencies applicable to combat situations. The first area of such activity was in continuation of work on ejection seats for escape from aircraft begun by the Germans. The third derivative of motion, or jolt, in relation to exciting resonant response in the low natural frequency and resonant response range of the human body, between 2 and 20 cps, was carefully investigated in determining an acceptable rise time for the ejection catapult stroke. Kroeger[42] developed a telescoping catapult with three concentric tubular components expanding in a 5 foot stroke to a velocity of 60 feet per second, required for the seat and occupant to clear the tail of a jet fighter at high subsonic speeds. The rate of change of acceleration during this expansion was a function of the burning rate of the gun powder exploding in the catapult. With a rise time of less than 90 milli-seconds to attain 16.0 g of acceleration, the seat cushion stored energy like a spring, adding to the catapult acceleration as it recoiled. An analagous compression at the lumbar spine due to the acceleration of the pelvic mass resisted by the inertia of the upper torso, reacted like a second spring. The subsequent amplified rebound localized high forces, at the first lumbar or twelfth thoracic vertebral bodies, combined with forward hyperflexion to produce the wedge fractures of vertebral bodies described by Ruff.[53] Slower burning gun powder and thinner, harder, cushions of energy-absorbing materials greatly improved the situation.

These findings led to extensive research on whole body mechanical impedance as an injurious factor in impact and vibration exposure. Considering it as a double mass spring coupled system with a highly damped visco elastic linkage, Latham[43] measured amplitudes of response to sinusoidal oscillations in the range of 2 to 20 cps for the seated human subject, tightly strapped to the seat. At 5 cps, there was a whole body resonance with respect to the seat; at 8 cps, maximum amplitude of shoulder displacement relative to hip occurred, and at 17 to 20 cps, oscillation of the head relative to shoulders was maximal. These frequencies correspond respectively to pulse durations of .1, .0626 and .025 to .0295 seconds. Dropping a subject in the seat 6 inches onto a concrete floor excited a predominant resonance of 5 cps, recorded by an accelerometer mounted on the subject's hip adjacent to the CG of the body in this position. Similarly, upward sledge hammer blows against the bottom of the seat caused impact pulses of shorter duration, which excited initial resonance at 8 cps on the hip and 17 to 20 cps recorded on the subject's head. Latham evaluated the 5 and 8 cps resonances to be subjectively more severe than the 17 to 20 cps resonance of the head-neck linkage.

Zigenrucker and Magid[89] exposed ten human subjects to voluntary duration limits of sine wave oscillations on a shake table at 3 to 15 cps, at increments of amplitude up to tolerance limits. Amplitude and frequency tolerance limits were less than 2 g at 5 and 8 cps, for less than a minute of exposure. At 15 cps, 7.5 g was tolerated for 20 seconds.

Mandel and Lowry[49] substantiated the subjective pain g-thresholds for resonant frequencies in 1 minute exposures of twenty-two subjects. Defining mechanical impedance as the ratio of applied force to resulting velocity, von Gierke[85] notes that it can be measured without interfering with the body, either on a shake table at sinusodial steady state, or by short duration impact pulse. Only at frequency less than the first resonance of 4 to 6 cps does the body react in accordance with rigid body mechanics. Near and above the resonance, the body is deformable, its impedance deviates from that of a pure mass, and the CG shifts dynamically under the force input. Mechanical energy is propagated in tissues in the form of transverse shear waves at low frequencies; where the shear wavelength is large compared to the dimensions of the body, at less than 100 cps, the propagation is characterized in terms of energy exchange between lumped elasticities and masses. When stretched beyond its elastic limits, tissue damage and breakage occurs. One gross measure for the body's overall mechanical reaction to external forces is the mechanical impedance measured by the body surface.

Edwards and Lange,[23] Nickerson,[51] Weis,[87] and Coermann[20] have measured the driving point impedance of sitting, standing and supine human subjects on the shake table and by single impact. The impedance of the sitting man exhibits a resonance between 4 and 6 cps, a range of maximum energy transfer determining both impact and vibration tolerance. Strain measurements on the circumference of chest and abdomen at this frequency range gives the quantitative resonant response of the thorax-abdomen system. Motions and deformations of organs within the thorax and abdomen can be observed during resonant response by x-ray techniques. Weiss and Mohr[88] observed and recorded organ responses of sixteen human subjects by means of an intensified image fluoroscopic screen, photographed at 60 exposures per second, by a high sensitivity television camera, during seated drop test at 8 feet per second, to an impact of 7.5 milliseconds duration. This is less than the resonant pulse duration at 4 to 6 cps; therefore the response amplitude is directly correlated with the area of the impulse. This amplitude corresponded with a subjective pain limit of voluntary tolerance for the subjects. A wave of radiographic density was observed to pass from the iliac wings to the lung apices, more clearly seen in the abdomen than in the thorax. Synchronous with it was a downward deviation of the liver, descending as much as 1.75 inches, measured at the diaphragm. The heart moved synchronously with the liver, and the lungs displaced downward on impact. The resonant frequency of the liver was 7 cps, damped to a 50 per cent decrement.

Impact, applied to anesthetized monkeys, at a velocity change of 55.7 feet per second, 149.8 peak g for 14 milliseconds pulse duration, while simultaneous high speed motion picture photography and radiography recorded responses, showed a surface wave and a shear wave involving general dilation of the torso diameter. The compression of the torso could be seen to meet this wave at the level of the nipples, corresponding, to the level of injuries occurring to the spine during the impact. Secondary injuries consisted of hemorrhages under the surface membranes of liver and lungs and inner lining of the heart, corresponding to the effects of a strain wave exceeding the elastic limits of tissues. The spinal injury was accounted for by Weis as a lumped parameter response. From the radiographic data, he deduces that a critical velocity change excites a strain wave associated with the density wave, amplified at resonance to exceed tissue elastic limits.

Bierman[12] recorded standing waves in the abdominal and thoracic walls of twenty-two human volunteer subjects supine on a narrow table after a vest weighted at the corners was dropped from a height of 3 feet onto the chest and abdomen. The voluntary tolerance limit for this impact exposure was about 3,000 pounds of force. No instrumentation, other than high speed motion picture cameras and load cells, was used. The subject, sandwiched between the table top and the weighted vest, sustained abrupt intra-abdominal and intrathoracic pressure change with lateral deformation of the body cavities, with the wave phenomena probably confined to the body wall, in contrast with the inertial excitation of internal masses and body wall during abrupt velocity change of the whole body.

It becomes evident that three modes of energy transmission to the whole body can produce subjective distress, and ultimately injurious effects as a result of impact deceleration: (1) abrupt pressure change and localized deformation proportional thereto by inertial displacement of the body against restraints applied to the body surface, or against resistant objects; (2) excitation of spring-mass responses characteristic of body mechanical impedance, with maxima at resonant frequencies of body segments or of particular organ masses, coupled with elastic linkages, with injurious interactions, and (3) propagation of strain waves, which at resonance, exceed the elastic limits of tissues.

THE PROBLEM

The driver's dilemma in the eminent motor vehicle crash predicament is outlined in Table 15-I. The distance travelled while the driver decides to act increases with vehicle speed, as does the distance in which he can complete a braking stop. An effective decision must initiate breaking action at any given speed soon enough to halt the vehicle short of the collision target. Delayed action results in collision at the remaining speed of the vehicle when it reaches the target. The majority of fatal and injurious crashes occur at about 40 mph, consequent to a belated braking decision by the driver. Crashes above this collision speed are less frequent, but more often fatal. Here the sum of the cubic function of velocity, or jolt, and the square function of velocity, acceleration, determined by the crash distance, and the consequent kinetic energy changes, increase formidably with speed. Protective measures for survival must be augmented and optimized correspondingly, within limits of human tolerance for the forces involved. Severy[59] observed in an experimental collision of a moving vehicle into the rear of a parked vehicle, up to 30 mph, that the rear of the stationary vehicle was penetrated incrementally with speed to 3 feet, beyond which the front of the moving vehicle collapsed progressively to

TABLE 15-I

Velocity		Distance in 2 sec.	Dry Brake Stop Average			Crash Stop Average			Force on 170 lb. man	Loading Restraint Area sq. in.	
mph	ft./sec.	ft.	ft.	g	sec.	ft.	g	sec.	lbs.	Seat Belt	psi
7.5	11	22	6	.31	1.0	1.0	2	.176	340	40	8.5
15.0	22	44	23	.33	2.1	1.5	5	.137	850	40	21.0
22.5	33	66	48	.35	3.0	2.0	9	.117	1,530	40	38.0
										3 point	
30.0	44	88	79	.38	3.6	2.5	12	.114	2,040	80	25.5
37.5	55	110	118	.40	4.3	3.0	16	.108	2,720	80	34.0
45.0	66	132	161	.42	4.9	3.5	19	.106	3,230	80	40.0
52.5	77	154	209	.44	5.4	4.0	23	.104	3,910	80	49.0
										Belt + 2 shoulder straps	
60.0	88	176	262	.46	6.0	4.5	27	.101	4,590	120	38.0
67.5	99	198	324	.47	6.5	5.0	30	.101	5,100	120	42.5
75.0	110	220	383	.48	7.0	5.5	34	.099	5,780	120	48.0
82.5	121	242	462	.49	7.7	6.0	38	.099	6,460	120	54.0
90.0	132	264	543	.50	8.2	6.5	42	.098	7,140	120	59.5

The Motor Vehicle Crash Problem: At driving speeds of 7.5 to 90.0 mph, the driver covers 22 to 264 feet while taking 2 seconds to react. He can come to a stop on dry pavement in 6.0 to 543.0 feet, during 1.0 to 8.2 seconds. Otherwise, he can crash in 1.0 to 6.5 feet of crushing and collapsing distance in 176 to 98 msec average impact duration, at 2 to 42.0 g deceleration. The average force, from his 170 pound mass times the average deceleration will be 340 to 7,140 pounds. He can sustain up to 9.0 g on the seat belt alone, averaging 38 pounds per square inch loading, up to 23.0 g against the three-point restraint, averaging 49 pounds per square inch, and up to 42.0 g against the seat belt and two shoulder straps averaging 59.5 pounds per square inch, provided the integrity of his enclosure is maintained.
Calculated from ideal assumptions with last digit smoothed.

an additional 3 feet 55 mph, so that the sum of collapsing distance between the two vehicles determined the crash distance. Calculated average decelerations are given in Table 15–I for estimated crash distances at given velocities, and resulting average forces on the restrained occupant are computed. Assuming the occupant compartment is not invaded by the colliding vehicle, or object struck, and that lethal or injurious flying objects are not contacted by the persons in the vehicle, the problem becomes one of human tolerance for the collision forces, while optimally restrained against secondary collision with vehicle interior, or perhaps, for attenuated collision with prepared areas of vehicle interior. The design criteria and performance requirements, under crash conditions for vehicle crash protection devices, are determined by human tolerance limits for vehicle crash force parameters. These can only be found by controlled increments of exposure to actual forces on human volunteer subjects, using vehicle crash simulators. Once determined with statistically valid numbers of humans up to voluntary exposure limits, substantiated by exposures of man-sized animal subjects to forces corresponding to those estimated for fatal and injurious human accidents, performance testing thereafter can be performed with anthropometric dummies up to actual and extrapolated limits for man.

HUMAN EXPERIMENTS

Experimental whole body exposures of human subjects to controlled increments of forces, corresponding to crash impacts and decelerations, have been accomplished by a number of investigators with reference to the following factors:

1. Initial velocity and velocity change.
2. Distances in which velocity change occurs.
3. Displacements of subject during impact or deceleration.
4. Rates of change of acceleration, or jolt, of subject and simulator.
5. Duration of impact or deceleration pulses, including rise time, plateau and decay.
6. Direction of velocity change relative to long axis of the subject in seated position.
7. Inertial force measurements of restraints or supports bearing against subject body areas.
8. Anthropometric dimensions, physiological responses, and subjective reactions of human subjects before, during and after impact deceleration exposure.
9. High speed motion picture and x-ray motion studies of human subjects before, during and after exposure to impact deceleration.

Recordings from experiments have included some or all of the foregoing factors. Available data from human experiments, found to be appropriately applicable to the range of human tolerance and crash protection under conditions of automotive crash exposure, have been compiled and reported in Tables 15-II, III, IV, V, VI, VII, VIIA and VIII. In addition, a limited number of vehicle barrier crashes with human volunteer occupants are reported by Ryan,[56] for testing effectiveness of energy absorbing front bumpers and collapsing steering wheel, in which modification of the vehicle crash forces and collision velocity kept the impact acceleration well below human tolerance limits to demonstrate effectiveness of a crash protection system.

The numerous records of measurements of vehicle crash forces on anthropometric dummy occupants reported by Severy[59] and many other in-

TABLE 15-II

DECELERATION OF HUMAN SUBJECTS SEATED FACING FORWARD, SUMMARIES OF 40 EXPERIMENTS

Run No.	Name	Sled Velocity In Brakes Entry MPH	Ft/Sec	Exit Ft/Sec	Change Ft/Sec	MPH	Sled Deceleration Ft	Sec	Calculated Sled Onset Plateau G/Sec	G	Subject Weight Lbs.	Force F × M Lbs.	Restraint Area Sq.In.	Body Loading P.S.I.	Observed Effects on Subject
96	JPS	148.0	217	115	-102	-69.6	48.8	.30	1,200	11.5	172	1,978	138	14.3	L 9th,10th,11th ribs tender for 4 weeks
119	JPS	138.5	203	95	-107	-73.0	48.8	.33	1,068	10.9	174	1,897	218	8.7	L 10th,11th ribs tender 1 wk.
94	JPS	147.3	216	128	- 88	-60.0	48.8	.21	1,068	15.4	172	2,649	261	10.1	No adverse effects
97	WAR	154.2	226	149	- 77	-52.5	48.8	.21	1,065	14.7	155	2,278	244	9.3	No adverse effects
98	WAR	146.0	214	116	- 98	-66.8	36.3	.21	1,130	16.5	154	2,541	208	12.2	No adverse effects
102	RHA	143.2	210	121	- 95	-64.8	36.3	.21	1,010	15.0	170	2,550	266	9.6	No adverse effects
106	DIM	150.0	220	126	- 94	-64.2	36.3	.21	1,168	16.6	176	2,922	271	10.8	No adverse effects
117	RHA	150.0	220	146	- 74	-50.4	36.3	.21	973	13.8	170	2,346	204	11.5	No adverse effects
118	RL	137.8	202	114	- 88	-60.0	36.3	.22	917	14.2	177	2,513	238	10.6	Harness stitches brake pain in upper abdomen
149	FHS	148.0	217	122	- 92	-62.8	36.3	.24	1,141	16.4	197	3,231	198	16.3	No adverse effects
150	HG	152.8	224	141	- 83	-56.6	36.3	.22	1,107	15.4	208	3,203	199	16.1	No adverse effects
164	WJAM	133.0	195	92	-103	-70.2	36.3	.22	954	15.1	142+21.0	2,461	168	14.6	Hysterical subject
178	JFF	146.6	215	131	- 84	-57.3	36.3	.24	1,021	14.8	149	2,204	201	11.0	No adverse effects
99	JFF	147.3	216	126	- 90	-61.4	27.0	.16	1,086	20.9	149	3,114	201	15.5	Bruised hand fm. flailing against sled windscreen
100	WAR	150.0	220	130	- 90	-61.4	27.0	.16	1,132	21.4	155	3,317	244	13.6	Chest belt caused painful hyperflexion of neck
142	WAR	147.3	216	134	- 87	-59.3	27.0	.18	1,011	19.5	155	3,022	176	17.2	Upper L back pain on inspiration for 30 min.
143	JFF	148.0	217	130	- 91	-62.1	27.0	.23	1,070	20.5	149	3,054	170	18.0	Narrow shoulder straps caused pain in shoulders - lasting 2hr
147	JFF	144.0	211	102	-109	-74.3	27.0	.18	1,175	23.2	155	3,457	170	20.3	Same
163	JPS	88.7	130	-	-130	-88.6	18.0	.17	-	-	170+21	-	-	-	
165	JPS	140.5	206	126	- 80	-54.6	27.0	.18	893	18.0	170+21	3,438	186	18.5	Tender lower sacrum
166	JPS	136.5	200	107	- 93	-63.4	27.0	.18	933	19.4	170	3,298	186	17.7	Fractured R wrist - coccyx sacrum bruised
103	JFF	152.8	224	140	- 84	-57.3	25.9	.16	1,118	26.0	155	4,030	240	16.8	Leg strap abrasions
104	WAR	141.5	209	122	- 87	-59.3	25.9	.16	983	24.4	152	3,709	208	17.8	Slight muscle soreness of neck & upper back - 1 day
122	JFF	139.0	204	126	- 78	-53.2	25.9	.16	857	21.8	152	3,314	201	16.5	No adverse effects
107	JFF	148.6	218	134	- 84	-57.3	24.9	.16	1,052	30.1	149	4,485	240	18.7	Strap abrasions of shoulders & inner thighs
108	WAR	144.5	212	129	- 83	-56.6	24.9	.16	980	28.9	153	4,422	208	21.2	R shoulder strap contusion
109	RHA	145.2	213	133	- 80	-54.6	24.9	.16	948	27.8	140	4,726	204	23.2	Mild cardiovascular shock, retinal reinular spasm, vision blurred
110	JPS	154.2	226	142	- 84	-57.3	24.9	.15	1,141	31.5	172.5	5,434	218	24.9	Mild cardiovascular shock, retinal reinular spasm, purple contusions of inner thighs
111	JFF	144.0	211	104	-107	-73.0	24.9	.16	1,160	34.3	152	5,214	240	21.7	No adverse effects
123	RHA	135.0	198	106	- 92	-62.8	24.9	.15	904	28.5	172.5	4,859	204	23.8	No adverse effects
124	JPS	143.2	210	134	- 76	-51.8	24.9	.15	896	26.6	170.5	4,642	217	21.4	Mild cardiovascular shock, dimning of vision
130	JFF	137.2	201	127	- 77	-52.5	24.9	.16	796	24.7	174.5	3,779	240	15.7	Headache for 15 min. after run
133	RL	145.2	213	87	-126	-85.8	24.9	.16	1,315	38.5	153	6,814	238	28.6	Cardiovascular shock with 2 episodes of fainting, severe contusions of all strap areas and head, 3 days to recuperate
135	JPS	150.0	220	106	-115	-78.4	24.9	.16	1,373	37.9	177	6,519	218	29.9	R wrist fractured, moderate cardiovascular shock, vision blurred, contusions of all strap areas.
210	PWS	143.2	210	116	- 94	-64.2	50.9	.24	347	15.6	172	3,214	280	11.5	No adverse effects
211	JPS	148.6	218	123	- 95	-64.8	47.8	.22	254	16.5	206	2,688	218	13.2	No adverse effects
212	PWS	143.2	210	90	-120	-81.8	45.7	.22	271	32.7	206	6,736	280	24.0	No adverse effects
213	JPS	156.8	224	71	-153	-104.3	47.8	.25	293	36.5	175	6,388	218	29.3	Vision disturbed for 30 minutes
214	PWS	152.0	223	41	-181	-123.4	47.8	.28	314	38.6	206	7,952	280	28.4	No adverse effects
215	JPS	154.2	226	50	-175	-119.3	42.6	.23	413	45.4	175	7,954	218	36.4	Retinal hemmorhage, severe frontal headache

vestigators also establish the pattern and parameters of dynamic stresses to which occupants are subjected in unmodified standard vehicles. The primary problem of human tolerance measurements has been investigated, with maximum control of exposure factors hazards, by use of crash simulators performing under carefully predetermined conditions, for safe increments, through limits of voluntary exposure and minor, recuperable injury. The experiments reported in Tables 15–II and 15–III include fifty-six human experiments out of a total of seventy-three that were accomplished with a rocket powered sled, decelerated by mechanical friction brakes. Although primarily related to aircraft crash velocity changes, these experiments demonstrate human responses and tolerances applicable to the range of automotive vehicle crash exposures. In some instances, the durations exceed those of automotive vehicle barrier crashes, attaining the same peak deceleration and rate of onset values. These experiments and the rocket powered decelerator are described in detail by Stapp.[71] The subject was secured in a steel-tubing seat that could be mounted facing forward, facing to the side, or facing backward, on a 1,500 pound chrome molybdenum steel tubing sled of welded truss construction, slipper mounted on 2,000 feet of precision rail track on a concrete bed. Either a metal enclosure or a windscreen protected the subject. Propulsion was by one to four solid fuel jato rockets of 1,000 pounds thrust for 5 seconds duration, enabling velocities of 90 to 243 mph to be attained in less than 750 feet. Deceleration was by pneumatic-hydraulic actuated friction brake shoes in a series of brake units mounted between the rails in the brake

TABLE 15-III

DECELERATION OF HUMAN SUBJECTS SEATED FACING BACKWARD, SUMMARIES OF 16 EXPERIMENTS

Run No.	Name	Velocity in Brakes Entry MPH	Ft/Sec	Exit Ft/Sec	Change Ft/Sec	MPH	Sled Decele-ration Ft	Sec	Calculated Sled Onset Plateau G/Sec	G	Subject Weight Lbs.	Force F = MA Lbs.	Restraint Area Sq. In.	Body Loading F.S.I.	Observed Effect on Subject
17	JPS	142.2	210	136	74	50.2	37.4	.23	586	11.6	172	1,995	260	7.7	No adverse effects
18	JPS	142.2	210	120	90	61.4	35.3	.23	582	17.3	172	2,976	260	11.4	Occipital headache - 1 min
19	JPS	143.0	211	91	120	81.8	30.1	.27	624	24.6	172	4,231	260	16.3	Brief occipital headache
24	JPS	141.8	208	122	86	58.6	30.1	-	428	21.4	172	3,681	260	14.2	No adverse effects
25	JPS	140.0	205	96	109	74.3	30.1	.23	488	24.8	172	4,266	260	16.4	Sacral contusion - 24 hrs.
27	JPS	142.2	210	74	136	92.7	30.1	.24	530	31.5	172	5,418	260	20.8	Headache, lassitude, sacral contusion
121	WAR	142.2	200	72	128	87.2	48.8	.37	575	11.9	152.5	1,814	207	8.6	
20	JPS	145.2	212	122	91	62.0	47.8	.30	1,061	10.4	172	1,789	260	6.9	Noticeable difference in abruptness of onset
21	JPS	140.5	206	124	82	56.0	37.4	.16	808	12.2	172	2,098	260	8.1	30 secs. of occipital headache
22	JPS	144.5	212	118	94	64.2	35.3	.23	954	18.7	172	3,216	260	12.4	Very abrupt onset sensations, teeth jarred painfully
26	JPS	139.0	204	79	125	85.2	28.0	.22	944	24.0	172	4,128	260	15.9	Headache - 30 secs.
112	WAR	141.8	208	100	108	73.6	36.3	-	1,130	17.0	152	2,584	260	9.9	No adverse effects
113	WAR	140.5	206	90	116	99.0	24.9	.16	1,155	35.0	152	5,320	260	20.5	Brief headache, lower lumbar spine tender - 24 hrs.
114	JFF	141.8	208	96	112	76.4	24.9	.16	1,156	34.7	153	5,309	252	21.1	Brief headache, lower lumbar spine tender - 72 hrs.
179	WAR	145.2	213	116	87	59.4	36.3	-	1,110	16.3	152	2,478	260	9.5	No adverse effects
40	LL	129.5	190	-	190	129.5	40.0	.40	-	-	-	-	260	-	Stopped in 40 ft. by brake failure, tender coccyx and lumbar spine - 3 days

318 *Impact Injury and Crash Protection*

area, 1300 to 1350 feet from the starting end of the track. These were in parallel rows in line with two parallel keels mounted lengthwise under the sled, which they clasped with an action similar to pulling a knife blade through a clamped vise, with a maximum of approximately 5 g friction drag for each such pair, thus determining magnitude of deceleration in 5 g increments. Deceleration time patterns were controlled by (a) the entry velocity of the sled into the brake system, (b) the number and sequence of brake units activated, and (c) the closing pressure of the brake shoes. Instrumentation included the following:

1. Time displacement measured by passage of a magnet, attached to a sled slipper, over coils in series at 10 feet intervals in the acceleration path and at 1 foot intervals in the brake area, recorded along with a 100 cps timer trace.
2. Four channels of AM-FM telemetry used variously for transmitting strain gauge accelerometer and load cell signals.
3. Sled mounted 128 frames per second motion picture camera.
4. Trackside motion picture and ribbon frame cameras to record acceleration events.
5. 1500 frame per second cameras in six overlapping profile sequences 35 feet from the braking area to record motion-study events during deceleration.

A total of thirteen subjects ranging from 142 to 206 pounds in weight, 66 to 74 inches in height, and 25 to 39 years of age were used in the fifty-four forward facing and nineteen backward facing experiments from which Table 15-II and 15-III data were selected.

In the forward facing experiments, at onsets of 1,010 to 1,200 g per second to peaks of 10 to 15 g, for durations of .21 to .33 seconds, (see experiments 96, 119, 97, 102, 117, 118 and 178) the only complaint was transient discomfort of restraint webbing impingement. In the range of 893 to 1,168 g per second onset, 15.4 to 20.8 peak g for .16 to .24 seconds duration, (runs 94, 98, 106, 149, 150, 164, 99, 142, 143, 165, 166, 210 and 211) there was increased discomfort due to restraint strap impingement, and two complaints of transient back muscle pain and lower pain due to forward scooting on the seat.

The subject of experiment 166 was seated on a seat pack parachute, which elevated him 5 inches; the arms were straight between the shoulders and the rigid hand holds, on which the palms of the hands were bearing down. At the peak inertial load of 19.4 g × the upper torso weight of 84 pounds, an estimated 1,630 pounds, the right wrist was fractured. In the range of 796 G per second onset to 1,175 g per second, peak g range of 21.4 to 24.7 total durations of .16 to .18 seconds, (see runs 100, 147, 104,

122 and 130), upper dorsal hyperflexion pains were experienced, in addition to more severe and persistent shoulder strap area muscle soreness. There were also two instances of headaches lasting several minutes. The next increment, in the range of 896 to 1,160 g per second onset, 26.0 to 34.4 peak g, and durations of .15 to .16 seconds, (see experiments 103, 107, 108, 109, 110, 111, 123 and 124). Visual changes and distinct signs of cardiovascular shock were observed. Opthalmoscopic examination of several subjects immediately post-run demonstrated pale retinas with marked veinular vasoconstriction. Several subjects reported bright, scintilating spots in the visual fields and intermittent darkening with blurred vision, lasting 2 or 3 minutes after exposure. Diminished blood pressure and bradycardia, with marked pallor and sweating, were observed as signs of cardiovascular shock.

The most severe immediate reactions to impact occurred in experiments 133 and 135, at 1,315 g per second onset, 38.5 peak g, duration .16 second; and 1,373 g per second, 37.9 g for .16 seconds respectively. In the first of these, within a minute after the run, the subject had a fainting spell, and after brief recovery of consciousness, relapsed for another minute or so, with blood pressure less than 50 systolic and 0 mm of mercury diastolic. Pain was very severe in all strap impingement areas. For the next 3 days, the subject was lethargic, preferred bed rest, moved with pain due to tender, livid, deep contusions of strap impingement areas in shoulders, hips and inner thighs. The subject of the second of these runs sustained a right wrist fracture from flailing the upright support of a rigid hand rest, with hematoma and extreme edema of the struck area; vision was blurred and dimmed to a smokey gray haze; blood pressure dropped below 50 mm systolic and consciousness was almost lost. Areas of strap impact were painfully abraded and contused, turning discolored by the following day. Visual fuzziness persisted for several hours after exposure. The subject was able to have the wrist fracture set on the way to the hospital. He completed all laboratory and clinical tests and observations.

The effect of rate of onset was evident by comparison with the last group of runs, (see runs 212, 213, 214 and 215) in which rates of onset ranged from 217 to 413 g per second, peak g from 32–7 to 45.4, and durations from .22 to .28 seconds. Only mild signs of transient cardiovascular shock were present, there were no strap contusions, and no interference with immediate recovery. Delayed effects were noted following run 215 at 413 g per second, 45.4 peak g, and .23 seconds duration. Minimal signs of shock, including pallor lasted less than a minute following the impact. Bright, scintillating pinpoint spots were seen in both peripheral fields of vision for approximately one minute after the run, followed by intermittent darkening at 20 or 30 second intervals for a few minutes, with

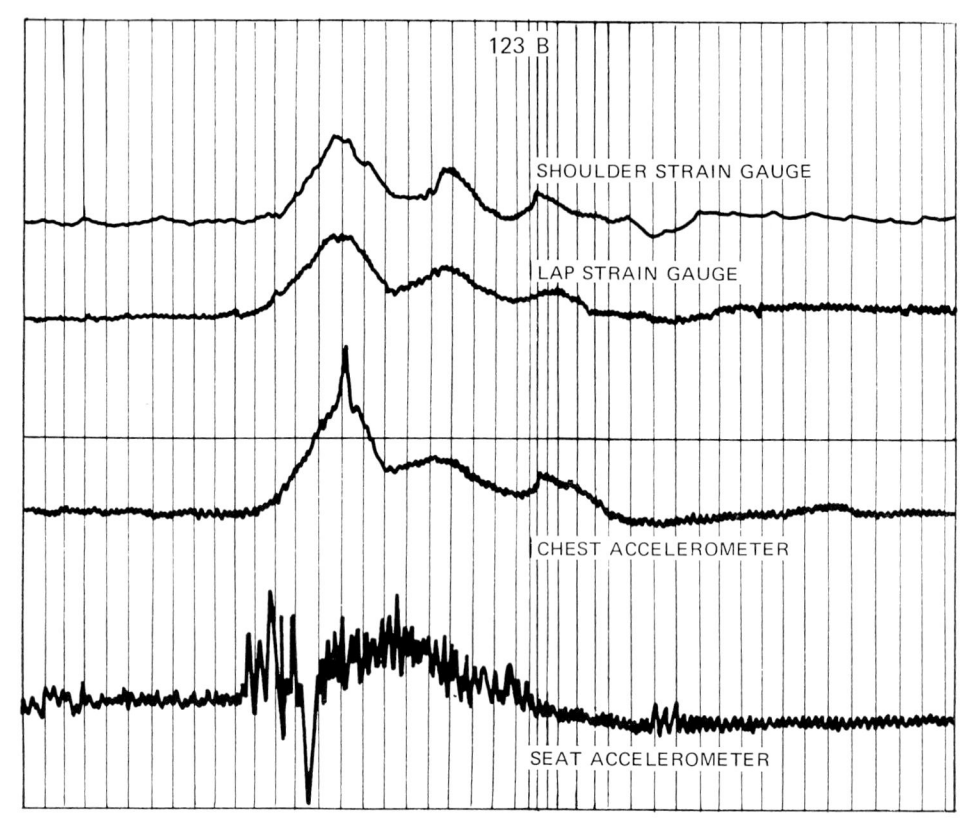

Figure 15-1A.

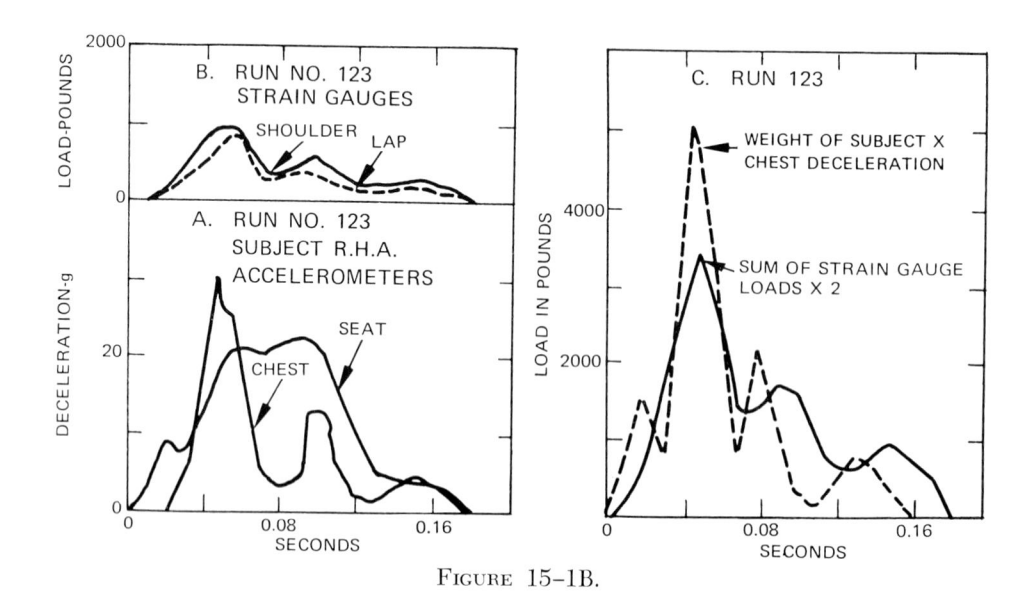

Figure 15-1B.

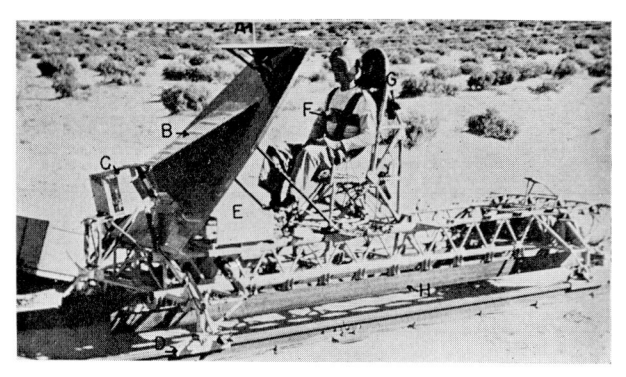

FIGURE 15–2. Decelerator with subject in position for forward facing run. A—Telemetering antenna. B—Windshield. C—Movie camera. D—Slipper. E—Telemetering equipment. F—Chest accelerometer. G—Shoulder strain gage. H—Braking keel.

continued blurring of vision, blurring and intermittent shadowing at longer intervals continued for about 4 hours, and the subject was progressively more fatigued. On the next morning the subject awoke with a severe frontaloccipital headache and noticed a gradually increasing blot in the right lateral half of the central field of vision of the right eye. Despite marked fatigue and lassitude, the subject was able to go about his duties. Opthalmoscopic examination revealed a horse-shoe shaped retinal hemorrhage from the tip of the nasal branch of the central retinal vein, involving apparently ruptured retinal veinules. Both eyes were painful on lateral and vertical movements. Petechiae of bulbar conjunctival veinules were still present from a previous run. The frontal headache disappeared within 24 hours. The irregular black blot in the right visual field cleared gradually during the following ten weeks, going from a black to an eggwhite opacity in the right central lateral visual field. There were no persistent contusions or strap marks after this run.

Out of nineteen runs with instrumentation in which subjects were exposed to deceleration in the backward facing position, sixteen have been completed with adequate records. With the seat back in the upright vertical position, uniform loading of the back body surface was observed, in runs 17, 18, 19, 24, 25, 27 and 121, in which rate of onset ranged from 428 to 624 g per second, with more intense pressure corresponding to increments of 10.4 through 31.5 g. Beyond 15 g, brief occipital headaches were felt for about 30 seconds post-run. Beyond 20 g peaks, the dull sensation in the occipital area began to resemble the after effects of a few good blows to the chin in a round of boxing. Confusion and depression became noticeable at 31.5 g. During run 25, at 488 g per second and 24.8 peak g, the subject anticipated impact by muscular tension against hand holds and foot rest, enhancing the impact effect to a painful degree. The result

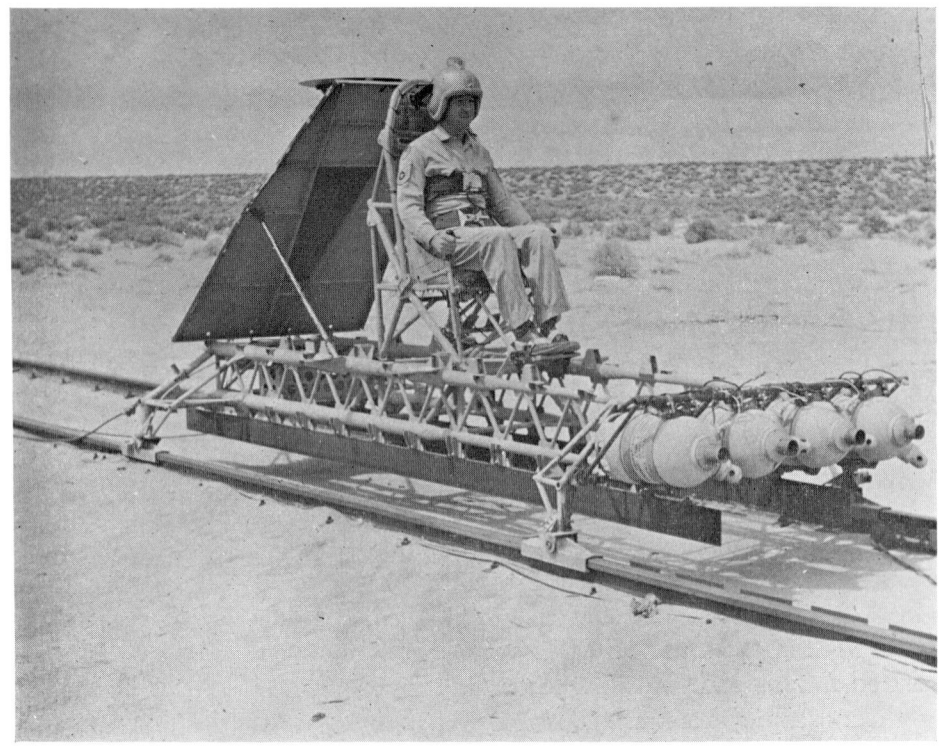

FIGURE 15–3. Subject Seated Facing Backward on Rocket Sled.

was a very hard impact to the lumbar spine and sacrum with soreness and stiffness in both hip and sacroiliac spine, and edema over the sacrum. The enhancing effect of muscular tension was avoided in run 26, at 944 g per second and 24 peak g. On the same day, the subject accomplished run 27, at 530 g per second and 31.5 peak g. The accumulative effect of two such runs in one day may have contributed to dullness, confusion and loss of control of fine movements, such as in writing, during 30 minutes following the last one. Riding a jeep over rough ground the following day excited twinges of headache. The area over the sacrum was discolored and slightly endematous.

Even a full stop in the brakes from 190 feet per second, or 129.5 mph in 40 feet after damage to a front right slipper attachment by a brake cam, did not exceed voluntary tolerance to impact in the backward facing seated position. Accelerometer traces were hard to decipher because of high frequency large amplitude vibrations, but appeared to exceed a mean 40 g peak. The subject of this run had tender coccyx and lumbar spine for 3 days, which was aggravated by a parachute jump in tennis shoes onto the hard surface of Muroc dry lake on the third day post run. The effects were not noticeably more severe than for the subjects of runs 113 and 114,

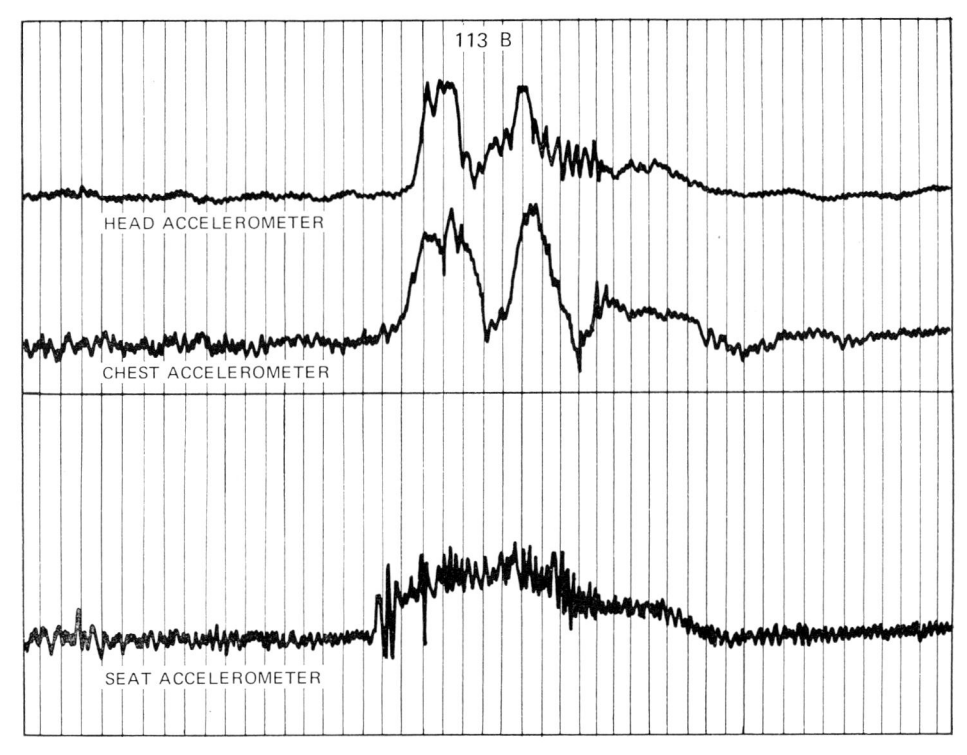

FIGURE 15–4A.

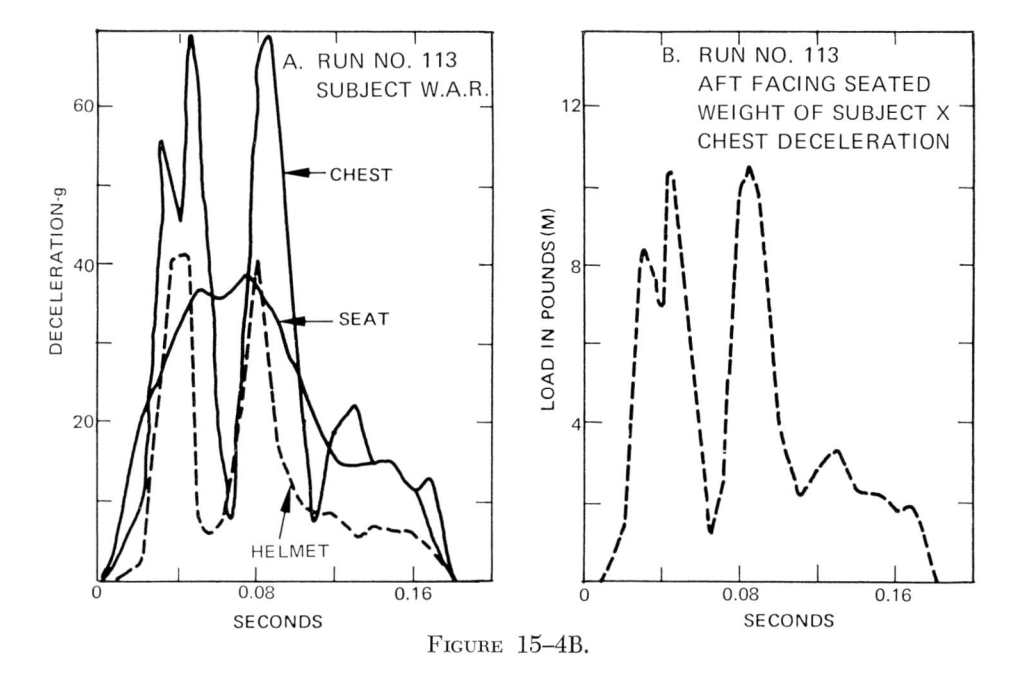

FIGURE 15–4B.

at 1,155 g per second and 35 g during velocity change of 79.0 and 76.4 mph respectively.

The most perceptible subjective difference observed in this backward facing series of runs was the striking increase in abruptness between 500 and 1,000 g per second onset at 10, 15 and 20 g, which exceeded the difference in sensation between 15 and 20 g at the same rate of onset at either 500 or 1,000 g per second. The magnitude of impact tended to diminish perception of this difference above 20 g. The only signs of injurious effects in the backward facing position in this series relate to minor contusions of coccyx and sacrum against the steel seat back, padded only with an inch thickness of felt. Despite a fiberglass shell helmet lined with cellular cellulose acetate against the felt seat back, fleeting headaches resulted from higher force impacts. With head and neck against the seat back and in line with the spine, higher than 40 g can be sustained at onsets of 500 to 1,000 g per second, according to these results.

Resonant responses* of the human body were sought in the actual motion of the body observed from 2,000 frame per second motion picture profile sequences, and in the periodicity of accelerometer and strap tension records, in response to the applied acceleration pulse. Such an analysis is presented for run 123 with subject seated forward facing, in Figure 15–5. This is a simultaneous plot, on a common time basis of the following: (1) calculated sled deceleration, and (2) the g force on subject measured by a chest mounted accelerometer during the braking period. Calculated sled deceleration was based on consecutive application of six brakes to a plateau value of 28.5 g sustained by adding two additional brakes to the front of the 11 foot long keels as the trailing end emerged from brakes 1 and 2, to maintain constant deceleration. The chest g force curve starts to rise about 40 milliseconds after theoretical entry of the sled into the brakes, due to delay in full bearing pressure of the first brake and transmission time for sled retardation to the seat and through restraints to begin deforming flesh and bones to the deceleration peak. This was followed by a peak-to-peak periodic rise and fall of the g force curve, corresponding to 20 cps of chest response. Figure 15–6 shows subject displacement, relative to sled, during braking, which reached a calculated plateau value of 24.3 g in 40 milliseconds, maintained for 50 milliseconds. Visual reference for analysis of 2,000 frame per second motion pictures of body displacements in profile was the subject's back, relative to a vertical frame member of the sled, to be determined and plotted as a function of sled position in the brakes, correlated with timing marks on the high speed film, for plotting displacement information as a function of time. The sled

* Unpublished analysis by C. F. Lombard, Northrop Space Laboratories Technical Report 65–152, Oct. 1965.

Voluntary Human Tolerance Levels 325

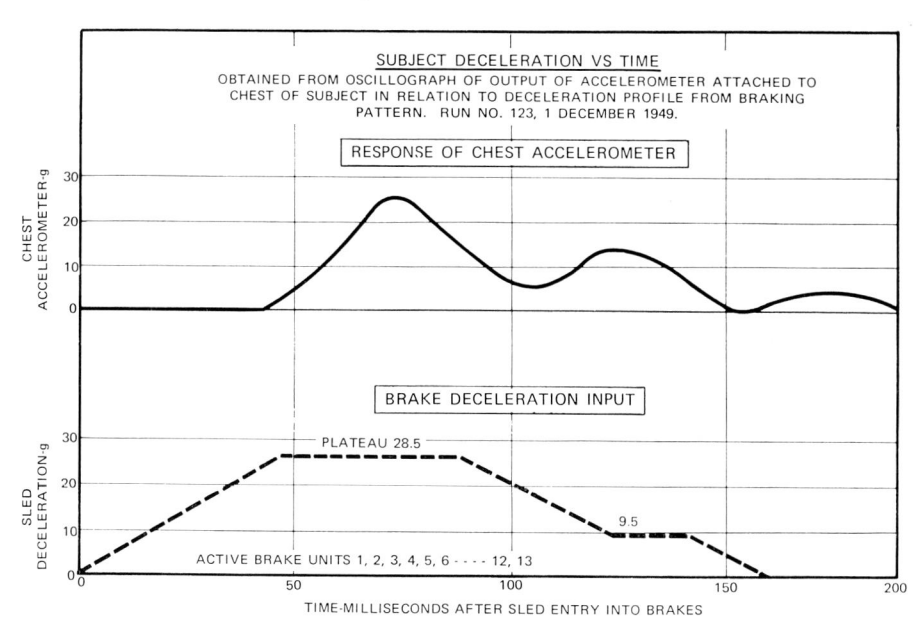

FIGURE 15-5. Human Subject Response to Abrupt Deceleration.

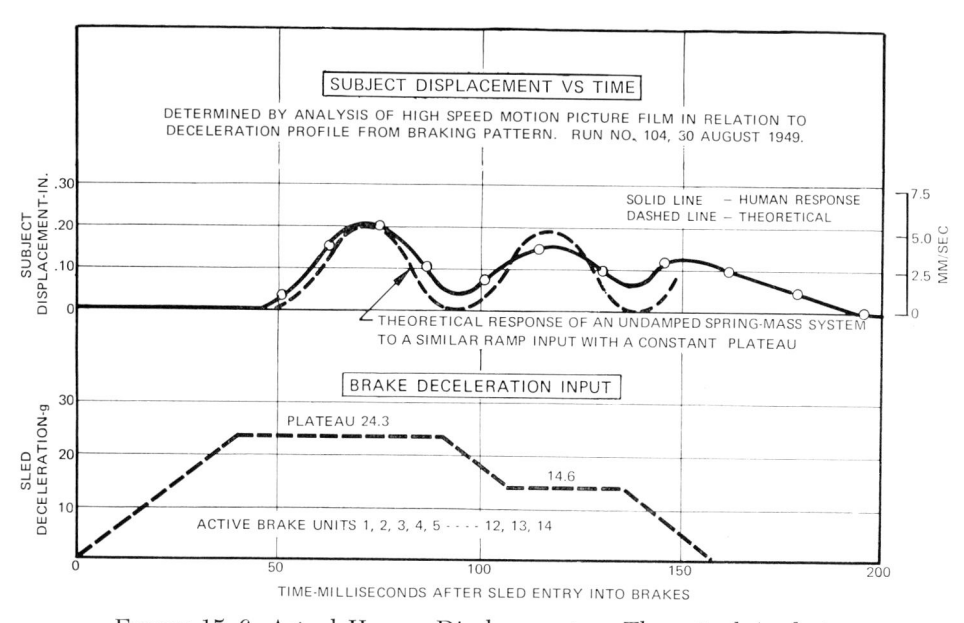

FIGURE 15-6. Actual Human Displacement vs Theoretical Analysis.

and body displacement curves are shown, along with a dashed line representing the theoretical curve of response of an undamped spring-mass system with characteristics approximating those of the human body in the type of strap used in this experiment. Inclusion of an effective damping co-

326   *Impact Injury and Crash Protection*

efficient would result in a damped response curve corresponding even more closely to the actual response curve shown.

All forward facing seated runs in this series were with either the standard Air Force Seat Belt and two shoulder straps, or with addition of the inverted V strap from the belt buckle, fairing around the thighs to the two rear corners of the seat. For backward facing seated exposures, a seat belt and a slack safety chest belt were used.

No evidence of cumulative effects due to repeated exposures to decelerative forces were found in any of the thirteen human subjects in this series, including one who sustained twenty-six exposures in a period of 50 months. This was verified by autopsy of one of the subjects who died 9 days after an automobile-train collision with a car he was driving, in which he was ejected, landing 135 feet from the vehicle. No sign of scars or old injuries were found either grossly or microscopically, other than recent trauma accounted for by the fatal accident. The fatality occurred 7 weeks after this subject's last experiment, and after a total of ten deceleration exposures in the previous 36 months.

Human response to impact force in the range of automotive vehicle collision speeds and crash distances at comparable velocity changes has been investigated with three simulators.

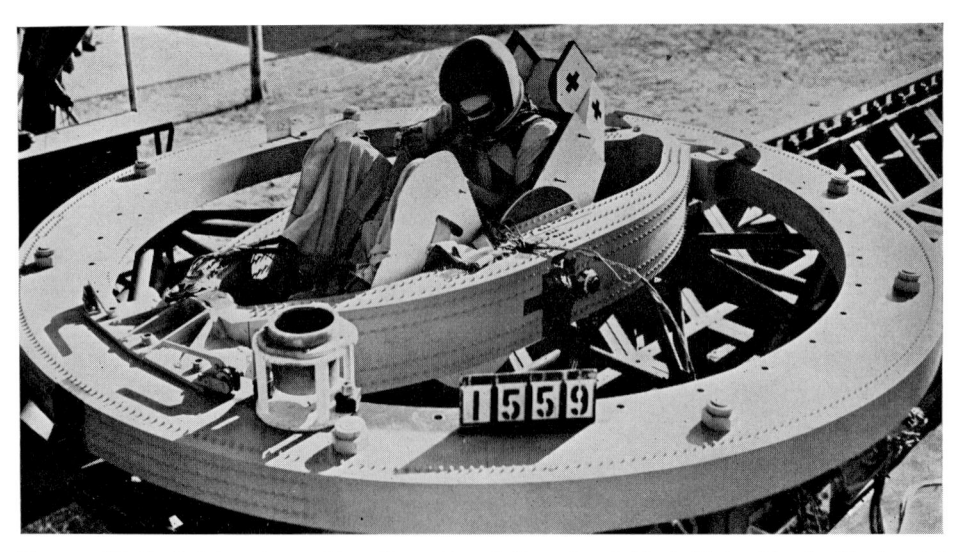

FIGURE 15-7. Subject in position 5, on Omni-directional Sled, Daisy Track. Horizontal ring, 3.05 meters in diameter, with bolt holes for 10 degree increments of yaw positioning of cradle, suspended between gimbals providing for 10 degree increments of positioning in roll; contained between gimbals in the cradle is the seat, locked in pitch position 45 degrees, tipped back from vertical, or 0 degree pitch. Trailing cable in lower right corner of picture links sled instrumentation to recording station in upper right.

EXPERIMENTAL INSTRUMENTS

The Daisy Decelerator

This decelerator has been described by Chandler[16] and in numerous papers reporting results of experiments with it, by Stapp,[76,77] Beeding,[5,6,7,8,9] Chandler[15] and Lewis.[44] Essentially, it consists of a test sled, a two-rail track, a propulsion device and a water inertia brake. It is capable of producing deceleration forces up to 200 g on human, animal and anthropometric subjects within a distance of 4 feet, and can attain speeds of 155 feet per second at brake entry. Many special purpose sleds have been developed for this track. Two that concern experiments reported here are as follows: (a) A rectangular, slipper mounted sled holding a seat that can be mounted facing forward or facing backward, with CG of occupant and sled aligned approximately between the elevated rails on either side. A brake piston 4½ feet long and 6 inches in diameter is mounted on the front. (b) An omnidirectional sled, on four slippers, of truss tubular welded design, carrying a horizontal ring of 10 feet outside diameter, concentric to which is a system of three sets of locking gimbal assemblies, enclosing a seat by pivot bearings at the center of gravity of seat and occupant. The three sets of gimbals are arranged to permit positioning in yaw by 10 degree increments through 360 degrees, in pitch through 180 degrees by 10 degree increments and likewise in roll. Within these limits, pre-selected pitch, roll, and yaw angles determine the axes of the test subject with respect to the fixed yaw line of motion of the sled on the rails. A piston for inertia water braking is carried on the front of the sled.

The two rail track was originally 120 feet in length, later lengthened to 240 feet. Two cylindrical solid steel rails 3 inches in diameter and 5 feet apart are mounted on concrete piers 3 feet tall, from a concrete base 18 inches thick. Provisions for thermal expansion and for realignment assure less than 2 g vibration in any direction during motion.

Propulsion was originally by MIAI ejection seat catapults thrusting horizontally with a 5-foot stroke to attain velocities in the order of 62 feet per second. One or two catapults simultaneously fired, provided a range of velocities adjusted for brake entry by the predetermined coasting distance. A more reliable method of propulsion was developed in the form of an air gun acceleration device, suitable for large payloads and high velocities. A pneumatically actuated piston with a 42-foot stroke smoothly pushes the sled at predetermined pressure up to the desired velocity and the sled coasts on beyond the stroke length to the water brake.

The water brake consists of a steel block securely mounted between the rails, with a 4-foot horizontal cylinder bore into which the piston on the front of the sled penetrates, breaking an occluding frangible membrane holding in a column of water. Inertial force of extruding the water through a variable area orifice results in retardation of sled motion, according to a predetermined pattern of onset and peak g, with duration determined by the sled velocity and the stopping distance for the piston.

Bopper

This device consists of a seat mounted on a small platform moving on rails 24 inches apart, mounted on a portable base 18 feet in length. Propulsion is accomplished by abrupt release of a stretched shock cord. A single row of spring loaded clasp type brake shoes bearing against a central steel keel under the seat platform provides friction brake action. Entrance velocity and stopping distance are the primary factors considered in establishing a deceleration pulse. A maximum deceleration of 22 g measured on the seat was obtained at maximum velocity in minimum stopping distance. The seat can be positioned facing forward or facing backward.

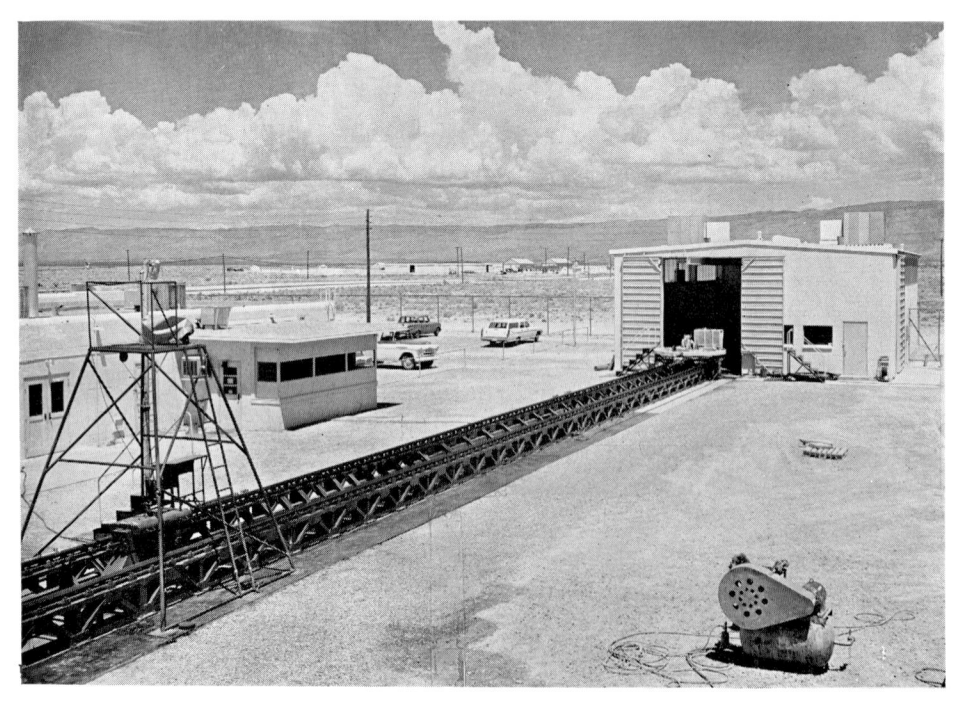

FIGURE 15-8. The Daisy Decelerator. This view shows the facility from the midpoint of the track towards the breech end. The airgun accelerator is housed in the building to the right. The tower to the left of the picture provides a firm stand for high speed overhead cameras, and is located over the waterbrake number 1, here mounted at the track midpoint. Instrumentation and fire control buildings are in the background.

The Swing Seat

An L shaped platform holding an aircraft seat, suspended like a garden swing to a boom with a pair of cables 18 feet and 11 inches from the bottom of the platform. An aircraft cable anchored by eye bolts at the center of gravity of the platform back, extending from the vertical position of the seat to the base of a crane, serving as a snub braking device when the seat is raised and allowed to drop back to the vertical position. The decelerative force is primarily a function of drop height and corresponding horizontal swing velocity. Berkeley counters measured swing velocity in the last foot of travel before snubbing. See Figure 15–9.

All three devices described above provided for direct trailing line connections for recording electronic sensors such as strain gauges, accelerometers and electrocardiogram. High speed motion pictures of head on, profile and overhead views of the subject during impact made possible motion studies. Clinical and laboratory procedures before and after recorded physiological changes in the subject.

Tables 15–IV and 15–V present data from human impact deceleration exposures in the forward and backward facing positions respectively, obtained from the Daisy Track Sled. Restraints on the subjects included seat belt and two shoulder straps in the forward facing position, seat belt only in the backward facing position. A typical range of velocity variation impact pulses are shown in Figure 15–9. With the sled propelled by two M 3 ejection seat catapults, thirteen exposures were accomplished in the range of 1,072 to 2,136 g per second onset, 23.8 to 40.4 peak g, at durations of .040 to .052 seconds. Two subjects experienced dyspnea for about 4 minutes immediately after impact.

Another subject, run 335, sustained 40.4 peak g at 2,136 g per second. The rise time of this rate of onset is .0832 seconds, equivalent to that for 12.02 cps of vibration. The accelerometer mounted on the subject's chest indicated 82.6 peak g at 3,826 g per second onset. The rise time of this rate of onset is .0864 seconds, which is equivalent to 11.6 cps. This would represent the period for rib cage deformation excited by the impact, with a $82.6/40.4 = 2.058$ amplification ratio. The effect on the subject was of a definite limit of tolerance reached with evidence of mild, recuperable injury. Immediately after impact the subject experienced severe back pain, extending from second lumbar to the coccyx, sweating, dizziness, vertigo, and loss of consciousness, with no blood pressure reading. Supine with legs elevated on a litter, five minutes post impact blood pressure registered 70 systolic over 40 diastolic, 100/70 ten minutes post impact, and 110/80 twenty minutes later. Pulse became steady at 70 per minute. The subject required 3 days hospitalization, with legs in traction the first day.

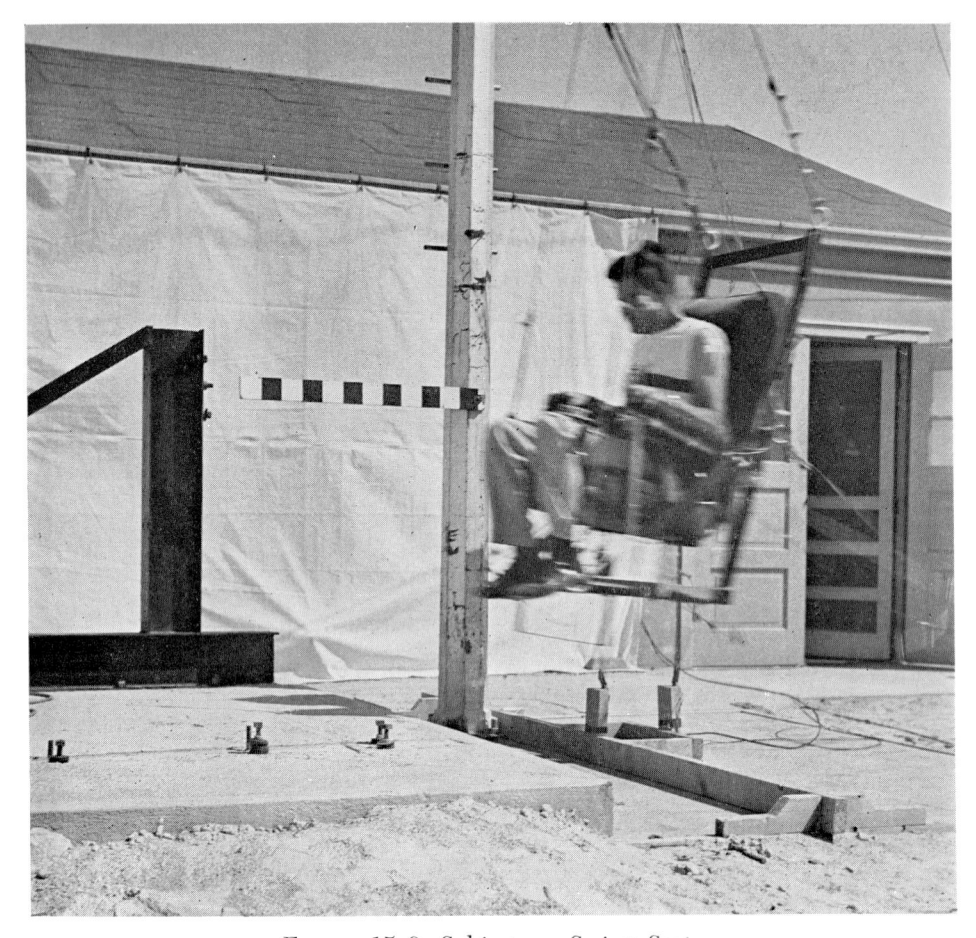

FIGURE 15-9. Subject on Swing Seat.

Stomach pains occurred during the first six meals after the run. A 150 pound black bear was exposed to 39 g at 1,779 g per second onset in the same body orientation. The chest accelerometer indicated 73.1 g and the rate of onset was 1,779 g per second. The rise time for the sled rate of onset is .0216 seconds, equivalent to 11.42 cps; that for the subject's chest is .0242 seconds, equivalent to 10.34 cps. The amplification of impact, $73.1/39.0 = 1.876$ for impact transmission through the bear's rib cage. The bear was anesthetized, indicating relaxation that would lower resonant frequency. The man had no such advantage. The bear was euthanized and autopsied. Congestion, hemorrhage and edema of the stomach were found, indicating corresponding difficulties in the human subject. An area of hemorrhage was observed at the third lumbar level lateral to the vertebral column, an area of back pain complaint in human subjects.

Fifteen human subjects were exposed to forward facing deceleration on

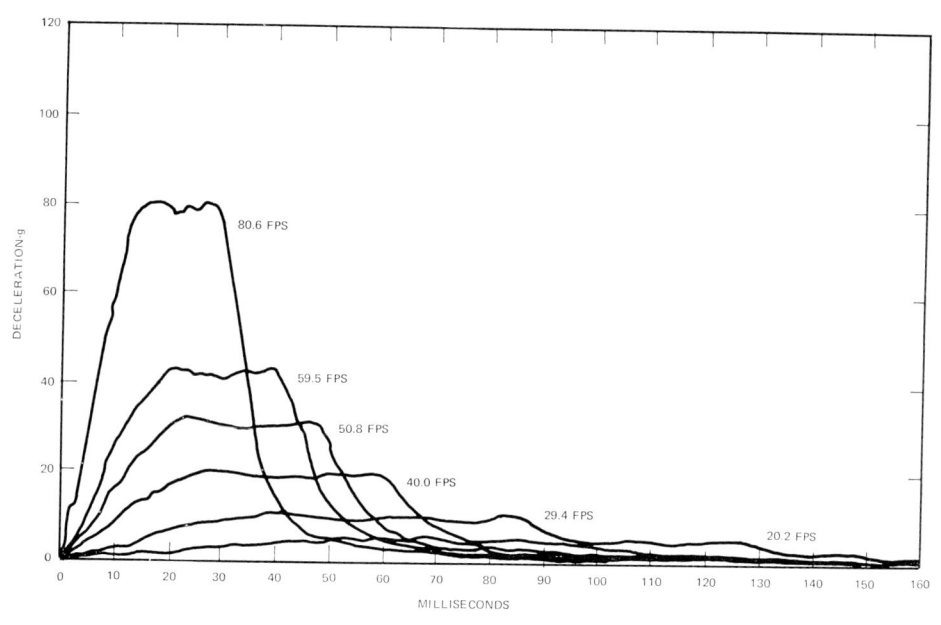

FIGURE 15–10. Overlay of velocity variation tests.

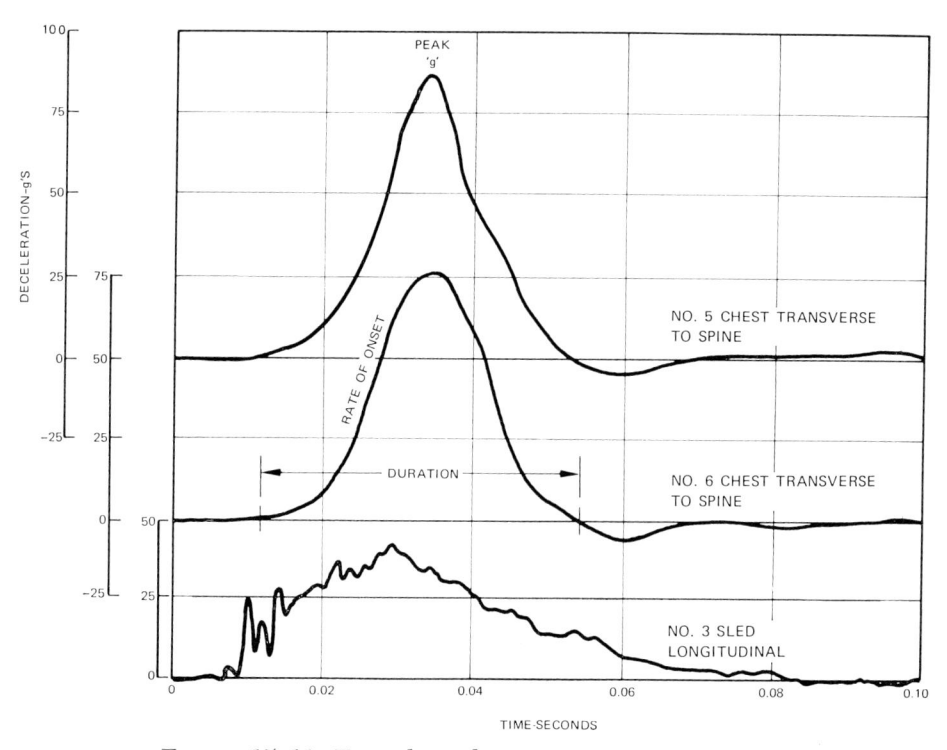

FIGURE 15–11. Typical accelerometer tracing (run 335).

TABLE 15-IV
BACKWARD FACING DECELERATION TEST RESULTS*

Run No.	Date	Subject	Sled g	Sled Onset g/sec	Forcing Function Vector Coefficients gx	gy	gz	Vector Sum. X,Y,Z g	Along Subject's X-Axis g	Duration (sec.)	Onset g/sec.
300	31 Mar	JA	25.5	1072	+.985	0	−.174	—	37.8	0.044	1740
318	31 Mar	ELB	25.5	1237	+.985	0	−.174	—	45.7	0.040	2427
319	31 Mar	JDM	25.4	1547	+.985	0	−.174	—	37.3	0.044	1724
320	10 Apr	RAG	23.8	1120	+.985	0	−.174	—	44.3	0.051	1888
321	10 Apr	KLL	25.8	1363	+.985	0	−.174	—	58.5	0.044	2324
322	10 Apr	DRC	26.9	1852	+.985	0	−.174	—	41.1	0.052	2102
329	7 May	DLE	31.1	1187	+.985	0	−.174	—	49.9	0.048	1653
330	7 May	AM	31.5	1224	+.985	0	−.174	—	52.4	0.042	1953
331	7 May	AWY	30.1	1224	+.985	0	−.174	—	39.3	0.052	1602
332	9 May	AVZ	37.5	1517	+.985	0	−.174	—	52.6	0.044	2156
333	9 May	JHW	35.4	1351	+.985	0	−.174	—	67.0	0.042	2594
334	9 May	LAG	34.3	1336	+.985	0	−.174	—	45.8	0.048	1637
335	16 May	ELB	40.4	2136	+.985	0	−.174	—	82.6	0.090	3826
337	19 May	BEAR	39.0	1779	+.985	0	−.174	—	73.1	0.044	3021

* Orientation fixed at 180° yaw, 0° roll, 10° pitch.
† Measured with chest mounted accelerometer package which was partially displaced during impact causing misalignment from subject axes.

TABLE 15-V
FORWARD FACING DECELERATION TEST RESULTS*

Run No.	Date	Subject	Sled g	Sled Onset g/sec	g_X	g_Y	g_Z	Vector Sum X,Y,Z g	Along Subject's X-Axis g	Duration (sec.)	Onset g/sec
661	18 Feb	ELB	34.0	743	−.985	0	+.174	38.4	32.0	0.071	959
662	19 Feb	JDM	28.2	768	−.985	0	+.174	32.2	30.5	0.070	768
663	19 Feb	RED	27.4	874	−.985	0	+.174	34.8	32.7	0.084	652
664	19 Feb	JAK	27.4	875	−.985	0	+.174	33.4	32.0	0.072	868
665	19 Feb	SFC	26.0	775	−.985	0	+.174	31.1	29.8	0.068	725
666	23 Feb	JF	28.7	859	−.985	0	+.174	34.1	32.3	0.076	966
667	23 Feb	RGH	30.4	942	−.985	0	+.174	36.0	32.3	0.066	974
668	24 Feb	HHB	30.5	813	−.985	0	+.174	35.3	32.9	0.080	521
669	24 Feb	RAG	29.8	776	−.985	0	+.174	30.3	29.5	0.076	654
670	24 Feb	KSF	18.0	480	−.985	0	+.174	19.6	14.9	0.086	278
671	24 Feb	GID	28.7	878	−.985	0	+.174	38.0	44.5	0.072	785
674	26 Feb	MCS	33.7	1036	−.985	0	+.174	31.4	35.2	0.066	849
675	26 Feb	TBK	34.4	1041	−.985	0	+.174	39.3	38.9	0.665	930
676	26 Feb	KMH	29.0	1073	−.985	0	+.174	32.9	29.9	0.065	808
677	26 Feb	PDJ	30.2	1111	−.985	0	+.174	36.3	33.4	0.065	110

* Orientation fixed at 0° yaw, 0° roll, 10° pitch.
† See same note for TABLE 15-IV.

the Daisy Track. The exposures ranged from 18.0 to 34.4 peak g at 480 to 1,111 g per second onset, .065 to .086 durations. Accelerometer measurements recorded on the subject's chest ranged from 14.9 to 38.9 peak g, at 278 to 1,100 g per second rate of onset. Restraints consisted of lap belt and two shoulder straps, with the inverted-V leg straps from belt buckle, fairing around the insides of the thighs to the rear corners of the seat. Two subjects (runs 662 and 664) submarined beneath the lap belts sufficiently to bruise the coccyx with tenderness persisting for three weeks.

The subject in run 661 experienced partial loss of vision in the left eye for 3 minutes post run; ophthalmoscopic examination was negative. The subject almost fainted right after impact. In run 675, the subject sustained 38.9 peak g measured on the chest at 930 g per second, with 34.4 peak g and 1,081 g per second measured on the sled. The impact pulse rise time for the subject was .0416 seconds, equivalent to 5.98 cps, and for the sled, .0318, equivalent to 7.86 cps. The amplification would be 38.9/34.4 = 1.13. The effect on the subject was the most severe of any in this series. One minute after impact the blood pressure dropped to 80 mm systolic and undetermined diastolic pressure. The EKG revealed a nodal rhythm post-impact, which became normal by 20 minutes later when it was taken again. X-rays revealed compression fractures of the body of the fifth thoracic, fracture lines in the sixth thoracic, and a linear fracture of the anterior superior border of the fifth lumbar. The effect of resonant response excited at 5.98 cps, within the sensitive range for whole body response, cannot be ruled out.

Table 15-VI presents twenty-five experiments in which subjects were decelerated in the forward facing seated position, restrained by lap belt only. Included are sixteen exposures on the Swing Seat, four on the Bopper and five on the Daisy Track. Other than localized strap contusions and abrasions of minor significance, there were no serious adverse effects in this series, although run 7 on the Bopper resulted in back muscle strain and transient abdominal pain of sufficient severity to attain the voluntary tolerance limit for that subject. In this instance, the peak g measured on the belt buckle attained 26.0 at 850 g per second onset, for a calculated force in pounds of 4,290 on the belt, or 89.5 pounds per square inch average over the presenting area of the belt. Subject # 126 on the Daisy Track sustained a localized right upper quadrant pain following impact which might have been related to incipient gall bladder troubles, at rate of onset of 500 g per second and 13.6 peak g. This subject was slightly obese and of sedentary habits. From these 25 experiments, there are indications that rates of onset between 280 and 1,600 g per second and 11.4 to 32.0 peak g can be sustained against a lap belt restraint up to approximately 90 pounds per square inch average load, with no significant injuries resulting.

TABLE 15-VI

HUMAN SUBJECTS DECELERATED SEATED FORWARD FACING LAP BELT ONLY
25 EXPERIMENTS

Run No.	Name	Drop Ht. Ft.	Velocity at Snub Ft/Sec	Seat Onset G/Sec	Seat Peak G	Chest Onset G/Sec	Chest Peak G	Abdomen Onset G/Sec	Abdomen Peak G	Knee Onset G/Sec	Knee Peak G	Strain Gauge Lbs.	Subj. Wt. Lbs.	Force F=MA Lbs.	Peak Duration Sec.	Belt Load P.S.I.	Observed Effects
Swing Seat																	
1	STL	3.0	15.4	1,200	24	170	12	-	-	300	12	600	165	-	.002	-	No adverse effects
2	DEP	3.0	15.6	1,800	24	250	15	370	15	250	15	500	160	2,400	.002	50.0	No adverse effects
3	AM	3.5	15.4	1,500	30	160	13	570	23	320	19	800	156	3,588	.001	74.7	No adverse effects
4	BT	3.5	15.4	1,450	29	200	12	400	17	310	19	700	140	2,380	.002	52.8	No adverse effects
5	AWY	3.5	15.4	1,600	32	250	18	500	22	300	19	600	160	3,520	.001	78.2	No adverse effects
6	HHK	3.5	15.4	1,203	24	250	18	420	17	220	13	800	187	3,179	.002	58.8	Hip contusions
7	GJAS	3.5	15.4	800	24	350	23	420	18	220	15	600	170	3,060	.001	56.6	Hip contusions
8	JJ	3.5	15.4	1,200	23	350	17	450	18	200	12	500	138	2,384	.002	61.0	No adverse effects
9	ED	3.66	-	600	27	200	18	300	19	250	20	800	178	3,382	.002	-	No adverse effects
10	JPS	4.0	-	700	28	200	20	360	22	200	19	900	165	3,382	.001	50.5	No adverse effects
14	JIM	4.5	19.6	450	27	250	17	300	15	250	17	1,100	150	2,250	.003	46.0	No adverse effects
15	BT	4.33	19.6	600	20	300	16	500	11	400	22	1,100	138	1,518	.002	31.0	No adverse effects
16	AM	4.16	19.6	1,300	26	300	17	600	13	600	20	1,100	152	1,976	.001	41.0	Lower rib margin tender 4 days
17	ELB	4.5	19.6	350	17	170	14	300	14	250	18	1,400	128	1,792	.001	42.6	Lower rib margin tender 4 weeks
18	AWY	4.0	16.8	600	25	250	17	-	4	-	4	1,800	162	-	.002	-	No adverse effects
19	JJ	4.5	19.6	500	26	350	22	-	-	250	16	1,500	136	-	.002	-	No adverse effects
Bopper		Stop Inches															
2	JR	6.3	19.0	524	18.9	320	25.0	478	15.0	-	-	-	163	2,445	.01	54.3	Transient abdominal pain
3	JJ	6.9	19.5	540	16.0	250	17.0	550	19.0	-	-	-	136	2,584	.004	66.2	Transient abdominal pain
4	AY	6.9	19.0	576	17.0	240	18.0	450	16.0	-	-	-	162	2,592	.002	57.6	Transient abdominal pain
7	STL	5.5	19.0	740	20.0	260	26.0	850	26.0	-	-	-	165	4,290	.002	89.5	Back muscle strain 48 hrs - transient abdominal pain
Daisy		Stop Inches															
120	DFP	18.9	24.0	280	12.4	300	14.3	370	10.8	327	12.5	1,421	159	1,717	.002	36.0	Chest pain
121	AM	19.6	28.7	300	11.4	250	8.5	300	11.2	270	11.2	1,143	155	1,736	.002	36.5	Persistent chest pain, hip contusions
122	BT	18.6	28.0	453	12.8	350	14.0	515	11.8	400	13.2	1,576	145	1,711	.002	38.0	Hip contusions
125	ELB	14.3	29.0	544	18.7	450	19.3	500	17.0	450	28.0	2,130	130	2,210	.002	52.6	Pain at lap belt area
126	HHK	14.1	25.0	500	14.8	328	13.0	500	13.6	886	23.0	2,468	185	2,516	.002	46.5	Severe upper abdominal pain. 3 days in hospital

Table 15–V presents one experiment in each of twenty-six orientations on the Omnidirectional Sled on the Daisy Track in pitch and yaw, selected from a total of 290 runs with seventy-eight different subjects. The entire series has been reported by Stapp,[78] Brown et al.[14] and in an anthropometric study of the subjects by Godby et al.[32] Pertinent measurements on the largest and smallest of these subjects will give an indication of their size range:

Name	LARGEST GAR	SMALLEST SMcD
Age, Years	26	22
Weight, Pounds	202	125
Height, Inches	72.5	66.0
Sitting Height, Inches	37.1	33.85
Sitting, Midshoulder Height, Inches	25.6	23.3
Height Above Hip Hinge Point, Inches	34.0	30.5
Height Below Hip Hinge Point, Inches	38.5	35.8
Calculated ¼ of Body Area, Sq. In.	808.0	620.0
Calculated Body Weight ¼ of Body Area, PSI	.25	.20

Test numbers to date for the subject:

LARGEST GAR	SMALLEST SMcD
1322	1226
1405	1342
1436	1466
1548	1536
1567	1598
1611	1757
1770	
1805	
1835	

Side panels on the seat contained the legs, thighs, shoulders and extended on each side of the head rest. A 4.5 pound helmet was worn, secured to a neck ring to simulate the Apollo pressure suit. The restraint system consisted of shoulder straps, arm pit straps, flank straps rising from the seat belt anchorages, all converging on a common chest buckle, and a lap belt with inverted-V and upper leg straps, all of 3 inch dacron webbing of 8,000 pound tensile strength.

Negative or inconclusive laboratory and clinical findings were found in most of the large variety of measurements made before, during and after exposure, with the exception of electrocardiograph records, in which fifty-five subjects showed significant slowing of heart rate immediately subsequent to impact exposure, usually within 15 seconds after impact of more than 15 g. Those body positions favoring a headward vector component of impact and consequent hydrostatic pressure pulse in the carotid arteries correlated its lower thresholds and larger values of decrease in heart rate. Only changes of more than 10 beats per minute were counted as significant. Positions with a footward vector which caused a drop in carotid hydrostatic pressure showed no significant decrease in heart rate at 50 per cent higher peak g than the observed threshold. Maximum decrease in heart rate post-impact occurred in the backward facing semi-supine seated position.

There were no complaints of significant pain, breathing difficulty, faintness or delay in recuperation beyond 12 hours for positions 7, 11, 13, 14 and 15. Positions 7, 11, and 15 are in five degree pitch, essentially upright, and at 40 degree yaw to right or left; position 13 is backward facing, bowing 45 degree from vertical, with vectors compressing the subject against the back and bottom of the seat.

Duration and magnitude of impact deceleration also were significant and relative to subjective complaints. Even at 2,000 g per second, the

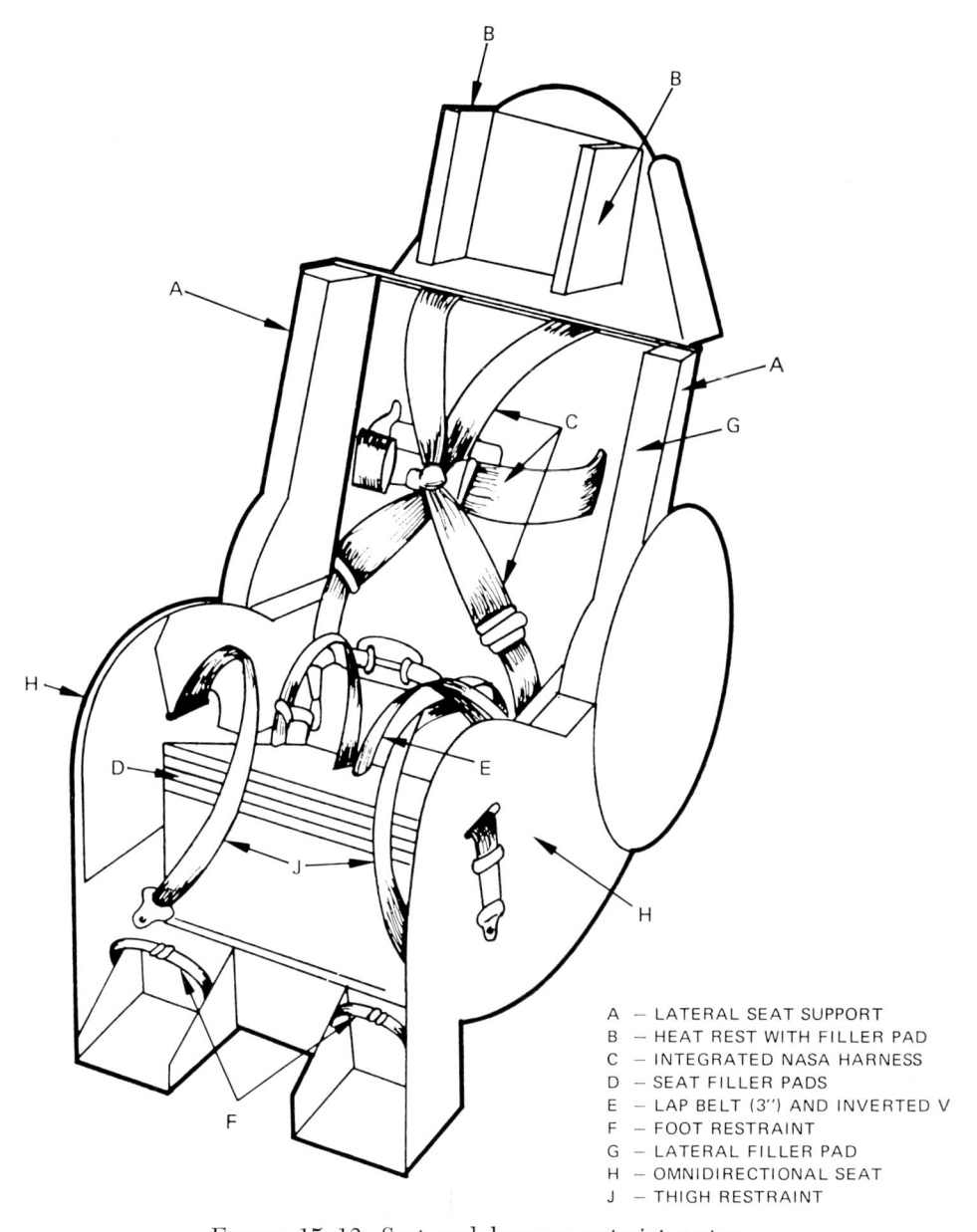

FIGURE 15-12. Seat and harness restraint system.

A — LATERAL SEAT SUPPORT
B — HEAT REST WITH FILLER PAD
C — INTEGRATED NASA HARNESS
D — SEAT FILLER PADS
E — LAP BELT (3") AND INVERTED V
F — FOOT RESTRAINT
G — LATERAL FILLER PAD
H — OMNIDIRECTIONAL SEAT
J — THIGH RESTRAINT

longer duration decelerations in 34 inches of water brake at entry velocities of 45 feet per second, the higher impacts in positions 9 through 16 were more tolerable than 22 feet per second entrance velocities decelerating in 17 inches of water brake. There were seventeen subjective complaints in the lower duration group, exposed to 75 to 100 millisecond duration im-

338   *Impact Injury and Crash Protection*

**DECELERATION FORCE VECTOR ORIENTATION
FOR APOLLO IMPACT TESTS**

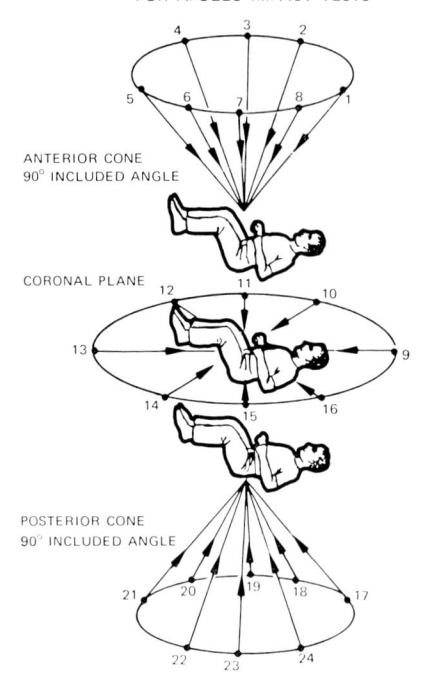

ANTERIOR CONE
90° INCLUDED ANGLE

CORONAL PLANE

POSTERIOR CONE
90° INCLUDED ANGLE

| SEAT POSITIONS ||||||||
| POSITION NUMBER | YAW | ROLL | PITCH | \multicolumn{3}{c}{DIRECTION COSINES} |||
				G_X	G_Y	G_Z
1	0	0	315	−0.707	0	−0.707
2	030	0	335	−0.785	−0.453	−0.423
3	040	0	005	−0.763	−0.640	+0.087
4	030	0	035	−0.772	−0.450	+0.571
5	0	0	045	−0.707	0	+0.707
6	330	0	035	+0.450	+0.571
7	320	0	005	−0.763	+0.453	+0.087
8	330	0	335	−0.785	+0.453	−0.423
9	180	0	085	+0.087	0	−0.996
10	140	0	085	+0.067	−0.643	−0.763
11	090	0	085	0	−1.000	0
12	040	0	085	−0.067	−0.643	+0.763
13	0	0	085	−0.087	0	+0.996
14	320	0	085	−0.067	+0.643	+0.763
15	270	0	085	0	+1.000	0
16	220	0	085	+0.067	+0.643	−0.763
17	780	0	045	+0.707	0	−0.707
18	150	0	035	+0.772	−0.450	−0.571
19	140	0	005	+0.763	−0.453	−0.087
20	150	0	335	+0.785	−0.453	+0.423
21	180	0	315	+0.707	0	+0.707
22	240	0	335	+0.785	+0.453	+0.423
23	220	0	005	+0.763	+0.640	−0.087
24	210	0	035	+0.772	+0.450	−0.571

FIGURE 15–13. Omni-directional seat force vectors, seat position angle, and direction cosine functions for g_X, g_Y, and g_Z determination.

TABLE 15-VII

HUMAN DECELERATION IN 26 BODY ORIENTATIONS

Run No.	Name	Orientation Pitch°	Yaw°	Sled Deceleration Velocity Ft/Sec	Stop In.	Duration Sec	Onset G/Sec	Peak G	Seat Vector Onset G/Sec	Sum G	Subject Vector Onset G/Sec	Sum G	Wt. Lbs.	Force F=MA Lbs.	Heart Rate/Min Base	Run	Post Impact Pre-Change	Observed Effects
1561	JPW	1	315	0	31.1	10.0	.120	980	24.6	540	24.6	580	31.5	175	4821.6	80	102	−36	P+; R 14 days
1578	JNP	8	335	330	29.7	10.0	.114	1,360	21.0	3,580	24.9	2,750	29.7	142	3129.0	80	126	+2	P+; R 5 min
1557	GOS	7	5	320	32.0	12.2	.101	1,030	25.6	1,920	26.6	1,190	35.5	167	4321.4	60	145	−18	P2+; R 24 hrs
1564	MDH	6	35	330	31.5	10.0	.092	1,020	25.0	1,330	25.1	1,350	41.5	168	4850.0	88	122	−26	P3+; R 3 min
1559	JCT	5	45	0	31.4	11.0	.120	960	25.0	720	27.4	500	37.5	165	4475.0	85	126	−68	P3+;B3+;F3+; R 60 days
1567	GAR	4	35	30	31.4	10.0	.112	1,000	24.5	1,520	27.0	1,380	39.5	202	5218.5	68	102	−14	P+, R 72 hrs
1555	TKC	3	5	40	31.3	10.0	.106	1,030	23.5	1,330	25.6	1,070	41.7	154	3760.0	90	150	−15	P+; R 36 hrs
1581	WCC	2	335	30	31.3	9.2	.130	1,600	24.7	3,070	24.6	2,000	33.9	170	4915.3	73	112	−32	P+; R 12 hrs
1646	FTC	17	45	180	45.8	26.4	.180	2,110	32.5	3,380	30.9	1,230	35.7	170	4140.0	105	150	−48	P+; B+; R 5 min
1639	BDN	24	35	210	45.5	26.4	.140	2,120	23.5	3,400	28.6	1,050	30.2	140	3478.0	82	145	−63	P+; B2+; R 3 hrs
1619	SBB	23	5	220	45.3	27.5	.150	1,450	19.3	1,833	24.3	1,470	31.3	125	2451.1	75	130	0	No adverse effects
1635	JDT	22	335	210	45.8	26.4	.197	1,860	21.9	3,220	25.8	2,130	49.2	175	3832.0	120	180	−13	P+; R 3 hrs
1644	GW	21	315	180	44.3	27.5	.190	1,970	20.0	3,000	26.7	1,500	35.7	172	3740.0	105	150	−48	No adverse effects
1627	GTB	20	335	150	45.6	25.3	.170	1,530	21.7	1,400	25.8	1,300	36.2	185	4079.6	118	150	0	P+; R 1 min
1436	GAR	19	5	140	43.9	24.4	.140	1,040	21.0	710	23.0	1,350	35.2	165	3570.0	120	135	0	No adverse effects
1638	FRS	18	35	150	45.9	25.3	.190	2,130	22.3	3,500	28.6	1,430	40.7	188	4370.8	110	150	−40	No adverse effects
1386	TTP	9	85	180	19.2	25.3	.170	360	11.8	450	17.6	400	22.4	160	1886.0	80	92	−23	No adverse effects
1805	GAR	16	85	220	34.6	25.3	.160	1,410	15.0	1,630	17.7	710	24.1	202	3060.0	86	120	−60	No adverse effects
1352	JNP	15	85	270	20.2	25.3	.150	800	17.4	710	18.2	840	26.8	142	2470.0	0	0	0	No adverse effects
1806	TWM	14	85	320	45.8	26.4	.197	1,420	14.7	1,810	17.7	900	27.5	158	2842.0	100	113	+14	No adverse effects
1388	JPW	13	85	0	16.2	25.3	.175	220	9.4	310	13.0	260	14.4	175	1860.0	80	83	+1	No adverse effects
1804	JPW	12	85	40	35.0	25.3	.162	1,400	14.6	2,000	18.6	710	20.8	175	2552.0	86	100	+20	No adverse effects
1355	EWS	11	85	90	16.8	25.3	.155	520	13.5	520	14.2	900	25.9	205	2770.0	0	0	0	No adverse effects
1793	JLP	10	85	140	33.0	25.3	.120	1,250	15.5	1,420	17.6	1,050	31.5	166	2570.0	80	96	−38	No adverse effects
1364	GTB	25	5	180	42.2	25.3	.140	780	14.5	1,130	19.0	660	18.7	185	2682.0	0	0	0	No adverse effects
1169	GTB	26	35	270	24.4	25.3	.158	525	15.4	350	16.9	550	24.0	185	2850.0	102	124	−36	No adverse effects

Subjective Reactions: Pain = P
Breathing Difficulty = B
Faintness = F
Recuperation = R and time to recuperate
Mild = +
Moderate = 2+
Severe = 3+

TABLE 15-VIIA
SIGNIFICANT POST-IMPACT PHYSICAL EXAM FINDINGS

Significant Physical Findings	Test Position	Test Numbers	Sled g
Harness burns	2	1537	20.0
(All First Degree)	7	1552	23.0
Dazed and disoriented	17	1163	17.4
(Lasting no longer than 2 min. post-impact)		1187	18.9
		1204	21.7
		1205	25.8
		1456	19.6
	19	1295	30.0
	24	1303	28.1
		1182	24.6
		1403	16.5
	9	1387	9.8
	1	1517	17.2
	21	1610	10.0
Respiratory difficulty	17	1187	18.9
	23	1191	19.5
	18	1215	24.6
		1216	23.2
	24	1217	23.7
		1403	16.5
Blood pressure difference (20 mm at pre- and post-run physical exam)	19	1295	30.0
Pulse difference (20 beats/min. at pre- and post-run physical exam)	23	1192	19.4
	17	1456	19.6
	24	1441	20.2
	12	1819	19.5
Engorged retinal vessels	17	1204	21.7
	3	1487	9.2
Back and/or neck pain and decreased range of motion	17	1205	25.8
	1	1517	17.2
	5	1559	25.1
		1591	21.0

pact pulses, compared with five complaints among those exposed to 145 millisecond pulses at higher entry velocities.

In experiment 1559, with the subject facing forward and reclining 45 degree in pitch, a slack harness contributed to excessive rebound from extreme forward flexion during exposure to equal downward and forward vectors. The subject was in shock from the pain of localized compression at about the sixth through eighth thoracic levels. There was tenderness and limitation of motion for about 60 days following the exposure, although all x-rays were negative for fractures. Deceleration of the sled in this run was from 32.5 feet per second in 17 inches, attaining 25.14 g measured on the sled frame in line of motion.

Two categories of most frequent types of complaints relate to two general orientations of the seated anatomy. With the body facing the direction of motion or within 40 degrees of yaw to either side, and the trunk reclining up to 45 degrees, vectors simultaneously compressing and

TABLE 15-VIII
SIGNIFICANT POST-IMPACT PHYSICAL EXAM FINDINGS

Significant Physical Findings	Test Position	Test Numbers	Sled g
Harness burns	2	1537	20.0
(All first degree)	7	1552	23.0
Dazed and disoriented (lasting no longer than 2 min. post-impact)	17	1163	17.4
		1187	18.9
		1204	21.7
		1205	25.8
		1456	19.6
	19	1295	30.0
	24	1303	28.1
		1182	24.6
		1403	16.5
	9	1387	9.8
	1	1517	17.2
	21	1610	10.0
Respiratory difficulty	17	1187	18.9
	23	1191	19.5
	18	1215	24.6
		1216	23.2
	24	1217	23.7
		1403	16.5
Blood pressure difference (20 mm hg at pre- and post-run physical exam)	19	1295	30.0
Pulse difference (20 beats/min at pre- and post-run physical exam)	23	1192	19.4
	17	1456	19.6
	24	1441	20.2
	12	1819	19.5
Engorged retinal vessels	17	1204	21.7
	3	1487	9.2
Back and/or neck pain and decreased range of motion	17	1205	25.8
	1	1517	17.2
	5	1559	25.1
		1591	21.0

flexing the head, neck and vertebral column resulted in complaints of muscle spasm or strain in the neck, back and lower extremities. These effects were, no doubt, accentuated by the weight of the 4.5 pound helmet. With the body facing away from the line of motion or within 40 degrees to either side of rear facing, with the trunk reclining up to 45 degrees, upward and chest-to-back vectors resulted in unpleasant sensations of abdominal viscera plunging against the diaphragm and compressing the chest contents, with transient chest pains, difficult and painful breathing, and pains in abdominal viscera. Position 24 and 18 produced the most numerous complaints of breathing difficulties, positions 17 and 24 were associated with repeated observations of disorientation and stunning after impact.

In general, it would appear that low pain thresholds and injury vulnerability are associated with simultaneous flexion and compression of head, neck, and vertebral column, related to body positions generating forward

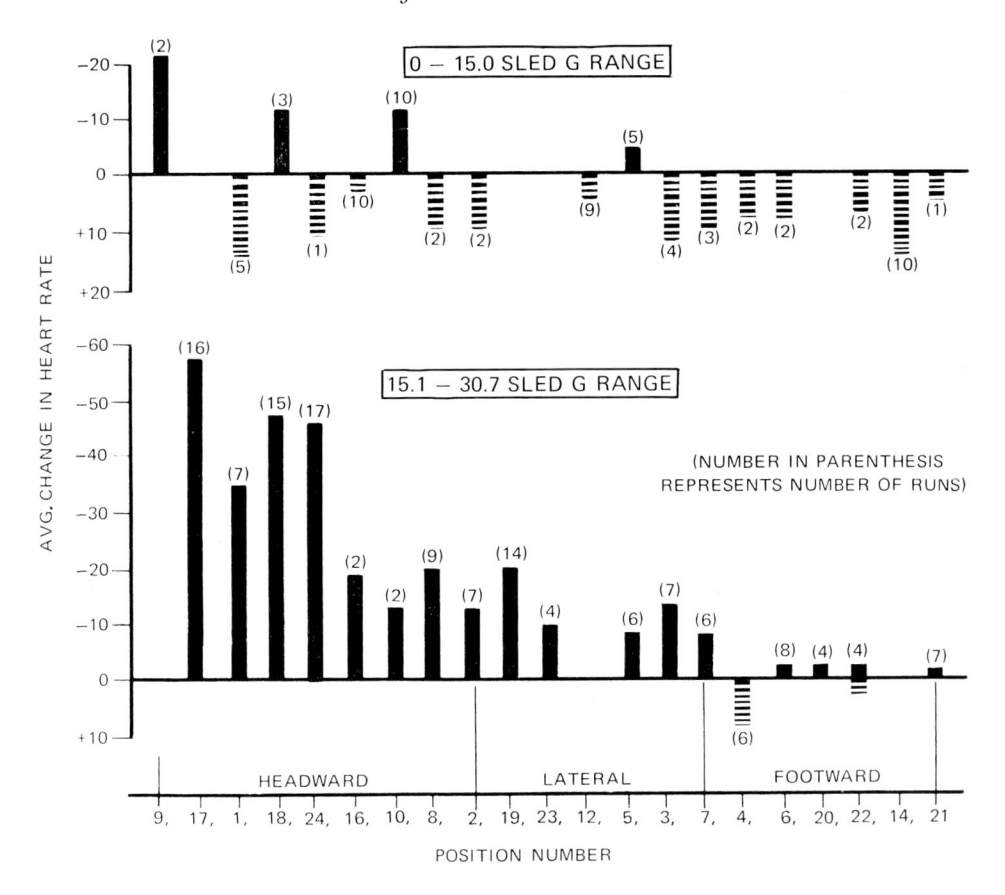

FIGURE 15–14. The average change in heart rate is plotted against subject impact position at two ranges of impact force. Subject position numbers are arranged from left to right in descending order of $-g_z$ vector component.

and downward vectors acting simultaneously, and with headward displacement of abdominal and thoracic viscera, resulting from body positions having upward and chest-to back vectors. The reflex slowing of the heart by stimulation of the carotid sinus due to hydrostatic distention of the carotid arteries has no pathological significance in the range of decelerations reported in this series.

Tables 15–II, 15–III, 15–IV and 15–V present a total of 147 human experiments selected from 428 reported on in this paper out of several series performed at Edwards, California and Holloman Air Force Base, New Mexico. Personal communications from Armstrong[2,3] indicate that an additional seventy-five human experiments have been accomplished to compare seat belt restraint effectiveness with that of seat belt and diagonal upper torso restraint. These unpublished results will be reported on in the near future. Other research on human exposures to impact acceleration include those of Cooper and Holmstrom,[21] Evans et al.,[25,26,27,28] Gurdjian et al.,[33,34] Hirsch,[36] Hodgson et al.,[37] Holcomb,[38] Hueey et al.,[40] Patrick,[52] Ryan,[55] Shaw,[60,61,62] (60,61,62), Swearingen et al.,[80,81,82,83,84] and Weis et al.[86,87,88] These include whole body tolerance to stresses not directly applicable to the automotive crash situation and studies on particular parts of the anatomy.

It is evident from these results of seated human exposures to impact deceleration in twenty-six body orientations, that adequate webbing restraints and head rests can assure survival and minimize injury for healthy males between 19 and 48 years of age, through the range of automotive crash experience outlined in Table 15–I. It is apparent from reports of Snyder[66,68] on injuries produced by seat belts in vehicle crashes, that webbing restraints are subject to the vicissitudes of human error in their use, and that they can be less than adequate for the protection of the pregnant. Clark et al.[17,18] has proposed pneumatic air bag restraints in place of webbing. In preliminary tests with pregnant baboons, Snyder found evidence of effectiveness of air bag restraints, but difficulties have been encountered in adapting them to the automobile.

To supplement webbing restraints, Ryan[54,55,56] has tested hydraulic energy absorbing bumpers to attenuate and prolong onset and peak deceleration of the vehicle, thus reducing abruptness and magnitude of forces reaching the occupant through body restraints.

Another approach to the problem is suggested by Lombard et al.[46,47] who finds that it is better to restrain or support the semifluid mass of the torso in a manner which prevents distortion rather than to hold the body by the skeleton. In experiments with 128 one-pound guinea pigs and ten monkeys weighing 10 pounds each, he found that injury from impact deceleration is minimized by decreasing distortion of internal organs and tissues, with an approach to isovolumetric containment of the torso which prevents large volume shifts, bending and bulging around restraints. In all positions except footward, survival limits were markedly increased by a relatively simple isovolumetric containment of the torso as opposed to the harness system of restraining the torso by holding the pelvic and pectoral girdles. This was done with broad webbing or fabric and fixation of head and neck as well as with a padded cocoon restraint. For these small animals, threshold of survival was reached in the best orientation and containment, with velocity change of 40 feet per second in excess of 400 g at onset of over 200,000 g per second. Prevention of distortion of the torso during impact, particularly in sidewise deceleration, increased survival limit by fourfold. Sonntag[70] has followed up on this finding in a report presented at the Aerospace Medical Convention of May 6–9, 1968, in Miami, Florida. He and Dr. Sidney Leverett of the School of Aerospace Medicine exposed two chimpanzees to impact deceleration on the Daisy Track in the forward facing seated position, sandwiched between 4 inch layers of ensolite in one case, and styrofoam in the other, against an eighth of an inch thick aluminum shield in front, and ⅜ of an inch plywood panel behind, strapped tightly together. The aluminum shield was strongly anchored to the front of the seat, extending from above the head to the tops of the thighs, with room for the legs in front. At head height was an opening for the face, from eyebrows to chin, padded with ensolite at forehead and chin. Restrained by this essentially insovolumetric containment, each of the subjects was decelerated from almost 90 mph to a stop in 28 inches with no concussion, evidenced by eye corneal and ear pinnal reflexes still present after impact, despite light nembutal anesthesia; and no fractures, no evidence of internal organ injuries or other damage. Both animals survived, one was autopsied five experiments later, the other survived in good condition. Results were as follows:

TABLE 15-IX

Run no.	Chimpanzee weight lbs.	Sled Velocity ft./sec.	mph	Stopping Distance in.	Accelerometer Location, in Line of Motion	Onset g/sec.	Peak g	Duration sec.
3849	55	131.5	89.8	28	Sled #1	12,743	147.45	.0157
					Sled #2	13,005	147.57	.0162
					Subject's Head	19,955	238.79	.0212
3850	50	130.0	88.8	28	Sled #1	11,881	149.62	.0152
					Sled #2	12,549	149.04	.0155

The aluminum shield buckled 3 inches in the middle, there were bending failures in the extensive angle steel supports, and in the case of the styrofoam, the material was crushed and cracked considerably.

Considering the report of Kiel[41] including the case of a paratrooper falling from 1,200 feet and landing in 3½ feet of snow on his back at free fall velocity of 120 mph, sustaining 140.5 peak g estimated with no significant injury, and similar high falls into snow described by Snyder,[67] in which the material against which deceleration took place behaved in the manner of an isovolumetric containment during impact, as well as the reports of De Haven[22] on falls into soft earth, the extrapolation of Lombard and of Sonntag and Leverett's findings to human tolerance, while isovolumetrically contained, might well fulfill De Haven's 1942 prediction that "structural provisions to reduce impact and distribute pressure can enhance survival and modify injury within survival limits of 200 g in aircraft and automobile accidents."

SUMMARY

The vertebral column is a flexible mast on which are suspended all the structures of the human body. Injuries result from exposure to impact deceleration which bends or compresses the mast, or flails structures attached thereto, or distorts vulnerable body areas by localized compression, tension or shear, or imparts hydraulic pressure displacement to body fluids, beyond strain limits, and particularly at rates of application that excite resonant response. The method of restraint against impact deceleration determines largely the parameters of exposure that can be sustained in any given body orientation.

1. Healthy, adult male volunteer subjects exposed to impact deceleration in the seated forward facing position can withstand velocity changes corresponding to automobile crash up to 30 peak g at rates of onset below 1,500 g per second while restrained by a 3 inch dacron or nylon seat belt bearing against the pelvic girdle, with minor, reversible injurious effects.

2. Impact decelerations exceeding 1,000 g per second at higher than 25 g become progressively more difficult to withstand, even in the backward facing position, or with pelvic and shoulder girdle restraints, eliciting transient musculoskeletal or visceral pain, visual and cardiac changes and breathing difficulties, depending on body orientation and resultant force vectors.

3. At more than 1,300 g per second and more than 38 g in the forward facing seated position, immediate effects of impact deceleration are more severe than at less than 500 g per second and 45 g peak.

4. At 2,000 g per second and 40 g peak in the backward facing seated position, a distinct limit to voluntary human tolerance with transient but severe subjective and physiological effects is encountered.

5. With optimum restraint applied to the pelvic and pectoral girdles by webbing belts and straps, the entire range of vehicular crash forces described in Table 15–I can be survived with minimal reversible injurious effects.

6. Restraint by isovolumetric containment rather than by traction on the skeletal system can provide more effective protection to corresponding impact deceleration exposures than is obtained by webbing harness.

REFERENCES

1. ALDMAN, B.: Biodynamic studies on impact protection. *Acta Physiol Scand* 56 suppl 192, Stockholm 1962.
2. ARMSTRONG, R.W.: Occupant Restraint Conference, National Bureau of Standards, Gaithersburg, Md., Aug. 14, 1967.

3. ARMSTRONG, R.W.: Personal communication, March 28, 1968, Vehicle Systems Research, National Bureau of Standards, Washington, D.C.
4. BARTER, J.T.: Estimation of the Mass of Body Segments, WADC TR 57–260, April 1957, ASTIA Document #118222.
5. BEEDING, E.L. Jr.: Daisy Track Tests. Test Rpt. #6, Sept. 10, 1957, Proj. 7850, Task 78503; Aeromed. Field Lab, ARDC, AF Missile Dev. Center, Holloman AFB.
6. BEEDING, E.L. Jr.: Daisy Track Tests, Aeromed. Field Lab, ARDC, AF Missile Dev. Center, Holloman AFB, Proj. 7850, Task 78503, Test Rpt. #7, March 1958.
7. BEEDING, E. L. Jr: Human forward facing impact tolerances, *Aerospace Med 32;* p. 241, 1961.
8. BEEDING, E.L. Jr.: Daisy Track Tests—May 22, 1958—July 9, 1959. Test Rpt. #59–14, AF Missile Dev. Center, Holloman AFB, NM, Dec. 1959.
9. BEEDING, E.L. Jr., and HESSBERG, RUFUS R.: ARDC, AF Missile Dev. Center, Holloman AFB, NM.—Daisy Track Tests 271–337, Run—Feb. 4–Mar. 19, 1958, Proj. 7850, Task 78503, Test Rpt. #8, Nov. 1958.
10. BEEDING, E.L. Jr., and MOSELY, JOHN D.: Human Deceleration Tests—Tech. Note AFMDC–TN–60–2, Holloman AFB, Jan. 1960.
11. BIERMAN, H.R.: Test and evaluation of experimental harness under controlled crash conditions. Nav. Med. Res. Institute, Bethesda, Md. Proj. X-630, Rpt. #11, April 10, 1947.
12. BIERMAN, H.R.: Protection of the human body from impact forces of fatal magnitude. *Military Surgeon, 100:* 2, Feb. 1947.
13. BIERMAN, H.R.; WILDER, R.H. Jr., and HELLEMS, H.K.: The principles of protection of the human body as applied in a restraining harness for aircraft pilots. Naval Institute, Bethesda, Md., Proj. X–630, Rpt. 6, May 1946.
14. BROWN, W.K.; ROTHSTEIN, J.D. and FOSTER, P.: Human response to predicted apollo landing impacts in selected body orientations. *Aerospace Med, 37:* 4, p 394–98, April 1966.
15. CHANDLER, R.F.: Determination of equivalent natural frequency indicated by accelerometers mounted over the sternum during human impact in the G_x direction. Tech. Doc. Rpt. #ARL–TDR–62–29, Dec. 1962.
16. CHANDLER, R.F.: The Daisy Decelerator Tech. Doc. Rpt. #ARL–TDR–67–3, Holloman AFB, NM, May 1967.
17. CLARK, C. and BLECHSCHMIDT, C.: The Analytical Performance of an Airstop Restraint System in an Automobile Crash, ER 14005, Oct. 1965.
18. CLARK, C., and BLECHSCHMIDT, C.: *Human Transportation Fatalities and Protection Against Rear and Side Crash Loads by the Airstop Restraint.* 9th Stapp Car Crash Conference Proceedings—1965, p 19–64, U. of Minnesota Press—1966.
19. COERMANN, R.R., *et al.*: The Passive Mechanical Properties of the Human Thorax Abdomen System and of the Whole Body System. *J Aerospace Med, 31:* 443, 1960.
20. COERMANN, R.R.: The mechanical impedance of the human body in sitting and standing positions at low frequencies. *Hum Factors, 4:* 227, 1962.
21. COOPER, K.H., and HOLMSTROM, F.M.C.: Injuries during ejection seat training. *Aerospace Med, 34:* 139, 1963.

22. DE HAVEN, H.: Mechanical analysis of survival in falls from heights of fifty to one hundred and fifty feet. *War Medicine, 2:* 586–596, July 1942.
23. EDWARDS, R.G., and LANGE, K.O.: *A Mechanical Impedance Investigation of Human Response to Vibration.* AFSC TR AMRL–TR–64–91, WPAFB, Ohio, Oct. 1964.
24. EIBAND, A.M.: *Human Tolerance to Rapidly Applied Accelerations.* A Summary of the literature. NASA Memo #5–19–59E, June 1959.
25. EVANS, F.C.: *Studies on the Anatomy and Function of Bone and Joints,* Springer-Verlag, New York 1966.
26. EVANS, F.C., and LISSNER, H.R.: Biomechanical studies on the lumbar spine and pelvis. *J Bone Joint Surg, 41-A:* 278–290, Mar. 1959.
27. EVANS, F.C., and LISSNER, H.R.: *Studies on the Energy Absorbing Capacity of Human Intervertebral Discs,* 7th Stapp Car Crash Conference Proceedings, p 386, 1965.
28. EVANS, F.C.: LISSNER, H.R. and PATRICK, L.M.: Acceleration induced strains in the intact vertebral column. *J Appl Physiol, 17:*405, 1962.
29. FRIEDE, R.L.: Experimental concussion acceleration. *Arch Neurol, 4:*449, 1961.
30. FRIEDE, R.L.: Specific cord damage at the atlas level as a pathogenic mechanism in cerebral concussion—*J Neuropath Exp Neurol,* V XIX #2, April 2, 1960.
31. FRIEDE, R.L.: *The Pathology and Mechanics of Experimental Cerebral Concussion.* WADC Tech. Rpt. 61–256, Mar. 1961.
32. GODBY, R.O.; BROWNING, S.B.; BELSKI, D.S., and TAYLOR, E.R.: *Anthropometric Measurements of Human Sled Subjects.* Tech. Doc. Rpt. #ARL–TDR–63–13, Holloman AFB, NM, April 1963.
33. GURDJIAN, E.S.; LISSNER, H.R., and PATRICK, L.M.: *Concussion, Mechanism and Pathology,* 7th Stapp Car Crash Conference Proceedings, p 470, 1965.
34. GURDJIAN, E.S., ROBERTS, V.L., and THOMAS, L.M.: Tolerance curves of acceleration and intracranial pressure and protective index in experimental head injury. *J Trauma, 6:* 5, p 600–604, May 1966.
35. HANSEN, R.E., and CORNOG, D.Y.: *Annotated Bibliography of Applied Physical Anthropology in Human Engineering,* WADC Tech Rpt. 56–30, ASTIA Document AD–155622, WPAFB, Ohio, May, 1958.
36. HIRSCH, A.E.: *Man's Response to Shock Motions.* ASME Publication 63–WA–283, May 26, 1963.
37. HODGSON, V.R.; LISSNER, H.R., and PATRICK, L.M.: Response of the seated human cadaver to acceleration and jerk with and without seat cushions. *Hum Factors,* Oct. 1963, p 505–523.
38. HOLCOMB, G.A., and HUHEEY, M.: A Minimal Compression Fracture of T–3 as a Result of Impact. *Impact Acceleration Stress.* National Research Council Publication 977, 191, 1962.
39. HOLLISTER, N.R.; HORNE, R.G.; JOLLEY, W.P., and FRIEDE, R.: *Biophysics of Concussion.* WADC Tech. Rpt. 58–193, ASTIA Doc. AD–203385, Sept. 1958.
40. HUHEEY, M., and SIMMONS, C.F.: Investigations to determine human tolerance to short duration accelerations. Stanley Avn. Corp, Denver, Colo., Doc #127, Nov. 2, 1960.
41. KIEL, F.W.: Hazards of military parachuting. *Milit Med, 130(5):* 512–521, 1965.

42. KROEGER, W.J.: Internal Vibrations Excited in the Operation of Personnel Emergency Escape Catapults, Frankford Arsenal Lab Div, Memo. Rpt. MR–340, Nov. 26, 1946.
43. LATHAM, F.: A Study in Body Ballistics: Seat Ejection. Proceedings of the Royal Society B, 147: 121–139, 1957.
44. LEWIS, S.T. and STAPP, J.P.: Human tolerance to aircraft seat belt restraint, *J Aviation Med*, 29: 187–196, Mar 1958.
45. LOMBARD, C.F.: Human Tolerance to Forces Produced by Acceleration. Feb. 27, 1948.
46. LOMBARD, C.F., and ADVANI, S.H.: Impact Protection by Isovolumetric Containment of the Torso. 10th Stapp Car Crash Conference Proceedings, SAE Reprint 660796, p 117–124, Nov. 8–9, 1966.
47. LOMBARD, C.F.; BRONSON, S.D.; THIEDE, F.C.; CLOSE, P. and LARMIE, F.M.: Pathology and physiology of guinea pigs under selected conditions of impact and support-restraint, *Aerospace Med*, 35:9, p 860–865, Sept. 1964.
48. LYLE, D.J.; STAPP, J.P., and BUTTON, R.R.: Opthalmologic hydrostatic pressure syndrome. *Amer J Opthal*, 44:652–657, 1957.
49. MANDEL, M.J., and LOWRY, R.D.: One Minute Tolerance in Man to Vertical Sinusoidal Vibration in the Sitting Position. Tech. Doc. Rpt. AMRL-TDR-62–121, Oct. 1962.
50. MORRIS, J.M.; LUCAS, D.B., and BRESLER, M.S.: Role of the trunk in stability of the spine. *J Bone Joint Surg (Amer)*, 43-A:3, April 1961.
51. NICKERSON, J.L., and DRAZIC, M.: Internal Body Movement along Three Axes Resulting from Externally Applied Sinusoidal Forces, Tech. Rpt. AMRL-TR-66–102, WPAFB, Ohio, July 1966.
52. PATRICK, L.M.: *Human Tolerance to Impact—Basis for Safety Design*. SAE Reprint #1003B, International Automotive Engineering Congress, Jan. 1965.
53. RUFF, S.: Brief Acceleration—Less than one second. German Aviation Med. WW II, V I–US Govt Printing Office 1950.
54. RYAN, J.J.: *Reduction Crash Forces*. 5th Stapp Car Crash Conference, p 48, 1961.
55. RYAN, J.J.: Human crash Deceleration tests on seat belts. *Aerospace Med*, 33, p 167–174, Feb. 1962.
56. RYAN, J.J.: *Automotive Human Crash Studies. Impact Acceleration Stress*, p 345–353, Natl. Academy of Sciences/Natl. Research Council, Publication 977, 1962.
57. SCHNEIDER, R.G., PAPO, M., and ALVAREZ, C.S.: The effects of chronic recurrent spinal trauma in high d.ving, a study of Acapulco's divers. *J Bone Joint Surg*, 44-A, 648–656, 1962.
58. SENDROY, J. JR., and CECCHINI, L.P.: The Determination of Human Body Surface Area from Height and Weight. Research Rpt. NM 004 006.05.01, 1/19/54, Naval Medical Research Institute, Bethesda, Md. ASTIA #AD-44829.
59. SEVERY, D.M.; BRINK, H.M., and BAIRD, J.D.: Backrest and Head Restraint Design for Rear End Collision Protection. Automotive Engineering Congress, Detroit, Jan. 8–12, 1968, SAE Paper 680079.
60. SHAW, R.S.: Ruptured Intervertebral Disc from Positive Acceleration, *J Aviation Med*, 19:5, p 276, Sept. 1948.
61. SHAW, R.S.: Human Tolerance to Negative Acceleration of Short Duration, *J Aviation Med*, 19:2, p 39, Feb. 1948.

62. SHAW, R.S., and SAVELY, H.E.: Acceleration-Time Diagrams for Catapult Ejection Seats, Memo. Rpt. TSEAA-695–66D, Feb 11, 1947.
63. SIMMONS, C.F., and HERTING, D.N.: Strength of the Human Neck, Life Sciences Dept., North American Aviation, Rpt. SID 65–1180, Sept. 22, 1965.
64. SNYDER, R.G.: Human tolerance to extreme impacts in free-fall, *Aerospace Med, 34:8*, p 695–709, Aug. 1963.
65. SNYDER, R.G.: Human tolerance limits in water impact, *Aerospace Med, 36:10*, p 940–947, Oct. 1965.
66. SNYDER, R.G., et al.: *Impact Injury to the Pregnant Female and Fetus in Lap Belt Restraint.* 10th Stapp Car Crash Conference Proceedings, p 151–155, SAE Publication 660801, 1966.
67. SNYDER, R.G.: Terminal velocity impacts into snow. *Milit Med, 131:10*, p 1290–1298, Oct. 1966.
68. SNYDER, R.G.; SNOW, C.C.; YOUNG, J.W., PRICE, G.T., and HANSON, P.: Experimental Comparison of Trauma in Lateral ($+G_y$), Reward Facing ($+G_x$) and Forward Facing ($-G_x$) Body Orientations when restrained by Lap Belt Only. *Aerospace Med, 38:9*, Sept. 1967.
69. SNYDER, R.G.; YOUNG, J.W.; SNOW, C.C., and HANSON, P.: *Seat Belt Injuries in Impact.* Proceedings of Symposium April 19–21, 1967. *The Prevention of Highway Injury.* HSRI–The U of Michigan Press 1967.
70. SONNTAG, R.W.: Personal communication April 3, 1968, 6571st Aeromedical Res. Lab, Holloman AFB.
71. STAPP, J.P.: WADC AF Tech Rpt. 5915, Part 1, June 1949, Human Exposure to Linear Deceleration, Part 1. Preliminary Survey of Aft-Facing Seated Position. Part 2. The Forward Facing Position & Development of a Crash Harness, Dec. 1951.
72. STAPP, J.P.: Crash protection in air transports. *Aeronautical Engineering Review, 12:71*, April 1953.
73. STAPP, J.P.: Trauma Caused by Impact and Blast, *Clin Neurosurg, v 19:* p 324–343, 1965.
74. STAPP, J.P.: *Review of Air Force Research on Biodynamics of Collision. Review of AF Research on Biodynamics of Collision Injury.* 10th Stapp Car Crash Conference Proceedings, SAE reprint #660805, p 204–210, Nov. 8–9, 1966.
75. STAPP, J.P., and ENFIELD, D.L.: Evaluation of the Lap-type Automobile Safety Seat with reference to Human Tolerance. SAE preprint 62A, SAE Summer meeting, June 8–13, 1958.
76. STAPP, J.P., and LEWIS, S.T.: Criteria for Crash Protection in Armed Forces Ground Vehicles, HADC Tech Note, April 1956, Holloman AFB, NM.
77. STAPP, J.P., and LEWIS, S.T.: *Human Factors of Crash Protection in Automobiles.* Proceedings SAE Summer Meeting, Atlantic City, June 6, 1956, V 65, p 489–492.
78. STAPP, J.P., and TAYLOR, E.R.: Space cabin landing impact vector effects on human physiology. *Aerospace Med*, v 35:12, p 117–1133, Dec. 1964.
79. STAPP, J.P.; TAYLOR, E.R., and CHANDLER, R.F.: *Effects of Pitch Angle on Impact Tolerance.* 7th Stapp Car Crash Conference Proceedings, p 1–3, Charles C Thomas, Publishers, 1965.
80. SWEARINGEN, J.J.: Tolerance of the Human Face to Crash Impact. AM 68–20, FAA Office of Aviation Med. CARI, July 1965.

81. SWEARINGEN, J.J.: Determination of Centers of Gravity of Man. Federal Aviation Agency, Aviation Med. Service, CARI, Oklahoma City, Rpt #62–14, Aug. 1962.
82. SWEARINGEN, J.; HASBROOK, A.H.; SNYDER, R.G., and MCFADDEN, E.B.: Kinematic Behavior of the Human Body during Deceleration. Federal Aviation Agency, Aviation Med. Service, ARD, CARI, Oklahoma City, Rpt. #62–13, June 1962.
83. SWEARINGEN, J.J.; MCFADDEN, E.B.; GARNER, J.B., and BLETHROW, J.B.: Human voluntary tolerance to vertical impact. *J Aviation Med*, p 980, 1960.
84. SWEARINGEN, J.J.; WHEELWRIGHT, C.D., and GARNER, J.D.: An Analysis of Sitting Areas and Pressures of Man 62–1. Civil Aeromed Res. Institute, Oklahoma City. Jan. 1962.
85. VON GIERKE, H.E.: Response of the Body to Mechanical Forces. Tech Rpt AMRL-66–251, Wright-Patterson AFB, Oct. 66.
86. WEIS, E.B. JR.; CLARKE, N.P., and BRINKLEY, J.W.: Human response to several impact acceleration orientations and patterns. *Aerospace Med*, 34:1122, 1963.
87. WEIS, E.B. JR.; MARTIN, P.J., and CLARKE, N.P.: Analysis of Force and Acceleration Data from Human Impact Experiments. Proceedings of 16th annual conference on Engineering in Medicine and Biology, V 5, 1963 and in abstract form in *Aerospace Med*, v 35:4, April 1964.
88. WEIS, E.B., and MOHR, G.C.: Cineradiographic analysis of human visceral responses to short duration impact. *Aerospace Med*, Oct. 1967, p 1040–1044.
89. ZIEGENRUCKER, G.H., and MAGID, E.B.: Short Time Human Tolerance in Sinusoidal Vibrations, WADC Tech Rpt. 59–391, July 1959.

DISCUSSION

Channing L. Ewing

I must agree wholeheartedly with Col. Stapp's premise that the primary instrument for measuring the effects of mechanical force on man is man. His further statement concerning the inadequacy of surrogates, living or dead, is at once a clear indication of future directions for research in biomechanics and a challenge to a considerable portion of recent work in the field. The validation of any dummy, mathematical model or even cadaveric response to impact acceleration must await measurement of the dynamic response of the living human.

This seems to be a propitious time to announce that a joint Army-Navy-Wayne State University study entitled "Determination of the Dynamic Response of the Living Human Head and Neck to Impact Acceleration" has recently gotten underway.

Experimental design was performed by an interdisciplinary joint Army-Navy team, while design and construction of the accelerator and acceleration sled was conducted by Prof. Lawrence Patrick and his staff at Wayne State University. The experimental subjects are active duty Army and Navy volunteers and include two flight surgeons.

Human tolerance information is not being collected. Instead, only

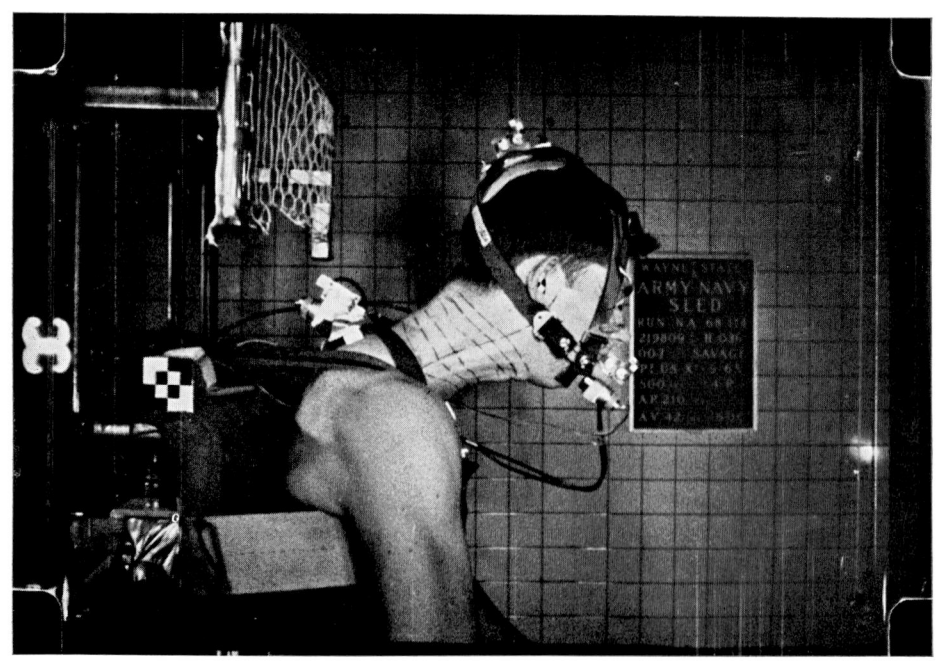

FIGURE 15–15. Maximum neck stretch on run Ho36, peak sled acceleration 6G, rate of onset 250 G/sec side camera 500 frames/sec.

dynamic response is being measured, well within the tolerance limits established by Col. Stapp and others. Information being collected includes photographic and transducer data, with transducers mounted on the subject. However, discussion of experimental design or results is beyond the purview of today's discussion.

Figure 15-15 is an enlarged single frame of 16mm film from our 36th human acceleration experiment. The camera is a pin-registered, 500 frame per second model which is sled mounted to obviate the parallax problem. The human subject with unrestrained head and neck is using torso and pelvic restraint and is facing to the right. The sled suddenly is accelerated to the left, causing the head and neck to appear to move forward (i.e. to the right) as a unit until a limit is reached, and the head is snapped somewhat, followed by the neck moving thru an arc almost to the horizontal. Peak sled acceleration reached on this run was 6 g.

Chapter XVI

TOLERANCE OF SUBHUMAN PRIMATE BRAIN TO CEREBRAL CONCUSSION

Arthur E. Hirsch, Ayub K. Ommaya, and Richard H. Mahone

INTRODUCTION

In recent years, both military and civilian sectors have become concerned with the prevention and management of trauma resulting from impact during explosions, airplane crashes and highway accidents. From the standpoint of frequency of occurrence and probability of fatality or serious disability, head injuries rank high. As a consequence, protection of the head is receiving increased attention. It becomes apparent on searching the literature that in spite of much having been written, there exists no universally satisfactory description of the mechanism of brain concussion and closed head injury. Because of the deficiency of such data, designers of helmets and head restraint systems must resort in a large part to guess work, past experience, and incomplete biomechanical data.[1]

In recognition of this problem, the Naval Air Systems Command has sponsored a cooperative program conducted by the Naval Ship Research and Development Center, and the Institute of Neurological Diseases and Blindness, National Institutes of Health. The aim of the program is a thorough understanding of the concussive process and other fundamentals of trauma to the nervous system.

In this chapter, we will compare the plausibility of several theories of brain injury and concussion mechanics in the light of our data from current experiments and our earlier efforts.[2-5]

There are three relatively independent hypotheses of the mechanics of head injuries. First, the pressure gradient hypothesis, which suggests that accelerative impacts set up pressure gradients which result in either "flow" initiated shear stresses in the craniospinal junction, or negative pressure induced cavitation lesions at the antipole of the point of impact.[6-15] The second hypothesis suggests that bending and/or stretching of the upper cervical cord during head and neck motion is the primary injurious mechanism.[16-19] The third hypothesis states that there are *two* main causes of brain injury: (1) deformation of the skull with or without fracture, and

(2) sudden rotation of the head causing shear stresses within its contents due to the "inertia effect" of these soft materials.[20,21]

Our work has been developed to test particularly the third hypothesis, first advanced by Holbourn in 1943, because it is capable of explaining most of the available experimental and clinical observations.

THEORY

In the brief descriptions of this hypothesis, Holbourn emphasizes the importance of head rotation-induced shear stresses in producing "contre-coup injuries . . . some intracranial hemorrhages, and probably . . . concussion." He states "for blows of long duration the injury is independent of the time for which the force acts . . . the injury is proportional to the acceleration." He goes on to say that

> for very short blows the injury is proportional to the force multiplied by the time for which it acts—hence—the injury is proportional to the *change of velocity* of the head and not to the rate of change i.e. acceleration—the change-over from one law of injury to the other occurs gradually somewhere in the region between ½ and ½₀₀ of a second.

Implicit in this analysis is an assumption that the brain and its restraints are following the physical laws governing the action of a spring-mass system. In a discussion of the response of such a single degree of freedom system to transient accelerations, Kornhauser states that this crossover occurs at about ⅓ or ¼ of the natural period and the damaging velocity can be related to the damaging acceleration as follows:[22]

$$\dot{\theta}_D = \frac{\ddot{\theta}_D}{W} \qquad (1)$$

Where

$\dot{\theta}_D$ is damaging rotational velocity (Radians per second)
$\ddot{\theta}_D$ is damaging rotational acceleration (Radians per second²)
W is natural frequency of rotation of brain (Radians per second)

From this equation, it would appear that depending on the time period of the initial maximum head response an acceleration dependence or a velocity dependence of cerebral concussion can be demonstrated.

METHODS

An experimental program designed to test the head rotation aspect of Holbourn's hypothesis requires several parts: first, one would need to know the natural frequency of the brain; second, the rotational acceleration levels at which injury occurs and lastly the rotational velocity levels at which injury occurs. In addition, some consideration should be given to the statement that skull deformation is also an injury producing mechanism albeit less significant for the onset of cerebral concussion and only causing local contusions.

A series of such experiments were conducted at the Naval Ship Research and Development Center and at the Clinical Center of the National Institutes of Health. Rhesus monkeys (*Macaca mulatta*) were employed as the experimental animal. During all tests, the animals were under sedation (Brevital ½ to 1 cc) in accordance with our previously published protocol and standard regulations regarding treatment of experimental animals.[23] The criteria for onset of experimental cerebral concussion were as previously reported.[2]

Natural Frequency of Brain Motion

Two series of experiments were performed to discover the rotational frequency of the monkey brain. The first involved a cinefluoroscopic technique in which small radiopaque spheres of a density equivalent to that of cerebral tissue were imbedded at several points in the monkey brain (Fig. 16–1). The head was then shaken briefly by hand and the resultant brain motion relative to fixed screws on the skull were recorded cineradiographically at 60 to 80 frames per second.

In the second series of experiments, monkeys were outfitted with a transparent plastic calvarium according to our modification of an earlier technique (Fig. 16–2). High-speed motion pictures of the cerebral cortex motions relative to a fixed point on the Lexan calvarium were made during impact loading at 3000 to 9000 frames per second.[24]

Whiplash Tests

A relatively simple and effective method of exposing the head to a violent rotational motion without significant head deformation is the generation of "whiplash." This is a commonly observed phenomenon associated with automobile read-end collisions. When the car is struck from the rear, it is suddenly propelled forward carrying the occupant's body with it while the head, on the relaxed neck, momentarily left behind, is then whipped around and forward as the neck takes hold. Figure 16–3 shows the car and propelling device designed to produce this motion. Our experimental method for this test procedure has been described in some detail previously.[3,25] Records of head rotation versus time were obtained from high speed cinematography of the monkeys. Force, linear acceleration and

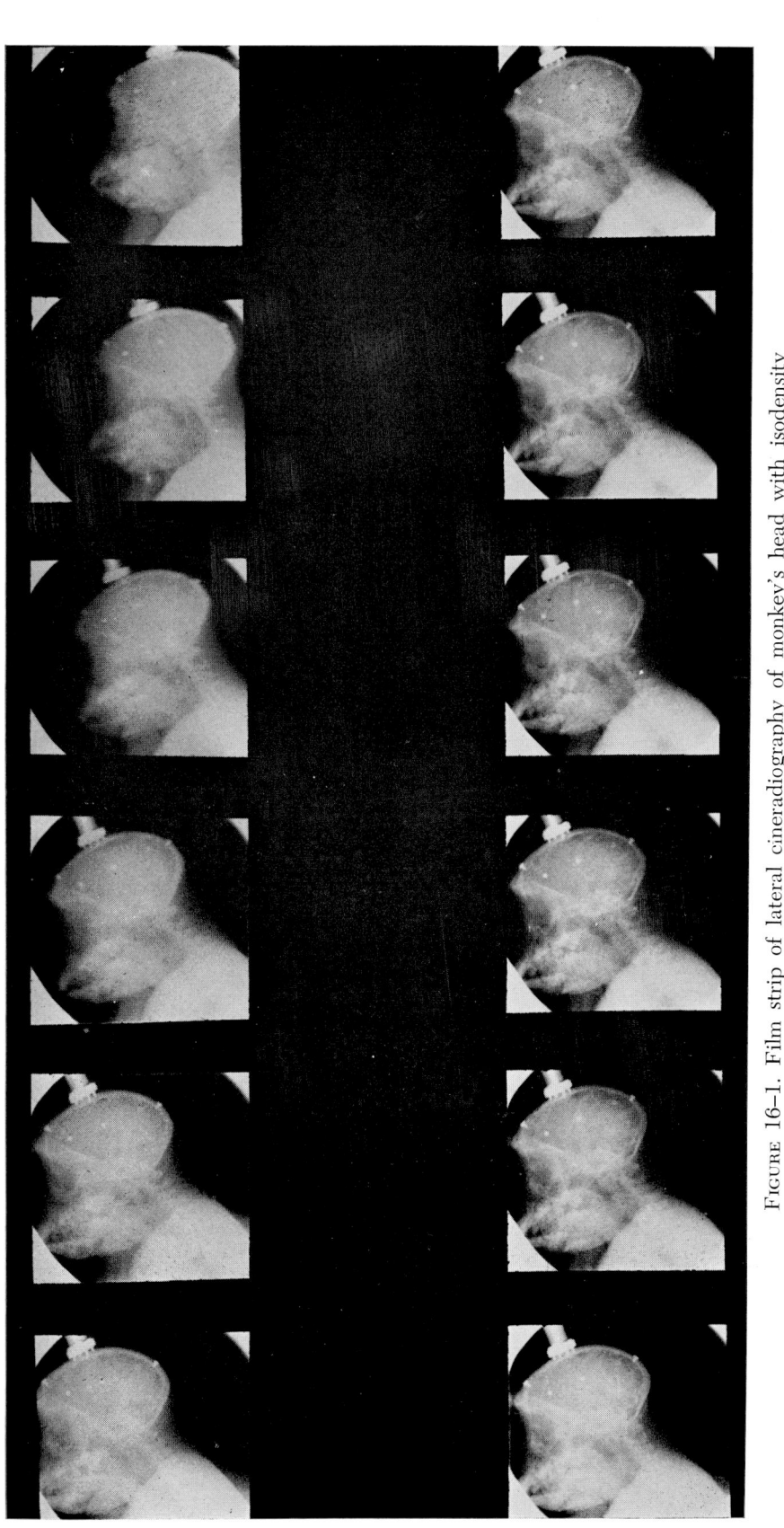

FIGURE 16-1. Film strip of lateral cineradiography of monkey's head with isodensity pellets embedded in brain during abrupt head rotation. Displacement of these radiopaque markers with the brain relative to the skull when the head is shaken allows measurement of the rotational frequency of brain.

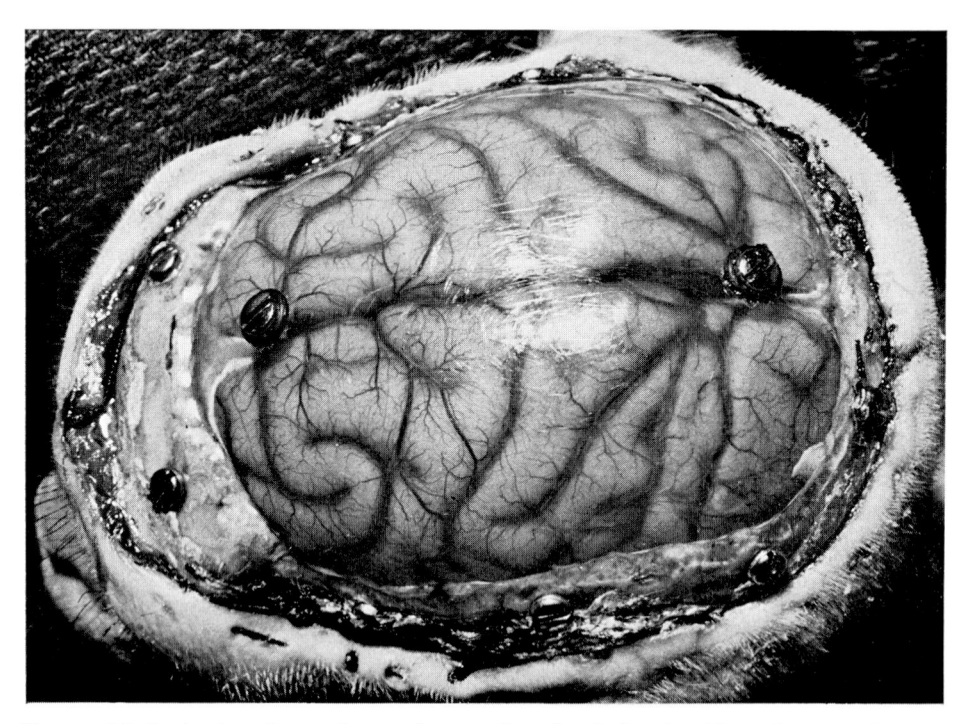

FIGURE 16–2. A view from above of a monkey head fitted with a Lexan calvarium taken approximately 3 weeks after surgery. Note the clarity of details of the cortical surfaces as seen through the thermoformed polycarbonate sheet. Displacement of sulci relative to the vent-hole screws (in the sagittal plane of the calvarium) during occipital impact provided the data for the second source of measurement of rotational frequency of the brain. (Data recorded by high-speed cinecamera at 3000–9000 frames per second.)

time measurements of the propelled cart were recorded on a FM tape recorder at 30 ips and then played back at 1⅞ ips onto a direct writing oscillograph for viewing and analysis. A typical record is shown in Figure 16–4.

Impact Tests

According to Holbourn, rotation of the head was the primary cause of cerebral injury and probably of concussion. If this is correct, then the method of inducing such rotational motion should be relatively unimportant, and concussion due to head blows should occur at the same levels of head rotation as concussion due to whiplash.

In an earlier series of tests developing our model of experimental cerebral concussion, we had studied the effects of measured impacts to the occipital region of the monkey head.[2] The apparatus is shown in Figure

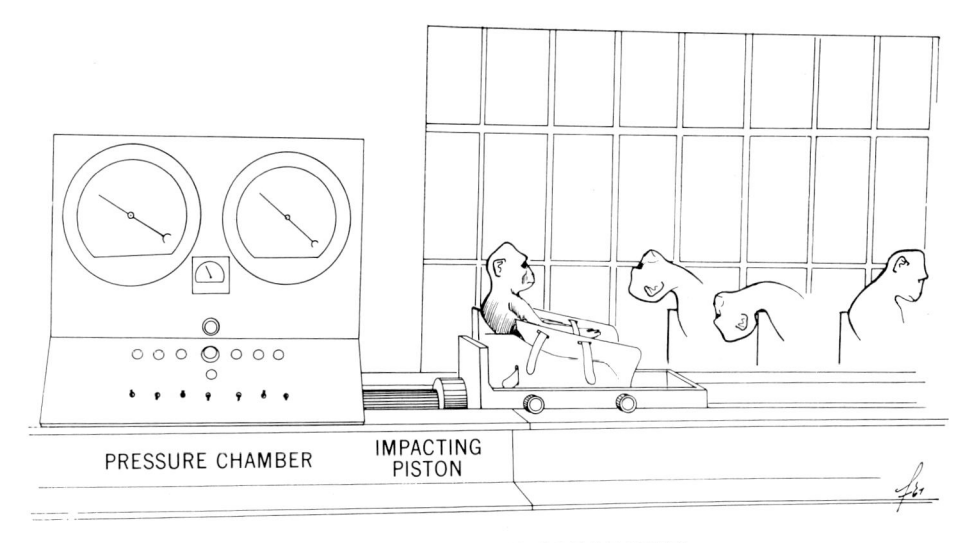

Tolerance of Subhuman Brain to Cerebral Concussion

PRESSURE CHAMBER   IMPACTING PISTON

WHIPLASH INJURY APPARATUS

FIGURE 16–3. View of whiplash apparatus showing the monkey seated in a fiberglass cart which is suddenly accelerated on roller skate wheels down the track by rear-end impacts produced by a Hy-G. apparatus. Displacements of the monkey are recorded by the high-speed cinecameras in the foreground.

WHIPLASH TEST W-60
IMPELLER PRESSURE RATIO 1500/300
CONCUSSIVE

Acceleration of Cart — 250 g's — Area of Accel-Time is Velocity – 68 fps

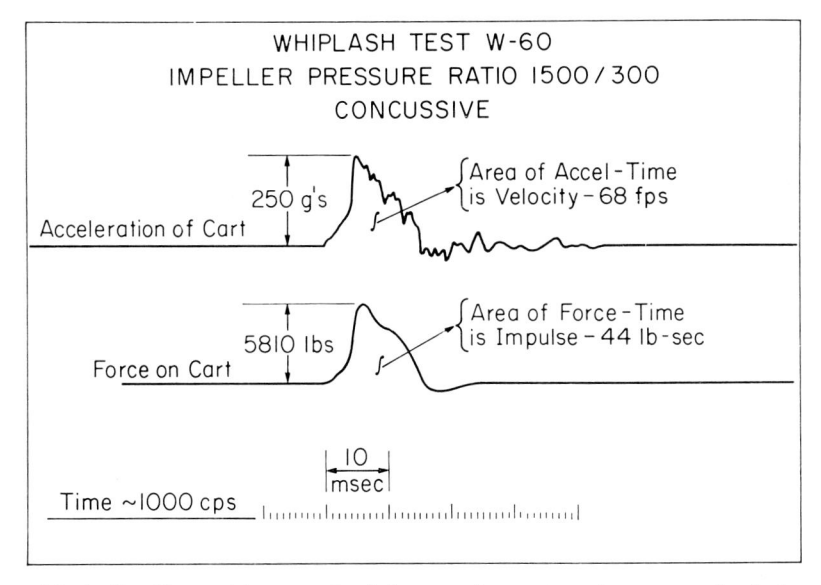

Force on Cart — 5810 lbs — Area of Force-Time is Impulse – 44 lb-sec

Time ~1000 cps   10 msec

FIGURE 16–4. Oscillographic record of impact force (to the rear-end of the cart), linear acceleration of cart and time signal obtained during a typical whiplash experiment.

16-5. The monkey is seated in a special chair with arm and leg restraints. The pneumatic gun propels a piston containing a strain gage dynamometer the output of which permits a measurement of the force applied to the head as a function of time. The piston ends in a firm rubber pad with an impacting area of about 1 square inch. High speed cinematography also provided the record of head motions during each impact from which rotational velocity and acceleration data were calculated in the same way as with the whiplash tests. The impact force, head linear acceleration and other data were recorded from subsequent analysis in a manner similar to that described for the whiplash experiments. A typical record is shown in Figure 16-6.

Several head impact tests were also made in which the piston impact was against a hard skull cap which fit snugly and distributed the load over a large area of the monkey head. This will be described as the distributed load head impact situation.

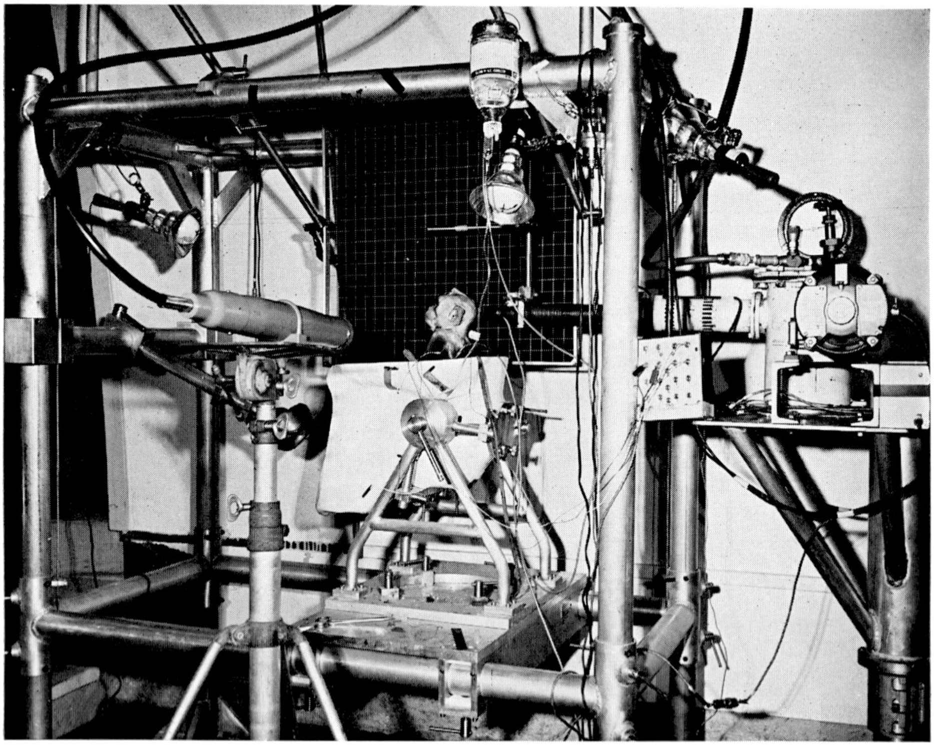

FIGURE 16-5. View of head impact apparatus. The seated animal can be positioned so that blows may be struck to any aspect of the head by a compressed air driven piston, the tip of which contains a dynamometer to record the impact force. Displacements of the monkey's head are recorded by high-speed cinematography.

**TEST V-71 SHOT I
HEAD FREE, CONCUSSIVE
ENERGY OF IMPACT 21.1 FT.-LB.
EBI**

TIMING 1000 CPS

VELOCITY OF IMPACTING HAMMER

23.3 FPS ← *130g's*
ACCELERATION OF HEAD

FORCE APPLIED TO HEAD
← 212 LBS. *(0.575 LB.-SEC., IMPULSE)*

INTRACRANIAL ← +23 PSIG
LEFT MOTOR CORTEX

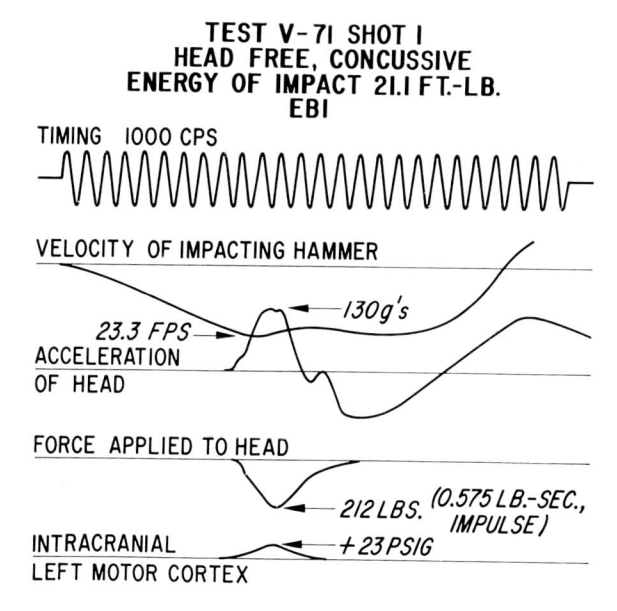

FIGURE 16–6. Oscillographic record of velocity of impacting piston, impact force (to the occipital region of the head), linear acceleration of the head (from a miniature accelerometer screwed into the skull vertex), intracranial pressure changes (measured at the brain surface with miniature semiconductor strain gage transducers) and time signal, obtained during a typical head impact experiment.

RESULTS

Natural Frequency

Analysis of the brain motions during impact were made from the 60 to 80 frames per second cineradiographic measurements and the 3000 to 9000 frames per second cinephotography of the brain through the Lexan calvarium. Figure 16–7A is a plot of the displacement of the radiopaque spheres relative to a fixed point on the skull. It can be seen that the frequency is about 10 Hz. Figure 16–7B shows the motion of a cortical sulcus relative to a fixed point on the Lexan calvarium. It can be observed that there are two frequencies present, a high frequency of about 50 Hz superimposed on a low frequency of about 5 Hz. This high frequency may be a surface perturbation generated by the piston impact or a translational wave which did not show up in the cineradiographic study because of the low time resolution of the camera. If the above measurements are correctly interpreted, then the rotational frequency of the monkey brain can be estimated to be between 5 and 10 Hz and the period 100 to 200 milliseconds. The transition region between acceleration and velocity sensitivity to injury should be ⅓ or ¼ this period or about 25 to 50 milliseconds.

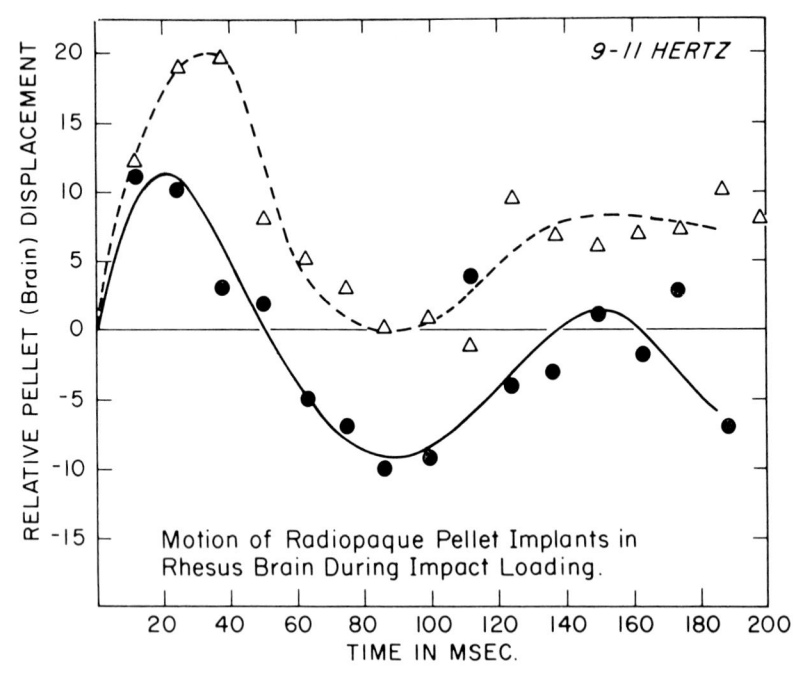

FIGURE 16–7A. Calculated relative displacement (in arbitrary units) of radiopaque pellets in monkey brain as seen in Figure 16–1 during sudden head movement (two experiments plotted). Total amplitude of such brain displacements (equated to pellet displacement because of equal densities) usually does not exceed 3 to 4 mm under these conditions. Approximate frequency (rotational movement) of brain = 10 Hz with a period = 200 milliseconds.

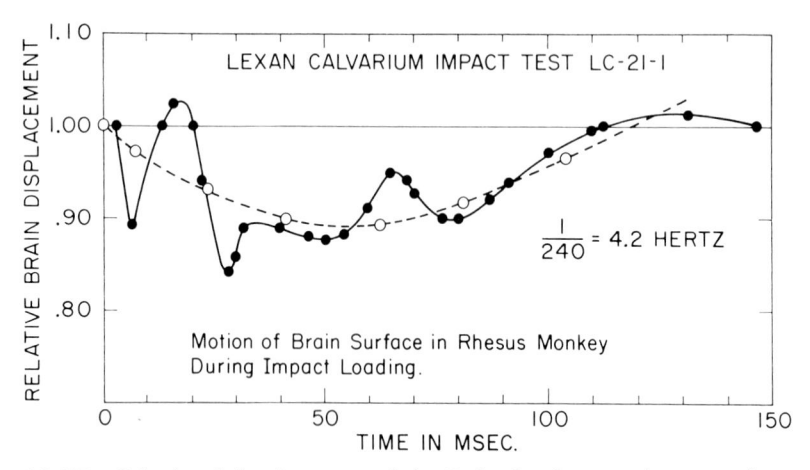

FIGURE 16–7B. Calculated displacement of the Rolandic fissure relative to the posterior vent-hole screw as seen in Figure 16–2. Note that *two* frequencies were recorded; a high one at about 50 Hz superimposed on a low one of about 5 Hz. The lower frequency was taken as the rotational frequency under these conditions, with a half period = 120 milliseconds.

Whiplash Tests

The data obtained for the whiplash tests are shown in Figures 16-8A and 16-8B. It can be seen that the monkey head is accelerating for durations between 1 and 20 milliseconds. This time range is below the predicted transition zone of 25 to 70 milliseconds, and hence a velocity dependence of injury should be expected. This is indeed indicated in the data. It appears that 300 to 350 radians per second is the angular or rotational velocity beyond which whiplash will produce cerebral concussion. Implicit here is a whole range of rotational accelerations ranging from about 10,000 to over 300,000 radians per sec.² Figure 16-8B illustrates this dependence. Insofar as these data are concerned, Holbourn's hypothesis that for "very short blows the injury is proportional to the change of velocity of the head" has been verified.

It is possible at this point to speculate on further implications of the theory. If we can assign the empirically determined values of 300 to 350 radians per second as the change in velocity at which concussion will occur and if we use the values of 5 to 10 Hz as correct for the natural frequency of the brain in rotation it is possible by employing equation

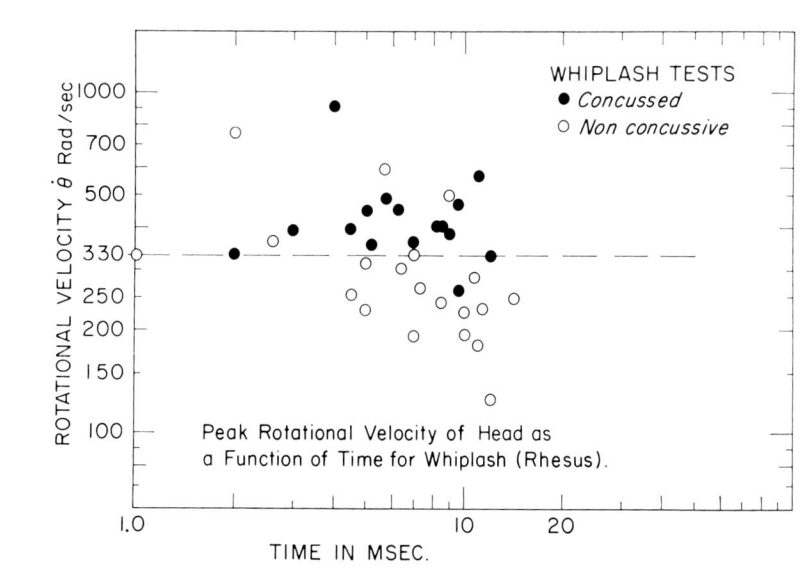

FIGURE 16-8A. Rotational velocity of the head during whiplash injury. Plot of rotational velocity of the monkey head (calculated by differentiating once, the angular displacement of an axis on the head relative to a horizontal axis), versus time in milliseconds. Both concussed and nonconcussed points are shown. The probable 50 percent concussive threshold level is indicated at about 330 radians per second and indicates that cerebral concussion in this time regime is velocity dependent.

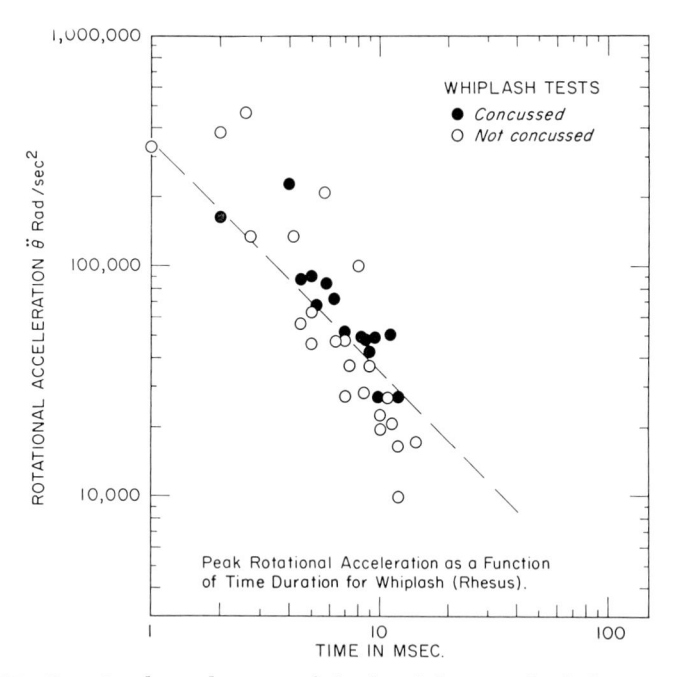

FIGURE 16–8B. Rotational acceleration of the head during whiplash injury (calculated by double differentiation of angular displacement data recorded by high-speed cinematography). The acceleration versus time data clearly indicates a time dependency for the occurrence of cerebral concussion.

(1) to compute the long duration acceleration injury response in whiplash by simple substitution

$$\ddot{\theta}_D = 2\pi(5 \text{ to } 10) \times (300 \text{ to } 350) \text{ radians per second}$$
$$\ddot{\theta}_D = 10{,}000 \text{ to } 20{,}000 \text{ radians per second}^2 \text{ approximately}$$

These values have been plotted in Figure 16–9 which is a tolerance curve relating concussive rotational velocity to concussive rotational acceleration. Of course this extrapolation has not been verified, and our current head rotation experiments are seeking to explore this long duration (20 to 100 milliseconds) time regime. It should be noted that time increases from right to left in this type of plot.

Impact Tests

As has been mentioned, if Holbourn's hypothesis is correct and the rotational response of the brain is the primary factor in determining the concussion level, then it should make little difference as to the method used in exciting this response provided significant skull deformation does not occur. Concussion should occur at approximately the same levels of

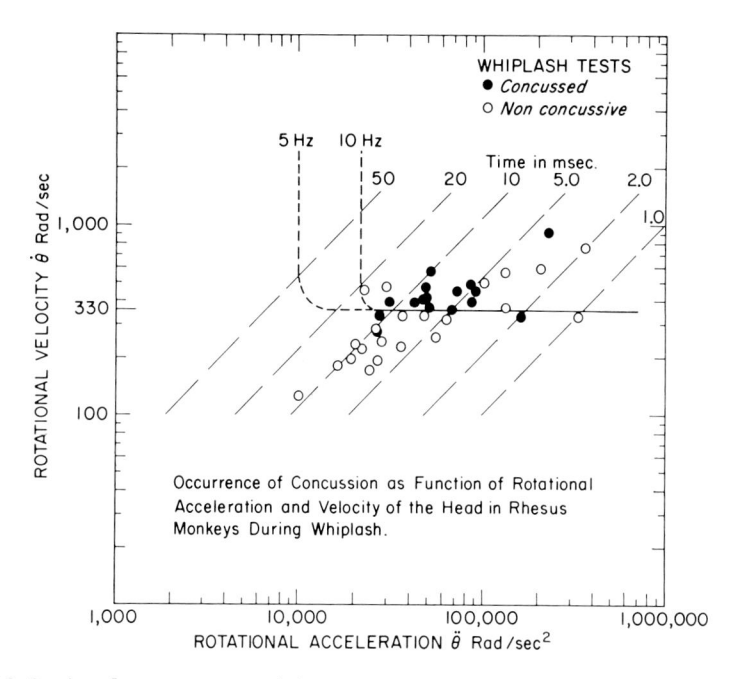

FIGURE 16–9. A tolerance curve (after Kornhauser) relating rotational velocity and rotational acceleration for cerebral concussion in whiplash injury. Note that time increases from right to left at a 45 degree slope to the abscissa in this type of plot. Theoretically predicted tolerance levels for long duration rotations (25 to 100 msec.) have been indicated at the two brain frequencies measured experimentally (5 and 10 Hz). It is predicted that such acceleration dependent concussions will result in data points falling mainly to the right of the vertical asymptotes of the tolerance curve. The horizontal asymptote is similar to the data plot seen in Figure 16–8A.

rotation when the head is struck a blow or when it moves during whiplash.

The data from our impact experiments are shown in Figures 16–10A and 16–10B. Again it can be clearly seen that the concussion level is a velocity rather than acceleration dependent function. It should be noted however that the concussive level is about 140 radians per second. This is only 40 per cent the amplitude required to concuss a monkey by whiplash. It is obvious that the local skull deformation and accompanying phenomena play an important role in the concussion process during impact. Unless it can be shown that the brain rotates more violently within the skull during impact than it does during whiplash, the rotational-motion-shear stress hypothesis does not account for the whole concussion complex.

The importance of this local impact effect has been tested by several additional experiments in which a skull cap was fitted over the occipital area in order to distribute the impact load over the entire skull. Figure 16–10C suggests that distribution of the loading by minimizing local skull

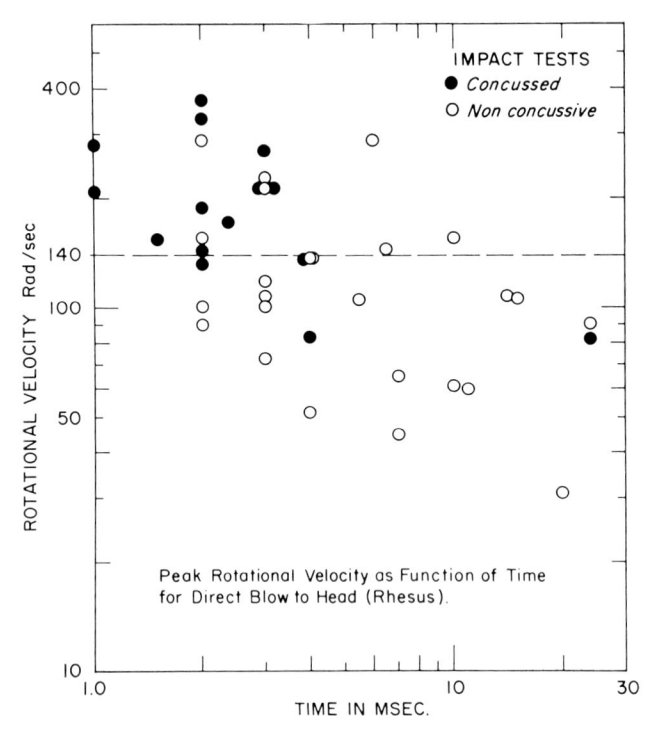

FIGURE 16–10A. Rotational velocity of monkey head during occipital impact plotted versus time. Note that the 50 percent probability of concussion threshold is at about 140 radians per second. This should be compared to the similar data for whiplash trauma where the threshold was almost 60 percent *higher,* suggesting significant local effects of impact for the genesis of cerebral concussion in head injury.

deformation effects may raise the tolerance to impact up to the whiplash values. The data are insufficient to conclude that local deformation alone is responsible for the decrease in tolerance to rotation observed during head impact and further investigation in this area is in progress.

A prediction can be made now concerning the long duration response of the monkey to head impact. Employing the same equation used for the whiplash example, we see in Figure 16–11 that a blow producing an average rotational acceleration greater than about 5000 to 9000 radians per second squared for more than 20 to 50 milliseconds, or rotational velocity change greater than 140 radians per second (for duration < 20 milliseconds) is likely to produce cerebral concussion in about 50 per cent of adult Rhesus monkeys.

SUMMARY

Our current experimental data provide supporting evidence for Holbourn's theory that brain concussion is related to the shearing strains de-

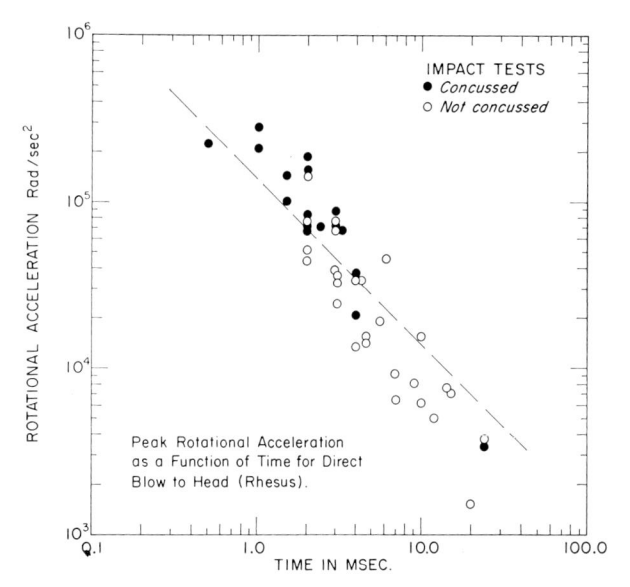

FIGURE 16–10B. Rotational Acceleration of monkey head during occipital impact plotted versus time. Note the time dependency of the data in the whiplash situation as seen in Figure 16–8B.

veloped by severe rotational motions of the brain. There is doubt however whether this is the whole explanation since the local skull deformation which Holbourn describes as a minor contributor to rotational motion and hence concussion seems to play an important role in increasing the brain sensitivity to concussion, since 60 per cent less rotational response is required when local deformation effects are experienced. The injurious significance of rotational motion of the brain is however well brought out by our experimental production of cerebral concussion as well as significant surface brain hemorrhage by whiplash (when no significant head impact occurs).[25]

We have shown that cerebral concussion occurs in Rhesus monkeys at a lower threshold value of rotational velocity of the head after direct head impact as compared to that required to produce cerebral concussion during whiplash. This observation may be explained by any of a number of hypothetical local factors, some of which may be as follows:

1. That the brain rotation during head impact is much more violent than the brain rotation resulting from equivalent head rotation in whiplash. There is as yet no experimental evidence in favor of this possibility, and we would not support it.

2. That skull deformation (even without fracture) is a significant factor in enhancing the impact induced pressure gradients resulting in either

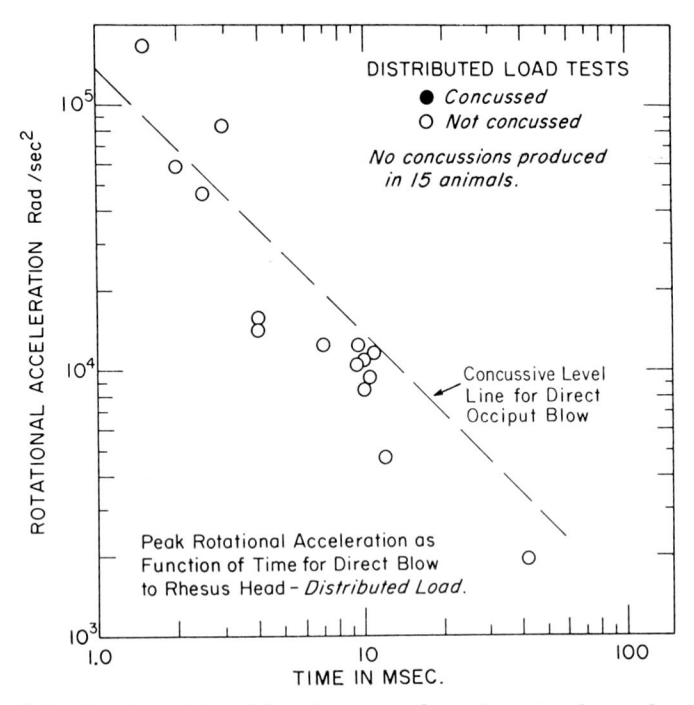

FIGURE 16–10C. Distributed Load head impact data. Rotational Accelerations of the head plotted versus time. A dotted line is drawn along a path indicating where the 50 percent concussion probability for the direct (nondistributed) impact experiment would be seen as in Figure 16–10B. It should be noted that none of these animals were concussed, suggesting that reduction of the *local* effects of the impact, under these conditions, tends to raise the threshold of cerebral concussion (in terms of rotational velocity) to a level closer to that of the whiplash situation.

"flow" initiated shear stresses at the craniospinal junction, as suggested by Gurdjian et al., or "cavitation" as an injurious concomitant of the negative pressures. We are planning to test these and related hypotheses directly in our animal model.

3. The theory that tensile or bending stresses on the upper cervical cord and brain stem are the cause of "acceleration concussion"[17-19] cannot explain either the observed time dependency or the discrepancy between the concussive thresholds for head rotation in whiplash and after impact. In addition to thus failing to explain the increased sensitivity to impact any better than the rotational theory, the neck-stretching (cervical cord bending and stretching) hypothesis is not compatible with our demonstration that the wearing of a cervical collar (reducing rotation of the head but *not* limiting stretching of the neck) *raises* the threshold for cerebral concussion by impact much in the same way as observed in animals subjected to the distributed load impact tests.[3,25] Moreover, the experiments

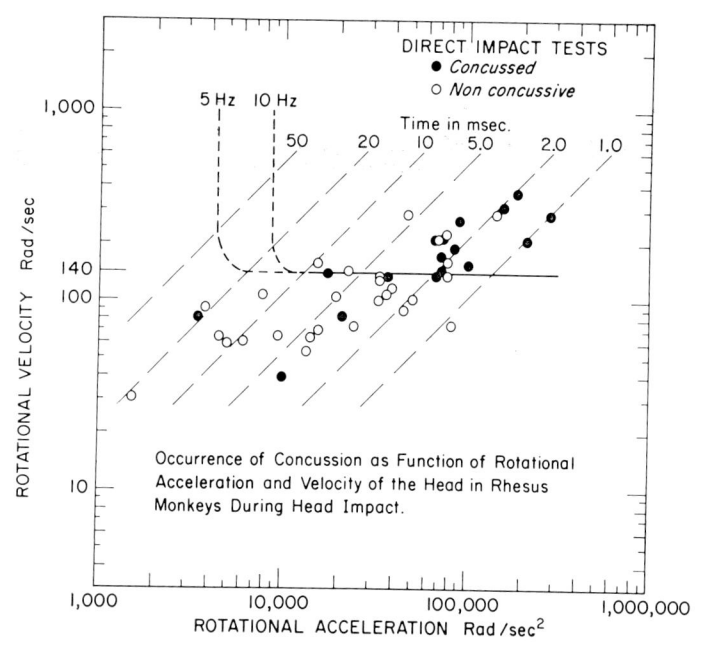

FIGURE 16–11. A tolerance curve relating rotational velocity (ordinate) to the rotational acceleration (abscissa) of the monkey head during occipital impact head injury with time increasing from right to left along 45 degree slopes. This curve is similar to that seen in Figure 16–9 although the actual values for the velocity and acceleration dependent concussions are significantly different.

of Hollister et al.[17-19] (and before them, of Douglas Wright[16]) with cats may be explained also in terms of the head angulation or rotational hypothesis.[3]

It would therefore seem quite feasible to suggest a synthesis of most observations on the mechanics of experimental cerebral concussion and to draw together the apparently unrelated hypotheses listed in the introduction. When the freely movable head is subjected to an impact, there are *two* injurious mechanisms immediately responding; rotation of the head and deformation of the skull, each contributing about equal amounts to the injury potential of the blow. When the head is suddenly accelerated indirectly as in a "whiplash," skull deformation effects may probably be neglected and rotational effects become highly significant. When the relatively immobile head is subjected to impact, skull deformation effects predominate and head rotation becomes the minor factor. However, because this latter case is a relatively rare occurrence in nature, the measurement of the head rotation response to injurious inputs, as a more easily measured common denominator to head impact and whiplash injury than intracranial pressure gradients, would appear to be a useful approach.

What is also needed in the understanding of all these varieties of mechanical trauma to the nervous system is the time duration of the injurious inputs and their responses. Our current work is directed towards completing the experimental fitting of our data to the tolerance curves predicted in Figures 16–9 and 16–11, particularly in the long duration time regime, and the completion of our scaling experiments to fit such tolerance levels for impact and whiplash in the squirrel monkey, rhesus monkey and chimpanzee to a theoretically derived inverse two-thirds brain mass relationship allowing tentative prediction of concussive tolerance of man.[4] Finally, we are conducting specific investigations of the skull deformation effects of head injury including a direct experimental test of the pressure gradient and cavitation hypotheses. It is hoped that in this way, all the hypotheses and experimental observations made in various laboratories will be finally evaluated in a uniform experimental model for head injury.

REFERENCES

1. HIRSCH, A.E.: Current problems in head protection. In Caveness, W.F., and Walker, A.E. (Eds.): *Head Injury, Conference Proceedings*. Philadelphia, Lippincott, 1966, Chapt. 3, pp. 37–40.
2. OMMAYA, A.K.; HIRSCH, A.E.; FLAMM, E.S., and MAHONE, R.H.: Cerebral concussion in the monkey: an experimental model. *Science*, 153:211–212, July 1966.
3. OMMAYA, A.K.; HIRSCH, A.E., and MARTINEZ, J.: The role of whiplash in cerebral concussion. *Proceedings of the Tenth Stapp Car Crash Conference*. New York, Soc. Automotive Engineers, 1966, pp. 197–203.
4. OMMAYA, A.K.; YARNELL, P.; HIRSCH, A.E., and HARRIS, E.H.: Scaling of experimental data on cerebral concussion in sub-human primates to concussion threshold for man. *Proceedings of the Eleventh Stapp Car Crash Conference*. New York, Soc. Automotive Engineers, 1967, pp. 47–52.
5. This research program has been supported by funds from the Naval Air Systems Command. *BuWep Task WF 0121011 FC7–41–07* and *BuMed Task MR–005–04.0037*. (Experiments have been conducted with the assistance of E.S. Flamm, P. Yarnell, F. Faas, P. Corrao, D. Gainsburg, F. Whitten and N. Pickford.
6. GURDJIAN, E.S., and LISSNER, H.R.: Mechanism of head injury as studied by the cathode ray oscilloscope. Preliminary report. *J Neurosurg*, 1:393–399, 1944.
7. GURDJIAN, E.S., and LISSNER, H.R.: Photoelastic confirmation of the presence of shear strains at the craniospinal junction in closed head injury. *J Neurosurg*, 18:58–60, 1961.
8. THOMAS, L.M.; ROBERTS, V.L., and GURDJIAN, E.S.: Impact-induced pressure gradients along three orthogonal axes in the human skull. *J Neurosurg*, 26:316–321, 1967.
9. EDBURG, S.; RIEKER, J., and ANGRIST, A.: Study of impact pressure and acceleration in plastic skull models. *Lab Invest*, 12:1305–1311, 1963.
10. GOGGIO, A.F.: The mechanism of contrecoup injury. *J Neurol Psychiat*, 4:11, 1941.

11. WARD, J.W.; MONTGOMERY, L.H., and CLARK, S.L.: A mechanism of concussion: a theory. *Science, 107*:349–353, 1948.
12. GROSS, A.G.: A new theory on the dynamics of brain concussion and brain injury. *J Neurosurg, 15*:548–561, 1958.
13. SELLIER, K., and UNTERHARNSCHEIDT, F.: *Mechanik und Pathomorphologique der Hirnschaden nach Stumfer Gewalteinwirkung auf den Schadel.* Berlin, Springer, 1963, pp. 1–40.
14. UNTERHARNSCHEIDT, F.: *Die Gedecten Schaden des Gehirns.* Berlin, Springer, 1963, pp. 1–124.
15. LINDGREN, S.O.: Experimental studies of mechanical effects in head injury. *Acta Chir Scand* (Suppl. 360), 1966, pp. 1–100.
16. WRIGHT, D.R.: Concussion and contusion. *Surgery, 19*:661–667, 1946.
17. HOLLISTER, N.; JOLLEY, W.P., and HORNE, R.G.: Biophysics of concussion. *WADC Technical Report, 58–193, ASTIA Document No. AD 203305*, Sept. 1958 (Armed Services Technical Information Agency, Arlington Hall Station, Arlington, Virginia).
18. FRIEDE, R.L.: The pathology and mechanics of experimental cerebral concussion. *WADD Technical Report, 61–256, ASTIA Document No. 266210*, March 1961 (Wright Air Development Division Air Research and Development Command, U.S. Air Force, Wright Patterson Air Force Base, Ohio).
19. FRIEDE, R.L.: Specific cord damage at the atlas level as a pathogenic mechanism in cerebral concussion. *J Neuropath Exp Neurol, 19*:266–270, 1960.
20. HOLBOURN, A.H.S.: Mechanics of head injuries. *Lancet, 2*:438, Oct. 1943.
21. HOLBOURN, A.H.S.: Mechanics of brain injuries. *Brit Med Bull, 3*(6):147–149, 1945.
22. KORNHAUSER, M.: Prediction and evaluation of sensitivity to transient acceleration. *J Appl Mech, 21*:371, 1954.
23. The experiments reported herein were conducted according to the principles enunciated in Guide for Laboratory Animal Facilities and Care prepared by the Committee on the Guide for Laboratory Animal Resources, NAS-NRC.
24. OMMAYA, A.K.; BORETOS, J.W., and BEILE, E.E.: The lexan calvarium: an improved method for direct observation of the brain. *J Neurosurg* (submitted to in March 1968).
25. OMMAYA, A.K.; FASS, F., and YARNELL, P.: Whiplash injury and brain damage: an experimental study. *JAMA, 204*:285–289, April 1968.

DISCUSSION

Elisha S. Gurdjian

In their chapter, Drs. Hirsch, Ommaya and Mahone have emphasized the importance of rotational acceleration in the production of concussion in the subhuman primate. I get the impression from reading their paper that nothing else but rotational acceleration may be the cause of a concussive effect. We feel that rotational acceleration and linear acceleration co-exist in most impact injuries of the head along with some deformation of the skull. In recording rotational acceleration with the triaxial accelerometer, one also gets a record of translational acceleration at the same time. Our records of rotational acceleration show lower figures than those of the authors. Possibly calculating angular acceleration photographically may be different than by the accelerometer. There is no doubt that relative movements of the brain do occur during impact and we have been able to show them with the help of the flash x-ray technique. The inserted pellets not only move during impact but also return to their original position indicating a degree of elasticity of the brain *in situ*. The relative movements are caused by pressure gradients through the brain resulting from inertia forces. Angular acceleration probably functions in the more peripheral portions of the brain resulting in tears of connecting vessels and contusions of the brain surface. It is our present impression that concussion is an acceleration sensitive phenomenon and when apparent acceleration is computed by dividing the force by the mass of the concussed head in the Rhesus monkey, increasing severity of concussion is noted with the higher figures of apparent acceleration.

I think that it's about time to consider together the various parameters of injury rather than to discuss one parameter disregarding other parameters. Many of us over the years have been one parameter experts. It seems to me that we can now analyze the effects of an impact and rightly conclude that translational and angular accelerations co-exist in an impact injury, that the magnitude of the energy and the size of the head impacted are all very important in the resultant effect.

The effects of deformation of the skull without fracture are interesting to analyze. As suggested by Unterharnscheidt and Sellier, in certain directions, the static loading of the head causes a slight increase in volume rather than a decrease. In the fronto-occipital direction, some increase in the skull volume follows static compression. Many years ago, in the cadaver head, we recorded negative pressures in the temporal area from a frontal impact. A static loading of the parietotemporal region causes a decrease in the volume of the skull. What differences may be expected from impacts in various regions of the head is a problem that we are studying at the present time.

I am very interested in their findings of whiplash effects in the subhuman primate. First, one should emphasize that the usual whiplash injury in the human does not cause concussion, if one includes in the definition of concussion a state of unconsciousness following the impact. On the other hand with more severe rear end collisions, injuries may involve the spinal column, the blood vessels of the spinal cord, the spinal cord. Peripheral nerves, muscles and bones may be stretched in the hyperextension-hyperflexion effect.

Chapter XVII

TOLERANCE OF THORAX AND ABDOMEN

Harold J. Mertz, Jr. and Charles K. Kroell

In general, trauma to the thorax and abdomen can be classified as either penetrating or nonpenetrating depending on whether the impacting object pierces the thoracic or abdominal wall. This paper will be mainly concerned with nonpenetrating trauma of the thoracic and abdominal regions and specifically with the dynamic responses and tolerance levels of these areas to blunt impact loading.

Statistics relating to the relative frequency of occurrence and severity of thoracic and abdominal injuries resulting from traffic accidents differ according to the source and the criteria for comparison. Generally, however, thoracic injuries are encountered more frequently, although with a lower mortality, than is the case for abdominal injuries.[1,2,3,4,5] Kihlberg[1] (1965) presents data covering 992 accident vehicles in which the front seat was occupied by at least two people, the driver and the right front seat passenger, and injury was sustained by either one or both of these occupants or, in the case of additional rear seat passengers, by one of them. This data sample was obtained in 1964 and involved only those automobiles which were manufactured after 1958. For the 992 accidents, the total number of injuries to the drivers and passengers were 1704 and 1953, respectively, of which 311 (18.0%) and 305 (15.5%) were injuries to the thorax and 103 (6.0%) and 146 (7.5%) were injuries to the abdomen. The entire injury spectrum from minor to fatal is represented.

Table 17-I gives a comparison of the degree of severity of the thoracic and abdominal injury for the driver and his passenger. The statistics given in this table indicate that the passenger received more serious injuries to the thorax and to the abdomen than the driver.

In another accident survey, Huelke and Gikas[6] (1966) studied in detail 139 fatal automobile accidents which occurred in the Washtenaw County area of Michigan during the period of 1961 to 1965. In these accidents, 177 people were killed. Examining the statistics given by these investigators as related to the areas of the body which were injured, the thorax, abdomen, or a combination of both were principally involved in 106 of

TABLE 17-I
COMPARISON OF THE DEGREE OF SEVERITY OF THORACIC AND ABDOMINAL
INJURY FOR THE DRIVER AND HIS PASSENGER (KIHLBERG[1])

	Minor	Nondangerous	Dangerous	Fatal	Other	Number of Injuries
Thoracic Injury						
Driver	62.7	18.6	5.8	7.4	5.5	311
Passenger	45.2	28.5	10.5	9.8	5.9	305
Abdominal Injury						
Driver	55.3	22.3	11.7	3.9	6.8	103
Passenger	50.7	26.0	14.4	4.1	4.8	146

the fatalities (or 60%). Omitting the fatalities due to ejection, the thorax and abdomen were involved in eighty of 120 fatalities (or 62%).

Nahum et al.[2] (1966) studied 150 accidents involving 222 vehicles occupied by 374 motorists, of which 239 were afflicted with 496 "significant injuries," i.e. injuries other than minor or fatal. Ejection was excluded and, although all accident configurations and seating locations were included, the sample was strongly biased to the driver and frontal impacts. The reported distribution of significant injuries included 16 per cent for the chest and 8 per cent for the abdomen.

These accident surveys were completed prior to the 1967 model year and, consequently, do not reflect the performance of safety innovations characterizing the current automobiles. However, statistics such as those from these reports do exemplify the need for quantitative thoracic-abdominal tolerance levels so that safety design criteria related to these vital body areas can be more intelligently specified.

ABDOMEN

The serious nature and diagnostic elusiveness of intra-abdominal injuries resulting from blunt trauma have been emphasized repeatedly in the clinical literature. Reports of the significance of abdominal trauma as related to the overall accidental injury picture as well as of the frequency with which the various abdominal organs are involved differ markedly among the various investigators.[3,7,8] In large part, this is due to differences in personal clinical experience, the specific criteria upon which such comparative studies are based and the differences in diagnostic practice. Regarding this matter, Baxter and Williams[8] comment: "These findings suggest that the varying percentages of abdominal visceral injuries reported clinically may result from differences in opinion of the criteria for surgical exploration of the abdomen." These authors themselves rank the kidney, spleen, liver and pancreas in that order of injury frequency among the solid abdominal organs on the basis of their study of "158 patients with blunt abdominal trauma." The associated mortality, if any, was not presented. Others have ranked both the liver and the spleen as the most frequently injured organ. For example, Kennedy[3] (1960) points out that "Pathologists usually report rupture of the liver as the most common nonpenetrating injury to the abdomen" and that "clinicians usually place rupture of the spleen as more frequent." The matter is rendered even less clear by the fact that, frequently, multiple injuries occur and the cause of death cannot be discreetly attributed.

Virtually no experimental work has been uncovered in the literature with the expressed objective of quantifying abdominal impact tolerance and/or response. Clinical studies abound with detailed accounts of the nature, frequency, seriousness, and treatment of injuries resulting from blunt trauma to the abdomen, as well as hypotheses for the pathogenic mechanisms of such injuries. However, only fragmentary data have been presented expressing abdominal tolerance in the meaningful terms required by designers of protective impact environments—forces; rise time; duration; area, shape, and conformability of contact interface; and location and direction of blow.

Roberts[9] (1967) cited the works of Hellstrom,[10,11] Grimelius and Hellstrom,[12] Baxter and Williams,[8] and Williams and Sargent[13] in this area. A brief review of these studies will be given.

Hellstrom and Grimelius[10,11,12] (1965 to 1966) administered multiple dosed traumas to the right flanks (half way between the xiphoid process and the umbilicus) of twenty-three adult dogs ranging in weight from 29 to 77 pounds. The supine animals were impacted with a 34-pound pendulous hammer at velocity levels of 8.5 and 14.4 feet per second, representing energy levels of 38.6 and 110.6 foot-pounds, respectively. The hammer was a cylinder 3.15 inches in diameter with a spherical striking surface of 4.72-inch radius. The corresponding forces of impact ranged from 120 to 239 pounds at the lower velocity level, producing lateral compression of the dogs' bodies of from 50 to 70 per cent, to 290 to 580 pounds at the higher level, producing compressions of 70 to 80 per cent. The times required to develop maximum force were reported to vary from 30 to 90 milliseconds at the lower velocity level and from 30 to 50 milliseconds at the higher level. In general, the maximum body compression lagged the peak force by 30 to 45 milliseconds, indicating a substantial viscous contribution to the resisting force developed by the dogs' bodies. Of the twenty-three dogs used, only four were subjected to a single trauma prior to autopsy. One of these, exposed to an 8.5 feet-per-second blow, suffered "a solitary, deeply penetrating rupture of the liver," while the other three, after exposure to single blows of 14.4 feet per second, all suffered only "small capsular lacerations with superficial parenchymal damage." The dogs exposed to multiple traumas (as many as thirty-five blows per dog) in general suffered more severe liver damage, as well as damage to the spleen, lungs, and right adrenal gland. However, the significance of the extent of the injuries suffered as the result of the multiple traumas is difficult to assess.

Baxter and Williams[8] (1960) administered both anteroposterior and flank trauma to eighty dogs (weight range not given) constrained in a human-like sitting position. The pendulous impactor was "a solid weight, approximately the size of a steering wheel, in comparison with the relative dog size," and delivered 200 to 300 foot-pounds at impact. The striking velocities were not specified, although the inference was made that the 300 foot-pound blow corresponded to 7 mph. No data were given relating to the impact waveforms or to body compression. The numbers of injuries produced per impact were determined and associated with impactor area (6 versus 36 square inches), energy of impact (200 versus 300 foot-pounds), and site of trauma (A-P versus flank). Surprisingly, the number of injuries per dog was reported to increase with increasing area of contact. However, as noted by Roberts,[9] overall injury severity was not reported and may have actually decreased. The number of injuries also increased, as expected, with input energy level. Flank blows were reported to produce a fivefold increase in liver injury and a twofold increase in kidney injury compared to A-P trauma. Although not made clear in the original work, Roberts[9] indicates that all flank trauma was to the right side, consistent with the high increase in liver injury.

Williams and Sargent[13] (1962), in a study of the mechanism of traumatic intestinal injury, administered A-P trauma to forty-five dogs (weights not given). A 400-foot-pound dose was delivered by dropping a 50-pound weight 8 feet onto a board laid across the abdomen of the supine animal. The size, shape, and exact location of the board were not specified; nor were data relating to the force and time parameters. In ten cases, the A-P compression was limited by arresting the loading board 2.5 to 4 inches "anterior to the animal's posterior skin." What this represented in terms of percentage compression, however, was not given. The objective of this work was to investigate the validity of three long-standing hypotheses of the normal mechanism of intestinal rupture resulting from blunt abdominal trauma: (1) tearing at the intestinal "fixed points," (2) a sudden excessive increase in intraluminal pressure, and (3) crushing between the loading interface anteriorly and the vertebral column posteriorly. To simulate the human intestinal fixed points, a segment of ileum was sutured transversely across the spine in twenty dogs, and in four of these this segment was ligated bilaterally and filled, in two instances, with water and in two with air. Of the ten animals exposed to limited compression, two were provided with a fixed ileal segment. During the impact, pressures within the peritoneal space, stomach, small intestine, and sigmoid colon were recorded in various tests. Although other abdominal injuries were produced in this study, only intestinal lesions were reported. These ranged from serosal and mesenteric tears to complete luminal ruptures. The general character of the latter was not specified; i.e. whether the tears were oriented transversely, longitudinally, etc.

All of the injuries were located in the midline, intraperitoneal pressures actually exceeded intraluminal pressures and, when abdominal compression was limited, injuries either did not occur or consisted of minor membranous tears. All of the foregoing led the authors to conclude the following:

1. pressure plays little part in intestinal injury
2. compression with tearing between two opposing surfaces such as the abdominal wall and spine appears to be the most likely cause of intestinal and mesenteric injury
3. It would appear that a severe sudden blow to the abdomen by an object capable of compressing the anterior abdominal wall against the spine is required.
4. In both patients and dogs the site of injury cannot be related directly to intraluminal pressure, the usual fixed points or to the presence or absence of air and fluid in the intestinal lumen.

These findings are in sharp contrast to some prior opinions, as for example those expressed by Kennedy[3] as follows:

The most frequent sites of injuries to the intestinal tract are near points of fixation—the ligament of Treitz, the ileocecal junction and the area adjacent to the attached portions of the large intestine—where shearing force may be exerted. These portions of the bowel cannot move as readily in an acceleration type of accident and so are more likely to be torn. Gas and fluid, usually present in the gastrointestinal tract, particularly in the ileum, make this tract vulnerable to rupture from bursting pressure.

Probably the most meaningful reported abdominal data, from the standpoint of a justifiable, assumed link with human tolerance, are those deriving from the limited study of Winquist, Stumm and Hansen[14] (1953). Using a monorail decelerator device at the Edwards Air Force Base, traumas were administered to upright-seated, forward-facing hogs weighing from 63 to 197 pounds. One of the expressed objectives of this study was "to study the magnitude of forces required to produce internal injury under various conditions of deceleration." Two basic types of exposure were used: (1) impingement of the free moving animal against load cell supported targets both in the thoracic and abdominal areas and (2) abrupt whole body deceleration imposed by restraining belts.

The impact forces on the body were developed against three configurations of impingement block and, in the case of abdominal loading, were applied to both the midriff and the lower abdominal regions. Complete details of the impingement blocks were not given, but were described by the authors as follows: "Three impingement blocks were used, each resembling roughly an object likely to be struck in an aircraft cockpit during a crash. Block number 1 resembles a control wheel; number 2, a stick or lever-like projection; number 3, a large flat surface such as a radio box." The latter was further described as being 10 inches square. If a very rough scaling of the projecting peg is made from an illustration in the report, this would appear to be a rod 1 to 2 inches in diameter and 4 to 6 inches long with a rounded tip, and protruding from an 8 to 10-inch-wide (dimension in the plane of motion) surface. The rod was aligned along the axis of impact, i.e. aimed directly at the target site on the animal's body.

A reasonably complete account of the experimental procedure, test data and resulting injury pathology was provided and has enabled compilation of Tables 17-II and 17-III summarizing the midriff and lower abdominal loadings, respectively. Copies of the actual oscillograph records were given, from which the tabulated values of maximum force rise times and pulse durations were estimated. Also, illustrative plates prepared from selected frames of the high speed motion pictures for certain tests enabled a rough approximation to be made of the per cent body compression in these cases. For the lower abdomen, in addition to the control wheel impingment block tests, Table 17-III includes two snubs from a 3-inch-wide abdominal belt. The assumption that this represents essentially a concentrated abdominal loading is justified on the basis of the following statement by the authors: "The abdominal belt application used in these experiments does not parallel the lap belt application in aircraft unless one considers the case wherein the lap belt is worn, or is displaced, so as to become an abdominal belt."

Impact velocities near 20 feet per second were termed low velocities and those near 40 feet per second high velocities. Following each test the animal was autopsied and the injuries judged either survivable or fatal. As shown in the tables, all of the high velocity exposures—with forces ranging from 2360 to 6660 pounds—were fatal. A force of 1080 pounds against the 10-in-square target, a force of 893 pounds against the projecting peg, and a 750-pound loop load through the abdominal belt were all considered survivable. This study was limited and few experimental animals were used. The authors acknowledge that, ". . . the hog

TABLE 17-II
MIDRIFF LOADING Winquist et al.[14]

Type of Exposure	Hog Weight lb.	Impact Velocity ft./sec.	Maximum Force Applied lb.	MFRT*/PD† msec msec	Approx. Body Compression % of normal thickness	Description of Injuries
Control Wheel Impingement Block	95	20.7			40	*Survivable*—small subpleural and subendocardial hemorrhages; incomplete defect in anterior wall of stomach.
	100	40.7			80	*Fatal*—massive internal injuries including bilat. fract. disloc's at costochondral junct., ruptured diaphragmatic hernia, large inguinal hernias, perforation of stomach and intestines and laceration of spleen.
	166.5	39.1				*Fatal*—multiple comp. rib fract. bilaterally; destruction of liver; lacerations of pericardium, heart, right lung, diaphragm, colon and peritoneum.
Ten Inch Square Impingement Block	104	20.3	1080	48/95	30	*Survivable*—small subpleural and subendocardial hemorrhages; subserosal hemorrhage of the colon.
Ten Inch Square Impingement Block	95	39.5	2360	22/85		*Fatal*—massive internal injuries including multiple rib fract. and disarticulation, lacerations of pericardial sac, heart, pulmonary artery, stomach and intestines.
	156.5	40.3	6660	38/72		*Fatal*—massive internal injuries including multiple rib fract., hemorrhage and emphysema of lungs, multiple lacerations of liver and spleen, multiple ruptures of colon.
Projecting Peg Impingement Block	175	17.0	893	68/135	70	*Survivable*—Single rib fracture.
	149	39.7	3085	27/95	90	*Fatal*—massive internal injuries including puncture into right pleural cavity, comp. rib fract. bilaterally, laceration of pericardium, heart, right lung, diaphragm, liver, intestines, stomach and peritoneum.

* Maximum force rise time.
† Pulse duration.

TABLE 17-III
LOWER ABDOMINAL LOADING (Winquist et al.[14])

Type of Exposure	Hog Weight lb.	Impact Velocity ft./sec.	Maximum Force Applied lb.	MFRT*/PD† msec msec	Approx. Body Compression % of normal thickness	Description of Injuries
Control Wheel Impingement Block	185	23.6	2365	68/100	80	*Fatal*—petechiae over lungs, subepicardial ecchymosis over anterior portion of interventricular septum, hemorrhage in diaphragm, subcapsular hemorrhage of liver, multiple ruptures of wall of colon.
	187	39.6	5080	46/88	80	*Fatal*—massive internal injuries including laceration of rectus abdominus muscle, ruptured diaphragmatic hernia, lacerations of liver and spleen, pericapsular hemorrhage about left kidney, ruptures of colon.
Three Inch Wide Abdominal Belt	62.8	19.3	750 (loop load)	28/52		*Survivable*—subendocardial hemorrhage over septal portion of left ventricle and multiple subserosal hemorrhages of mid portion of jejenum.
	69.8	44.2	4700 (loop load)	38/60		*Fatal*—massive internal injuries including ruptured diaphragmatic hernia, ruptures of stomach and colon, fragmentation of spleen, lacerations of kidneys and liver.

* Maximum force rise time.
† Pulse duration.

differs markedly from man in bony structure and weight distribution." They also note, however that there is a gross resemblance of the internal anatomy of man to that of the hog. Furthermore, the hogs used approximated human weights; and the test conditions (i.e. impact or snub of the upright-seated free-moving animal) were very similar to those encountered by man in many accidental exposures. Therefore, it is felt that the results of this study, as summarized herein, and in the absence of more applicable data, might well be regarded as a starting point for approximating human tolerance to abdominal loading under similar conditions.

Definitive studies involving man as the test subject do not appear to have been carried out. Goldman[15] (1946) has reported a table of "Estimated Tolerances of Unprotected Human Body to Various Mechanical Forces" in which a "localized" abdominal exposure of 2000 pounds for 10 milliseconds, with syncopal response as the criterion, has been listed. No details were given regarding the method of loading, contact interface geometry, waveform of applied load, etc.

Very recently, the January 5 issue of *LIFE* magazine reported the record-breaking, unprotected underwater descent to 217½ feet made by a naval petty officer. At this depth, his entire body was exposed to a uniform external hydrostatic pressure of 96 psi above atmospheric. Under such conditions, one might expect severe abdominal compression and high diaphragmatic loading. The voluntary tolerance level was reached, however, because of painful pressure upon the ears. The subject in this experiment was reported to have an abnormally high lung capacity— some 34 per cent greater than average. These conditions were, of course, essentially static and the loading uniformly distributed as compared to the more concentrated impact loading with which this paper is mainly concerned.

A rather unusual investigation has been reported by Fryer[16] (1961) in which seated, restrained, forward-facing human subjects were propelled, underwater, at velocities up to 32.6 feet per second to simulate the ram pressures experienced at much higher velocities in air, as during ejection from a high velocity aircraft. In these tests, the subject held his breath and probably was in a state of high muscle tension. The loading situation was essentially static, with the subject forced against the surface of a high contoured seat back by a complex pressure gradient acting over the thoracic and abdominal areas with maximum pressures acting at stagnation points. An attempt was made to measure, at two locations, the changes in trunk thickness associated with the applied ram pressures. The transducer employed consisted of a pair of coils attached, one anteriorly and one posteriorly, to the body. A current was passed through one of the coils. The induced current in the second coil was monitored and related to the change in trunk thickness. No mention of linearity is made, but the accuracy was judged to be of the order of ±.1 inch. The two locations of measurement were at the level of the second intercostal space (where the normal respiratory excursion was found to be only about .15 inch), and at the umbilicus. At ram pressures of from 4 to 5 psi, the reported A-P deformation of the chest and abdomen were similar and were of the order of ¾ to 1¼ inches.

THORAX

Injuries to the thorax and their prophylaxis comprise a major problem area, especially as related to automobile accidents. Of the more serious thoracic injuries, extensive skeletal damage and pulmonary lesions (pneumothorax, hemothorax, hemopneumothorax, "wet lung," pulmonary contusions and lacerations, etc.) appear to be the most common.[4,5,17,18,19] Several studies, however, have sharply focused attention upon the incidence of injuries to the cardiovascular system—both of the dangerous/fatal and reversible/survivable types. Leinoff[20] (1940) reported the results of a study undertaken to "determine the frequency of acute cardiac damage following fatal automobile accidents". The autopsy records of fifty nonselected and consecutive traffic fatalities in New York City demonstrated "definite macroscopic findings of damage" in 16 per cent of the victims. More recently Greendyke[21] (1966) has reported that of 218 autopsied traffic accident fatalities during the four-year period 1961 to 1965 in Monroe County, New York, 16 per cent had suffered rupture of the aorta. Bright and Beck[22] (1935) were the first to suggest a high incidence of reversible/survivable cardiac injury associated with trauma but generally overlooked by the standard diagnostic procedures. Sigler[23] (1945) attributes the first attempt to determine the incidence of such injury to Barber[24] (1942), who conducted EKG studies on a series of thirty-three cases of chest trauma and found that eight of this group manifested abnormalities. Sigler himself conducted a similar EKG study on forty-two cases of patients who had sustained "rather serious accidental injuries to the body," not limited to the chest as with Barber. In 76 per cent of Sigler's patients there was "demonstrable evidence of some cardiac damage, clinical, electrocardiographic, or both." The most recent study of this type has been that of Lasky et al.[25] (1968). The important results of this work are twofold. First, the problem of frequent traumatic cardiovascular injury is reiterated. Secondly, the protective benefits deriving from the performance of the recently incorporated energy-absorbing steering assemblies in traffic accidents are demonstrated. This will be treated in more detail later.

Although still very limited in extent, there has been more experimental injury work done concerning the thorax than the abdomen. As previously indicated, thoracic injuries are well represented in the clinical literature, and various studies of injury mechanisms have been reported. There remains, however, only limited quantitative data related directly to the response and tolerance of the human thorax to impact loading.

Mechanistic studies using animals have specialized on injury to the tracheobronchial structure and, to a greater extent, the cardiovascular system. Considerable attention has been directed to the latter, especially with regard to the heart proper and the thoracic aorta. In their classic experimental work, Bright and Beck[22] traumatized the exposed hearts of dogs by administering mechanical impacts directly to the myocardium. They expressed surprise at the resistance to trauma which the heart demonstrated and, as noted, pointed out the probability of a relatively high frequency of reversible heart injury.

Clinically the most frequent site of aortic rupture is at the ismuth, in close proximity to the ligamentum arteriosum. That a localized weakness is represented by this area was suggested as early at 1924 by Letterer[26] and has been reemphaized often by others, most recently, Lasky et al.[25] Both the hypothesis advanced by Cammack et al.[27] (1959) and the more recent experimental findings of Roberts[9] (1965) have indicated that excessive intrathoracic displacement of the heart relative to the major points of fixation, and not sudden excessive increases in intraluminal pressure, is the chief cause of aortic tears. This would seem to be borne out by the clinical observation that aortic tears, practically always, are of a transverse rather than a longitudinal orientation.

In a study of the mechanism of traumatic vascular injuries Roberts et al.[9] administered blunt thoracic trauma to fifty-five dogs weighing from 18 to 34 pounds. The dogs were supported dorsally in the erect, seated position, and blows to the midsternum were delivered with a 14-pound rotary hammer. The latter was a 3½ inch in diameter steel cylinder with a flat striking surface. Impact velocities ranging from 17 to 25 feet per second with associated energy levels of 57 to 120 foot-pounds, respectively, were used. The investigation consisted of an acute series and a chronic series, the development of post-traumatic aneurysms being of interest in the latter. Injuries produced in the acute series were severe and included tears of the pericardium and major vessels as well as ruptures of the right atrium, pulmonary hematomas and fractures of the liver. Surprisingly, no rib fractures were produced by any of the anteroposterior blows, even though the sternum is reported to have been depressed hard against the vertebral column. The vascular tears produced were invariably located posterior and usually biased to the right side of the vessel involved. Aortic tears were always at the base of the ascending aorta, and those of the brachial-cephalic and subclavian arteries occurred at the points of bifurcation from the aorta. Roberts concludes, and offers confirmation from Lloyd,[28] that the heart was displaced into the left chest under load. This, of course, would be necessary to establish sternovertebral contact. Lloyd calls attention to the fact that the highly cartilaginous canine thorax can undergo severe distortions, the lateral diameter nearly doubling when the sternum is pressed against the spine.

Roberts concluded that this complex heart motion, mainly into the left chest, gave rise to tearing stresses in the vascular walls which produced the lesions. It is interesting that no tears near the ligamentum arteriosum were reported and suggests the possibility of a somewhat different stress environment than that frequently existing in the human. Roberts himself suggests this possibility and points to three pertinent anatomical differences between the dog and man: (1) differences in shape and cartilage content of the thoracic skeleton, (2) different number of great vessels branching from the aorta (human—3, dog—2), and (3) different size and shape of the mediastinum. These experiments, however, demonstrate convincingly that, for the experimental conditions used, the mechanism of vascular tearing resulting from blunt thoracic trauma to the dog was one of displacement loading and did not involve excessive intraluminal pressures.

The typical hammer deceleration-time history presented by Roberts is somewhat surprising in that the inferred dynamic load-compression characteristic of the chest is found to rise rapidly to a level which is then maintained constant throughout practically the entire compression stroke until sterno vertebral contact occurs. The impact force values were not given. It is stated that hammer acceleration, pulse duration and impact velocity could not be correlated with the degree of injury. However, increasing net input energy did show a positive correlation with increased injury.

Other studies, however, have indicated that hydraulic pressure, per se, can be the predominating mechanism in cardiac damage. Bright and Beck,[23] from a clinical analysis of 152 fatal heart rupture cases, proposed as injury mechanisms both anteroposterior compression between the sternum and spine as well as an indirect sudden compression of the abdomen and/or legs. With regard to the former, it was stated: "It would seem that this compression would be more destructive if it were applied at the moment when the heart is filled with blood and is beginning to contract as at the end of diastole and at the beginning of systole." Leinoff[20] also noted: "During systole the heart wall is under tension and trauma at that moment may rupture or damage this organ."

Very recently Life and Pince[29] (1968) have reported the results of experimental research "performed to determine if cardiac injury, as a consequence of thoracic impact, is related to the contractile state of the myocardium at the time of the impact." Twenty-six male dogs weighing from 44 to 55 pounds were supported dorsally in the supine position by a deep V-block cradle. A 40.15-pound weight with a 4-inch diameter steel disc as the striking surface was dropped from 6.5 feet (260 foot-pounds at 20.4 feet per second) through a guide tube aimed at the animal's midsternum. All dogs were subjected to the same exposure, and the measured responses were reported to vary only a few per cent over the entire series, despite variations in animal weight and whether or not skeletal damage was produced. Typical impact characteristics were reported as a maximum force of approximately 1040 pounds developed in 20 milliseconds with an overall pulse duration of 50 milliseconds. A-P body compressions were estimated to be 50 per cent of the exterior A-P diameter or greater, but were not actually measured.

Under these experimental conditions and at this energy level, a remarkably high frequency of cardiac damage was reported:

> Summarizing the results, all animals impacted during either ventricular diastole or systole had rupture(s) of one or both atria. Eighty-five per cent of the animals impacted during ventricular systole had ruptures of one or both ventricles while none of the animals impacted during ventricular diastole had ventricular ruptures.

In addition, five cases of aortic ruptures were reported, with the lesions all occurring in the arch, generally in proximity to the ligamentum anteriosum. Minor rib fractures were reported to have occurred in about 26 per cent of the cases. Although in these experiments, the energy level used was great enough to produce cardiac rupture (either atrial or ventricular) in 100 per cent of the cases, the authors conclude that their findings "suggest that the contractile status of the heart is perhaps the single most important factor in rupture injury."

The results of this study differ in several respects from those reported by Roberts[9] and by Lloyd.[28] Mainly, these differences are as follows: (1) the 100 per cent frequency of cardiac ruptures with limited vascular damage, (2) location of the vascular damage which did occur, (3) the occurrence of rib fractures in 26 per cent of the cases, and (4) the apparent absence of sternovertebral contact. It may be that the deep V-block cradle used introduced the element of lateral constraint, thus limiting the extent of lateral diametral increase. It would be expected that heart movement under such circumstances would be inhibited but that the organ would be subjected to more severe anteroposterior compression with increased vulnerability to rupture. Also, lateral constraint might well be a factor predisposing the thoracic skeleton to fracture damage.

Heart damage from sudden compression of the lower body has also been indicated clinically and produced experimentally. Bright and Beck[22] cited cases from the literature and also investigated this hypothesis experimentally. The cases of a man suddenly engulfed to the waist in a sandbank and of a boy loaded against the anterior trunk by a heavy tube swinging from a crane are cited. Both instances were characterized by fatal heart rupture. The experiments reported consisted of encapsulating the legs and abdomen of dogs within a rubber bag connected to an air supply. Body compression was effected by inflating the bag to pressures of 2.3 to 11.6 psi. However, this was essentially a static loading as it was reported that "It required about 15 seconds for the pressure in the bag to rise to 120 mm Hg." Concerning the results the authors state the following:

> In these experiments, we found that acute cardiac dilation and failure could be produced, but in none of the experiments was the heart actually ruptured. Small hemorrhages in the epicardium and myocardium were not uncommon. The right auricular pressure showed a marked rise when the legs and abdomen were compressed, and it is probable that under certain circumstances actual rupture takes place in this way.

Later, Joffe[30] (1949) and Fasola et al.[31] (1955) both reported experiments in which dogs were snubbed through an abdominal belt placed at the level of the chondrocostal arch. A line was attached to the belt and the snubbing action delivered in a more or less caudocephalad direction as if the subject had fallen from a ledge with the line tethered. Again, the quantitative data provided is sparse and cannot be adequately specified. Dilation of the heart was observed both by autopsy and with high speed x-rays. The animals not deliberately sacrificed died eventually of congestive heart failure attributed to myocardial damage. Associated lesions included potentially fatal liver injury and acute passive congestion of vital organs.

Fasola et al.[31] cite Potain (1894) as having proposed a vascular pressure mechanism of heart damage and actually demonstrating heart rupture experimentally "with pressure differentials of 896 mm Hg." The specific paper by Potain is not identified, however.

In a study of the mechanism of rupture of the main bronchi in closed chest injury Lloyd et al.[28] (1958) administered trauma to sixty-four dogs (weighing apparently 25 to 30 pounds) by impacting the animals with a 50-pound sandbag. The bag was both dropped onto the chest of supine animals and swung, pendulum fashion, against the chest of animals supported in the upright-seated position. A 12 to 14-inch length of 2 × 4 lumber was laid across the sternum and transmitted the blow to the dog's body. The input energies and forces developed in this manner are not clear. It is implied that the 50-pound mass was dropped from both 5 and 10 feet elevations and at other times was swung from a 5-foot elevation. Forces of 750 and 1500 pounds were said to have characterized the drops when the weight was arrested in 4 inches. However, these are simply the force relationships computed using square wave (constant force) deceleration theory, and would be expected to bear little relationship to the actual resisting forces developed by the dogs' bodies.

The input energies used, however, were sufficient to bottom the sternum against the vertebral column, for one group of tests was run in which sternovertebral contact was deliberately precluded by as little as ¼ inch.

To test the theory that a closed glottis increases bronchial vulnerability to blunt trauma, both patent and occluded airways were investigated. Although the frequency of bronchial ruptures was increased fivefold (74% versus 14%) with a closed airway, the authors attribute the damage not to blowout from excessive endobronchial pressure but to the effects of laterally directed equal and opposite forces acting upon the trachea at the carina. These forces, it is affirmed, are developed as the result of the extensive increase in transverse diameter of the chest concomitant with extreme A-P compression. If the lungs remain fixed to the chest wall, their lateral spacing is increased, loading the bronchi in tension and inducing failure in the proximity of the carina. It is stated that a tensile force of approximately 6.5 pounds acting in this way through the bronchi (presumably canine) is sufficient to induce failure. These impact exposures were severe in general, and in addition to the bronchial lesions, major damage to the cardiovascular system and liver was produced. Of the sixty-four dogs used in the investigation, bronchial ruptures were produced in twenty-four (75% on the left side). However, thirty-nine dogs died as the result of injuries other than rupture of the bronchus. It is interesting to note that in Roberts'[9] study no bronchial damage was produced. The method of loading differed somewhat and open airways were apparently used, although as noted previously, extreme chest compressions were the rule in both studies.

Surprisingly, when the sternum was deliberately arrested during compression by as little as ¼ inch short of vertebral contact, even with the airway occluded, five out of five dogs survived the trauma with neither bronchial nor fatal vascular injuries. In addition, when the 2×4 interface board was replaced by one 6 inches wide, still with a closed airway, only minor mucosal bronchial tears are reported to have resulted. The incidence of other than bronchial injuries is not given; nor is the extent of A-P chest compression which was developed using the 6-inch wide board. Likewise, when the loading interface was made a 1½-inch wide board and the airway maintained closed, bronchial ruptures were also absent but severe damage to the lung parenchyma resulted. It is assumed that no deliberate limitation of compression was used with either the 1½-inch or the 6-inch interface boards, but this is not stated in the paper.

In a recent clinical study, Chesterman and Satsangi[32] (1966) lend support to Lloyd's theory of failure by noting that 80 per cent of their case ruptures have been located within 1 inch of the carina. These authors, however, also note that there are occasional cases of posterior tracheal and bronchial blowout indicating excessive sudden internal pressure. Infrequent tracheal rupture above the carina is attributed to a shearing failure between adjacent tracheal rings. The authors further note the following: "No evidence of rupture of the trachea has been found in a patient who survived, which could be attributed to direct compression between the spine and the manubrium sterni."

In the study of Winquist et al.,[14] previously referred to, three tests were conducted during which thoracic impacts were administered to the hogs. In all cases, the control wheel impingement block was used. The animals weighed 168, 178, and 197 pounds, and the impact velocities were approximately 40, 16, and 22 feet per second, respectively. The high velocity impact was fatal, whereas both low velocity runs were judged survivable. Only in the 22 feet-per-second run was a force measurement made. This was reported as having a peak of 1320 pounds. Massive internal injuries were produced by the high velocity impact including laceration of the heart and transection of the great vessels, trachea and right main bronchus. The 16 feet-per-second run resulted in a simple sternal fracture, emphysematous blebs and subpleural hemorrhages of both lungs, subepicardial petechiae and superficial hepatic lacerations. These injuries were judged survivable. The 22 feet-per-second, 1320-pound impact resulted only in bilateral disarticulation of the first ribs from the sternum and minor pulmonary damage.

In 1946, a study, (Research Project X-630) was carried out at the United States Medical Research Institute* during which young (19 years average) male volunteers were subjected to both static and impact load applications to the torso through various configurations of restraint harness. Several reports by Bierman et al.[33,34,35,36] provide a well documented account of this work. Loads were applied to the body through the following: (1) the conventional aviator's safety harness of that time—a pair of suspender-like shoulder straps passing over the clavicular area bilaterally, converging slightly, and buckled into a lap strap in the vicinity of the umbilicus (approximately 76-square-inch body contact area); and (2) a

---

* National Naval Medical Center, Bethesda, Maryland

nylon "vest-type garment" of approximately twice the body contact area of the conventional harness. Superiorly this vest blended into bilateral shoulder straps and, inferiorly, into lap straps.

The experimental procedure consisted of supporting the volunteer in an essentially supine orientation and passing the shoulder and pelvic straps over supports to direct the pulls approximately 90 degrees to the longitudinal body axis at the shoulders and essentially as a lap restraint below. The four strap segments were then brought together at a common point below the subject and attached, in series with a force-measuring link, to the loading apparatus. The latter consisted of a rod suspended from the force link and terminating at the free end in a flange for intercepting and arresting weights dropped from a desired elevation and guided by the rod.

Using the conventional harness, loads as high as 2500 pounds were sustained by volunteers. However, it was reported that, ". . . the usual level of the subject's tolerance was about 2000 pounds." Tolerance here was based upon pain and such minor injuries as "bone bruises, small costochondral or ligamentous separations, or even hemorrhage into the abdominal rectus muscles." An estimate of about 2.2 inches for body compression under a 2500-pound load was given. This was an overall compression made up from several contributions associated with the different strap segments comprising the harness and bearing upon the body in different areas. It was shown that the pressure distribution to the body through this conventional harness was highly nonuniform with highest values existing in the abdominal region where the shoulder and lap straps were buckled together.

From the reports available, it was not clear whether the lap strap portion of the "vest-type garment" truly was directed so as to substantially load the pelvic girdle, or whether this load was applied for the most part to the lower thoracic or upper abdominal areas. The latter would seem to be inferred by the authors' remark: "The subjects were placed in a supine position on the impact decelerator, and static loads or impact forces were applied to the anterior chest wall and abdomen by a vest-type restraining harness. . . ." However, an illustration in one of the reports[42] suggests the possibility of some pelvic support.

With this vest restraint, the authors reported that volunteers were subjected to impact loads of up to 3300 pounds without injury. This maximum load was developed by dropping 165 pounds from 5 feet, approximately 12 mph. The times to peak load varied from 50 to 70 milliseconds and the total pulse durations averaged 150 milliseconds. It was stated as follows: "Attempts to exceed this force [3300 pounds] have led to injuries." However, what maximum forces were developed and the extent of the injuries produced were not given.

In addition to the impact loads, maximum static forces of 550 pounds applied through the vest were repeatedly tolerated for periods of from 10 to 80 seconds, although in several instances during the period of load application both the radial pulse and respiration of the volunteer were absent. It was further reported that, in several of the maximum load static tests (550 pounds), a single measurement of pressure was made under the vest in the right pectoral area and that these averaged 2.7 psi.

It is suspected that the table presented by Goldman[15] may have been derived from studies of this type. In addition to the 2500 pounds, 10 milliseconds, figure suggested for the abdomen, the following "estimated tolerances" for the chest were given: >600 pounds static load with respiratory distress as the tolerance criterion; and >1000 pounds for 10 milliseconds dynamically with pain as the criterion. However, in none of the Project X-630 tests reported were loads applied exclusively to the abdomen.

Experimental work in which thoracic response and tolerance levels were determined using human cadavers is presented in two publications by Patrick et al.[37,38] (1966 to 1967). In this research program, embalmed human cadavers were seated on the sled of a horizontal accelerator and accelerated to a specified velocity. After reaching the desired velocity, the sled was abruptly stopped. During the deceleration of the sled, the cadavers slid forward relative to the sled and impacted knee, chest and head load cell supported targets which were rigidly attached to the sled. A 6-inch diameter, flat padded surface was used as the chest impactor. For each run, a time history of the total load applied to the thorax was obtained. The corresponding displacement of the sternum relative to the thoracic vertebrae was obtained by photographically monitoring the movement of a probe attached to the sternum and passed through the thoracic cavity. Cross plotting the load-time and the displacement-time data, dynamic load-deflection curves for the chest were obtained.

The dynamic load-deflection curves resulting from these studies are presented in Figures 17–1 and 17–2. The curves shown in Figure 17–1 are for the same cadaver subjected to increasing severities of sled impact. The first rib fracture, as determined by radiological examination, occurred during the 16.8 mph sled impact. Additional rib fractures were noted after the 19.5 mph sled impact. The sudden increase in load (400 pounds) without apparent deflection of the chest probe for the 16.8- and 19.5-mph impacts was caused by the angulation of the chest load cell. In the loading sequence, the inferior portion of the sternum was the first part of the thorax to contact the chest target. Since the chest probe was attached to the thorax above midsternum, the initial load applied to the lower end of the sternum resulted in only a very small movement of the probe. The unusual shape of the unloading cycle of these curves was conjectured to

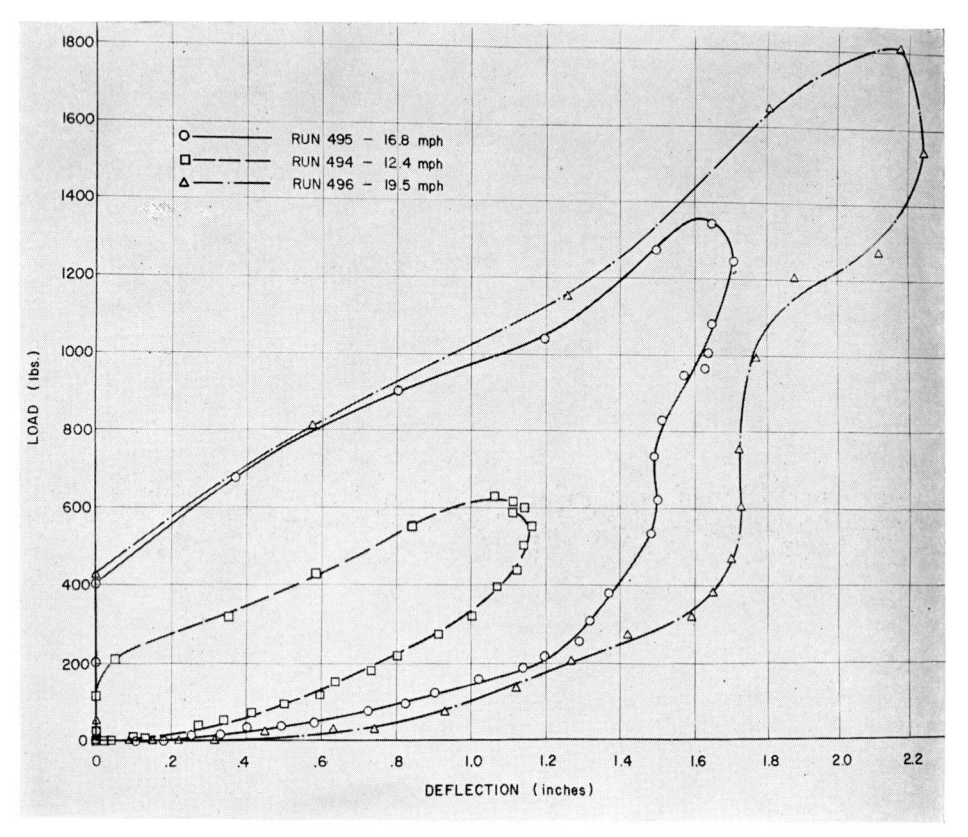

FIGURE 17-1. Dynamic load-deflection characteristics of the thorax of a cadaver for increasing impact severity (Patrick et al.[38]).

reflect a combination of probe distortion and frictional forces acting on the probe during retraction into the body.

The thoracic load-deflection characteristics for three different cadavers, whose thoraxes were initially intact, are depicted in Figure 17-2 for the same severity of sled impact (approximately 16.5 mph). The pertinent chest impact parameters for these runs are listed in Table 17-IV. Several interesting points are immediately apparent from this set of curves and the corresponding tabular data: (1) The rib fracture patterns of all cadavers were similar, (2) The initial thoracic stiffnesses for the cadavers of Runs 386 and 389 are approximately 1000 pounds per inch, and (3) The maximum chest load (1340 and 1400 pounds) and the corresponding maximum chest deflections (1.7 and 1.5 inches) for the cadavers used in Runs 495 and 389, respectively, are of the same order of magnitude. An additional observation was that for Runs 386 and 389, the "knees" in the curves, occurring between the 900 to 1000-pound load level, may well have corresponded to the initiation of rib fractures.

TABLE 17-IV
COMPARISON OF THORACIC IMPACT RESULTS FOR THREE CADAVERS SUBJECTED TO IDENTICAL SLED IMPACT CONDITIONS
(Patrick et al.[37,38])

Run No.	Cad. Wt. lb.	Sled Vel. mph	Max. Chest Load lb.	Max. Chest Defl. in.	Initial Chest Stiffness lb./in.	Radiological Examination
386	195	16.5	1600	2.5	1000	Strong suspicion of incomplete fracture of right second, third, and fourth ribs just distal to the costochondral junction.
389	160	16.5	1400	1.5	1000	Fractures of right third, fourth, fifth, and possibly sixth rib in the anterior axillary line and questionable fracture of left fourth rib in A–A line.
495	140	16.8	1340	1.7	*	Fracture of left third, fourth, fifth ribs in anterior axillary line.

* No initial stiffness measurement because of poor angulation of chest target; however, after this angulation effect is negated by torso rotation, the load corresponding to a 1-inch deflection is approximately 1000 pounds.

Static thoracic stiffness measurements were also made using three embalmed human cadavers with previously undamaged thoracic skeletons. For these cases, the static loads were applied through a 4-inch wide, weighted bar (25 to 30 square inches contact area) suspended from a spring scale and lowered onto the mid-chest with a chain fall. A-P move-

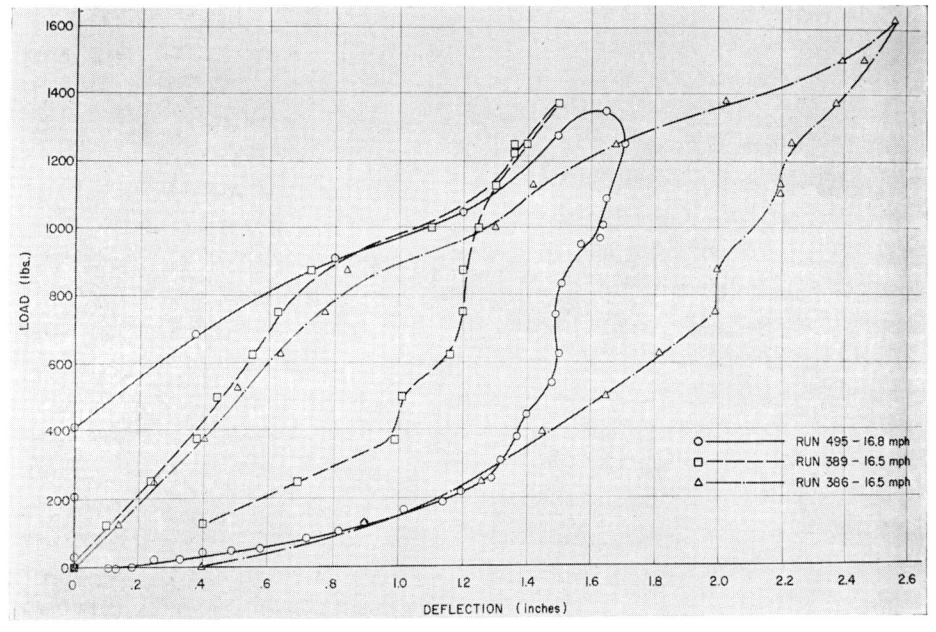

FIGURE 17-2. Dynamic load-deflection characteristics for three different cadavers at approximately the same impact speed, 16.5 to 16.8 mph (Patrick et al.[38]).

ment of the loading bar, corresponding to chest deflection, was measured with a dial indicator. The resulting static thoracic load-deflection characteristics for the three cadavers are depicted in Figure 17–3. At an applied load of 100 pounds, the range of static stiffness extended from 185 to 400 pounds per inch. It was noted that these stiffnesses represent only stabilized measurements made following three or four previous loadings, and, in general, the stiffness associated with the first load application was somewhat less than that determined from successive loadings.

In addition, Patrick[37] conducted a series of tests in which volunteers applied static chest loads using their own muscular power. In each case, the loading surface was the same 6-inch diameter target used for the cadaver impact tests. The maximum force developed by pulling the chest against the load cell was 400 pounds with padding and 300 pounds without padding. Neither one of these loads produced injury or excessive discomfort to the thorax.

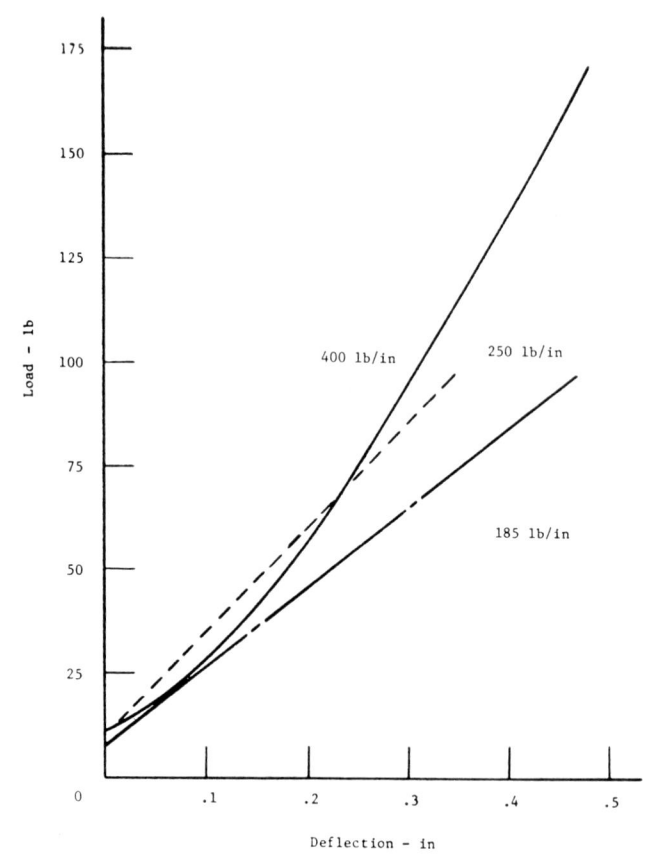

FIGURE 17–3. Static force-deflection characteristics of the undamaged thoraxes of three cadavers (Patrick et al.[37]).

Jude et al.[39] (1964) report that during external cardiac resuscitation on an average adult, a force of 60 to 100 pounds is required to depress the lower third of the sternum 4 to 5 cm, which gives a thoracic stiffness of 50 to 60 pounds per inch. It is important to note that the load is applied with a small area (the heel of the hand) on the lower third of the sternum (the least rigid portion of the bony thorax). Both of these conditions are conducive to maximum deflection for minimum applied load which is ideal for external cardiac resuscitation. Consequently, this static thoracic stiffness range of 50 to 60 pounds per inch is less, as would be expected, than the range given by Patrick[37] of 185 to 400 pounds per inch.

The appreciable difference between the static (185 to 400 pounds per inch) and dynamic (1000 pounds per inch) thoracic stiffness for embalmed cadavers is the result of the fundamental difference between loading the thorax by a blow delivered in a matter of milliseconds and compressing the chest less rapidly between rigid surfaces. In the latter case, a force is applied to the front of the body and an equal and opposite reaction is developed at the back, with resulting deformation determined by the static stiffness and fracture characteristics of the body. On the other hand, when the chest is subjected to an impact loading on the sled, there is no force reaction developed upon the back. Rather, an inertial force gradient, due to the forces required to decelerate the internal organs, viscera, and bony structure of the thorax, extends across the thickness of the body and diminishes from a maximum value at the site of loading to zero at the surface of the back. Owing to the complexity of the body mass distribution and the presence of flexibly attached thoracic viscera, this force gradient is not a simple relationship. Also, the dynamic force-deflection characteristics are influenced by the viscous behavior (sensitivity to rate of loading) of the fluid-filled body tissues and organs which tend to increase the thoracic stiffness.

The data given by Patrick et al.[37,38] guided the General Motors Corporation in selecting the crush level for its energy-absorbing steering assembly designated the "EA column." An evaluation of this column using embalmed cadavers as subjects is given by Gadd and Patrick[40] (1968). The setup for their evaluation consisted of mounting an automobile body buck on the sled of a horizontal accelerator. A steering assembly with an EA column was mounted in the body buck. In two of the three tests, the wheel and column were instrumented so that the force on the steering wheel rim could be distinguished from the force on the steering wheel hub. Two cadavers with undamaged thoracic structures were used as subjects. For a given run, the cadaver was placed on a standard automobile bench seat directly in front of the steering assembly and lap belted in position. The sled, body buck, and cadaver were accelerated to the desired velocity and then decelerated according to a prescribed pulse. During the deceleration, the cadaver rotated around the lap belt and impacted the steering assembly.

The EA column was evaluated using two different sets of sled speeds and corresponding stopping distances: (1) 24.4 mph and 18 inches, and (2) 29.4 mph and 24 inches. The shape of the deceleration pulse in each case was approximately rectangular. The crush of the energy-absorbing elements of the columns ranged from 4 to 5¾ inches. The results of the evaluation, shown in Table 17-V, indicate that the total loading developed against the steering system was quite consistent, ranging from 1630 to 1810 pounds independent of initial conditions. The chest loading against the hub plate was 740 and 550 pounds and the net body loading against the rim and spokes was 1070 and 1080 pounds, respectively, for the two tests in which instrumentation permitted separation of loads. The radiologist found no evidence of thoracic skeletal damage after the first test on each of the two cadavers. However, Cadaver 1085 was impacted a second time at the higher sled speed of 29.4 mph. After this impact, x-rays indicated fractures of three, possibly four, ribs and fracture of the lower half of the sternum. In all runs, chest deflection, as measured using the chest probe technique previously described, was less than 1 inch, corresponding to the low values of measured hub loads. The relatively high values of net rim-spoke loads were attributed to the "wrap around" effect of the shoulders and upper limbs.

The basis for the design of the EA column is further substantiated through the evaluation of actual automobile accidents in which an EA column was involved. In their analysis of cardiothoracic injuries resulting from frontal impact accidents, Lasky et al.[25] (1968) present statistical findings relating to the effectiveness of the EA column. A rating system was developed to classify the degree of severity of cardiovascular injury. The classification consisted of four groupings: (1) Minimal—disorder of rhythm, (2) Moderate—contusion, (3) Severe—laceration, (4) Fatal. Regarding the relationship between cardiovascular injury and other thoracic injury, the authors state, "Cardiovascular injury appeared to be associated frequently with injury to the thoracic cavity, especially in the more severe cardiovascular injuries, but it could still occur with no evidence of thoracic damage." As a verification of this statement, the authors present one case where a moderate cardiovascular injury occurred without thoracic lesions. Other investigators[20,22,23,27,41] have also noted that cardiovascular injury can occur without fracturing of the bony thorax, particularly in young people, whose chests are more flexible and consequently can undergo greater deformations without rib fracture. The authors state further, "In a large proportion of the cases, the thoracic injury consisted

TABLE 17-V
PEAK LOADS OBTAINED FROM ACCELERATOR TESTS OF STEERING ASSEMBLY (Gadd and Patrick[4])

Test Conditions	Run No.	Cad. No.	Chest Load on Hub Plate lb.	Net Force on Wheel Rim Alone lb.	Force Through Crush Element lb.	Total Force of Upper Body on Wheel and Hub lb.	Lap Belt Load on Subject lb.
24.4 mph 18 in. stop		840			1130	1680	1360
24.4 mph 18 in. stop	488	1035	740	1070	1160	1810	1280
29.4 mph 24 in. stop	489	1035	550	1080	1200	1630	1340

of fracture of the bony thoracic cage . . . usually of one or more rib fractures but occasionally a fracture of the sternum was seen."

In twenty-four cases, in which column collapse ranged from ¼ to 5½ inches, there were only two cases in which a moderate cardiovascular injury was found, and both of these cases involved rib fracture. An additional note—one of these two cases involved a paraplegic with special accessory hardware attached to the steering column. In a comparable group of fifteen frontal accidents involving cars with a rigid steering column and standard steering wheel there were ten cases in which there was cardiovascular injury (seven moderates, one severe, and one fatal) and rib fracture occurred in nine out of ten of these cases. In the one case without rib fracture, a moderate cardiovascular injury occurred. These first published field statistics demonstrate that the EA column has significantly mitigated thoracic injuries. This conclusion in turn implies a degree of confidence in the preliminary thoracic tolerance data upon which the impact performance of the EA column was based.

CONCLUSION

In view of the foregoing summary of reported experimental studies concerning thoracic/abdominal tolerance and response to mechanical loading, there is an obvious need for much more work to be done. The coming years will undoubtedly see substantial strides made until, ultimately, sufficient quantitative data have become available to enable the designer of protective environments to intelligently approach optimization.

In the course of conducting this literature search, one outstanding problem became apparent. In many carefully planned and executed investigations, the potential usefulness to persons with a need for tolerance and response data is not fully realized. Frequently, the objectives, per se, of such studies are rather specialized in nature and require only a minimum of quantified impact parameter data. For example, studies of the general relationship of trauma to physiological responses exemplify this. If, however, such experiments were designed with more awareness of their full potential usefulness and some added effort applied to instrumentation and detailed reporting, the store of meaningful human tolerance and response data could be increased significantly.

As the result of both the foregoing observations and a critical evaluation of personal work, the following recommendations for instrumentation and reporting practice are given as guidelines for the design and documentation of research investigations of this type of maximize utility of results:

1. Measurement and presentation of the impact amplitude (force, pressure, acceleration)—time histories comprising the test event, given

in sufficient quantity to truly typify the study, and clear indentification of the location of all such measurements.
2. The impact velocity and, if an impacting "hammer" is used, the geometric and inertial properties.
3. Detailed description of the geometry and conformability (e.g., padding type and dynamic stiffness characteristics) of the impact interface.
4. Clear description of the site of loading and direction of load application.
5. Compression-time history of the test specimen at the site of loading or, better yet, a load-compression relationship covering both the loading and unloading phases.
6. An indication of the distribution of pressure over the loading interface, if possible.
7. Description of the geometry, weight and condition (physical, physiological, anatomical) of any experimental animals or other biological specimens employed.
8. A description of the geometry of any resulting injuries, e.g., location of lesion, whether ruptures were longitudinal or transverse, dimensions of lacerations and whether they were superficial or deeply penetrating, etc.
9. Description of the instrumentation used including performance characteristics—specifically, manufacturers identification and frequency response.
10. A clear, descriptive verbal and photographic documentation of the test apparatus and setup conditions used.
11. Illustrative high-speed movie sequences illustrating the test kinematics, if available.
12. When computed data are presented, a statement of the computational techniques employed and any assumptions made.

The foregoing list is comprehensive, and will be impractical to follow in many cases, but any investigation documented to such an extent would provide the interested reader the fullest opportunity for analysis of the work in accordance with his own specialized needs. Many questions would thereby be anticipated and answered in advance.

REFERENCES

1. KIHLBERG, J.K.: Driver and his right front passenger in automobile accidents. *Proceeding of the Ninth Stapp Conference.* 1965, pp. 335–354.
2. NAHUM, A.M.; SIEGEL, A.W., and TRACHTENBERG, S.B.: Causes of significant injuries in nonfatal traffic accidents. *Proceedings of the Tenth Stapp Conference.* 1966, pp. 182–196.

3. KENNEDY, R.H.: *Nonpenetrating Injuries of the Abdomen.* Springfield, Thomas, 1960.
4. PACE, W.G.; PASSARO, E., JR., and KLASSEN, K.P.: Experience with intrathoracic injury following automobile accidents. *Amer J Surg*, 99:827–832, 1960.
5. PACE, W.G.: Thoracic trauma. *J Mississippi Med Assoc*, 3:540–542, 1962.
6. HUELKE, D.F., and GIKAS, P.W.: Causes of deaths in automobile accidents. Final Report U. of Mich. ORA Project 06749, 1966.
7. STEPHENS. G.L.: Steering wheel blunt abdominal trauma. *J Kentucky Med Assoc*, 59:131–139, 1961.
8. BAXTER, C.F., and WILLIAMS, R.D.: Blunt abdominal trauma. *J Trauma*, 1961, pp. 241–247.
9. ROBERTS, V.L.: Experimental studies on thoracic and abdominal injuries. Proceedings of a Symposium—The Prevention of Highway Injury. Ann Arbor U. of Mich. 1967, pp. 211–215.
10. HELLSTRÖM, G.: Intra-vascular pressure response to closed liver injury: an experimental study in dogs. *Acta Soc Med Upsal*, 70:167–190, 1965.
11. HELLSTRÖM, G.: Electrocardiographic, blood pressure, respiratory and electroencephalographic responses to closed liver injury, an experimental study in dogs. *Acta Soc Med Upsal*, 70:152–166, 1965.
12. GRIMELIUS, L., and HELLSTRÖM, G.: Patho-anatomical changes after closed liver injury: an experimental study in dogs. *Acta Chir Scand*, 131:485–494, 1966.
13. WILLIAMS, R.C., and SARGENT, F.T.: The mechanism of intestinal injury in trauma. *J Trauma*, 3:288–294, 1963.
14. WINDQUIST, P.G.; STUMM, P.W., and HANSEN, R.: Crash injury experiments with the monorail decelerator. *AF Technical Report No. AFFTC 53-7*, April 27, 1953.
15. GOLDMAN, D.E.: Mechanical forces acting on aviation personnel. *J Aviation Med*, Oct. 1946, pp. 426–430.
16. FRYER, D.I.: The effects upon man of exposure to high ram pressure loads. *Flying Personnel Research Committee Report No. 1167*, Royal Air Force Institute of Aviation Medicine, Farnborough, Hants, 1961.
17. SAMUEL, E.: Deceleration injuries of heart and lung. Postgrad Med J, 39:695–704, 1963.
18. KEMMERER, W.T.; ECKERT, W.G.; GATHRIGHT, J.B.; REEMTSMA, K., and CREECH, O., JR.: Patterns of thoracic injuries in fatal traffic accidents. *J. Trauma*, 1:595–599, 1961.
19. RUSHMER. R.F., and HASS, G.M.: A comparison of crash injuries in man and in laboratory animals. *Report No. 1, Project No. 471*, 27th AAF Base Unit, AAF School of Aviation Medicine, Randolph Field, Texas, 1946.
20. LEINHOFF, H.D.: Direct nonpenetrating injuries of the heart. *Amer Int Med*, 14: 653–666, 1940.
21. GREENDYKE, R.M.: Traumatic rupture of aorta. *JAMA*, 195:119–122, 1966.
22. BRIGHT, E.F., and BECK, C.S.: Nonpenetrating wounds of the heart: a clinical and experimental study. *Amer Heart J*, 10:293–321, 1935.
23. SIGLER, L.H.: Traumatic injury of the heart. *Amer Heart J*, 30:459–478, 1945.
24. BARBER, H.: Electrocardiographic changes due to trauma. *Brit Heart J*, 4:83, 1942.
25. LASKY, I.I.; SIEGEL, A.W., and NAHUM, A.M.: Automotive cardiothoracic injuries: a medical-engineering analysis. Paper No. 680052 presented at SAE Automotive Engineering Congress, Detroit, Michigan, January 8–12, 1968.

26. LETTERER, E.: Beiträge zur entstehung der aortenruptur an typischer. *Stelle Virch Arch Path Anat*, 253:534–544, 1924.
27. CAMMACK, K.; RAPPORT, R.L.; PAUL, J., and BAIRD, W.C.: Deceleration injuries of the thoracic aorta. *Arch Surg*, 79:244–251, 1959.
28. LLOYD, J.R.; HEYDINGER, D.K.; KLASSEN, KARL P., and ROETTIG, L.C.: Rupture of main bronchi in closed chest injury. *Arch Surg*, 77:597–605, 1958.
29. LIFE, J.S., and PRINCE, B.W.: Response of the canine heart to thoracic impact during ventricular diastole and systole. *J Biomechanics*, July 1968. (In print. Also, personal communication with the author.)
30. JOFFE, M.H.: Anatomical and physiological factors involved in the tolerance to rapid deceleration. Doctorial Dissertation, Ohio State University, 1949.
31. FASOLA, A.F.; BAKER, R.C., and HITCHCOCK, F.A.: Anatomical and physiological effects of rapid deceleration. *WADC Technical Report*, 1955, pp. 54–218.
32. CHESTERMAN, J.T., and SATSANGI, P.N.: Rupture of the trachea and bronchi by closed injury. *Thorax*, 21:21–27, 1966.
33. BIERMAN, H.R., and LARSEN, V.R.: Distribution of impact forces on the human through restraining devices. Naval Medical Research Institute *Project X–630, Report No. 4*, Feb. 18, 1946.
34. BIERMAN, H.R., and LARSEN, V.R.: Reactions of the human to impact forces revealed by high speed motion picture technic. *NMRI Project X–630, Report No. 5*, April 25, 1946.
35. BIERMAN, H.R; WILDER, R.M., JR., and HELLEMS, H.K.: The principles of protection of the human body as applied in a restraining harness for aircraft pilots. *NMRI Project X–630, Report No. 6*, May 10, 1946.
36. BIERMAN, H.R.; WILDER, R.M., JR., and HELLEMS, H.K.: The physiological effect of compressive forces on the torso. *NMRI Project X–630, Report No. 8*, Dec. 19, 1946.
37. PATRICK, L.M.; KROELL, C.K., and MERTZ, H.J., JR.: Forces on the human body in simulated crashes. *Proceedings of the Ninth Stapp Conference.* 1966.
38. PATRICK, L.M.; MERTZ, H.J., JR., and KROELL, C.K.: Cadaver knee, chest and head impact loads. *Proceedings of the Eleventh Stapp Conference.* 1967.
39. JUDE, J.R.; KOUWENHOVEN, W.B., and KNICKERBOCKER, G.G.: External cardiac resuscitation. *Monogr Surg Sci*, 1:59–117, 1964.
40. GADD, C.W., and PATRICK, L.M.: System versus laboratory impact tests for estimating injury hazard. Paper No. 680053 presented at SAE Automotive Engineering Congress, Detroit, Michigan, Jan. 8–12, 1968.
41. LUNDEVALL, J.: Traumatic rupture of the aorta. *Acta Path Microbiol*, 62:29–33, 1964.
42. EVANS, F.G., and PATRICK, L.M.: Impact damage to internal organs. Proceedings of a Symposium on Impact Acceleration Stress. *Publication 977*, National Academy of Sciences, National Research Council, Washington, D.C., 1962, pp. 159–171.
43. SHEFTS, L.M.: *The Initial Management of Thoracic and Thoraco Abdominal Trauma.* Springfield, Thomas, 1956.

DISCUSSION

F. GAYNOR EVANS

This excellent review of the present state of knowledge about the tolerance of the human thorax and abdomen to impacts reveals areas in which future research is needed.

1. Data obtained from controlled impact experiments are badly needed in order to determine what the mechanisms of various types of serious or fatal injuries of the human thorax and abdomen actually are. At present, most of the explanations of the mechanics of such injuries are very speculative.

2. Most serious or fatal injuries from impacts to the thorax and abdomen result from trauma of the viscera rather than from trauma of the musculoskeletal system. Current knowledge of the mechanical properties of thoracic and abdominal viscera is inadequate. Much more is known about the behavior of bones and of bone under a variety of conditions than about viscera and soft tissues in general. The most extensive studies, as far as I am aware, of the strength characteristics of soft tissues and of organs are those made under the direction of Professor H. Yamada in the Department of Anatomy, Kyoto Prefectural University of Medicine, Kyoto, Japan. However, all the material was obtained from Japanese subjects. Similar studies should be made on non-Japanese material to determine if there are any statistically significant racial differences in the mechanical properties of various tissues and organs.

3. The majority of studies of the strength characteristics and other mechanical properties of biological material have been made under static conditions in which the load is slowly applied to the specimen in a materials-testing machine. The probable reason for this situation is that, until quite recently, there were no testing machines with which loads could be applied at controlled high strain rates. However, testing machines are now available with which loads can be applied at strain rates of several thousand inches per minute.

Investigations made with such machines show that the ultimate compressive stress and strain of compact bone increase with the speed of loading while the energy absorbed by the bone decreases. Similar studies of the behavior of the thorax and abdomen and their viscera under controlled high strain rates of loading are essential for a clearer understanding of the effects of impact injuries.

4. The physiological state of the viscera at the instance of impact should be considered in these studies. Mention has already been made of the different effects of impacts to the heart when it is in systole or diastole.

Perhaps the phase of respiration of the lungs or the amount of food in the stomach or intestines would affect the tolerance of these organs to impacts.

5. For obvious reasons, destructive impact tests cannot be made on living human subjects; therefore, we must depend on data obtained from experimental animals. However, caution should be exercised when interpreting human impact tolerance from animal data. For example, the thorax of quadrupedal mammals is quite different in shape from that of man. In an animal such as a dog or a cat, the diameter of the thorax in the sagittal plane is considerably greater than that in the frontal plane, while the human thorax is wider transversely than it is anteroposteriorly. Consequently, the radius of curvature, the slope, and the length of the ribs are quite different in a quadruped and in man. There are also differences in the structure of the animal and the human sternum. These factors would influence the behavior of the intact thoracic cage under impact loading. Species differences in the strength characteristics and other mechanical properties of the animal and the human thoracic cage, organs, and tissues may also play a part. Mesenteric supports of abdominal viscera in animals and in man are also different and may influence the tolerance of the organs to impacts.

The factors mentioned above may have little or no significant effects as far as the transferral of data obtained from impact studies on animals to man is concerned. However, until this is proven to be the case, these factors should be considered when designing an experiment and evaluating its results.

Chapter XVIII

IMPACT TOLERANCE OF HUMAN PELVIC AND LONG BONES

F. Gaynor Evans

INTRODUCTION

The tolerance of a body to an impact or a load that has been applied to it is a function of the size and shape of the body, and the mechanical properties of the material composing the body. This is true of a bone as well as of inorganic bodies.

It is common knowledge that a large piece of wood (e.g., oak) will support a greater load before breaking than will a small piece of the same type, shape, and dimensions. This, of course, is the result of differences in the size of the two pieces of wood. It is also well known that a steel rod requires a larger load or force to break it than does a wooden rod of exactly the same size and shape because of differences in the mechanical properties of steel and of wood.

Fractures usually arise from impacts or suddenly applied loads and thus are problems in energy absorption. Consequently, in studying impact tolerance of intact bones, the speed of loading must be considered because some of the mechanical properties of bone (compressive stress, modulus of elasticity, energy absorbing capacity) change with high strain rates of loading (McElhaney and Byars, 1965; Bird, Becker, Healer, and Messer, 1968; Burstein and Frankel, 1968). Similar behavior occurs in some engineering materials.

Although there is a considerable literature on the mechanical properties and limits of tolerance of whole bones and of standardized specimens of bone, practically all of the studies have been with materials testing machines under static or slowly applied loads. As far as I am aware, there are only a few investigations on the limit of tolerance of intact bones and of bone specimens under impact.

Most of the information on impact tolerance of bones has been obtained from studies of automobile and airplane crashes or impacts from free falls. The majority of crash injury studies are concerned with evaluation of the

Editors Note: This research was supported (in part) by Research Grant AM-03865-09 from NIH, USPHS.

injuries in terms of the part of the automobile or plane presumed to be responsible for the injury. In some cases, there are estimates of the g forces or accelerations acting on the vehicle at the time of the impact but there is little data, obtained under controlled experimental conditions, of the impact tolerance of various human bones.

TOLERANCE OF PELVIC BONES TO IMPACT

Tolerance of the intact human pelvis to static and dynamic loading under controlled experimental conditions has been investigated by Evans and Lissner (1955). Two series of tests were conducted.

In the first series of tests, twenty-two pelves, sixteen from embalmed dissecting room cadavers and six from fresh unembalmed bodies, were used. The pelves were obtained from sixteen white males, three Negro males, two white females and one Negro female. One of the Negro males was 29 years of age, but all the other specimens were from individuals between 50 and 85 years of age.

The pelvis and lumbar spine were removed from the body and defleshed. In some specimens, the sacrospinal and the sacrotuberal ligaments were also removed but in others they were preserved until ready for testing. The pelves from embalmed bodies were kept in embalming fluid and those from unembalmed bodies in a deep freezer.

The day before each test, the pelvis was coated with Stresscoat®, a brittle strain sensitive lacquer, and immediately before testing was covered with a sensitizing liquid. As soon as a test was completed, the liquid was wiped off and the specimen was sprayed with Statiflux® powder. During the spraying, the powder was given an electrostatic charge so that it collected in the cracks of the Stresscoat lacquer making them visible. The cracks were then traced with India ink so they could be easily seen in a photograph.

The specimen was suspended over a 140-pound steel block and a force dynamically applied to the ischial tuberosities by burning the supporting string. The weight of the specimen multiplied by the distance through which it was dropped gave the inch-pounds of energy applied to it. In each test, the pelvis was dropped so that both ischial tuberosities struck the steel block simultaneously. The specimen was caught by hand on the rebound so that it struck the block just once. Because of the low magnitude of the energy used in the tests (33.12 to 112.50 inch-pounds) it was assumed that, for all intents and purposes, all the available kinetic energy of a test was expended in deforming and/or fracturing the pelvis. The amount of energy transferred from the specimen to the steel block and absorbed by it would be negligible.

In the second series of tests, eight almost intact bodies of persons 47 to 82 years of age were used to determine the effect of the mass of the head, the trunk, and the upper limbs on pelvic deformations and fractures. In these cadavers, all of which were embalmed, the lower limbs, pelvic musculature, and viscera were removed and the pelvis stresscoated.

The body was then suspended over the steel block and dropped as in the first test series. Care was taken so that the ischial tuberosities struck the block simultaneously and that no other part of the body contacted the block. In some specimens, a half-inch of soft tissue (mainly gluteus maximus muscle and skin) was left under the ischial tuberosities to determine what effect this might have on the strain patterns produced in the pelves. The energy applied to the pelves ranged from a minimum of 200 inch-pounds to a maximum of 450 inch-pounds.

In the first series of tests, a minimum tensile strain pattern was produced in the embalmed pelvis of a white male 64 years of age with 103.35 inch-pounds of energy. An extensive strain pattern occurred in the embalmed pelvis of a 29-year-old Negro male with 60 inch-pounds of energy. An equally extensive strain pattern was produced in the unembalmed (fresh) pelvis of a 63-year-old Negro man with 90.18 inch-pounds of energy. No fractures were produced in the first series of tests.

In the second series of tests, 240 inch-pounds of energy produced a fracture of the right ischiopubic ramus near the acetabulum in the embalmed pelvis of a 79-year-old white man. No other fractures were produced with applications of 200 to 450 inch-pounds of energy. The latter amount of energy, applied to a specimen with some soft tissue under the ischial tuberosities, produced a minimal tensile strain (stresscoat) pattern, indicating that soft tissue is a very good energy absorbing material.

Analysis of the tensile strain patterns produced in the first series of tests indicated that the patterns arose from oscillations, in the lateromedial direction, of the anterior-superior iliac spines and the ischial tuberosities. Thus, the opposite aspects of the iliac alae and of the ischiopubic rami were alternately subjected to tensile strain as the region was bent first in one direction then in the other. The symphysis pubis and the acetabulae were displaced posteriorly and anterolaterally, respectively, thus creating tensile strain in the acetabulae and the iliopubic rami.

The tensile strain patterns produced in the second series of tests showed a similar behavior of the pelvis. The sacrospinal and sacrotuberal ligaments had no apparent effect in preventing the displacements causing the strain patterns.

Of course, in the intact body the presence of the muscles surrounding the pelvis would dampen these oscillations, if not entirely prevent them, and absorb most of the energy of an impact before it ever reached the pelvis. This may explain, in part, the relatively low incidence of pelvic injuries which, according to Braunstein, Moore, and Wade (1957), occurred in only 3.2 per cent of eight hundred survivors of light-plane crashes and in 2.7 per cent of 1,678 persons injured in automobile accidents.

The tolerance of unembalmed adult human pelves to impacts, applied by a small drop tower or pile driver, has also been investigated by Fasola, Baker, and Hitchcock (1955). The pile driver consisted of a mass of known weight which could be accelerated by dropping it a measured distance. The mass slid on guide wires so that the decelerative force or impact could be applied to a precise target. A Statham strain gage accelerometer was rigidly mounted on the accelerating mass and the force in g's determined from oscillographic recording.

However, the pile driver was not actually a free-fall device because of the friction between the guide wires and the bar to which the weight was attached. Whether or not the authors corrected for the frictional forces is not stated. They also do not give the capacity of the Statham accelerometer used in their tests.

The pelves used in one series of tests were defleshed and the vertebral column cut at the level between the third and fourth lumbar vertebrae. The lower part of the pelvis (ischia and inferior pubic rami) and part of the femur were embedded in a cement mold. A 3 × 3 × 1 inch steel block was placed on the upper surface of the fourth lumbar vertebra, and a load was dynamically applied to it by means of the pile driver.

The authors give the results of their tests as "ultimate breaking strength" for static or dynamic loading. However, the data they present are actually the ultimate breaking load (i.e. the pounds required to produce fracture of the pelvis or dislocation of the associated joints), *not* the ultimate breaking strength, which can only be determined in terms of load per unit area (pounds of force per square inch or kilograms of force per square centimeter). Although the authors state that "the force in g's" was determined from oscilloscopic records, neither the actual values for g nor the energy applied to the specimens are given.

The force required to dislocate the sacro-iliac joint was determined in preparations consisting of the defleshed pelvis and femurs with the intact hip and sacro-iliac joints. The specimen was mounted in cement up to the distal third of the femur, as in the erect standing position, and forces of gradually increasing magnitudes were applied to the sacro-iliac joint until failure of the joint occurred.

A force of 830 pounds was required to produce bilateral disjunction of the sacro-iliac joint from failure of the bone at the point of attachment of the ligaments. The ligaments themselves were not ruptured.

The authors inferred that the results indicated that the combined strength of the femurs was greater than that of the weight-bearing arches of the pelvis. The latter are (1) the femorosacral arch and (2) the ischio-sacral arch.

In other tests, the specimen was mounted in the same way but the pelvic viscera, muscles, and ligaments were left intact. Forces of gradually increasing intensity were applied as before until fracture disjunction of the sacro-iliac joint occurred with a load of 775 pounds.

A force was then directly applied to the symphysis pubis of the same specimen until a fracture of the symphysis was obtained with a force of 350 pounds. This test was to demonstrate the support the anterior wall of the pelvis gives to the posterior wall.

The reverse situation, i.e. the support the posterior pelvic wall gives to the anterior wall, was determined by applying a force to the anterior surface of the symphysis pubis until bilateral fracture of the superior and the inferior pubic rami occurred with a load of 595 pounds. The specimen was then mounted in cement and a force applied dynamically to the sacro-iliac joint. A force of 480 pounds produced fracture of the joint. Again failure of the bone at the sites of ligament attachment, not of the ligaments themselves, occurred.

In an embalmed and somewhat dry specimen, a dislocation of the sacro-iliac joint was obtained with a load of 270 pounds. This was not considered a valid test.

Tests were also made to determine the force required to rupture the lateral wall of the acetabulum. This was done by applying force first to the greater trochanter in the dry pelvis and then to the soft tissues overlying the greater trochanter in the fresh pelvis. The load was applied in graduating intensities by means of the pile driver. It was found that a force of 800 pounds produced fractures of the medial wall of the acetabulum and the regions of the epiphysial junctions. The fractures were radiating in character and accompanied by bending of the central part of the acetabulum.

In one case, the head of the femur was driven into the pelvic cavity together with fracture and central dislocation of the acetabulum. However, the femorosacral arch and the sacro-iliac joint were not involved in the injury.

Fasola, Baker, and Hitchcock also investigated rupture of the hip joint by applying a force to the inferior aspect of the neck of the femurs. This was done via a cable around the neck of the bones to simulate the force applied to this area by a parachute harness.

In the first specimen, partially denuded of muscles, rupture of the hip joint capsule occurred with a dynamically applied force of 600 pounds. The rupture occurred in the weakest part of the anterior aspect of the joint capsule, i.e. the area that is reinforced by the iliopsoas tendon in an intact body.

In a second, completely intact specimen, a load of 7500 pounds was required to produce a unilateral fracture of the superior pubic ramus and a fracture disjunction of the sacro-iliac joint.

From their studies, Fasola, Baker, and Hitchcock drew the following conclusions: (1) Femoral fractures do not occur in the intact body from application of force to the inferior aspect of the femoral neck or to the base of the sacrum, (2) Fractures and disjunctions of the sacro-iliac joint do not occur from fractures of the lateral pelvic wall and acetabulum, and (3) Unilateral or bilateral fractures of the pubic rami cause secondary fractures or disjunctions of the sacro-iliac joint.

A more recent study of tolerance of the human pelvis to impacts was made by Patrick, Kroell, and Mertz (1966). In these studies, intact human cadavers were placed in a car crash simulator and impact forces were applied (essentially along the femoral axis) to the patella.

The cadaver was placed in an automobile seat mounted on a sled which could be given accelerations of various magnitudes. The knees of the cadavers were impacted against a structure kinematically representing the impact against the lower surface of an instrument panel such as occurs in a frontal automobile collision. The impact was applied to the knees through a padding conforming to the target surface in order to prevent highly localized forces at the site of impact.

The knee-thigh-hip complex consisted of the three skeletal elements of each region. Ten cadavers were tested. The maximum force applied to the right hip varied from a minimum of 950 pounds to a maximum of 3850 pounds. The forces applied to the left hip varied from a minimum of 1400 pounds to a maximum of 2650 pounds.

Fractures of the right hip were obtained with loads of 1900, 1400, 2550, and 3850 pounds. Severe multiple fractures of the right hip were produced in one cadaver by a load of 1900 pounds and in another cadaver by 3850 pounds. A third cadaver sustained severe multiple fractures with a load of 2550 pounds. An impact of 1400 pounds produced a possible mild fracture of the right ischium.

Fractures of the superior and inferior rami of the left pubis were produced with a load of 1600 pounds, and severe multiple fractures with 2650 pounds. A possible fracture of the superior ramus of the pubis was produced with a load of 1950 pounds.

The authors believed their data were somewhat conservative in view of the fact that the subjects tested were all more than 50 years of age and embalmed. They also concluded that it was impossible to predict with certainty whether fracture would occur first in the patella, the femur, or the pelvis. They suggested, however, that the femur was the most vulnerable, since more fractures occurred there at a lower average load than in the patella or the pelvis. On the basis of available evidence, they concluded that a load of 1740 pounds was a reasonably conservative one for an overall injury threshold level.

As a corollary to this study, a series of tests on human volunteers was performed. In these tests, the volunteer impacted his leg by muscle action against one of the knee impact targets on the stationary sled in approximately the same kinematic manner as the cadaver knee was impacted during a dynamic test.

Eight volunteer males (from 18 to 45 years of age) subjected their knees, without pain or injury, to maximum forces varying from 450 pounds to 850 pounds for the right knee and from 400 pounds to 1050 pounds for the left knee. The maximum volunteer load of 1050 pounds compared to the suggested threshold load of 1400 pounds from the cadaver studies indicates that the latter tolerance load may be conservative.

Human tolerance to extreme impacts in free fall has been investigated by Snyder (1963). In ten individuals who landed buttocks first or in a seated position, fractures of the pelvis occurred in 31 per cent of the cases. It is, however, extremely difficult to accurately determine the magnitude of the force, the distribution of the force, the direction of the force, and the time of the deceleration in such accidents. Other factors are the material against which the impact occurred, the clothing worn by the victim, the age, the sex, and possibly the race of the individual as well as the individual's mental condition at the time of the accident. An additional factor is that many times the injuries are produced by a secondary impact rather than the initial one. Meteorological conditions may also affect the result of the fall, e.g., whether or not the ground was softened by rain, etc.

IMPACT TOLERANCE OF LONG BONES

The mechanical properties of the femur have been studied more extensively than those of any other bone. However, most of the experimental investigations on the limits of tolerance of the femur have been made under conditions of static loading.

Küntscher (1935) investigated the mechanical behavior of the femur under both static and dynamic loading by means of a strain sensitive lacquer called colophonium. None of the investigations under dynamic loading was carried to failure because the investigator was primarily interested in seeing the distribution of tensile strain produced in the bone under various loading conditions.

More recently, an extensive series of investigations on the biomechanical behavior of the femur with another strain sensitive lacquer, Stresscoat, has been made by Evans, Lissner, and their associates. Again the focus of interest was the extent and distribution of tensile strain produced in the bone by static loading.

In one of their studies (Pedersen, Evans, and Lissner, 1949), stress-coated femurs in various orientations were subjected to dynamic loading by dropping a 7.9 pound brass weight through various distances onto the bone. In one series of tests, the femur was placed in what was called the "abduction" position, in which the medial side of the head of the femur rested on a 160 pound steel block, while the brass weight was dropped on the greater trochanter. The weight multiplied by the distance through which it was dropped gave the inch pounds of energy dynamically applied to the bone. In a few cases the femur was tilted at a considerable angle by putting a larger block under the head of the bone. In both cases, the femur rested on the medial aspect of the head and the medial condyle. In one test, in which the head of the femur was raised 290 mm above the floor and 344.1 inch-pounds of energy were applied to the greater trochanter, a horizontal fracture extending across the trochanteric region was produced.

Although the fracture occurred far too rapidly to see exactly what happened, it probably arose from failure of the bone from the tensile stresses and strains within it. This was indicated by comparison with Stresscoat patterns and fractures produced by static loading in a materials testing machine of other bones in the "abduction" position. Fractures thus produced were initiated on the inferior aspect of the neck and were gradually propagated across the bone in the trochanteric region.

Patrick, Kroell, and Mertz experimentally produced fractures of the femur in cadavers by impacting the knees against a target with the automobile simulator previously mentioned.

In a series of tests with ten cadavers, impacts to the right knee produced a supracondylar fracture of the femur with 950 and 1650 pounds, a mid-shaft femoral fracture with 1500 pounds, and a comminuted fracture of the distal third of the femoral shaft and the intercondylar notch. A bone defect was suspected in the fracture produced with 950 pounds.

Impacts to the left knee of the cadavers resulted in an intertrochanteric femoral fracture through a bone screw with 1400 pounds; supracondylar femoral fractures with 1650, 2250, and 1850 pounds; and a dislocated trochanteric fracture with 2650 pounds.

In the cadaver tests, the right patella in the unpadded condition was fractured with loads of 1550, 1800, 1950, and 2150 pounds. Comminuted fractures of the patella were produced with loads of 2050 and 2250 pounds and a linear fracture of the patella with a load of 3850 pounds. In the left knee, a complete fracture of the patella, when unpadded, was produced with loads of 1500, 1800, 2000, and 2100 pounds. A comminuted fracture of the left patella was produced with a load of 2000 pounds. The above fractures of the patella were the only ones produced in the ten cadavers.

In a series of tests with human volunteers, loads of 800 to 1000 pounds were tolerated with only minor pain in the knee. Impacts were applied to the knee, through voluntary muscular activity on the part of the subject, by striking the same target used in the cadaver tests.

Experimental impact torsion tests of intact human tibias, both in the embalmed and unembalmed (fresh) condition, have recently been made by Burstein and Frankel. The tibia was rigidly fastened to a pendulum and the unit was allowed to gain kinetic energy at the expense of its potential energy. When maximum velocity was attained, the grip on the distal end of the tibia struck a stop and the pendulum, with the proximal end of the bone, continued to rotate. By measuring the energy remaining in the pendulum after fracture occurred, the energy lost by the pendulum, hence absorbed by the bone, was determined. This was done by recording the height to which the pendulum recovered. The tests were made in such a way that the loading duration was maintained at $\frac{1}{10}$ of a second. A comparable series of tests was conducted at a loading duration of 1 minute in order to determine if there were significant differences in the energy absorbing capacity with different loading durations.

Whenever possible, paired specimens of tibias were used and a combination of fresh and preserved bones were tested. All bones were kept wet throughout preparation and testing. It was found that the energy required for fracture of the fresh specimens was within the limits of the results obtained from preserved specimens. Because of the nature of the tests, the strain rates could not be maintained constant.

The tests showed a considerable variation among the individual bones but the investigators were able to obtain three paired specimens thus making direct comparisons possible. A strong correlation was found between the bone size and the energy required to fracture it.

In the three pairs of tibias tested, the energy at the low strain rate varied from a minimum of 38.4 kg–cm to a maximum of 154 kg–cm. At the high strain rate the energy absorbed ranged from a minimum of 96 kg–cm to a maximum of 375 kg–cm. The average energy absorbed for all specimens at the low strain rate (0.00003 to 0.0003 second^{-1}) was 103 kg–cm compared with an average of 229 kg–cm for all the specimens at the high strain rate (0.09 to 0.13 second^{-1}).

McElhaney and Byars, using standardized specimens of beef and of human cortical bone, found an energy ratio of 80 per cent in comparing energy absorption at strain rates of 0.001 second^{-1} and 0.1 second^{-1}. The whole-bone experiments of Burstein and Frankel exhibited a greater difference in the energy absorbing capacity (45%) which they believe may be explained by two factors.

First, whole bones contain spongy bone, which has not been investigated as far as time dependent and energy absorbing properties are concerned. Secondly, the resulting stress field in whole-bone experiments is more complex than in experiments with standardized specimens. Consequently, extrapolation of the data obtained in compression tests may not be accurate.

The effects of static and impact loading in forty-four pairs of fresh, unembalmed adult human femora were recently investigated by Mather (1968). One member of each pair of femurs was tested under static loading; the other member under impact loading. In both types of tests, the femur was supported at the ends and the load applied to the middle of the anterior aspect of the shaft.

The energy absorbing capacity of the femur under static loads was determined in a 22,000 pound (10,000 kg) capacity Mohr and Federhaff materials testing machine, in which the 1,100 pound range (500 kg) was used. The deflection occurring in the bone during a static loading test was measured with a dial gage calibrated in 0.001 inch (0.025 mm) attached to the test bed of the machine. Load deflection readings were taken at intervals as the load was increased to failure of the bone. From this data, load deflection graphs, to the point of failure, were drawn. The energy absorbed by the specimen was determined by measuring the area beneath the load deflection graphs.

In the impact loading tests, the energy absorbing capacity of the bone was measured by means of a drop-weight test. The apparatus consisted of a pair of vertically mounted guides and a striker or tuppet which fell freely between them. In each test, the bone was placed transversely between the guides, 2 feet above the base of the apparatus, and the tuppet struck the specimen with a velocity of 32 feet per second (22 mph, 35 km per hour). When the tuppet fell freely from the top of the columns, the energy with which it struck the base plate could be calculated. The reduction occurring in the energy when the bone is placed between the columns represented the energy expended in fracturing the bone. In each test, the residual energy was computed by allowing the tuppet to fall in a small cylindrical slug of annealed copper on the base plate of the testing apparatus. The compressive deflections produced in the slug were then compared with deflections occurring in a series of similar slugs which absorbed known amounts of energy.

The apparatus was calibrated by allowing the tuppet to fall from increasing heights on a series of slugs and constructing a graph of height of fall vs compressive deflection. Each point on the graph was the mean of two or three readings. The mean value of the standard deviation of a single reading was 0.0018 inch (0.0047 cm). This is a very small figure when compared with the magnitude of the deflections, 0.062 to 0.035 inch (0.16 cm to 0.60 cm), occurring during the tests. Consequently, it was concluded that the method used gave consistent results.

A series of impact tests was made on both members of twelve pairs of femurs in order to establish the symmetry of the energy absorbing capacity of paired bones. Of the remaining thirty-two pairs of femurs, one member of each pair was selected at random and tested statically while the other pair was tested under impact.

The magnitude of the energy required to fracture the femoral shaft varied with the rate of application of the load. In the static loading tests, a mean energy of 20.50 foot-pounds was required to fracture the bone. In the impact tests, made under the same geometry and an impact loading velocity of 32 feet per second, the mean energy absorbed to failure was 31.33 foot-pounds.

The author concluded that reliable estimates of the ability of an individual to withstand impact forces cannot be deduced from static loading studies of the individual bones. The impact energy absorbing capacity of the femur varied with the dimensions of its cross section but was not affected by variation in either the values of the material constants of bone tissue or by the age of the subject. However, the number of bones tested was too few for detailed statistical analysis of the findings.

The author pointed out that structures are more sensitive to the effects of discontinuities or flows under impact than under static conditions of loadings. Discontinuities in a structure act as stress raisers or sites where the stress concentration is higher than the surrounding material. It was suggested by the author that the variation in the distribution of anatomical discontinuities might contribute to widen the variations found in the values of impact of energy absorbing capacity of the femur.

The effects of high velocity impacts (spheres and bullets) on fractures have recently been the subject of a series of studies by Huelke and his associates. In the first study, Huelke and Darling (1964) investigated fractures produced in sixty-seven femurs, seven tibias, and three intact limbs by 4.5 automatic, 320 grain, or .22 long rifle standard velocity 40 grain cartridges. Some of the bones were dry museum specimens and others recently removed from cadavers. The proximal end of the femur, or the distal end of the tibia, was embedded in plaster of paris to hold the bone in place. The target sites were the middle of the shaft or the broad area near the knee.

The velocity of the bullets was determined with an Avtron Chronograph and the impact-fracture phenomena recorded with a high speed Fastax WF-1 camera. The framing rate at the time of bullet-bone impact was 10,000 to 14,000 frames per second.

Bullet impacts to the distal end of dry femurs produced "drill hole" fractures with a smooth-walled tract throughout the bone. Cadaver bones sustained many fractures around the point of exit of the bullet in this area.

Bullet impacts to the shaft of the bone shattered it with "butterfly" fragments on the side of the shaft perpendicular to the bullet tract. The same types of fractures were found in cadaver bones, thus complementing the results of bullet impacts to dry and to cadaver bones.

In a second study, the effect of high velocity impacts of spheres on femoral fractures was investigated (Huelke, Buege, and Harger, 1967). One-quarter inch, 16.1 grain steel spheres were used as projectiles and the popliteal surface of 122 embalmed adult human femurs as the target. The spheres were fired from a specially designed helium operated gun at velocities varying between 500 and 1700 feet per second. High speed motion pictures were taken of the projectile–bone impact phenomena and of the projectile's passage through the bone. The exit velocity of the projectile was calculated from the camera framing rate and the distance traveled by the projectile between each frame. The energy expended in producing the fracture was determined by electronic monitoring and by high speed photography.

Spheres were used in this study instead of bullets to eliminate problems of pitch and yaw of the projectile. The nondeformable spheres presented the same surface area to the target at all times whereas the nose of a bullet tended to flatten or mushroom, thus changing the surface area presented to the target.

It was found that "drill hole" fractures were produced in the low velocity range with low energy expenditure. With increasing velocity, the diameter of the "drill hole" also increased. At higher impact velocities, the bone exploded with violent displacement of the material surrounding the path of the projectile. The energy required to produce a fracture increased with increasing impact velocities.

In a third study (Huelke, Harger, Buege, Dingman, and Harger, 1968), using the same techniques employed in the second one, femoral fractures produced by smaller spheres (0.050 inch in diameter and 16.1 grains in weight) were compared with those resulting from impacts with larger spheres (0.406 inch in diameter and 69.1 grains in weight). Muzzle velocities of 200 to 2200 feet per second were used. A total of 222 embalmed adult human femurs was tested with the smaller projectiles and 173 with the larger ones. An additional fifty unembalmed femurs were tested with the smaller projectiles. The popliteal surface of the femur was the target area. The femurs were classified by a radiologist on the basis of x-rays as "normal," "mildly osteoporotic," and "osteoporotic."

The results of the study showed that at any given impact velocity, the larger (0.406 inch) sphere lost a markedly greater energy in producing a fracture than did the smaller (0.250 inch) sphere. However, the percentage of the impact velocity lost by the larger projectile was less than that lost by the smaller one at the same impact velocity.

In the 19 tests with the smaller spheres, the impact velocity varied from 200 to 2200 feet per second, the energy loss from 1.5 to 72.3 foot-pounds, and the percentage loss from 100 to 42.2. In fourteen tests with the larger spheres, the impact velocity varied from 200 to 1550 feet per second, the energy loss from 6.3 to 103.8 foot-pounds, and the percentage loss from 100 to 28.3.

No significant differences were found between the curves obtained from impacts with the smaller spheres on embalmed and on fresh femurs. Cavitation phenomena first occurred at a velocity of 600 feet per second with the larger spheres but not with the smaller spheres until a velocity of 800 feet per second was attained. The cavitation produced by the larger spheres at impact velocities of 1000 feet per second or higher were so great that the femoral condyles were almost completely separated from the rest of the bone. Comparable cavitation damage was not seen with the smaller spheres until a velocity of 1700 feet per second was attained.

The authors explain the differences in the cavitation phenomena found with the two types of spheres as follows. The impact velocity with the larger spheres collides with more of the fluid in the spongy bone than does the smaller sphere. Consequently, the larger sphere sets more fluid in motion which produces greater cavitation damage. The larger sphere presents a leading surface area of 0.259 inches^2 to the bone compared with an area of only 0.098 inches^2 for the smaller sphere. Thus, cavitation damage appears at lower impact velocities with the larger spheres than with the smaller spheres. Severity of cavitation damage is dependent upon two variables: impact velocity and projectile size. Normally calcified bones produced significantly greater energy loss by the projectile than osteoporotic bones, presumably because the latter were weaker.

The strength of intact human metatarsal bones under repetitive loading was investigated by Lease and Evans (1959). The specimens were loaded to failure in a Sonntag Flexure Fatigue machine equipped with an automatic counter and shutoff.

In order to hold the bones in the fatigue machine, the ends were embedded in a rectangular block of Selectron® 5026 Plastic. During a test, one end of the bone was held stationary while the other end was rapidly bent up and down in a direction perpendicular to the long axis of the bone. The bone was oriented in the machine so that its dorsal aspect faced upward. In some of the tests, water was allowed to drip on the specimen during the entire test to dissipate any heat that might have been generated. Other specimens were tested in the air-dried condition to determine what difference this might make in the fatigue life of the bone.

The fatigue life of fifty-one intact human metatarsal bones from eight adult males and from three females was determined under a uniform load of 15 pounds, the largest that could be applied with the fatigue machine available for the study. Only metatarsals two through five were tested because the first metatarsal was too large to be put into the testing machine.

The maximum number of cycles to failure varied from 150,000 to 13,908,000 for the wet-tested specimens and from 1000 to 10,297,000 for the dry ones. The lower fatigue life of the latter specimens was very probably a consequence of their increased modulus of elasticity (stiffness) as the result of drying. A similar phenomenon was found by Evans and Lebow (1951) for standardized specimens of embalmed human cortical bone from the femur. Metatarsals two and three had the longest fatigue life when tested wet, and metatarsals four and five when tested dry.

No consistent relations were found between the fatigue life of the bones and their general size or the age of the individuals from whom they were obtained. The types of fractures produced in the tests were comminuted and oblique, similar to those reported in the clinical literature.

CONCLUSION

In evaluating the significance of the experiments described previously, it should be remembered that bones in the living body contain fat, blood, marrow substance, and water all of which influence its behavior under impact. When a bone is subjected to an impact, except in the case of high velocity projectiles such as bullets, the bone is bent. As a consequence of this bending, the bone is subjected to a combination of tensile, compressive, and shearing stresses none of which is uniformly distributed over the cross-sectional area of the bone. Experiments with strain sensitive lacquers (see Evans, 1957, for review) show that linear types of fractures of the skull, the pelvis, and the long bones arise from failure of the bones from the tensile stresses and strains within it. There are also fractures, e.g., in the talus, calcaneum, and vertebral bodies, which arise from the compressive stresses and strains within the bone, and others (stress, march, or fatigue fractures) which are produced by failure of the bone under repetitive loading.

Practically all of the analyses of the mechanics involved in the production of these various types of fractures have been obtained from tests made under static loading. As previously discussed, relatively few studies under controlled experimental conditions have been made of fracture mechanics during impacts. Presumably the mechanism is not too different from that which occurs with static loading, but more experiments of the behavior of bone under impact are needed. The fact that some of the mechanical properties of bone are changed by high strain rates of loading may alter the picture.

The majority of studies on the limits of tolerance of human bones have been made on bones removed from the body. Consequently, less force is required to fracture them, than in the intact body where the surrounding soft tissues would absorb much of the energy of an impact before it reached the bone. The energy absorbing capacity of a relatively thin layer of soft tissue, e.g., the scalp, was clearly demonstrated in some studies of head injury under impact made by Gurdjian, Webster, and Lissner (1949). These investigators found that the least energy required for skull fracture in intact cadaver heads was in the neighborhood of 400 inch-pounds while dry skulls could be fractured with as little as 40 inch-pounds of energy. In the latter case, drying was undoubtedly a factor because it is known (Evans and Lebow, 1951) that drying of human cortical bone increases its tensile strength (in the long axis of the bone), its modulus of elasticity, and its hardness (Rockwell number). However, the shearing strength (perpendicular to the long axis) and the energy absorbing capacity of cortical bone are decreased by drying. The reduction in the energy absorbing capacity of bone by drying is especially important in the fracture mechanism because most fractures arise from impacts and, hence, are problems in energy absorption.

The chief conclusion to be drawn from a survey of the available literature is the need for more controlled studies of the impact tolerance of human bones in the intact body. This is especially important with respect to relatively low velocity impacts, as in the "second collision" in car and airplane crashes. Such data is badly needed by the safety engineer in many different fields.

BIBLIOGRAPHY

BIRD, F.; BECKER, H.; HEALER, J., and MESSER, M.: Experimental determination of the mechanical properties of bone. *Aerospace Med*, 39:44–48, 1968.

BRAUNSTEIN, P.W.; MOORE, J.O., and WADE, P.A.: Preliminary findings of the effect of automotive safety design on injury patterns. *Surg Gynec Obstet*, 105:257–263, 1957.

BURSTEIN, A.H., and FRANKEL, V.H.: The viscoelastic properties of some biological materials. *Ann NY Acad Sci*, 146:158–165, 1968.

EVANS, F.G.: *Stress and Strain in Bones*. Springfield, Thomas, 1957.

Evans, F.G., and Lebow, M.: Regional differences in some physical properties of the human femur. *J Appl Physiol,* 3:563–572, 1951.

Evans, F.G., and Lissner, H.R.: Studies on pelvic deformations and fractures. *Anat Rec,* 121:141–166, 1955.

Fasola, A.F.; Baker, R.C., and Hitchcock, F.A.: Anatomical and physiological effects of rapid deceleration. *WADC Tech. Report,* Wright-Patterson Air Force Base, Ohio, 1955, pp. 54–218.

Gurdjian, E.S.; Webster, J.E., and Lissner, H.R.: Studies on skull fracture with particular reference to engineering factors. *Amer J Surg,* 78:736–742, 1949.

Huelke, D.F., and Darling, J.H.: Bone fractures produced by bullets. *J Forensic Sci,* 9:461–469, 1964.

Huelke, D.F.; Buege, L.J., and Harger, J.H.: Bone fractures produced by high velocity impacts. *Amer J Anat,* 120:123–131, 1967.

Huelke, D.F.; Harger, J.H.; Buege, L.J.; Dingman, H.G., and Harger, D.R.: An experimental study in bio-ballistics: femoral fractures produced by projectiles. *J Biomech,* 1968, vol. 1 (in press).

Küntscher, G.: Die Bedeutung der Darstellung des Kraftflusses im Knochen. *Arch Klin Chir,* 182:489–551, 1935.

Lease, G.O'D., and Evans, F.G.: Strength of human metatarsal bones under repetitive loading. *J Appl Physiol,* 14:49–51, 1959.

Mather, B.S.: Observations on the effects of static and impact loading on the human femur. *J Biomech,* 1968 (in press).

McElhaney, J.H., and Byars, E.F.: Dynamic response of biological materials. *Amer Soc Mech Eng Publication* 65–WA/HUF–9:1–8, 1965.

Patrick, L.M.; Kroell, C.K., and Mertz, Jr., H.J.: Forces on the human body in simulated crashes. In Cragun, M.K. (Ed.): *Proceedings of the Ninth Stapp Car Crash Conference.* Minneapolis, U. of Minn., 1966, Chap. 12, pp. 237–259.

Pedersen, H.E.; Evans, F.G., and Lissner, H.R.: Deformation studies of the femur under various loadings and orientations. *Anat Rec,* 103: 159–185, 1949.

Snyder, R.G.: Human tolerances to extreme impacts in free-fall. *Aerospace Med,* 34: 695–709, 1963.

DISCUSSION

VICTOR H. FRANKEL

An impact is the striking of one body against another. It is one of the common mechanisms of injury of the locomotor system. In contradistinction to the degenerative disorders due to age change, impact injuries would seem to be avoidable through environmental control. As a model study, let us consider fractures of the neck of the femur. When a person falls down, an energy problem is created. This energy must be dissipated through the mechanisms available to the body and through alterations in the environment. The rate of energy input and dissipation is important in the viscoelastic biological tissues.

Force and Energetics of Femoral Neck Fractures

Some combination of trauma, general constitutional condition and metabolic bone weakness has been implicated as the cause of fracture of the femoral neck in the aged.

Gross stated that as early as 1795, it was known that fracture of the collum femoris was due to a twisting injury, a fall on the knee, or a fall on the hip.

Bone fails because of some combination of stress, strain, and energy absorption. Bone is a complex, anisotropic, nonhomogenous material with time dependent viscoelastic properties. The measurement of the stress level and strain at failure is difficult. The measurement of the energy absorbed at failure is relatively easy. We have determined experimentally that 20 to 60 kg–cm of energy are required to fracture the neck of the elderly femur.

Now consider the energetics of a fall on the hip. A 50 kg female 160 cm tall falls on her hip. Her c.g. originally 64 cm from the floor is lowered to 10 cm. As she falls, the potential energy possessed by her body is converted into kinetic energy. This kinetic energy must be absorbed by the body and the floor as strain energy and heat, and must be dissipated.

The energy available to fracture the femoral neck is many times greater than the energy needed to fracture the bone. The body possesses a number of mechanisms for distributing the energy produced by a fall.

Contact of the body with the ground is made at a number of areas. Of primary interest are the outstretched upper extremity, and the region of the hip and buttock.

Energy is absorbed in the upper extremity by muscle activity, by elastic strain in the bones and joint cartilage, and by plastic strain in the skeletal members resulting in fracture.

Energy is absorbed by resisted motion of the elbow and shoulder joints. The energy absorbing capacity of the triceps and shoulder girdle musculature, has been studied by noting the maximum load that can be lifted 30 cm. The energy absorbed by this maneuver is of order of 300 kg–cm.

The magnitude of the energy absorbed as elastic strain can be approximately calculated by multiplying the volume of cancellous bone at the wrist, elbow, and shoulder by 2 kg–cm per cm^2 which is the amount of energy that a cubic cm of cancellous bone can absorb. This will be approximately 230 kg–cm.

Plastic strain in the bones of the upper extremity of sufficient magnitude to cause fracture occurs concomitantly in 6 to 7 per cent of all fractures of the femoral neck. Since the volume of cortical bone is small, the additional energy dissipated by this mechanism will be small.

The mechanisms for energy absorption in the lower extremity are muscle activity about the knee and hip, elastic and plastic strain in the soft tissues, and elastic and plastic strain in the upper end of the femur.

The muscles in the lower extremity may absorb all of the energy if contracted in time. Up to 1,000 kg–cm is average.

The elastic strain in the soft tissue was measured by loading subjects and measuring the compression of the tissues over the greater trochanter and buttock. Loading was carried out to the threshold of pain in these subjects. In no case was a bruise noted. It was noted from the load deflection curve that unless a major change in the nature of the tissue elasticity occurs at higher loads, little additional energy will be absorbed at higher load levels. Up to 50 kg–cm of energy can be absorbed through this route.

Plastic strain in the soft tissues great enough to cause tissue disruption is frequently observed. Though not measurable, it will not significantly exceed the energy absorbed by the elastic strain due to the small amount of tissue involved and the nature of the load deflection relationship. This demonstrates that at the high load levels necessary for soft-tissue rupture, little additional deflexion will occur.

The elastic strain energy absorbing capacity of the greater trochanter has been measured by loading femoral specimens until failure of the cancellous tissue of the trochanter occurs. Up to 550 kg–cm of energy are absorbed in this manner including the energy absorbing capacity of the femoral head and neck.

As noted previously, the head and neck of the femur can absorb 60 kg–cm before failure occurs.

Plastic strain in the neck of the femur absorbs energy. When the energy is of sufficient magnitude, a clinical fracture will result. Larger amounts of plastic strain energy will result in displacement and comminution of the bone.

Energy will be absorbed by the floor. The amount will depend upon the type of floor and the covering material. It will average about 135 kg–cm.

It would seem that since the energy developed during a fall on the hip is many times the energy needed to fracture the neck of the femur, attention should be directed to other mechanisms of energy dissipation. Of great importance is the ability to absorb a large proportion of the energy in the upper extremity where muscle strength and coordination are important.

Rolling and tumbling are important methods of energy dissipation. These require good coordination.

It has not been shown that the osteoporotic bone is weaker than normal bone. Evans and King have noted some decrease in the energy-absorbing capacity in elderly cancellous bone.

In considering the causes of fracture of the neck in the aged, attention must be directed to such factors as neuromuscular reflex time, muscle strength and coordination. From the standpoint of prevention, it is important to develop energy-absorbing floor, materials, and clothing, to protect the group most prone to this injury: the thin elderly female.

PART IV
PRINCIPLES OF IMPACT INJURY MITIGATION

Chapter XIX

FUNDAMENTALS OF KINETICS AND KINEMATICS AS APPLIED TO INJURY REDUCTION

Joseph L. Haley, Jr.

INTRODUCTION

People are injured daily in automobile accidents. The medical treatment of such injuries is generally excellent. However, the prevention or mitigation of such injuries can surely be improved. Much remains to be done to reduce the degree and severity of injuries in these accidents. This chapter outlines the fundamental laws of physics used in designing to prevent or mitigate human injuries associated with vehicle impacts. The reduction of injuries by the use of improved restraint systems and interior padding is also discussed. Some of the terms and symbols in this chapter are defined below:

DEFINITION OF TERMS

Abbreviations and Symbols

F = force (pounds)
R = reaction force (pounds)
t = time (seconds)
s = distance (feet)
m = mass (slugs)
V = velocity (feet per second)
a = acceleration (feet per second per second)
g = acceleration of gravity

G = acceleration expressed in G-units
w = weight (pounds)
K. E. = kinetic energy
Δ = Delta, used to indicate a change in magnitude or quantity
Σ = summation
C G = center of gravity

Definitions and Basic Relationships

Force. The cause of the acceleration of any mass. A vector quantity, having magnitude, direction and location. F = ma (pounds).
Weight. A force caused by gravity, acting toward the center of the earth. W = mg (pounds).

Mass. The quantity of matter in a body. Mass remains constant.

$$m = \frac{W}{g} \text{ (pound-second}^2 \text{ per foot, or slugs)}$$

Velocity. Rate of motion, a vector quantity having both magnitude and direction. (The velocity of a body changes if there is a change of speed, or direction, or both. $V = \frac{\Delta s}{\Delta t}$ (feet per second).

Acceleration. Rate of change of velocity. $a = \frac{\Delta V}{\Delta t}$ (feet per second per second. Acceleration may increase or decrease speed and/or change the direction of motion. For ease of understanding an acceleration which produces a decrease in speed will sometimes be called a deceleration.

Acceleration of Gravity. Acceleration caused by the mutual attraction between masses. A free falling body, subjected only to this attraction, will accelerate at the rate of 32.2 feet per second per second on earth. $g = 32.2$ feet per second^2

G-Units—The ratio of acceleration to the acceleration of gravity. $G = \frac{a}{g}$

Kinetic Energy—Energy, or ability to do work, due to motion of a mass or masses.

$$\text{K.E.} = \tfrac{1}{2}mV^2 \text{ (foot-pounds)}$$

Work. Work is the expenditure of energy: the product of force multipled by the distance through which the force acts. $W = Fs$ (foot-pounds)

Change in Momentum.

$$m(V_2 - V_1) = \Sigma R \cdot \Delta t = \int_{t_1}^{t_2} R \cdot \Delta t$$

Momentum Conservation Law =

$$m_1 V_1 + m_2 V_2 + \cdots = m_1 V_1' + m_2 V_2' + \cdots$$

e = coefficient of restitution

$$e = \frac{\text{Relative velocity of a mass or masses after impact}}{\text{Relative velocity of a mass or masses before impact}}$$

BASIC CONCEPTS

Work—Energy Principle

Newton's first law of motion may be stated as follows: "Bodies in motion will remain in motion unless acted upon by an opposing or unbalanced force." The "body in motion" possesses *energy* while the "opposing force" does *work* on the body to decrease its velocity; this is the work-energy principle. This principle can be expressed by the equation

Fundamentals of Kinetics and Kinematics in Injury Reduction

$$\int_{S_1}^{S_2} F \cdot \Delta S = \frac{m}{2}(V_2^2 - V_1^2)$$

where:

F = opposing force acting on the CG of the mass (m).
S = distance traversed by CG of mass (m) while force (F) is acting.
m = mass of body on which force (F) is acting.
V_2 = velocity of mass (m) subsequent to the opposing force application.
V_1 = velocity of mass (m) prior to the opposing force application.

If the force (F) acting on the mass (m) is constant, the equation becomes the following:

$$F \cdot S = \frac{m}{2}(V_2^2 - V_1^2)$$

This equation is very helpful in determining the force-distance relationship when the velocity difference is known. The work-energy equation is less cumbersome to use when the opposing force is expressed in terms of the mass being decelerated. The equation is converted from a Kinetics to a Kinematics equation as follows:

$$F(S) = \frac{m}{2}(V_2^2 - V_1^2), \text{ and } F = ma; \text{ therefore,}$$

$$ma(S) = \frac{m}{2}(V_2^2 - V_1^2)$$

$$S = \frac{V_2^2 - V_1^2}{2a} \quad \text{and } a = gG = 32.2G$$

$$\text{finally: } G = \frac{V_2^2 - V_1^2}{64.4S}$$

The above equation is illustrated by three simple examples:

Example 1: An automobile is suddenly braked from a velocity of 41 mph (60 fps). The auto has excellent brakes and the stop occurs on dry level pavement. The distance (S) required to stop the car under these conditions is known to be about 70 feet, after the brakes are applied. The decelerative G level involved may be calculated by the above simplified equation:

$$G = \frac{V_2^2 - V_1^2}{64.4S}$$

where:

G = the ratio of the frictional force between the tires and pavement and the gravitational force acting on the car; i.e., the ratio of the braking force to the car's weight.
V_2 = initial velocity = 60 feet per second
V_1 = final velocity = zero
S = stopping distance required from instant brakes are applied

hence:

$$G = \frac{(60)^2}{64.4(70)} = 0.8$$

Example 2: The automobile from example 1 is again moving under the same conditions as before. The driver dozes; the car leaves the road and enters a row of sapling trees growing alongside the highway. The trees are sheared off just below the bumper level of the car and the remaining tree masses drape backward over the car. The car is decelerated by a nearly constant force level because the trees are closely spaced. The front of the car is not deformed significantly and the car is brought to rest in a distance of 15 feet. The average decelerative G level is:

$$G = \frac{(60)^2}{64.4(15)} = 3.7$$

Example 3: Again, the automobile from example 1 is moving under the same conditions. The driver dozes, the car leaves the road, hurtles across a small creek, and strikes the snow-covered opposite bank. The car comes to rest essentially intact after compressing the snow and mud to a depth of four feet. The average G level sustained by this vehicle would be approximately:

$$G = \frac{(V_2^2 - V_1^2)}{64.4S} = \frac{(60)^2}{64.4(4)} = 14G$$

The above comparison illustrates the application of the work-energy principle; the comparison also shows that the average G level is inversely proportional to the stopping distance. It should be noted that the second example represents a moderate crash of a vehicle while the third example represents a severe crash. The work-energy equation is accurate only so long as the following conditions apply:

1. The mass or masses do not become grossly deformed so that a large portion of a body is completely stopped while the remainder is still in motion.
2. The mass or masses do not disintegrate to the point that more than one mass is formed.

   Thus, it was assumed in the three examples above the mass of the vehicle remained essentially undeformed, i.e. sustained very little deformation of the front-end structure.

Momentum Exchange Principle

In certain impact situations, it is difficult to determine the *distance* moved by the moving mass or masses because of excessive deformation in

Fundamentals of Kinetics and Kinematics in Injury Reduction

the masses. In these cases, where a mass or body is deformed extensively, and stops in a distance only a fraction of its own depth, it is convenient to determine the force versus time relationship. If the total reaction force (R) is desired due to an impact by mass (M), it may be obtained from Newton's second law as follows:

$$R = ma \quad \text{and} \quad a = \frac{\Delta V}{\Delta t}$$

Eliminating a: $\Sigma R \cdot \Delta t = \Sigma m \cdot \Delta V$

The expression $\Sigma R \cdot \Delta t$ is known as the resultant *linear impulse* while the expression $\Sigma m \cdot \Delta V$ is called the resultant *linear momentum* change

Since all impact problems involve at least two masses even though one mass may be stationary, it is useful to express the above impulse-momentum equation for two masses in terms of their momentum before and after the impact. Newton's third law states the following: "Action and reaction forces between two particles are always equal and oppositely directed." This principle applied to the momentum problem indicates that the total momentum of two masses before impact must be identical to their momentum after impact. This relationship is called the Momentum Conservation Law and is stated as follows:

$$m_1 V_1 + m_2 V_2 + \text{---} = m_1 V_1' + m_2 V_2' + \text{---}$$

where:

m_1 and m_2 = mass of bodies under study
V_1 and V_2 = velocity of masses prior to impact
V_1' and V_2' = velocity of masses after impact

Common examples of the application of this equation include the following: (1) A bowling ball impacts a tenpin, (2) A cannon rebounds as the cannonball is ejected, and (3) An automobile impacts the rear end of a parked automobile and rebounds backward after the impact.

The velocity of impacting masses prior to impact and their velocities after impact is an important relation to study. This relation is expressed by,

$$e = \frac{\text{Relative velocity between two masses after impact}}{\text{Relative velocity between two masses before impact}}$$

$$e = \frac{V_2' - V_1'}{V_1 - V_2} = \text{coefficient of restitution}$$

This coefficient is really a measure of the elastic properties of a body. For example, perfectly elastic bodies would have exactly the same relative velocity after impact as before, and the value of (e) would be unity. On the other hand, perfectly inelastic (plastic) bodies would cling together after impact and the final relative velocity between the bodies would be zero and the value of (e) would be zero. Thus, actual values of (e) always lie between zero and unity. Severe impacts of vehicles usually result in very low values of (e) because of the plastic deformation which occurs in the bending and crushing of sheet metal. An example approaching an inelastic (plastic) impact is the "locking" together of two automobiles in a rear-end collision. Although some elasticity is involved in the deformation of the structures, the fact that the two masses are physically "locked" together simplifies the momentum calculation. The rear-end collision case of two "locked" cars is illustrated by the following example.

Example Momentum Problem: A 2500 pound car is stopped at an intersection, a 5000-pound car approaches the intersection, is unable to stop, and rams the stopped car at a velocity of 27 mph (40 feet per second). What velocity do the "locked" cars attain at the completion of impact? The momentum conservation equation is applicable:

$$M_1V_1 + M_2V_2 = M_1V_1' + M_2V_2'$$

where:

$$M_1 = \text{Mass of stopped car} = \frac{2500 \text{ lb}}{g}$$

$$V_1 = \text{Velocity of stopped car} = \text{zero}$$

$$M_2 = \text{Mass of moving car} = \frac{5000 \text{ lb}}{g}$$

V_2 = Velocity of moving car = 40 feet per second
V_1' = Velocity of stopped car after impact
V_2' = Velocity of striking car after impact

as stated, the cars "lock" together; therefore,

$$V_1' = V_2' = V_{1,2} \text{ or common velocity of both cars,}$$

substitution yields:

$$\frac{2500}{g}(\text{zero}) + \frac{5000}{g}(40) = \frac{(2500 + 5000)(V_{1,2})}{g}$$

The g is cancelled from the equation, and

$$V_{1,2} = 26.7 \text{ feet per second}$$

This example hopefully illustrates the reason for "whiplash" neck injuries. The small car has been accelerated to a velocity of about 18 mph in a distance of 2 to 4 feet (i.e. the crush depth of the small vehicle's trunk). The effect of such a velocity change on the occupant without a head support needs no discussion. A summary of the kinematics relations discussed thus far are graphically illustrated in Figure 19–1. This figure reveals the interaction between stopping distance, average G level, velocity

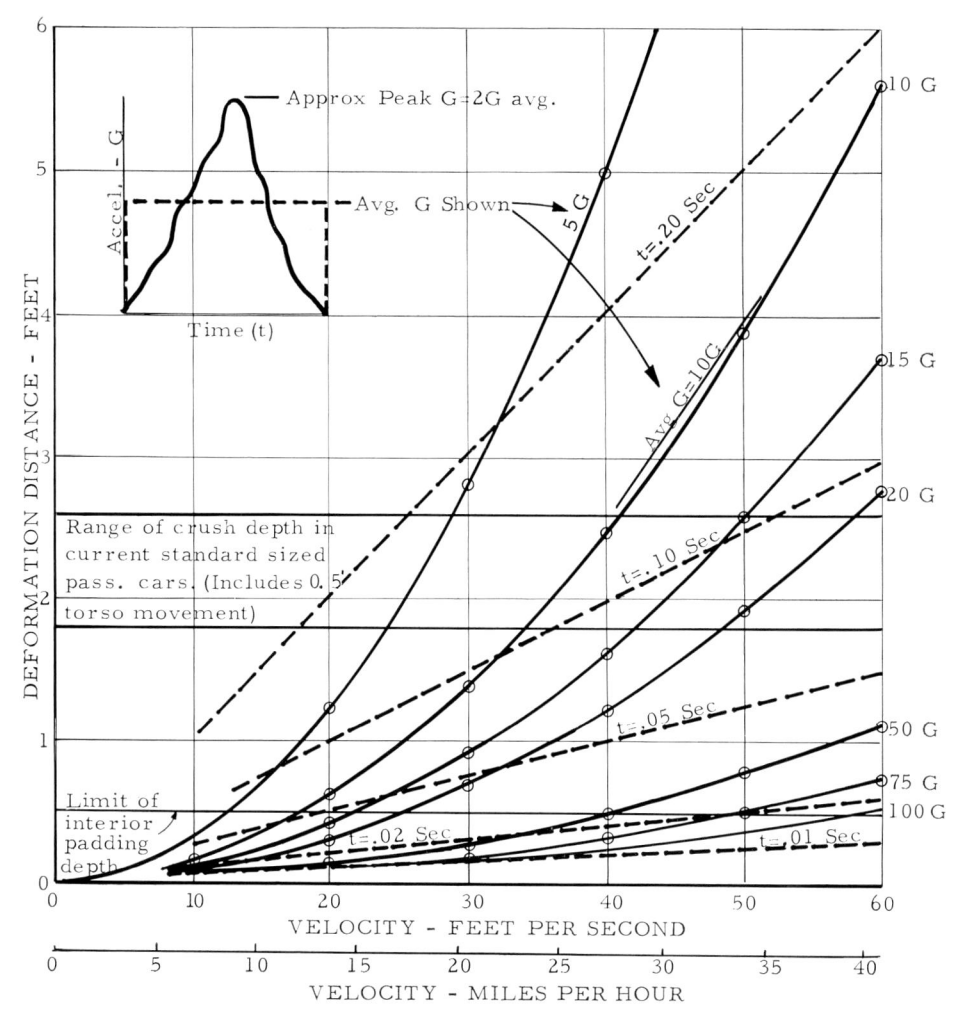

Fundamentals of Kinetics and Kinematics in Injury Reduction

FIGURE 19-1. Graphic portrayal of deformation distance, average g level, velocity change, and time duration for survivable impact conditions.

change, and pulse duration. The curves reveal that for a selected average G level, the distance required to absorb the energy is increased fourfold for a twofold velocity increase. The curves also show the proportional trade-off between stopping distance and average G level, i.e. doubling of the stopping distance will halve the G level. The acceleration pulse duration (t) for the assumed rectangular pulses presented are included as constant time lines. The time lines simply illustrate the fact that a larger velocity change must be accompanied by a proportional increase in the average G level, i.e. a larger impulse is required. The peak G value illustrated as being twice the average G level is shown for educational reasons only; experimental tests with dummies, however, indicate that this is a good approximation. The limit of interior padding depth and exterior deformation believed reasonable are superimposed on the figure to show the degree of protection possible with existing vehicles. The 50 to 100-G values are included primarily to illustrate the range of values appropriate to head impacts.

"Dynamic Overshoot" Phenomena

If the human body is rigidly attached (restrained) to a decelerating vehicle, the deceleration sustained by the human skeletal structure is about equal to that of the vehicle. This condition can only be achieved in experimental work, however, because humans are generally very loosely restrained. Restraint by only a lap belt with several inches slack permits a large relative movement of the body's center of gravity with respect to the vehicle. Restraint by a snugly fitted, nonelastic, upper and lower torso harness still permits up to 4 inches relative movement to occur between the seated occupant and the decelerating vehicle. The relative *movement* results in a relative *velocity* between occupant and vehicle, and this relative velocity must be reduced to zero. It is the reduction of this relative velocity to zero in a very short time span that causes the occupant deceleration to *exceed* that of the vehicle for a portion of the crash pulse. This phenomena is illustrated in Figure 19–2. The results shown in Figure 19–2 are test results taken from a sled run with a 200-pound dummy mounted on a U.S. Army experimental crew seat. Note that the forward-facing seat is accelerated in an opposite direction to simulate deceleration. Thus the velocities can be seen to increase rather than decrease.

It can be seen in Figure 19–2 that the occupant does not begin to accelerate until the initial elastic harness stretch and body compression is removed at about 0.04 second; the velocity of the seat is about 6 feet per second at this time while the dummy's velocity is only about 0.2 foot per second. Beyond 0.04 second, the slope of the velocity-time curve for the dummy increases rapidly as its velocity approaches and equals that of the seat. The dummy's acceleration can be seen to be double that of the seat at about 0.08 second and the slope of the dummy velocity-time curve is also maximum at this time. As one would expect, the velocity of the seat and dummy are nearly equal when the seat acceleration becomes zero at 0.21 seconds. The distance moved by the dummy is shown to be about 0.7 foot less than that of the seat; this distance consists of dummy deformation and harness elongation as the seat initially moves away from the dummy. The hysteresis of the harness webbing causes it to remain "stretched" as is shown by the relatively constant 0.7 foot differential between the dummy and seat movement. This differential distance dis-

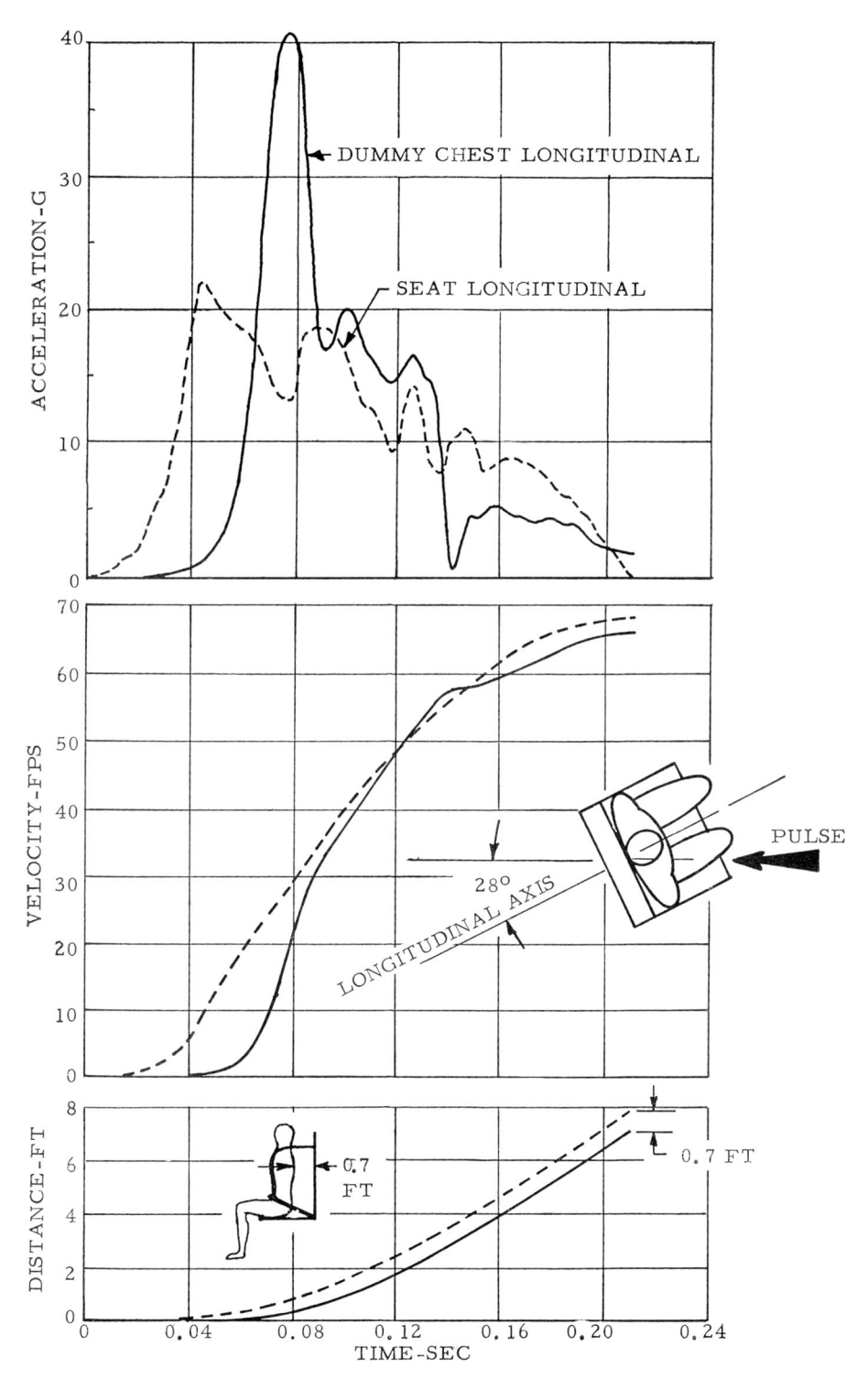

FIGURE 19–2. Illustration of "Dynamic Overshoot" effect for occupant restrained by an elastic nylon harness.

appears after the dummy's acceleration is reduced to zero; however, this did not occur until approximately ½ second later and is not shown in this figure.

The dynamic overshoot effect is not significant for situations in which any of the following conditions exist: (a) The body is *very* tightly restrained with a nonelastic harness, (b) The acceleration pulse rise time is relatively large (0.15 second or more) and, (c) The total pulse duration is relatively short, say 0.03 second or less. Since none of these situations are applicable for most severe accidents, it appears that some dynamic overshoot will be present, and allowance must be made for this factor in restraint system design.

INJURY REDUCTION TECHNIQUES

The tolerance of the human body to decelerative forces is proportional to the area over which the force is applied. This principle has been proven by so-called "miraculous" survivals of persons having impacted the earth after falling from heights over 100 feet.[1] Needless to say, the lap belt alone offers only a bare minimum of restraint because of the small area it covers. The addition of shoulder straps improves the situation; however, the lap belt and shoulder strap still fall far short of providing maximum force distribution (minimum pressure) on the torso. The astronaut's molded couch approaches an optimum pressure distribution system. Some of the most significant human test data on the tolerance of humans for decelerative forces transverse to the spine are summarized in Figure 19–3. It should be noted that the volunteers restrained only by lap belts did have clearance to "jackknife" forward until their chests contacted their legs.

Figure 19–3 is presented only to summarize significant human test data, which to the writer's knowledge has not been published before. The subject of human tolerance is covered by Col. Stapp, et al. in other chapters of this book. A review of Figure 19–3 quickly shows the demonstrated value of increased area of body contact with the restraint system. Several techniques of providing the best known restraint methods for a given area of body contact are discussed below.

Lap Belt Only Restraint

The lap belt should provide the following features: (1) Maximum contact area consistent with the occupant's torso. The existing two inch width belt in autos is probably adequate because it must be used by children with small pelvic bones; however, a 2.5 to 3.0 inch width is preferable for adults. (2) Optimum angle of belt to pelvis—pelvis rotation and "sub-

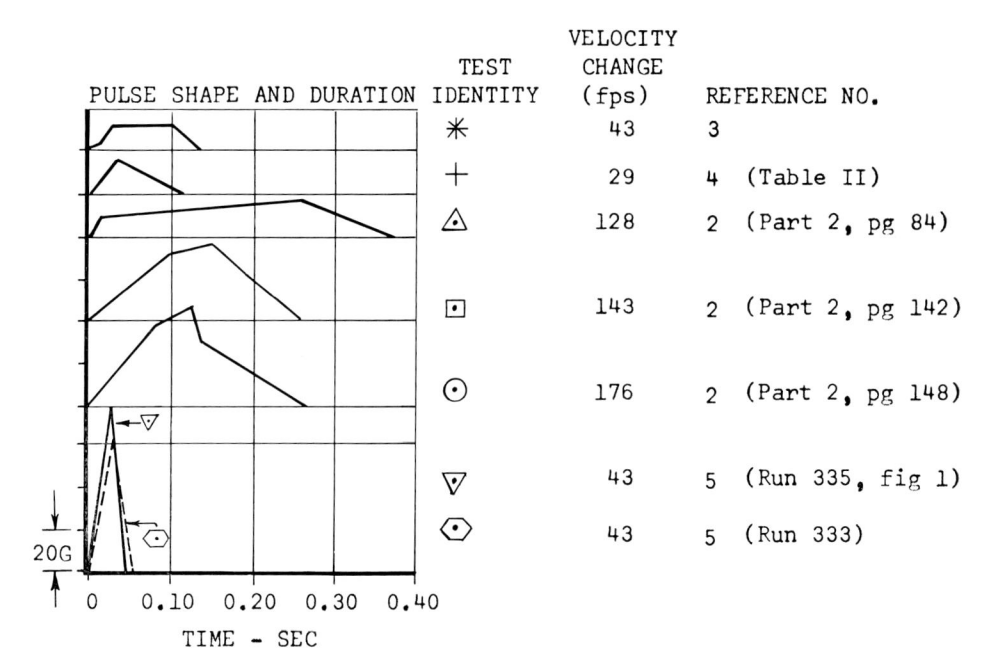

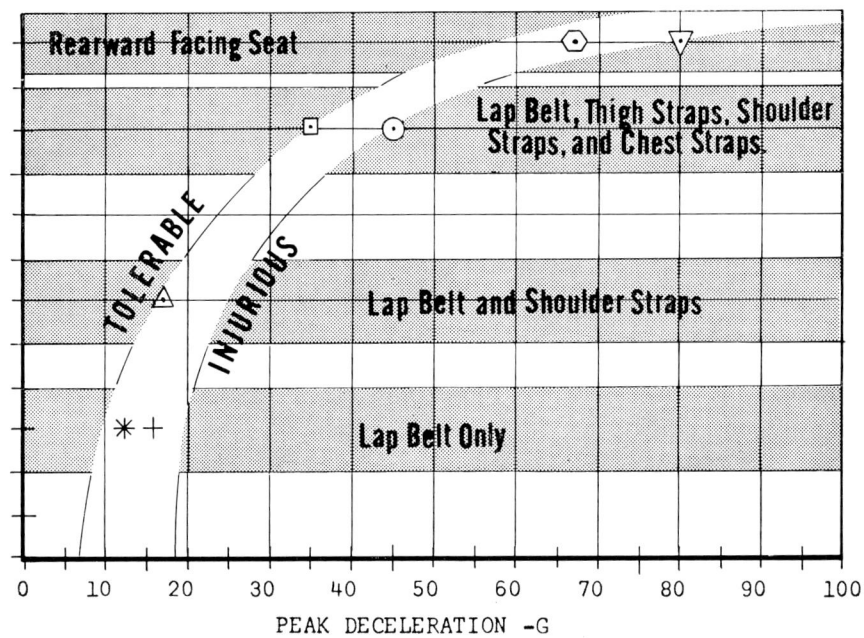

Fundamentals of Kinetics and Kinematics in Injury Reduction

PULSE SHAPE AND DURATION	TEST IDENTITY	VELOCITY CHANGE (fps)	REFERENCE NO.
	✳	43	3
	+	29	4 (Table II)
	△	128	2 (Part 2, pg 84)
	⊡	143	2 (Part 2, pg 142)
	⊙	176	2 (Part 2, pg 148)
	▽	43	5 (Run 335, fig 1)
	⬡	43	5 (Run 333)

FIGURE 19–3A, B. Approximate tolerance to abrupt acceleration transverse to the spine (eyeballs out or in).

marining" as shown in Figure 19–4 can occur when the belt angle to the seat bottom is too flat.² The movement shown is encouraged when a very soft seat cushion permits the buttocks to move downward easily. If "submarining" occurs, the belt applies pressure to the soft tissues of the abdomen. In the writer's opinion, based on static pull tests on humans up to 2 G, the angle to the cushion should be between 45 and 50 degrees to alleviate this problem. Most belts passing between the seat back and bottom cushion, in bench-type automotive seats result in an angle of 35 to 40 degrees on the average size motorist. (3) Adequate thickness in critical location over pelvis iliac spine bone to prevent creasing or "roping" of the belt webbing as the pelvis rotates. A minimum webbing thickness of 0.09

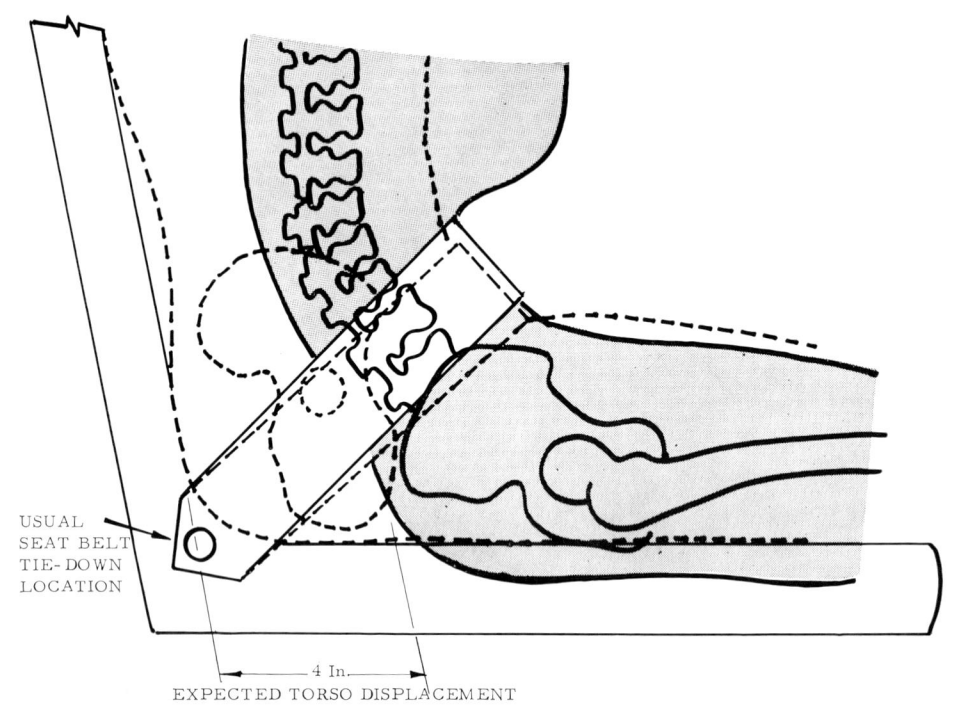

FIGURE 19–4. Illustration of pelvis slippage "Submarining" under seat belt.

inch appears to be a reasonable recommendation. A corollary benefit of increased thickness is increased webbing stiffness which decreases dynamic "overshoot" effects. (4) Adequate strength and flexibility in the attachment fittings to prevent failure due to a lateral impulse. (5) Minimum webbing elongation. It is recommended that the belt webbing as loaded end-to-end in a tensile test not elongate more than 3.0 inches at the SAE, (Society of Automotive Engineers) load of 3000 pounds. This will result in only 1.5 inches per side under the normal loop loading; however, the abdomen compresses another 2 to 2.5 inches for a total pelvis movement of about 4 inches.

Lap and Shoulder Strap Restraint

In general, the same factors stated for the lap belt are also applicable to the shoulder straps. In addition, the location of the shoulder strap attachment to the lap belt must be carefully considered. The double shoulder straps used by crew members in military aircraft are attached at the lap belt center release buckle. This arrangement gives reasonable upper torso restraint, but the upward load on the belt release buckle promotes the "submarining" of the pelvis.[2] This problem may be alleviated by the addition of a center "tiedown strap" to which the release buckle is attached as illustrated in Figure 19-5. This arrangement is being used in new U.S. Army helicopter aircraft. Double shoulder straps, of adequate width and thickness to prevent excessive pressure in the collarbone and neck area, used in conjunction with a tiedown strap, constitute a practical, single-release-point restraint harness for seated occupants. Nonetheless, it is unlikely that the general public is ready to accept a "tiedown" strap harness; however, it should be readily accepted and worn by all racing drivers, especially if it is equipped with an inertia reel as illustrated in Figure 19-6.

In the writer's opinion, either the three-point single diagonal shoulder strap harness attached to a lap belt or the inverted "Y" harness as described by Snyder, Young, and Snow[6] will be used for the forward-facing passenger position in the near future. This statement is based on the simplicity and ease of donning and doffing of either of these harnesses. Regardless of the type shoulder strap or straps used, the following are some important factors for consideration in their design:

1. Adequate pressure distribution in collarbone and neck area. This factor may be especially important where only one strap is used. Additional width should be provided over about ten inches length in the collarbone and neck area. The additional area could be provided by movable pads to adjust for different shoulder heights.
2. Location of shoulder strap intersection with lap belt. This point should be located as near as possible at the *side* of the pelvis (over the femur-to-pelvis pivot point) rather than over the pelvis as is the current practice on some models of the diagonal harness. The side location appears to be desirable for three reasons:
(a) The diagonal shoulder strap is placed higher on the chest so that the torso does not tend to rotate out of the harness in a crash, (b) Improved lateral restraint is provided for the 3-point, diagonal

436   *Impact Injury and Crash Protection*

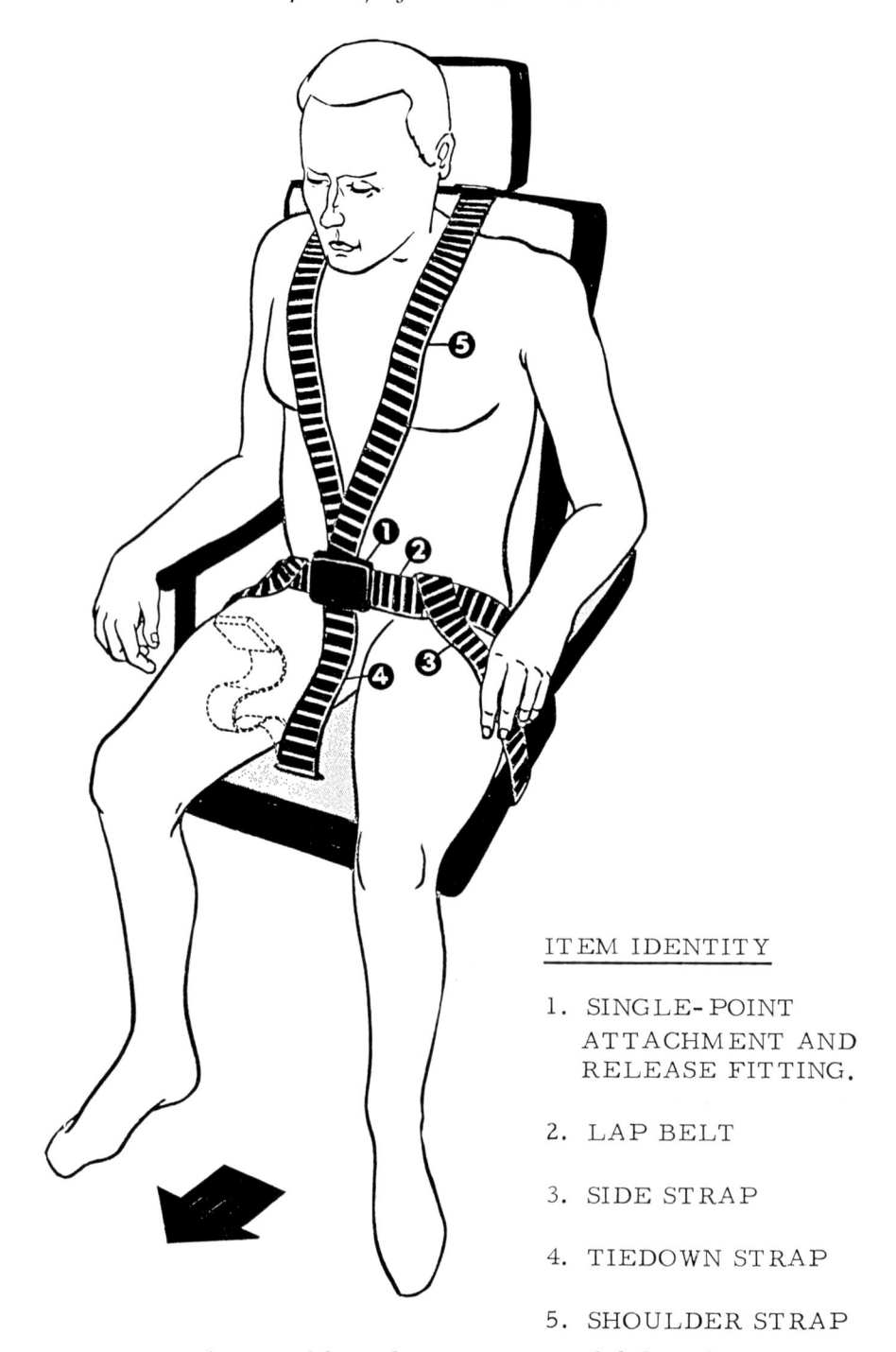

ITEM IDENTITY

1. SINGLE-POINT ATTACHMENT AND RELEASE FITTING.

2. LAP BELT

3. SIDE STRAP

4. TIEDOWN STRAP

5. SHOULDER STRAP

FIGURE 19–5. Forward-facing harness concept with belt tie-down strap.

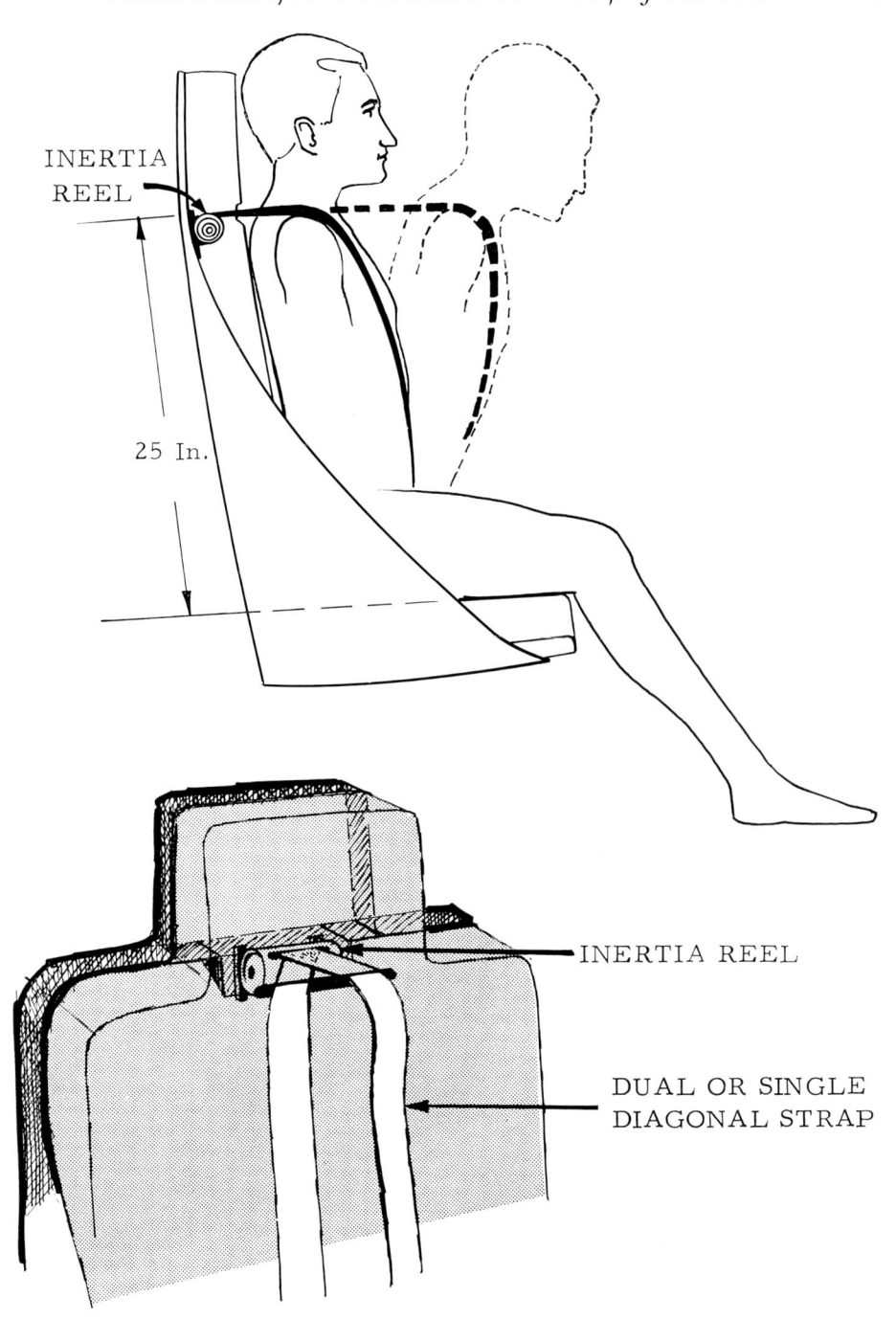

Fundamentals of Kinetics and Kinematics in Injury Reduction 437

FIGURE 19-6. Inertia reel located in seat back to permit normal movement of upper torso.

shoulder strap because of the increased diagonal angle, and (c) The release buckle is placed flat against the side of the pelvis rather than edgewise to the pelvis as is otherwise the case.

Of course, for the three-point harness, it is assumed that the release buckle will be located at the *inboard* hip, so that the single shoulder strap rests on the *outboard* side of the neck; thus, some protection is provided for lateral impacts.

3. Inertia reel provision. An inertia reel is definitely desirable for the driver's position of an automobile. The inertia reel permits normal shoulder movements, while locking in the event of rapid movements. Without it, the driver cannot turn to look backward when parking or turning to the right (unless a very slack harness is worn). An inertia reel installation concept for a dual strap is shown in Figure 19–6; however, the location would be similar for a single diagonal installation. The inertia reel could be an optional, extra cost, item for other positions in the automobile. One very nice operational advantage of the reel is its ability to store the webbing. Inertia reels, by the way, are already in use on the GT-500 version of the Mustang.

4. Location of shoulder strap pull-off point. The strap should pass through a slot in the seat back, or into the inertia reel, at a point about 25 inches above the deflected seat bottom cushion as illustrated in Figure 19–6. This location will result in the strap pulling upward at about 45 degrees for a small woman. Straps mounted to the ceiling of an auto are certainly superior to none at all; however, a ceiling location provides little lateral restraint and also makes it easier to rotate and slide out of the diagonal strap. A shoulder strap attachment to the seat back, of course, requires a stressed seat structure; however, this should not be an insurmountable problem since it is already accomplished in aircraft seats. The seat could be hinged at its forward edge with a rear leg locking device to permit easy exit and entry to the back seat. The contoured bucket seat, with the restraint harness built into it, appears to be the best method of obtaining improved restraint against lateral impact.

Automatic Inflating Mechanisms

The theory of this concept consists of enveloping the seated occupant with a gas-filled bag of sufficient pressure to prevent excessive movement in a crash. To be effective, the device must be inflated automatically within the first 30 milliseconds after vehicle impact. Developmental work involving full-scale human experimental drop tests, and full-scale aircraft and automobile tests with dummies have been conducted.[7,8] Once inflated, there is a little doubt that this type device can offer adequate restraint for occupants in primarily longitudinal impacts; however, there seems to be room for doubt about its capability to properly restrain the occupant for a lateral impact since less torso profile area will dictate higher pressure (5 to 10 psi).

Reference 8 indicates that the inertia switch actuator for timely bag inflation is feasible. It[8] was noted that the gas-filling of the bag produced a noise level of about 160 decibels; thus, the long-term effect of such a high noise level on humans must be considered. Even so, all the evidence indicates that this type of emergency restraint device should be evaluated further.

Lining of Vehicle Interiors With Energy-Absorbing Material

Reduction of occupant injuries by the addition of padding material to the vehicle's interior is like "closing the barn door after the horse is out" because it is far more difficult to absorb the energy of the moving torso as it impacts the interior of the vehicle than it is to provide the extra time and force on the body by a restraint harness, inflated bag, or other device. In other words, the *resisting force* acting through a distance (the total distance used in the stretch of a restraining harness and crushing of exterior vehicle structure) has been lost if no restraint has been used and the occupant impacts the vehicle's interior at nearly the same velocity as the initial impact velocity of the vehicle. Thus, the occupant is decelerated at a very high deceleration level upon contact with the vehicle's interior because not more than ½ foot of deformation distance will be available even with optimum conditions, whereas, 2 to 3 feet of distance (harness, torso, and vehicle exterior deformation) are available when the occupant is restrained by a harness or other device.

Regardless of the limitations of interior padding materials, padding is necessary as long as the occupant's upper torso and head are free to impact interior structures. An ideal padding will, of course, compress or deform at a pressure level which will not exceed that which a human can endure. The skull can sustain higher nonlethal pressures than can other areas of the body; fracture of the skull and/or internal brain damage, however, are responsible for a large percentage of lethal occupant injuries in accidents. It seems logical, therefore, to provide crushable materials that deform at a pressure level below that necessary to result in head injuries in order to provide the maximum protection (energy-absorption) for the limited deformation space.

In order to provide a constant force on the head, regardless of the depth to which it deforms the padding material, the idea illustrated in Figure

19–7 is offered as a concept worthy of further evaluation. The basic idea is to provide a frangible outer membrane which would not carry significant diaphragm loads and would insure a constant total force as the head compresses a constant area of paper or aluminum honeycomb tubes. The design of crushable aluminum tubes is well advanced because of their use as the primary energy-absorbing device in astronaut couches. Plastic-impregnated paper honeycomb could also provide an economical material for this use.

The concept illustrated should be equally applicable to an impact by the head, shoulder, elbow, etc. The key point is that a constant force level could be maintained for the critical head impact.

Although it is clear that interior padding is second best to adequate torso restraint in a crash, it appears that padding requirements should be defined immediately. Recent history indicates that the driving public is not going to voluntarily wear a restraint harness (just look at how many belts you still see hanging outside cars); therefore, a really effective approach to the reduction of crash injuries must be one over which the automotive passenger has no control. Thus, automatically inflating restraint devices, and interior padding are examples of methods which should be effective to some degree in most crashes. Reasonable protection can be provided by padding materials *now* while inflatable devices require further study; therefore, it would appear that improved padding for lateral as well as longitudinal impacts should be developed and installed with all haste.

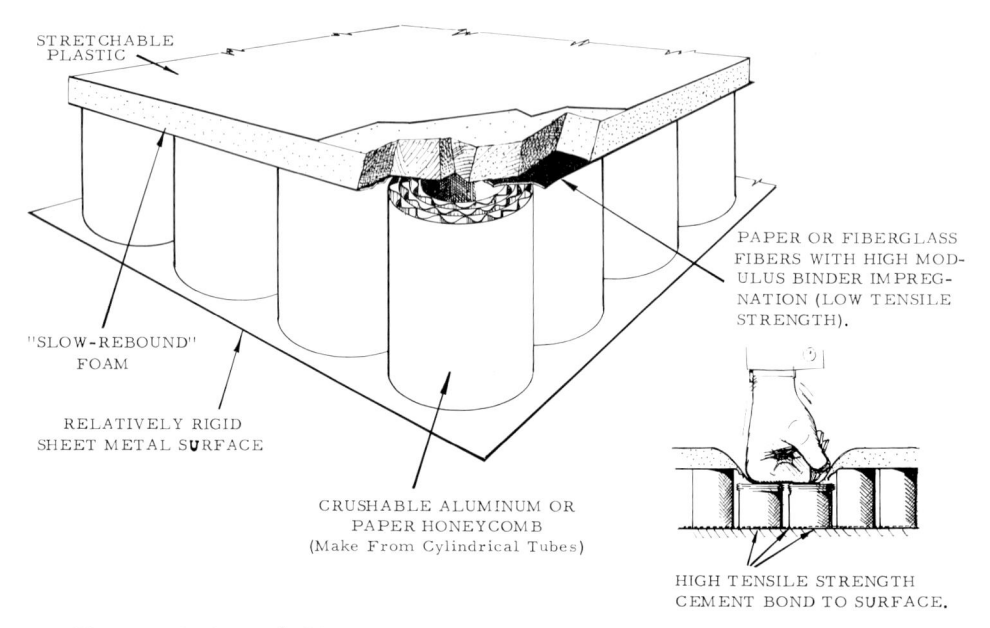

FIGURE 19–7. Crushable padding concept (similar to innerspring mattress).

CONCLUSIONS

The following conclusions have been reached:

1. Basic research is certainly needed in the human injury field; however, it is the writer's opinion that not enough application is made of the "ball park" knowledge already available.
2. A contoured bucket seat with a built-in restraint harness should be evaluated as soon as possible.
3. An automatic inflatable bag restraint system should be further evaluated for reliability and cost. This device could negate the need for a restraint harness.
4. Adequate energy-absorbing requirements for the interior padding of vehicles should be developed *until* the automobile passenger is protected by a fool proof restraint system.

REFERENCES

1. DeHaven, Hugh: Mean deceleration sustained by nine survivor's of free falls 55 to 185 feet. Design Data Sheet. Phoenix, Aviation Crash Injury Research, 1959.
2. Stapp, J.P.: The forward-facing position and the development of a crash harness. Air Force Tech. Rep. 5915, Wright-Patterson AFB, Wright Air Development Center, 1951, pt. II.
3. Carroll, D.F., et al.: Crashworthiness study for passenger seat design—analysis and test of aircraft seats. *NASA Report (AvSER 67–4)*. Phoenix, Aviation Safety Engineering and Research.
4. Lewis, S.T., and Stapp, J.P.: Human tolerance to aircraft seat belt restraint. *JAMA*, 1958, pp. 29–187.
5. Beeding, E.L.: Human deceleration tests. *AFMCD-TN60-2*, Holloman Air Force Base, 1960.
6. Snyder, R.G., et al.: Experimental impact protection with advanced automotive restraint systems. *Eleventh Stapp Car Crash Conference Proceedings*, New York, Soc. Auto. Eng., 1967, p. 271.
7. Clark, Carl, et al.: Human transportation fatalities and protection against rear and side crash loads by the airstop restraint. *Ninth Stapp Car Crash Conference Proceedings*. Minneapolis, U. of Minn., 1966, p. 19.
8. Kemmerer, R.M., et al.: Automatic inflatable occupant restraint system, Paper 680033. New York, Soc. Auto Eng., 1968.

DISCUSSION

Geoffrey Grime

Some of the basic principles which apply when vehicles are involved in crashes have been discussed.

I think that Mr. Haley oversimplifies the phenomenon of "dynamic overshoot," and in doing so conveys the impression that a belt wearer in a head-on accident may expect to experience twice the deceleration of the car. However, tests show that even with dummies this is not so. In dynamic tests at the British Standards Institution with dummies in belts with upper body restraint stopping from 30 mph in a distance of 24 inches (duration of deceleration about 0.1 second), the ratio of the maximum deceleration of the dummy's chest to that of the test vehicle ranged from about 0.8 to 1.5, the variation depending on type of belt, its arrangement on the dummy, and the type of dummy used. In barrier tests with cars at speeds in the range 30 to 38 mph, the ratios were between 1.0 and 1.8, values over 1.5 being exceptional. With humans, because of greater compressibility and flexibility, I would expect the ratios to be lower.

Theory[1,2,3] shows that this ratio depends on the relationship between the way in which the vehicle is stopped (duration and shape of deceleration/time curve) and the frequency characteristics of the restraint system.

Minimum webbing elongation is recommended. While this may be desirable for lap belts, in order to limit forward movement in jackknifing, it does not in general reduce dynamic overshoot. Again, both theory and practice indicate that it is best to use a webbing which allows as much elongation as possible, subject to the condition that when the restraint system exerts so great a force that some agreed injury threshold is exceeded, it shall be fully extended. The importance of using very extensible restraint systems has sometimes been over emphasized, but there is little doubt of the desirability of arranging that the extensibility is such as to make use of all the space available in the car immediately in front of the belted passenger. The car and restraint system form one whole protective system and should be designed as a whole.

Inertia reels are desirable, particularly for the driver of an automobile. Besides being more convenient, they afford improved safety. In Britain, where safety belts with upper body restraint are exclusively used, about one-quarter of the belts sold by a leading manufacturer (Britax Limited) are of the inertia reel type.

REFERENCES

1. Grime, G.: Seat harness. Effect of a harness on the movement of the occupant of a car during a head-on collision. *Auto Engr,* 53(1):12–18, 1963.

2. McHenry, R.R.: Analysis of the dynamics of automotive passenger restraint systems. Buffalo, New York, Cornell University, Cornell Aeronautical Laboratory, Inc., *Automotive Crash Injury Research Report No. V5–1823–R1*, 1963.
3. Neilson, I.D.: The dynamics of safety belts in motor car head-on impacts. *Symposium on Ergonomics and Safety in Motor Car Design*. Inst. of Mech. Engineers, Sept. 1966.

Chapter XX

APPLICATIONS OF HUMAN TOLERANCE DATA TO PROTECTIVE SYSTEMS:
Requirements for Soft Tissue, Bone and Organ Protective Devices

LAWRENCE M. PATRICK and GEOFFREY GRIME

The need for reducing injuries and fatalities from all types of accidents (home, highway, sports, industry, etc.) has long been recognized, and in some industries (mining and lumbering are outstanding examples) considerable progress has been made in reducing danger. This has been accomplished through the establishment of safety regulations, by personnel training and the installation of obvious and/or ingenious safety devices.

While one might argue that human error is the source of most accidents or that the danger of being injured or killed is small (less than six fatalities per 100 million miles), and therefore the danger to the individual is small, the arguments, though valid, must not be accepted as a reason for rejecting engineering improvements, since the gross number of U.S. accident fatalities is so large (over 100,000 per year from all causes) and the number of injuries is many times larger. All methods of reducing these terrible statistics must therefore be explored simultaneously and the findings implemented without delay.

One conclusion soon reached by most safety engineers is that people must be protected in spite of themselves, preferably with no action required on their part. The principal objective of this paper is to present a logical method of designing protective systems for maximum protection from impact using human impact tolerance as the design basis.

Emphasis over the past several years on automotive safety has resulted in considerable research on human impact tolerance. This, coupled with the large number of injuries in an environment which is well defined (the passenger compartment), permits a detailed analysis of a large number of impact conditions with known injury results. Consequently, much of the material presented herein is derived from automotive safety research, but the principles apply equally well to other impact situations. Impact trauma is of primary concern, as opposed to injury from temperature extremes, noxious gases, and similar nonviolent exposures.

Fundamentally, the problem of impact protection consists of reducing the relative velocity between the human, and the striking, or struck object, to zero without producing injury. The problem is complicated by the many variables affecting human tolerance including the following:

1. Relative velocity
2. Impact site
3. Mass of impactor
4. Area of contact
5. Geometry of the impacted area
6. Surface hardness
7. Surface roughness
8. Direction of impact
9. Impact duration

Fortunately, many of the variables are affected favorably by similar means. For example, padding tends to reduce injury from each of the variables except impact duration.

These parameters also affect the types of injury which are listed below in a general order of increasing severity:

1. Contusions
2. Abrasions
3. Lacerations
4. Bone fracture
5. Internal organ damage
6. Brain damage

Obviously, a single impact can result in several, or all, of the types of injury listed, and the degree of severity is not always in the order shown—a severe laceration can cause death from loss of blood or infection, while a mild brain concussion might have no lasting effect. The categories are chosen for easy classification by injury type commonly observed, with the brain isolated from other internal organs because of the frequency and severity of injury to it.

A list, of parameters affecting impact trauma and the type of injuries produced, provides a qualitative insight and understanding of the impact injury syndrome. However, efficient design of protective systems requires a quantitative interpretation of the injury phenomenon in terms of physical characteristics capable of being used in the design of structures. Acceleration, force, pressure distribution, and change of velocity, are some of the physical quantities that have been proposed as measures of injury with acceleration and/or force being the most widely accepted ones. With suitable precautions, these two parameters can be related through Newton's laws, but the indiscriminate use of the acceleration of a point on the body as the acceleration of the CG and hence proportional to force acting on the entire body will often lead to gross errors. Since force is usually difficult to measure when impacting the interior of a vehicle, acceleration appears to be the most suitable parameter with which to measure injury and will be used for the most part throughout this paper.

With acceleration as the primary injury criterion, some enlightening calculations can be made relating velocity, acceleration, and minimum stopping distance. For a minimum stopping distance from a given velocity without exceeding a given acceleration, a constant or uniform acceleration of the given value must be maintained in which case the simple, well-known equations for constant acceleration prevail.[1] An example of the relationship between velocity, acceleration and distance can be examined for the case of a tolerable head impact. Assuming 80 g as the tolerable impact level, the minimum stopping distance required from 30 mph is 4½ inches and from 60 mph is 18 inches under ideal, unattainable conditions. If the tolerance limit had been assumed to be 40 g, then the minimum stopping distance from 30 mph would have been 9 inches and from 60 mph, 36 inches. It should be emphasized that these are minimum or optimum distances which cannot be achieved, and about twice the distance given here is usually required. Thus, at 30 mph and 80 g, approximately 9 inches of deformation will be required for the usual nonuniform acceleration encountered in impact to engineering structures.

The foregoing example points out the necessity for establishing the human tolerance to acceleration at as high a value as possible. Even with the tolerance set at 80 g, the required stopping distance is not available in many parts of the vehicle such as the header, glazed area, and the A post, and it is impractical to provide sufficient distance without impairing visibility. In these instances, it may be possible to eliminate the problem by locating the components so they are not likely to be struck by the head.

If maximum utilization is to be made of the available stopping distance, it is essential that the structure be designed to approach the uniform acceleration condition as closely as possible, which means the component or part of the interior struck should deform at approximately the human tolerance force level over most of the available distance. It is necessary to put some load-distributing padding over the main structure, but this padding is generally too soft to be of major benefit decelerating the body during the impact so its thickness should be added to the effective stopping distance.

Details of the appropriate design procedures to use together with the human tolerance levels for various parts of the body will be discussed in appropriate sections herein.

HUMAN TOLERANCE TO IMPACT

Human tolerance to impact can be classified as voluntary, injury threshold, minor injury, and severe injury. The voluntary tolerance limit is that limit to which a volunteer is willing to be subjected and is usually well below the injury level. The injury threshold is the impact level at which injury is imminent but does not occur. Minor injury is based on a reversible injury level such as a mild concussion or soft tissue damage. Severe injury can be anything up to, and including, fatal injury. Obviously, this latter category is not a suitable impact tolerance level. The minor injury category is probably the best human tolerance value for use in automotive safety programs. With the minor injury, those least able to withstand an impact are likely to be injured rather severely, while the average will have minor or no injury and the strongest individual will be in the subinjury category. It should be pointed out that the human tolerance to impact is not an exact value. There are large physiological variations from individual to individual, and certain genetic or traumatic conditions can result in gross deviations in the tolerance to impact.

Impacts can be subdivided into whole body impacts, or impacts to individual body areas, or components. The whole body impact includes those encountered in falls, on centrifuges, impact sleds, and any other condition where the force is distributed over a large part of the body. An early attempt to establish human tolerance to impact was based on known conditions from survival of falls. DeHaven[2] found that falls in which the average deceleration was in the order of 140 g were survived without serious injuries, when the individual landed in a supine position, on garden earth, which distributed the load and provided several inches of deceleration distance. As a result of his work, he suggested 200 g as a survivable impact level, providing the load was adequately distributed.

Snyder[3] has investigated falls including those into water from great heights. In one case, the individual fell a distance of 178 feet and struck the water feet first at an impact velocity of 97 feet per second and was not injured. Another individual survived a fall of 275 feet with injury, after striking the water feet first at an impact velocity of 116 feet per second.

Kiel[4] reported on a paratrooper who fell 1200 feet, landing in a supine position on crusted snow. His impact velocity was about 178 feet per second and he produced a crater 3½ feet deep in the snow. The average deceleration for this condition was 140 g.

Stapp[5] in his ride on the Sonic Wind, in a forward-facing attitude, sustained a peak deceleration of 47 g for a change in velocity of 600 mph with minor injuries including retinal hemorrhages. This event was one of the early pioneering efforts to establish human tolerance.

Stapp[6] reports on a series of sled runs in which military volunteers in excellent physical condition were subjected to a 40 g acceleration in a rearward-facing seated position. At an onset of 310 g per second, the ride was considered tolerable, while, at the same 40 g level with an onset of 2090 g per second, severe shock resulted together with loss of consciousness. Based on this work, Stapp states ". . . protection of human occupants should be feasible up to 40 g at 1000 g per second onset in collision and rollover accidents."

A restraint system consisting of a lap and upper torso belt results in essentially whole body deceleration in a forward-force automobile collision, so the 40 g recommended by Stapp is reasonable. The vehicle frame reaches a 40 g peak for a short time in a barrier impact at about 30 mph. Barrier impacts at greater speeds can be sustained without exceeding the 40 g level on the occupant with a yielding restraint system which eliminates forces corresponding to accelerations over 40 g by allowing relative motion between the occupant and the passenger compartment whenever that force is reached. A much greater change in velocity can be safely accomplished by limiting the peak force or acceleration in this manner.

Some recommended human tolerance to impact levels and the reference for each item are given in Table 13-II. It is suggested that care be exercised when using these human tolerance values, and it should be especially noted that in some cases they are based on voluntary impacts, while in others they are inferred from cadaver impacts, animal impacts or clinical studies. Thus, some of the values are for human tolerance based on injury or skeletal damage, while others are voluntary limits and are probably well below the injury impact tolerance.

Impact to individual body areas or components occurs when some area such as the head strikes or is struck by an object with sufficient force to approach, or exceed, the tolerance level. There are two radically different approaches to head protection: All surfaces of the impact environment can be made energy absorbing or an energy-absorbing mechanism (helmet) can be worn on the head with the best results achieved if both are used. Padding the environment has the advantage of requiring no action on the part of the occupant, and in many areas, large decelerating distances permit protection from high velocity impacts. There are, however, locations where padding or energy-absorbing material cannot be used such as the glazed area, the "A" post where the small size requirement for visibility prevents the use of sufficient padding volume and those external to the vehicle in the case of ejection. Protecting the head with a helmet has an advantage in that it permits the most efficient utilization of the available stopping distance, but the stopping distance is limited to approximately 1 inch from a practical size consideration. The maximum normal impact velocity for which a helmet can provide protection is about 25 feet per second, but a well-designed helmet can protect the wearer at tangential velocities—such as encountered when sliding along the highway after a motorcycle accident—up to velocities of 70 mph.

Elimination of Excessive Relative Motion Between Body Components

Relative motion between body components can cause injury to joints, ligaments, muscles, bones, and internal organs. Adequate load distribution, over the entire body, will prevent such relative motions and eliminate the injury. Concentrated forces, occurring when the body is struck with an object of small cross-sectional area, can produce relative motion within internal organs such as liver or spleen or between the organ and its connecting tissue, thereby resulting in direct trauma to the organ or to the connecting tissues.

Tolerable relative motion is illustrated by the normal action of joints. Jackknifing, usually without injury, with considerable relative angular motion between the torso and the thigh due to seat belt loads, is a good example of large, noninjurious joint rotation. Other normal joint motion such as the elbow, knee, ankle, and neck, motions are also common without injury. On the other hand, if moments are applied to the joints, either after the end of the normal rotation is reached, or in the opposite direction to normal rotation, injuries to the joints often occur.

Untolerable relative motion is exemplified by the injury to the spine[7] observed when the seat belt is worn too high. In this case, the spine is subjected to a bending load, which often produces ligamentous and bone damage to the lumbar spine. Relative displacement of the internal organs from the force of the belt on the abdomen can also result in tissue-tearing and organ rupture. Excessive hyperextension of the head and neck results in soft tissue and, in extreme cases, bone damage.

Perhaps the most common relative motion seen in automobile accidents is the hyperextension of the head and neck, commonly referred to as whiplash. An analysis of the reactions at the juncture of the head and neck can be made using principles of mechanics with the head treated as a free body. The analysis[8] results in axial (tension), transverse (shear) and rotational (torque) reactions. Magnitudes of these reactions under voluntary conditions were obtained by applying a force to the head of a volunteer approximately through the center of gravity in five different configurations:

1. The head in normal position
2. The head flexed
3. The head extended
4. The head braced with hands clasped behind it
5. Hanging position

The results of these loadings together with the calculated shear, tension and torque values are provided in Table 20-I.

TABLE 20-I
MAXIMUM REACTIONS FOR FIVE DIFFERENT LOADING POSITIONS OF HUMAN VOLUNTEER IN WHIPLASH DIRECTION

Loading Condition	Applied Force lb.	Shear Force lb.	Tensile Force lb.	Torque ft.-lb.
1. Head upright, A-P force	41	40	22	10
2. Head and neck flexed, A-P force	64	57	34	11
3. Head and neck extended, A-P force	89	13	86	15
4. Head braced with hands*, A-P force	175			
5. Hanging attitude	330	192	254	0

* Not amenable to analysis for shear, tensile and torque reactions.

A series of simulated whiplash type accidents was conducted on an impact sled. The results[8,9] showed that the limiting value was the torque in the neck, rather than the shear or tensile load. An injury index, based on the ratio of the torque under the dynamic condition to the static voluntary torque, shows the shear and tensile injury indices to be less than half that of the torque index.

The injury index for 10 mph (stationary car struck in the rear end with a car traveling 10 mph) was 0.7 for the volunteer with an index of 1 estimated at 15 mph. The volunteer's muscles were tense during the simulated impact. With the muscles relaxed the maximum torque would have been higher, and the injury index would probably have been greater than one at 10 mph.

The maximum torque is a function of the angle of rotation. With the muscles relaxed, very little torque is required to produce an angular rotation of 45 to 60 degrees. At this angle, the tissues connecting the cervical vertebrae become taut, and the torque increases rapidly. Limiting the hyperextension angle to a value below the injury level will eliminate whiplash injury. Forty-five degrees is a conservative value for noninjurious rotation with 60 to 70 degrees probably safe, and injuries probably occurring in excess of 80 degrees. Ligamentous damage was observed in an aged cadaver at 83 degrees after several impacts. It should be pointed out that voluntary tolerance levels are usually well below the injury tolerance level, so the 10 to 18 foot-pounds of torque from the voluntary measurements are probably well below the injury level. However, there appears to be no reason why provision cannot be made in the design of the automobile seat back to limit the angular rotation of the head to a value well below the injury angle. This is different from most design requirements in automotive safety where it is necessary to design to some injury level in order to provide protection at the maximum possible velocity.

With a head support, the volunteer withstood an impact equivalent to a 44 mph rear-end collision without injury or even major concern for his head and neck. The head load was 340 pounds on a rigid head support with 5/8 of an inch of padding. The head support should prevent excessive head angulation without interfering with rear vision. This can be accomplished by supporting the head at the lower part of the occiput with a head support that is contoured to contact the neck and base of the skull.

PROVISION FOR DISTRIBUTING THE LOAD

The functions and properties of materials and structures used in constructing protective systems within the automobile are of the greatest importance in minimizing the occurrence and severity of injuries and have been the subject of a number of papers.[1,10,11] Their functions are twofold: 1. to distribute the load to best advantage (which usually means as evenly as possible) over the part of the body being decelerated, and 2. to decelerate the body within the available distance with the exertion of least force.

The components of the protective systems under consideration are as follows: 1. Padding materials and yielding structures (usually metallic), the most important of which are the instrument panel, the steering assembly and the windshield; (2) part or whole body restraint systems consisting of various arrangements of webbing; and (3) airbags (air-stop systems) which are included in whole body restraint systems, although they are not yet in general use.

PADDED AND YIELDING STRUCTURES

Previous studies have shown the importance of trying to achieve a load-deflection characteristic, which results in uniform deceleration of the body being arrested.[1] For the head, for which a tolerance level of 80 g has been established, the stopping distance required from given initial velocities can be calculated for various input pulses (the short duration spikes above 80 g are neglected). The shortest possible stopping distance results from

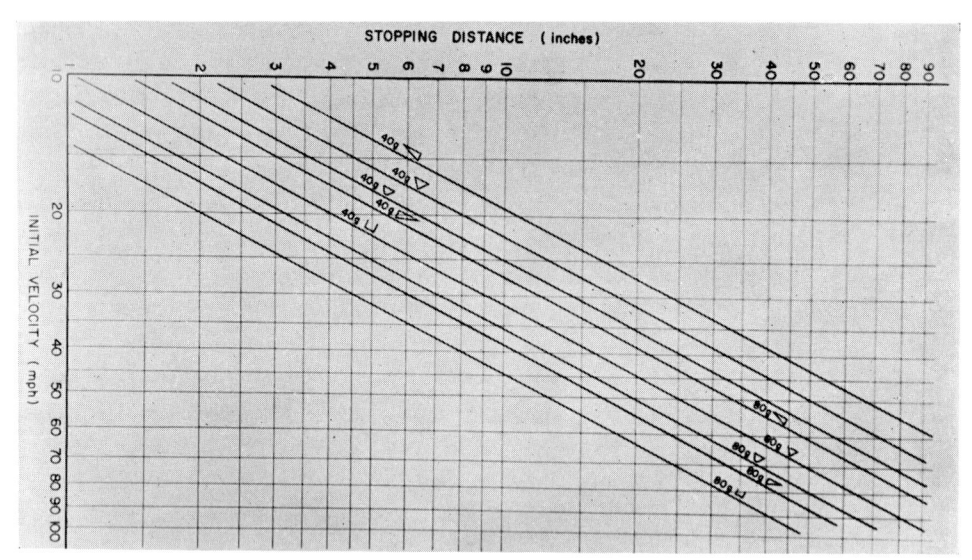

FIGURE 20–1. Stopping distance as a function of initial velocity with a peak deceleration of 80 g for the different acceleration pulse shapes of Figure 20–2.

constant (uniform) acceleration (deceleration is negative acceleration) at the maximum permissible value of 80 g. Any other pulse shape with the same maximum value results in greater stopping distance. The required stopping distances for constant or uniform acceleration and several other acceleration pulse shapes are shown in Figure 20–1. It is important to understand that if the maximum acceleration is stipulated (80 g in this case), there is no way that the head can be stopped from a given velocity in a shorter distance than shown for the constant acceleration curve of Figure 20–1. From a practical standpoint, this minimum stopping distance can never be achieved, but it does serve as a goal or base with which to compare actual deformations for efficiency of space utilization. The minimum stopping distance (constant acceleration) is tabulated along with other acceleration pulse shapes in Table 20-II for several initial velocity conditions.

Six different acceleration pulse shapes are shown in Figure 20–2 to illustrate the stopping distance required for them, and to provide insight into desirable design conditions. The area under each pulse is the same, if A_p (peak acceleration) is the same, and if the time is as shown for each. The area under the curve represents velocity change, so if the area is the same, the impact velocity is the same. The mathematical expression for stopping distance (S) is shown adjacent to each pulse shape, and can be used to find the stopping distance for any initial input velocity and peak acceleration. Data for these pulse shapes are shown in Table 20-II and Figure 20–2.

Application of Human Tolerance Data to Protective Systems

TABLE 20-II
STOPPING DISTANCE FOR DIFFERENT ACCELERATION PULSE SHAPES AND VARYING INITIAL VELOCITIES FOR PEAK ACCELERATIONS OF 40 AND 80 G UNITS

Initial Velocity V_o		Stopping Distance in Inches				
mph	ft./sec.	Constant Accel.	Softening Spring	Half Sine	Isosceles Triangle	Stiffening Spring
		$-.401 \frac{V_o^2}{A_p}$	$-.534 \frac{V_o^2}{A_p}$	$-.629 \frac{V_o^2}{A_p}$	$-.802 \frac{V_o^2}{A_p}$	$-1.07 \frac{V_o^2}{A_p}$
			for $A_p = -40$ g			
10	14.7	1.0	1.33	1.57	2.0	2.66
20	29.3	4.0	5.34	6.30	8.0	10.68
30	44.0	9.0	12.00	14.20	18.0	24.00
40	58.6	16.0	21.40	25.20	32.0	42.80
50	73.4	25.0	33.40	39.30	50.0	66.80
60	88.0	36.0	48.00	56.60	72.0	96.00
			for $A_p = -80$ g			
10	14.7	0.5	0.67	0.786	1.0	1.33
20	29.3	2.0	2.70	3.14	4.0	5.34
30	44.0	4.5	6.00	7.10	9.0	12.00
40	58.6	8.0	10.70	12.60	16.0	21.40
50	73.4	12.5	16.70	19.70	25.0	33.40
60	88.0	18.0	24.00	28.30	36.0	48.00

Figure 20–1 shows that an impact surface, which has a characteristic of a softening spring, requires 33 per cent more stopping distance than the minimum for uniform acceleration; the half sine pulse requires 57 per cent more; the isosceles triangle requires 100 per cent more; and the

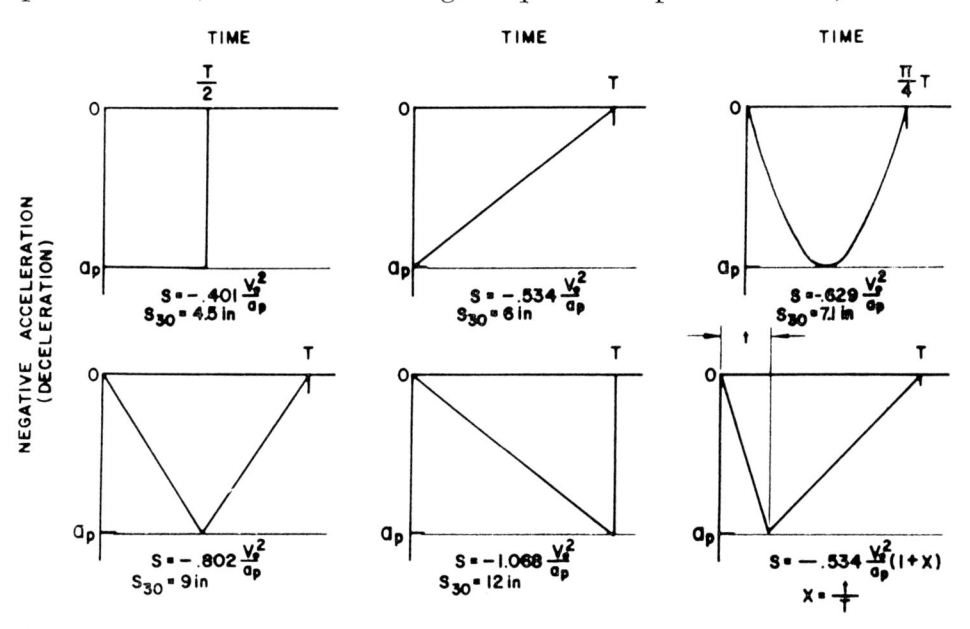

FIGURE 20–2. Stopping distance for various deceleration pulse shapes for the same maximum acceleration and initial velocity.

stiffening spring requires 166 per cent more. Many resilient foam padding materials have a characteristic impact acceleration pulse which approximates half of a parabola and requires considerably greater distance than the stiffening spring. Some rigid and semiresilient foams have characteristics which produce stopping distances about the same as the half sine acceleration-time pulse.

Assuming an 80 g maximum permissible head acceleration, (neglecting the permissible short term accelerations above the 80 g level) the stopping distance from 30 mph is 4.5 inches for constant acceleration, 6 inches for the softening spring, 7.1 inches for the half sine, 9 inches for the isosceles triangle pulse, and 12 inches for the stiffening spring. These values are rather large and present a formidable obstacle in the design of a safe vehicle interior in which the available stopping distance is severely limited. If the head strikes a surface with the required stiffness to provide minimum stopping distance, there is likely to be local injury, unless padding is provided to distribute the load over a large portion of the head. This padding adds little to the deceleration of the head, and consequently its thickness must be added to the required stopping distance.

At certain places inside an automobile, padding, or metal molding[12] has to provide protection—usually for the head. Examples of such places are the header, the sun visors, the corner pillars, the door pillars in 4-door cars, and the bodywork likely to be contacted by passengers in rear seats. At none of these places is it feasible to use more than 1 inch of padding. The designer has to decide whether to use material which initially deforms at a high pressure and therefore minimizes head injury at comparatively high impact speeds, but which may cause greater facial injuries at low speeds, or a softer padding which is less efficient at the higher speeds but gives more facial protection at lower speeds. It seems likely that the choice should always be the stiffer padding, since in frontal collisions, if no account is taken of the cushioning effect of the scalp, 1 inch of padding can only be expected to restrict the deceleration of the head to 80 g, which as we have already seen, experiment suggests as an upper limit for a relative velocity of about 14 mph, assuming the padding to have ideal characteristics and to compress to zero thickness. The performance of real materials will inevitably be considerably inferior to this. Twelve to 15 pound polyurethane has been suggested by one of the authors[1] as a suitable material for such positions, but it is important to realize the limited nature of the protection thus provided, particularly for an unrestrained occupant.

The characteristics, of real padding materials, are well illustrated in tests carried out by Moore in 1961.[11] The dynamic tests were conducted with a 3½ inch diameter specimen of the material mounted on a solid steel, 3½ inch diameter × 7 inch long, piezo-electric load cell located on a massive concrete block. A 10-pound striker was dropped from various heights to simulate the human striking an immovable object.

Blows of impact energies up to 100 foot-pounds (10 foot drop) were given to specimens of various materials of several different thicknesses and areas, and records of transmitted force against time were recorded with a cathode ray oscillograph. The results were exhibited as curves relating peak force to impact energy. An example showing the effect of varying the thickness of one type of padding is given in Figure 20–3.

Table 20-III gives an indication of the relative merit of a number of

TABLE 20-III
SPECIFIC ENERGY ABSORPTION OF DIFFERENT MATERIALS [after Moore[3]]

| Material | \multicolumn{5}{c}{Energy absorbed in ft.lb./cu.in. when peak pressure reaches:} |
	100 lb/ sq. in.	200 lb./ sq. in.	300 lb./ sq. in.	400 lb./ sq. in.	500 lb./ sq. in.
Foamed polysterene					
density 5 lb./cu.ft.		5	9	12	14
density 3 lb./cu.ft.	3	6	8		
Compressed cork	1	3	6	9	11
Natural cork	0.3	1.5	2	5	10
Sponge rubber (best specimen)					5
Felt (unperforated)	0.8	2	3	4	5
Foamed butadiene rubber	1.2	4.2	8.4	10.3	11.8
"Ideal" material					
(theoretical maximum)	8	17	25	33	42

materials tested. The values given are of the Specific Energy Absorption (foot-pounds per cubic inch); that is, the energy absorption of unit volume of the material given for a range of peak pressures.

The possibility of providing protection for all parts of the body is much greater when the underlying metallic structure of the impacted part can be designed to deform plastically. It is not always realized, by those who suggest alterations to the structure of cars to provide greater "energy absorption," that it is difficult to devise any better structure than one employing mild steel, of which all cars are constructed, deformed plastically by bending. The two important structures which can be designed in this way are the instrument panel and the steering assembly. The protective elements of both structures consist of two deforming components: (1) padding material to distribute the load—this is particularly important for the top of the instrument panel which is likely to be struck by the face of a lap-belted passenger; and (2) a metallic structure capable of much greater deformation than can be achieved by padding alone. Tests of a padded instrument panel and of an energy-absorbing steering assembly, both capable of deforming by about 6 inches, have been described.[1,12]

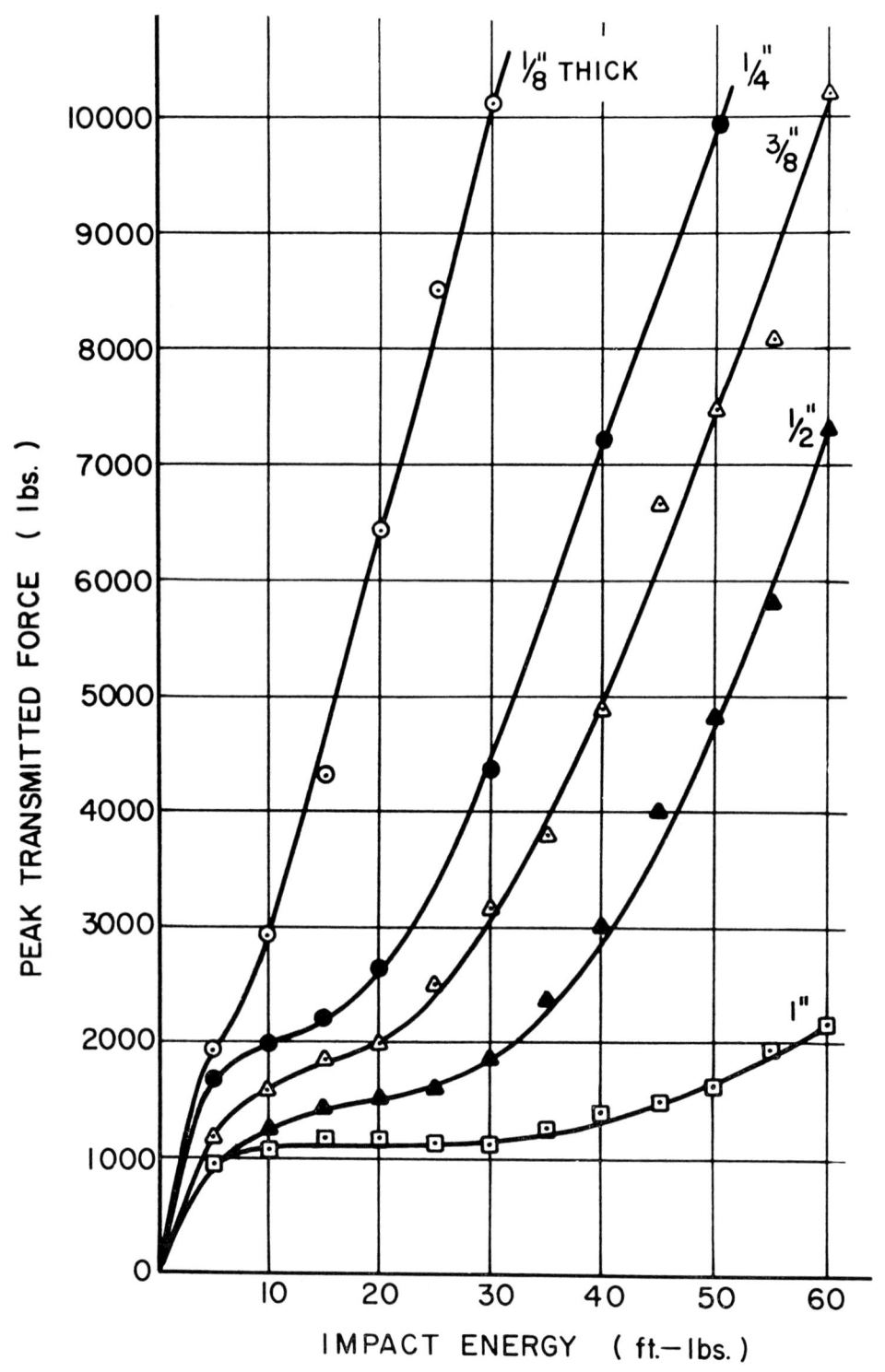

FIGURE 20–3. Peak transmitted force as a function of impact energy for increasing thickness of padding (after Moore[11]).

An example of a well-designed panel is shown in Figure 20–4, which is taken from Reference 13. This figure shows the undeformed panel and pad together with the permanent deformation of the panel at head impact speeds of 14, 19, 23 and 40 mph. Figure 20–5 shows the plastic panel deformation, the plastic panel plus pad deformation, and the plastic panel deformation plus pad deformation plus elastic panel deformation, as a function of head-to-panel impact velocity.

Tests of the energy-absorbing steering assembly were made with lap-belted cadavers impacting the steering assembly mounted on a sled which was stopped from speeds of 24 and 29 mph in distances of 18 and 24 inches, respectively. The energy-absorbing elements crushed from 4 to 5¾ inches and peak loads on the upper body of 1600 to 1800 pounds were recorded without any indications of serious danger to life injuries.

RESTRAINT SYSTEMS

The most important advantage, of body restraining systems over padded and deforming structures, is that the arresting distance may be much greater, not only because there is a substantial space for them to stretch into, but also because, as explained later, they make use of some of the stopping distance of the car.

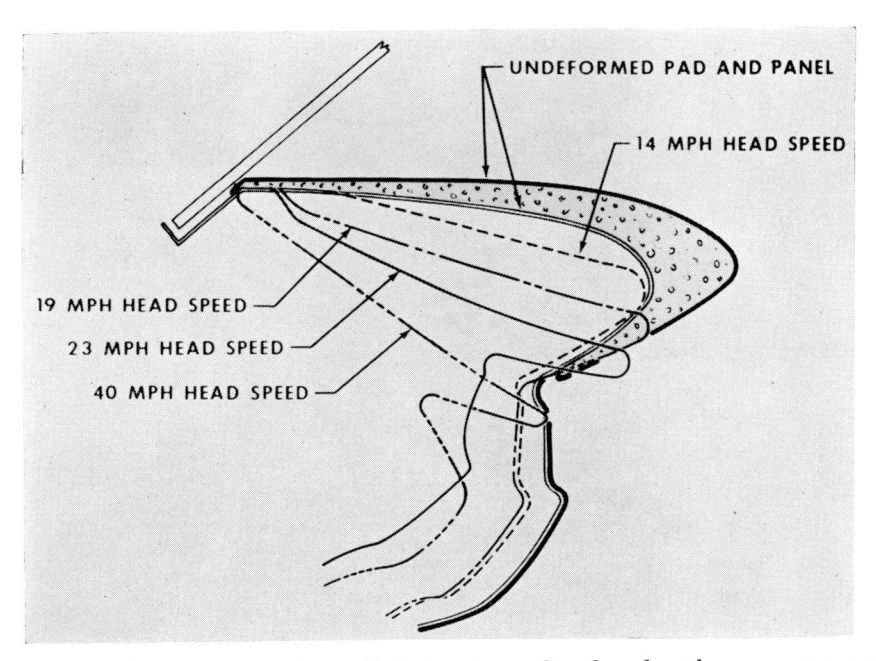

FIGURE 20–4. Cross section of a well-designed panel and pad with permanent panel deformation for head impacts at velocities from 14 to 40 mph.

Restraint systems in present use are generally constructed from nylon or terylene webbing usually 2 inches wide. As with all arresting devices, the ideal load-extension curve would be one in which all extension took place at a predetermined, constant load. This is far from being the case with existing systems. The restraint system characteristic is determined by two factors, the properties of the webbing, and the geometry of the system. A straight length of webbing may have a loading curve such that the force developed is approximately proportional to extension, but restraint systems always consist of one or more loops whose sides become more nearly parallel with the direction of action of the extending force as the load increases. The combined effect of webbing characteristics and geometrical arrangement produces a load-extension curve which resembles a spring of progressively increasing stiffness. Changing this characteristic to one approaching the ideal of a constant yield, would have greatest effect for whole body restraint systems, and it has often been suggested that the loops of the restraint system should be attached to the vehicle by means of links which would yield when a predetermined load was reached, the geometry of the system being arranged so that subsequent movement took place against a constant force. A development suggested by one of the authors[14] is to attach a very stiff restraint system to a strong seat which is arranged to slide forward in guides, its movement being controlled by a device yielding at a predetermined level of force.

The energy absorption of the restraint system webbing has, in the past, been given a great deal of attention, since the original and incomplete analyses, of the behavior of automobile restraint systems, assumed instantaneous stopping of the vehicle in head-on collisions, and in such circumstances, the whole of the wearer's kinetic energy is transferred to the webbing; the recoil velocity of the safety belt wearer is then proportional to the square root of the fraction of this energy that remains in the webbing. Figure 20–6 is an idealized load-extension curve for webbing under dynamic conditions. Area ABC represents the original energy required to extend it, and area DBC, the returnable energy. The early calculations equated area ABC with the kinetic energy of the car occupant, and area DBC with the energy available for his recoil into the seat. For the two webbing materials in current use, area DBC is about one-quarter of area ABC, so that the return or "sling-shot" velocity back into the seat would be expected to be one-half of the forward velocity. In practice, however, because the stop takes place over an appreciable time, (about $\frac{1}{10}$ second) much of the kinetic energy of the car occupant is transferred to the vehicle through the restraint system during the stop, and both theory and experiment[15] show the return velocity to be much lower than predicted from simple considerations; since the return velocities are so

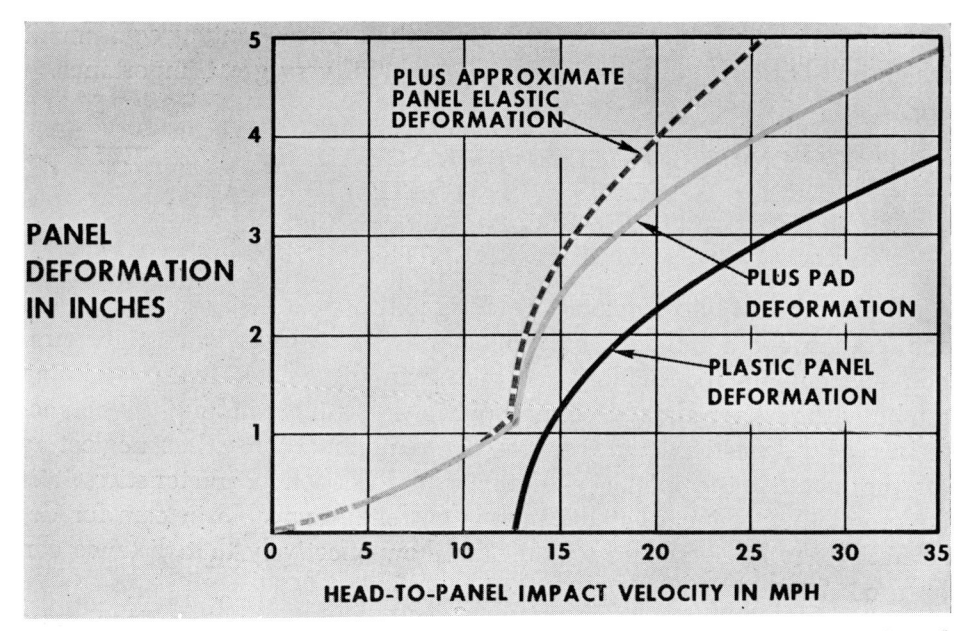

FIGURE 20–5. Plastic panel deformation plus approximate elastic panel and pad deformation as a function of head impact velocity.

low, differences in energy absorption between the commonly used webbing materials are of no practical importance.

Very little detailed investigation has been reported on the load-distributing properties of webbing restraint systems. The two types of greatest current interest are the lap strap and the lap-and-diagonal three-point belt. Extensive experience with lap straps, however, indicates that very large forces can be tolerated without any resulting injury more serious than bruising provided that the belt is properly worn. The area of the diagonal part of a three-point belt is large, about 40 square inches, and the doubts, which have sometimes been expressed concerning the possibility of injury due to the forces exerted by this diagonal strap, relate more to internal injuries resulting from excessive deceleration of the upper part of the body than to injuries caused by uneven distribution of force. This subject is dealt with briefly in the next section.

The "airstop" restraint system[16,17] would appear to hold out the possibility of the best distribution of load over the upper part of the body, since the inflated bag can be arranged to make contact with the whole of the body above the waist. As with webbing restraints, large stopping distances are possible, and the load-deflection curves appear to be similar to those of current webbing restraints.[16] It will be obvious, however, that there are formidable practical difficulties in inflating the bags quickly enough, and in bringing them very close to the car occupant, a requirement which will be shown in the next section to be of very great importance.

PROVISION OF SUFFICIENT DISTANCE TO ALLOW KINETIC ENERGY TO BE DISSIPATED WITHOUT EXCEEDING TOLERABLE IMPACT FORCES AND DECELERATIONS

All protective devices, which are designed to reduce impact forces and decelerations—other than those which provide strength against penetration—depend upon providing the maximum distance available to bring the body to rest. As already pointed out in discussing padding, the characteristic load-deflection curve is also of great importance; but neglecting for the moment the influence of the load-deflection characteristics, it is important to examine what distance is currently available in cars for decelerating the body of the occupant and how effectively that distance can be used.

In the first place, we shall consider only head-on impacts since these occur more frequently than any other kind of impact, and except for comparatively rare side impacts, are generally the most severe.[18] Such impacts occur not only in head-on collisions of two vehicles traveling in opposite directions on the same road, but also in single vehicle accidents when roadside obstacles are impacted, and in rear-end and intersection accidents, where there is always a striking car. The requirements for space to reduce impact forces apply for all directions of impact, and it is indeed fortunate that the head-on impact is the one for which protection has to be mainly designed, since there is, in general, more distance available in the fore-and-aft direction than in any other.

Of course, there is no doubt that the greater the amount of padding and controlled crushing of the underlying structure in a particular place in the car, the greater its protective value; but it is worth considering the effect of the positioning of the protective material or device in relation to the person who will strike it, since this is of comparable importance. The analysis is elementary and has been given elsewhere by one of the authors[18] and others,[19] but it brings out several points which are worth emphasizing.

It is well known that head-on impacts of both American and European cars at speeds between, say, 20 and 40 mph produce decelerations of the passenger compartment which, because of the large amount of crushing, last for about $\frac{1}{10}$ second (say, between 0.09 and 0.15 second). Examples of data from barrier collisions are given in Figures 20–7 and 20–8 (after Lundstrom[20]). In other types of head-on collision, durations may be a

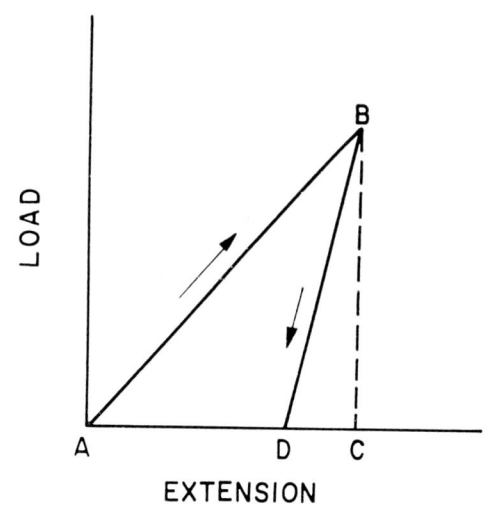

FIGURE 20-6. Idealized load-deflection characteristic for a linear webbing.

little longer; for example, in some rear-end collisions where the impacted rear-end may be relatively soft, but the difference is of little significance.

For convenience of analysis, it is usual to approximate these deceleration-time curves by half-sine wave shapes, triangles of various proportions or rectangles. Figure 20-9 shows a set of such curves, all of which give

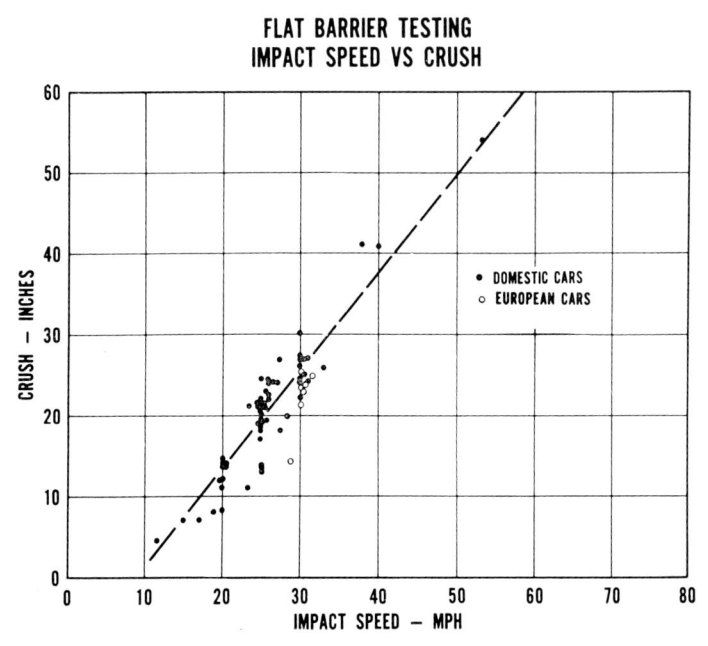

FIGURE 20-7. Front end crush as a function of barrier impact velocity for domestic and European cars (after Lundstrom[20]).

FRAME ACCELERATION VS TIME
30 MPH BARRIER

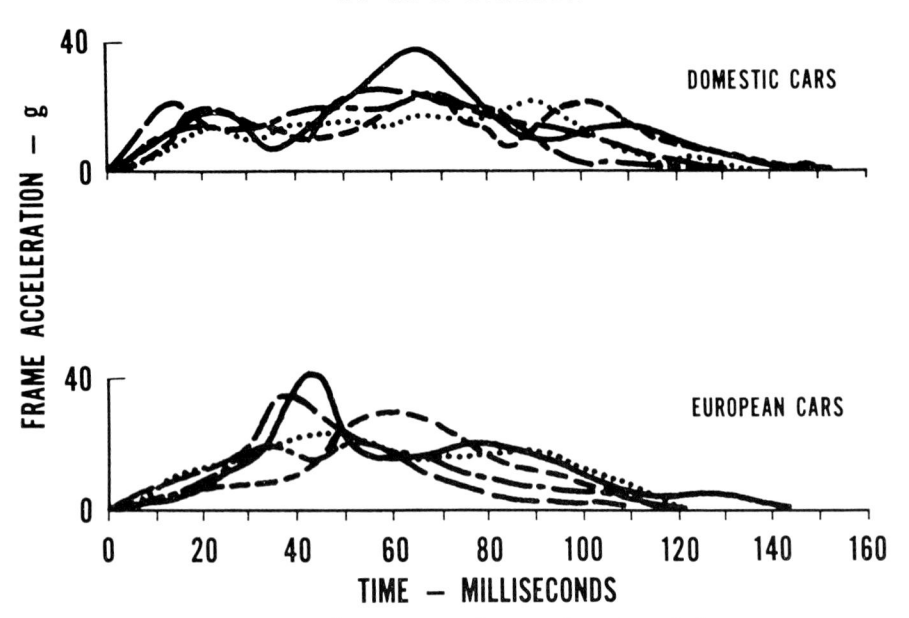

FIGURE 20–8. Frame acceleration time-history for 30 mph barrier impacts.

the same stopping distance (of the passenger compartment) from the same speed. (The condition for equal stopping distances from a given speed is that the centroids of the areas under the curves shall occur at the same time after the start of the impact.)

The effect of the distance at which protective devices are placed in front of the car occupant will now be considered, assuming a half-sine wave deceleration-time curve, an initial speed of 30 mph and a stopping distance of 24 inches. On impact, the passenger is assumed to move forward with the initial velocity of the car; that is, friction with the seat and forces exerted by the seat and floor are negligible.

In head-on impacts, most of the crushing happens in the early part of the impact; for example, half of the crushing takes place in a little over a quarter of the total time taken to stop. On the other hand, the forward movement of the passenger, relative to the car, develops only very slowly; in a quarter of the total stopping time, for example, the passenger moves forward relative to the car by only about 0.8 inch.

Figures 20–10 and 20–11, given in nondimensional form in Appendix 20-I, may be applied to any head-on impact. The five curves are drawn for the five deceleration-time curves of Figure 20–9.

These diagrams help in understanding the problem of protection in that

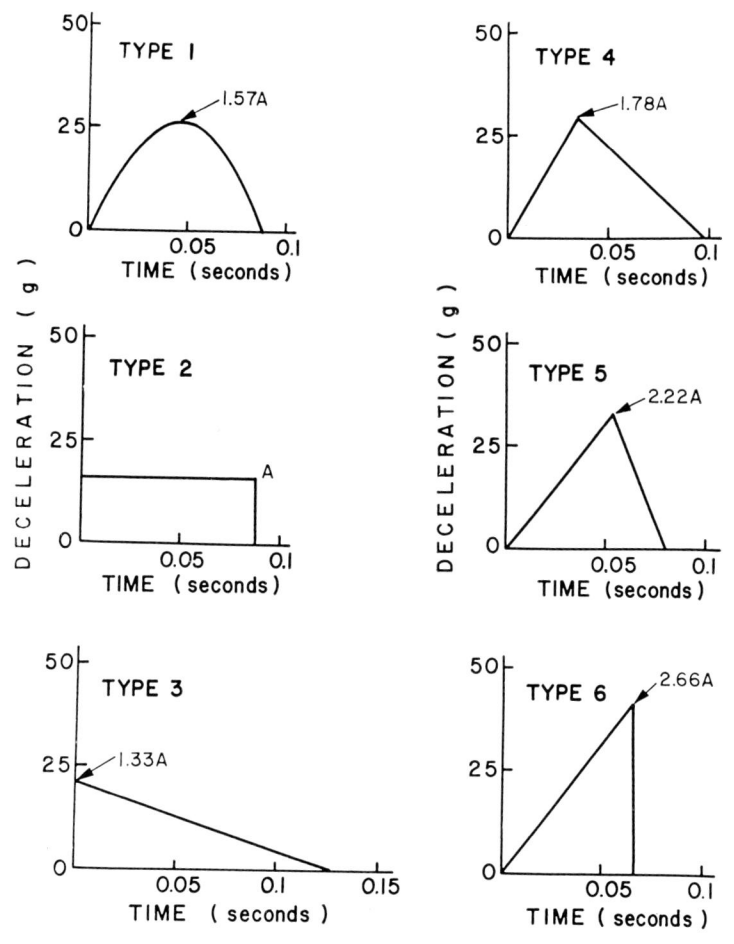

Application of Human Tolerance Data to Protective Systems 463

FIGURE 20–9. Acceleration pulse shapes all of which result in a stopping distance of 24 inches from 30 mph.

they explain the importance of having the protective device as close as possible to the car occupant. Arresting distance for the occupant may be obtained in two ways: (1) The occupant may be in close contact with the protective device and may decelerate with it; i.e. use may be made of at least some of the car's crushing distance, and (2) The device itself may deform or stretch. Table 20-IV[21] gives approximate distances from head to windshield, chest to instrument panel, chest to steering wheel and knee to nearest part of bodywork for some American and European cars. The sequence of events when a passenger moves forward in a head-on impact has been illustrated by one of the authors[13] in diagrams which are reproduced in Figure 20–12. It is clear that the car has almost stopped in some cases, before the knees make contact with the bodywork. For

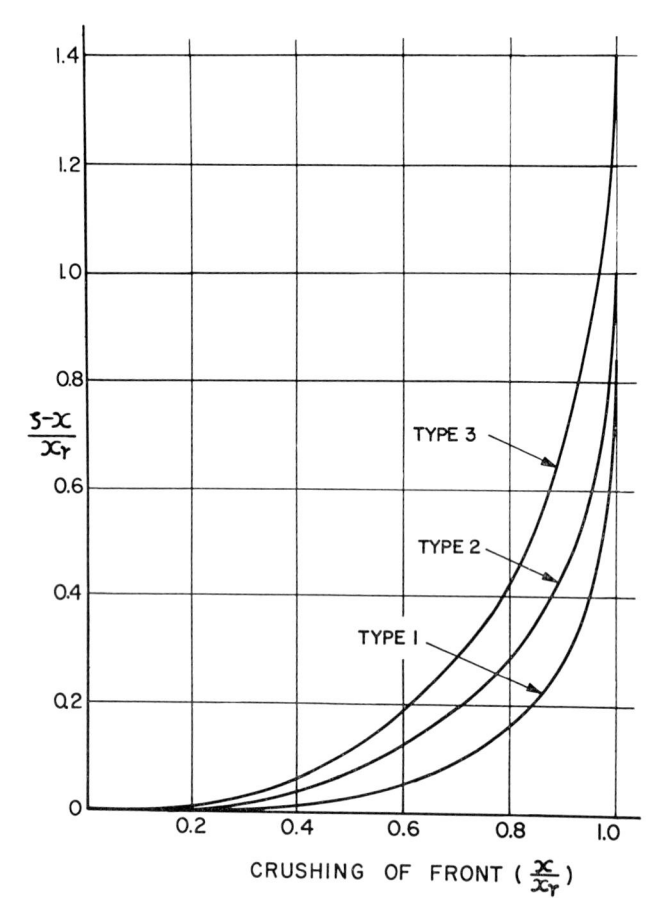

FIGURE 20–10. Half sine-wave approximation of crushing of front of car as a function of time after impact.

TABLE 20-IV

SPACE AVAILABLE IN SOME EUROPEAN AND AMERICAN CARS FOR A 5 FOOT 10 INCH, 170 POUND OCCUPANT

Vehicle	Clearance measurements, in. (car seat in mean position)				
	A	B	C	D	E
Austin Mini	19	22	28	16	7
Ford Cortina	14	18	24	13	7
Austin Cambridge	17	22	23	16	9
Citroen Safari	16	19	17	—	3
American Ford	13	22	24	15	2
Buick	15	27	25	16	7

Key:
A—From forehead to nearest point of car.
B—From forehead to windshield, horizontally.
C—From body to nearest point on car in forward direction.
D—From body to center of steering column.
E—From knee to nearest point on car in forward direction.

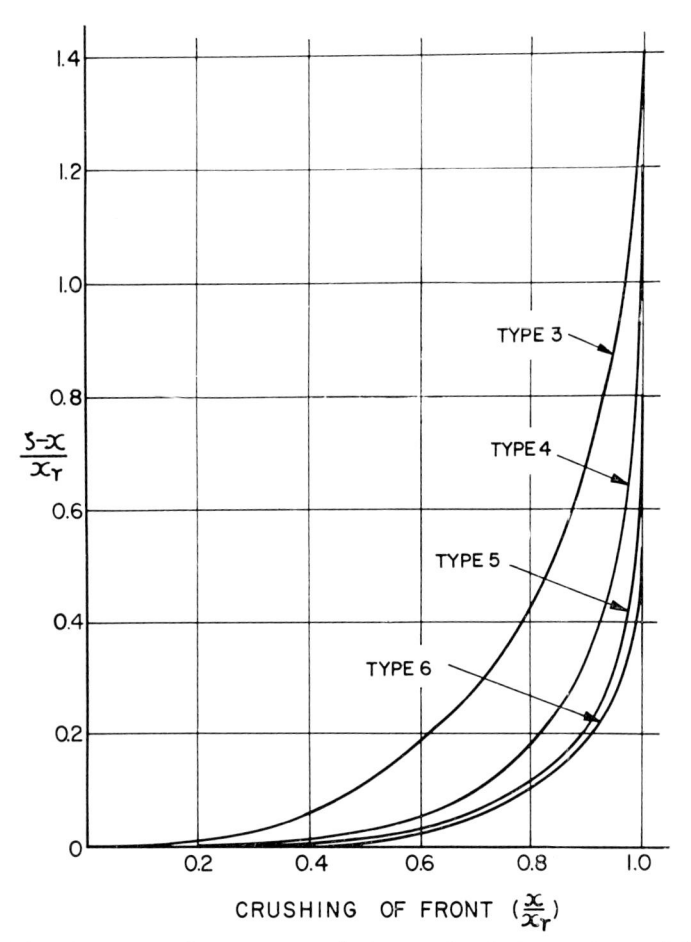

FIGURE 20–11. Movement of passenger relative to the instrument panel for crushing characteristics of Figure 20–10.

instrument panels and windshields, which are usually at much greater distances than the part struck by the knee, the car has to all intents and purposes stopped before the occupant strikes them; hence, the popular notion of the "second impact." A slight improvement is possible if the crushing of the front of the car produces uniform deceleration of the car structure, but the difference is small (see Fig. 20–10 and Ref. 18 for a more detailed discussion). Any cushioning for the head or body striking these forward components, the windshield and surrounding bodywork and the instrument panel, must all be provided by yielding of the structure impacted.

The only protective device presently in use, which clearly benefits from the movement of the car itself, is the seat belt, and particularly the belt with upper body restraint. This is usually worn with some slack, and in

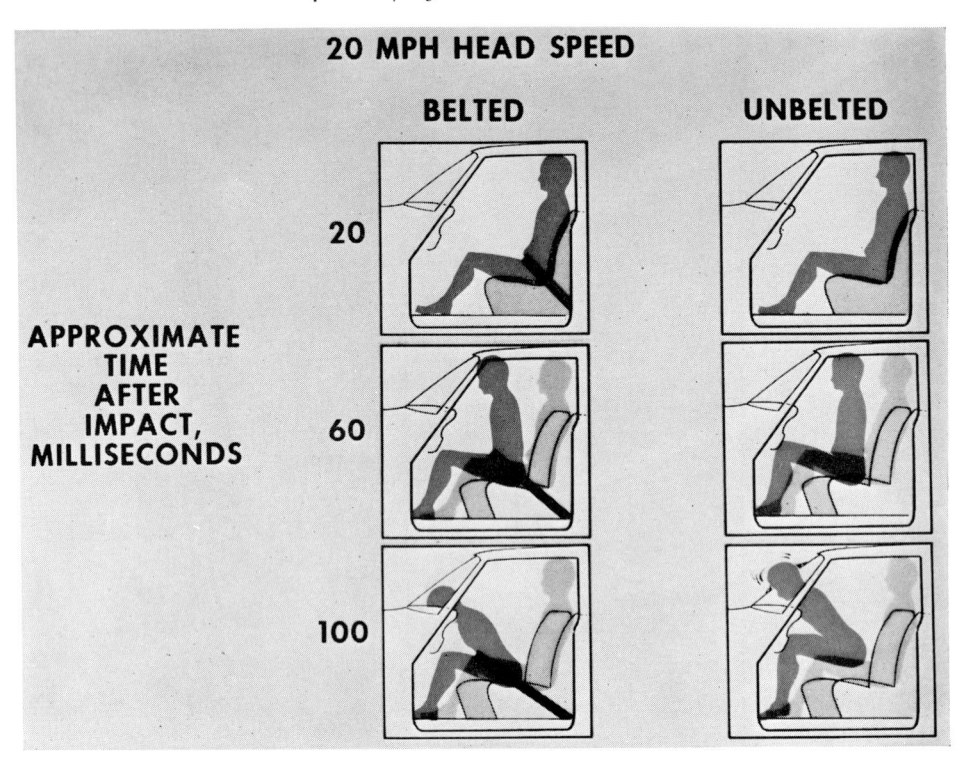

FIGURE 20–12. Movement of passenger relative to the instrument panel as a function of front-end crush.

any case, the flexibility of the body is equivalent to some slack; this will be assumed to be 1 inch of slack. The body, therefore, has to move forward this distance before it begins to be decelerated. At that instant in a 30 mph impact about 12 inches of the front remains uncrushed. Since the belt itself may also stretch up to 12 inches, in favorable circumstances, car movement may double the available stopping distance for a person in a safety harness involved in a head-on barrier collision at about 30 mph. The importance of wearing such harnesses tightly is also clear, and tightness of fit appears to be the main reason for the improved results obtained in Britain with automatic lap-and-diagonal safety belts compared with those of the ordinary three-point type.[22] With an automatic belt, the diagonal shoulder loop is held against the wearer by a spring-tensioned reel which locks against withdrawal almost instantaneously on impact from any direction.

The performance that may be expected from protective devices can now be estimated. There are three cases to consider: (1) the passenger or driver without belt, (2) the one wearing a lap belt, and (3) the one wearing lap-and-diagonal upper body restraint.

The movement of the unrestrained passenger has been shown to be forward as a whole until his knees contact the lower part of the instrument panel which stops the lower part of his body; the upper body then either jackknifes so that the head strikes the upper part of the instrument panel or, more probably, the windshield. The car will have stopped before this happens, and in most cases the speed at which the head is traveling is likely to be equal to, or greater than, the initial speed of the car. Since the head is the most important part of the body to protect, anything which can be done to reduce its speed or to reduce the likelihood of hitting the instrument panel or windshield is likely to be of value. One possibility is to allow enough room under the instrument panel for the body to move forward as a whole until the chest makes contact with a well-padded deformable structure, while the knees are simultaneously stopped by a similar structure under the instrument panel. However, this would necessitate bringing the instrument panel very much closer to the passenger's chest than it is at present, and it would probably be difficult to devise any acceptable permanent structure. A driver already has a steering wheel placed to receive his chest, and in his case, the padding to receive the knees should probably be so placed that contact is made with knees and chest at approximately the same time.

The forces on the chest of a lap-belted driver impacting an energy-absorbing steering assembly have been referred to in the last section. A very rough calculation of the movement of the upper part of the body can be made, assuming it to be an armless block held at the hips by a lap belt. The rotational velocity of the CG of the trunk at the end of the impact is found to be about 0.75 of the original impact velocity; the driver therefore gains an advantage by wearing a lap belt, since the velocity of the main mass of his upper body is reduced. On the other hand, the velocity of his head may be considerably greater than if he is unrestrained (30 per cent higher has been observed experimentally), and it is extremely important that the head should either be prevented from striking anything or should strike a suitably engineered surface.

Lastly, the design of restraint systems providing upper body restraint will be considered. These should include airbags, but the discussion will be limited to systems in use; that is, those using webbing although the calculations are similar in the two cases.

The performance that is theoretically possible with a three-point safety belt—that is, one having a lap loop plus a single shoulder loop—will now be considered; attention will be confined to the passenger, so as to avoid considering the complication of the steering wheel. It will be assumed that the object is to protect the passenger, as far as possible, from serious injury and death, rather than from slight injury. As a result of making this choice, there may be a greater risk of slight injury in minor accidents than would be the case if the primary consideration were to prevent slight injuries, but it will be assumed that this risk can be accepted. The performance is mainly determined by four factors:

1. The space for forward extension of the belt
2. The tolerance limit for the deceleration of the passenger's body
3. The load-extension characteristics of the belt
4. The amount of crushing of the front of the car, and its load-deformation characteristic

In designing whole body restraint systems, it is of first importance to regard the car plus safety belt as one single protective system, and to coordinate the design by taking account of all these factors. It will be assumed that 18 inches of forward movement is available for the restraint system to stretch, that the passenger can withstand a deceleration of 30 g, (giving a margin of safety on the 40 g postulated earlier in this paper that the restraint system has the ideal constant-yield characteristic and yields when the load exceeds the equivalent of thirty times the weight of the passenger) and that the front of the car will crush a distance of 36 inches to produce a half-sine wave deceleration-time curve; slack in the belt will be assumed to be 1 inch. In Figure 20–8 $x_T = 36$ inches $\xi - x = 1$ inch $\xi - x/x_T = 0.028$. This gives $x/x_T \sim 0.5$; that is, when the belt starts to tighten, about 18 inches of the front of the car remains to be crushed. This may therefore be added to the 17 inches available for the belt to stretch to give a total of 35 inches stopping distance for the passenger. At a deceleration of 30 g, this represents a stop from an initial velocity of about 51 mph; the strength of the front of the car must therefore be such that it decelerates the car from 51 mph in a distance of 36 inches.

Of course, the conditions assumed in this calculation are ideal ones, and serve merely to indicate the sort of performance which may ultimately be approached. On the other hand, the tolerance limit has been placed at 30 g, whereas in practice it may be 40 g or even more. In the meantime, however, a substantial body of evidence is accumulating on the performance in actual use of restraint systems of the lap-and-diagonal type. A recent paper to the Eleventh Stapp Conference[23] indicated that a spectacular reduction in deaths (a factor of about 5 to 1) might be resulting from their use in Swedish cars; however, the numbers of deaths were too small to be at all precise. Since 1962, the British Road Research Laboratory has collected and analyzed accident report forms filled up and returned by safety belt wearers who had been involved in accidents. These forms were enclosed with new belts sold by certain manufacturers; all belts provided upper body restraint. The evidence from these reports indicated that wearing safety belts of this type had reduced the risk of serious injury by a factor of about three.[13] Recently, a sample of about one thousand accidents reported in this way to one particular manufacturer (Britax Ltd.) has been examined in more detail by one of the authors, and, for a number of the more severe accidents involving head-on impacts, careful estimates have been made of the probable velocity change on impact. This part of the work is still at an early stage, but a number of instances of high velocity impacts can be listed with the resulting injuries; five are described in Table 20-V. They were selected not on the basis of injury, but because reliable estimates could be made of the minimum velocity changes at impact; these appear to have ranged up to at least 45 mph.

Most of the serious injuries were due to breaching of the passenger compartment; none of the eight belt wearers, in these particular accidents, suffered injury to internal organs due to forces exerted by the belt or to any other cause. A more extensive, but less detailed, investigation[22] has been made of 751 of the accidents, (involving 1096 belt wearers) and this confirms the rarity of internal injuries of this kind due to forces exerted by the webbing. In 1096 exposures to accidents, seven cases of injury to internal organs were reported; in two of these the injury probably occurred when the side or front of the car was pushed in; in another, a head-on collision, the driver with no passenger behind him was unhurt, but the front seat passenger had injuries to spleen, ribs, and lungs, probably by being crushed between the belt and the back of the seat by the impact of an unbelted passenger sitting behind him; in the remaining four cases, the injury may have been due to the belt, while performing its normal function; in two of these cases, the buckle was suggested as the cause of injury; and in the remaining two accidents, in both of which front seat passengers suffered injuries to the spleen, the injuries might have been due either to belt forces, or to impact with the instrument panel.

The next most serious injuries due to belt pressure were fractured sternums (six in 1096), fractured clavicles (nine in 1096) and fractured or cracked ribs (eighteen in 1096). It is worth noting that there were no instances of serious neck injury due to contact with the diagonal part of the belt, and of six injuries reported there were three burns, one cut and two bruises, all of which occured in severe accidents at high speeds. It may, of course, be objected that "dead men tell no tales." But it is inconceivable that if any appreciable number of deaths had been caused by contact with the diagonal strap, that they should not be accompanied by many more serious injuries; and belt wearers seriously injured in this way would be expected to be very vocal indeed. In the 1096 exposures,

TABLE 20-V
SEVERE HEAD-ON ACCIDENTS IN WHICH LAP-AND-DIAGONAL SAFETY BELTS WERE WORN[1]

Vehicles	Description of Accident	Velocity Change[2]	Sex; Age; Weight; Height	Particulars of Belt Wearers Injuries
A. 2-door sedan; 1680 lb. B. 2-door sedan; 1680 lb.	Head-on collision between A and B on bend	35 mph	D: Male; 20 yr; 189 lb; 75 in P: Male; 47 yr; 150 lb; 74 in	D: Bruises P: Bruises; cracked rib and small bone in back
A. 4-door sedan; 2016 lb. B. 4-door sedan; 2575 lb.	Head-on collision between A and B on bend; contact mainly from center to offside front. Engine and steering column pushed into passenger compartment	40 mph	D: Male; 44 yr; 168 lb; 66 in P: Male; 23 yr; 168 lb; 73 in	D: Broken right thigh and left shin due to engine intrusion. Facial bruising and concussion from steering wheel. P: Bruised knee, black eye
A. 4-door station wagon; 2670 lb B. 10-ton truck	Car A lost control on wet bend and hit B head-on; contact mainly on passenger side. Engine pushed back into car	45 mph	D: Male; 40 yr; 166 lb; 69 in	D: Left patella fractured and left leg lacerated by engine intrusion; slight facial laceration
A. 4-door sedan; 3000 lb. B. 8-ton truck	Car A lost control on icy bend and struck truck B head-on	35 mph	D: Male; age ?; 203 lb; 76 in	D: Minor facial injuries; fractured clavicle, patella, 3 ribs and 3 fingers
A. 4-door sedan; 2130 lb.	Car A ran off road and collided head-on with tree which penetrated about 48 in into front of car, level with windshield	More than 45 mph	D: Male; 21 yr; 217 lb; 69 in P: Male; 18 yr; 182 lb; 74 in	D: Facial and hand injuries; right leg broken in 3 places P: Fractured clavicle and ankle

[1] In the first three accidents the belts were of the automatic type; in the last two they were ordinary lap-and-diagonal belts.
[2] Estimated both from reported speeds and from damage.

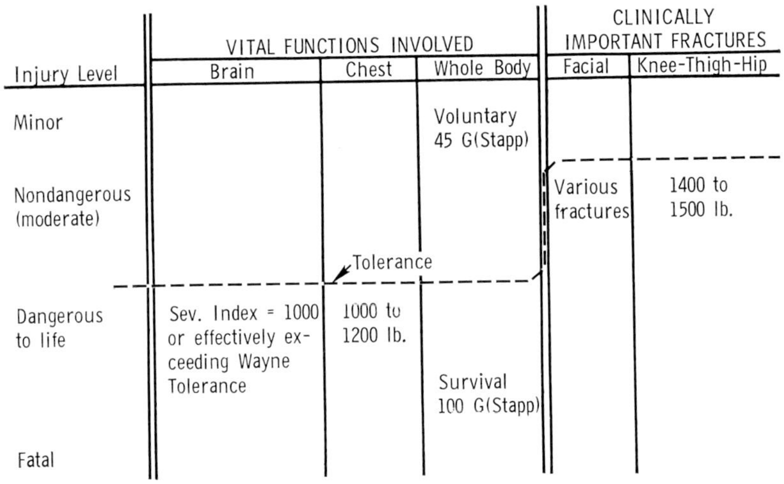

Application of Human Tolerance Data to Protective Systems 471

Injury Level	VITAL FUNCTIONS INVOLVED			CLINICALLY IMPORTANT FRACTURES	
	Brain	Chest	Whole Body	Facial	Knee-Thigh-Hip
Minor			Voluntary 45 G(Stapp)		
Nondangerous (moderate)				Various fractures	1400 to 1500 lb.
			Tolerance		
Dangerous to life	Sev. Index = 1000 or effectively exceeding Wayne Tolerance	1000 to 1200 lb.	Survival 100 G(Stapp)		
Fatal					

FIGURE 20–13. Nondimensional movement of passenger relative to vehicle as a function of front-end crush for types 1, 2 and 3 pulse shapes of Figure 20–9. (ζ is occupant, x is passenger compartment movement after impact and x_T is total front-end crush.)

there was only one serious neck injury, a fractured cervical disk, which occurred in a rear-end impact.

Finally, to determine whether the British accident reports were unduly concerned with minor accidents, a comparison has been made with accidents discussed in the recent report on Volvo cars.[23] Every Volvo car is guaranteed by the company against accident damage exceeding 80 U.S. dollars for the first 5 years after delivery, and the report is concerned with 37,761 accidents which occurred in Sweden in the period March 28, 1965, to March 28, 1966. During that time, 297,000 Volvo cars less than 5 years old were on the road, so that Volvo cars had, on the average, one accident in 7.9 years involving damage exceeding 80 U.S. dollars. Five and 3/10 per cent of the unbelted drivers were injured; therefore, on the average, under present conditions, a Volvo driver in Sweden could expect to be injured once in 149 years of driving. The corresponding figure for car drivers in Great Britain in 1964, deduced from Ministry of Transport data, was about once in 120 years. The risk, of injury to car drivers, was therefore not very different in the two countries, in spite of considerable differences in driving conditions. Figures, given in the Volvo report, indicate that Swedish safety belts in Volvo cars afford approximately the same degree of protection as British belts in Britain. But in the Swedish sample, only 3.32 per cent of belted drivers were injured, whereas in the accidents to drivers wearing safety belts in Britain, considered in this paper, about 40 per cent were injured. As conditions in the two countries appear to be roughly similar, it would appear that the British sample consisted of approximately the most severe one-tenth of the accidents similar in severity to those considered in the Volvo report.

REFERENCES

1. PATRICK, L.M.: Prevention of instrument panel and windshield head injuries. *The Prevention of Highway Injury.* 1967, pp. 169–181.
2. DEHAVEN, H.: Mechanical analysis of survival in falls from heights of fifty to one hundred and fifty feet. *War Med*, 2:586–596, July 1942.
3. SNYDER, R.G.: Human tolerance limits in water impact. *Aerospace Med*, 36: 940–947, Oct. 1965.
4. KIEL, F.W.: Hazards of military parachuting. *Milit Med*, 130:512–521, 1965.
5. STAPP, J.P.; MOSELY, D.; LOMBARD, C.F.; NELSON, G.; NICHOLS, G.; and LARMIE, F.: Analysis and biodynamics of selected rocket-sled experiments. Part I. Biodynamics of maximal decelerations. Part II. Dynamic response of restrained subjects during abrupt deceleration. USAF School of Aerospace Medicine, Brooks Air Force Base, Texas, July 1964.
6. STAPP, J.P.: The problem: biomechanics of injury. *The Prevention of Highway Injury.* 1967, pp. 159–164.
7. SCHNEIDER, R.C.; SMITH, W.S.; GRABB, W.C.; TURCOTTE, J.G., and HUELKE, D.F.: Lap seat belt injuries; the treatment of the fortunate survivor. *Mich Med* 67: 171–186, Feb. 1968.
8. MERTZ, H.J., JR., and PATRICK, L.M.: Investigation of the kinematics and kinetics of whiplash. *Proceedings of the Eleventh Stapp Conference.* 1967, pp. 175–206.
9. MERTZ, H.J., JR.: The kinematics and kinetics of whiplash. A Doctoral Dissertation submitted to Wayne State University, 1967.
10. SKEELS, P.C.: The energy absorbing steering column. *Proceedings of the Tenth Stapp Car Crash Conference.* 1966.
11. MOORE, R.L.: *Research on Road Safety.* London, H.M.S.O., 1963.
12. GADD, C.W., and PATRICK, L.M.: System versus laboratory impact tests for estimating injury hazard. *SAE Paper 680053*, Jan. 1968.
13. DANIEL, R.P., and PATRICK, L.M.: Instrument panel impact study. *Proceedings of the Ninth Stapp Conference.* 1966, pp. 165–179.
14. GRIME, G.: Automobile design in relation to passenger safety. *Inst Bull Brit Carr Mfrs*, 28 (new series) (592):21–32, 1964.
15. NEILSON, I.D.: The dynamics of safety belts in motor car head-on impacts. *Proceedings of Symposium on Ergonomics and Safety in Motor Car Design.* Institution of Mechanical Engineers, Sept. 1966.
16. CLARK, C.; BLECHSCHMIDT, C., and GORDON, F.: Impact protection with the "airstop" restraint system. *Proceedings of the Eighth Stapp Conference.* 1966.
17. KEMMERER, R.M.; CHUTE, R.; HASS, D.P., and SLACK, W.K.: Automatic inflatable occupant restraint system, parts I and II. *SAE Paper 680033*, Jan. 1968.
18. GRIME, G.: Safety cars. Principles governing the design of cars and safety devices. *Road Research Laboratory Report No. 8*, 1966.
19. MARTIN, D.E., and KROELL, C.K.: Vehicle crush and occupant behavior. *SAE Paper 670034*, Jan. 1967.
20. LUNDSTROM, L.C.: The safety factor in automotive design. Society of Automotive Engineers West Coast Meeting, August 1966.

21. GRIME, G., and LISTER, R.D.: The protection of car occupants in accidents. *Proceedings of Symposium on Ergonomics and Safety in Motor Car Design.* Institution of Mechanical Engineers, Sept. 1966.
22. GRIME, G.: Accidents and injuries to car occupants wearing safety belts. (unpublished).
23. BOHLIN, N.I.: A statistical analysis of 28,000 accident cases with emphasis on occupant restraint value. *Proceedings of the Eleventh Stapp Conference.* 1967.
24. LISTER, R.D., and NEILSON, I.D.: The effectiveness of safety belts. *Road Research Laboratory Report No. 16*, 1966.

DISCUSSION

Charles W. Gadd

The authors have done an excellent job of bringing together a great deal of useful information, and have included a good exposition of the general philosophy of trying to tailor a structure so that it will crush at a loading short of the bodily tolerance involved and thus make most efficient use of the available depth of crush. A question which has not been resolved as yet it is the degree of injury which is most logically representative of body tolerance. The authors suggest the use of the term "minor" to characterize a degree of injury to which one might try to design. In other papers, the Cornell Automotive Crash Injury Research organization terminology of nondangerous and dangerous to life are used. The writer feels that such descriptive terms, while valuable when applied to particular situations or types of injury, lead to difficulties if used too broadly, and that the other approach, also taken in the chapter, of developing a table of tolerances in detail for the many parts of the body is the preferrable way to summarize tolerance information. In order to bring all of these values into a form compatible with some of the descriptive terms which have been used, one might arrange them in a format as outlined briefly in the accompanying table. Thus all tolerances involving vital functions could be brought together as shown, and a horizontal line drawn for threshold of danger to life. For a second general class of injuries which do not usually involve vital functions, but which are nevertheless clinically significant (for example injuries of a cosmetic nature or which cause serious temporary disability or are difficult to correct) the tolerance line might logically be set between minor and nondangerous. While it may seem paradoxical at first glance to apparently be less conservative when danger to life is concerned, it can be argued that more lives can be saved by tailoring the structure in the range between nondangerous and dangerous. This is evidently the intent of the authors, who suggest in their table a number of tolerance values which are in this range. See Figure 20–13.

The charts used by the authors giving the relative position of the occupants and the car interior during the course of the accident are of considerable interest. With respect to the implications of this kind of analysis, one might also wish to refer to another recent paper.[1]

The writer is gratified that studies of effectiveness of harnesses are continuing in England. The results will be followed with a great deal of interest.

Reference

1. Martin, D.E., and Kroell, C.K.: Vehicle crush and occupant behavior. Paper No. 670034 presented at January 1967 Society of Automotive Engineers Annual Meeting.

Chapter XXI

THE EFFECTIVENESS OF CURRENT METHODS AND SYSTEMS USED TO REDUCE INJURY

WILLIAM A. LANGE and DONALD J. VAN KIRK

The Injury Risk Index published by Automotive Crash Injury Research (ACIR) of Cornell University shown in Table 21-I, rates the vehicle components in order of injury production based on the 1-2-4-8 weighting system. The four leading causes for all types of injuries are, in descending order: (1) Steering assemblies (20.5%), (2) Instrument panels (20.2%), (3) Ejection (18.0%), and (4) Windshields (13.7%). These constitute the majority of all injury or approximately 72.4 per cent.

During an accident or, more precisely, the "second collision," the driver

INJURY SCORE FOR LEADING CAUSES OF INJURY WITH CONTRIBUTION BY IMPACT TYPE
(1956 + CARS; 1-2-4-8 INJURY WEIGHTS)

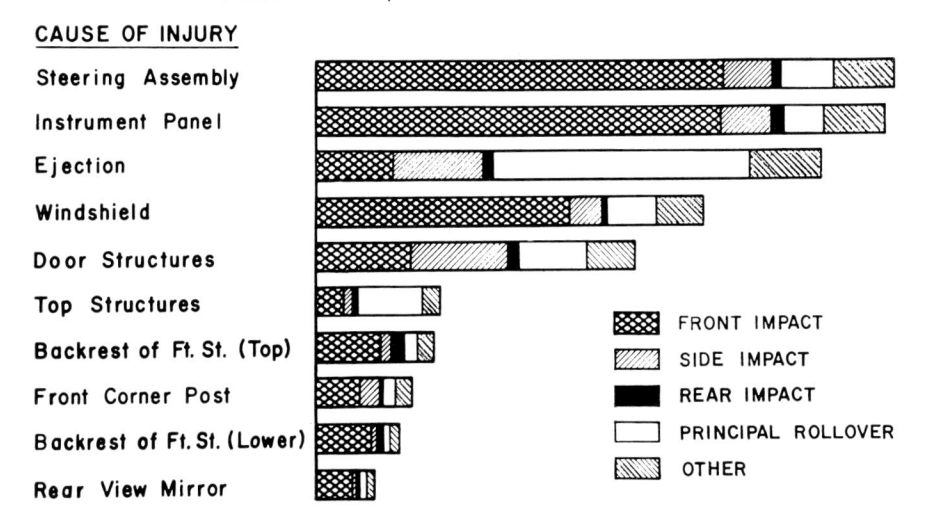

CAUSE OF INJURY
- Steering Assembly
- Instrument Panel
- Ejection
- Windshield
- Door Structures
- Top Structures
- Backrest of Ft. St. (Top)
- Front Corner Post
- Backrest of Ft. St. (Lower)
- Rear View Mirror

Legend: FRONT IMPACT, SIDE IMPACT, REAR IMPACT, PRINCIPAL ROLLOVER, OTHER

1-2-4-8 Injury Score

TABLE 21-I. From R. Wolf, *Leading Causes of Automobile Accidents.*

and front seat passengers are violently subjected to impacts with the interior components of the vehicle. To describe accurately what exactly occurs during this second collision has been the interest of research for many years. A typical example of what might occur to the driver during a second collision as a result of a frontal force accident may be described as follows:

The driver slides horizontally on the seat until his soft abdomen strikes the lower steering wheel rim. Upon impact, the rim begins to deform, causing displacement of the driver's internal organs resulting in a possible ruptured bladder or intestine with internal bleeding. The driver's knees then impact the instrument panel deforming the control knobs and heavy structured metal which supports the steering column. This impact causes contusions and abrasions or a fracture of the patellas. The upper part of his torso rotates at his hips or "jackknifes." His ribs strike the rest of the steering wheel rim and deform it until his sternum impacts the strong nonyielding center column. Two or more of his ribs may be broken and complicated with the puncture of his lungs. His head continues its pendulum motion striking the header with a velocity equal to, or in many cases greater than, the vehicle impact velocity. If the windshield is a pre-1966 model, his head punctures it and may cause a brain concussion. After penetration, his head "bobs" up and down on the jagged lower edge of the glass as his body retracts into the car causing severe facial lacerations. All of this action occurs in less than 0.5 of a second.

The horrible experience an occupant undergoes when the vehicle is accidentally impacted has been the constant reminder and basis with which the automotive safety engineers have made improvements in the design of the interior of modern motor vehicles. The largest single item which has reduced the severity of automobile impact injuries and, in many cases, has eliminated them completely is restraint systems.

Tourin and Garrett[1] compared seat belt users and nonusers for the California Highway Patrol and reported the following data:

1. Users of seat belts sustained approximately 35 per cent less of the major to fatal grade injuries than did nonusers.
2. Seat belt users sustained fewer fatalities than non-seat belt users.
3. Seat belts appear to function as a protective device chiefly in roll-over accidents or nonspecific (side angular or unusual) accidents.
4. The reduction of the "major to fatal" injuries is related largely to the performance of seat belts in preventing the occupant from being thrown out of the automobile under crash conditions.

In a second report to the California legislature on the same study[2] Tourin and Garrett stated that approximately 3.5 per cent of the automobiles involved in the accidents studied were equipped with one or more seat belts.

Among the cars having seat belts only one-third of the occupants wore them.

The California Highway Patrol overwhelmingly favors seat belts as a potential control of death and injuries in accidents, but their opinions are inconsistent in having influenced by the presence of belts and by the presence of injury in observed accidents.

In a study over a 2-year period in Adelaide, South Australia, by McLean, Robertsen, and Ryan[3] who investigated 542 cars involved in accidents in which there were 1,029 seated occupants, fifty-eight had seat belts available but only twenty-four were wearing them. They reported that thirteen had lap belts only, forty-two lap and sash belts, two diagonal belts only, and one not known. Fifty per cent of those wearing seat belts were injured and 49.7 per cent of those not wearing seat belts were injured. Twelve and five-tenths per cent wearing seat belts and 16.9 per cent not wearing seat belts sustained a greater degree of moderate to severe injury.

Many countries outside the United States have a greater percentage of small vehicles. In these smaller cars, the distance between the occupant and the interior components is greatly reduced. This necessitates the use of an upper torso restraint. Many use the upper torso belt alone, *not* in conjunction with a lap belt.

Lister and Neilson[4] reported in 1966 that the serious injury rate was reduced by 70 per cent when wearing safety belts. They compared the effectiveness of various safety belt configurations and concluded that the floor attached lap and diagonal belt is less effective in the "slight injury" class. They suggest the wearers would suffer fewer injuries if they were to wear belts tighter. They also suggest that lap belts *should not* be used in the front seat!! A comparison between the effectiveness of various belts is shown in Table 21–II.

TABLE 21-II

Belted Occupant	Overall	Head	Neck	Thorax	Abdomen	Upper Extremities	Lower Extremities
Less Severe	58	53	23	58	27	48	59
No Difference	121	119	182	130	176	125	122
More Severe	53	60	27	44	29	59	51

(*Courtesy* B. J. Campbell & J. K. Kihlberg from "Seat Belt Effectiveness on the Non-Ejection Situation.")

In an overall review of the relative merits of the various types of motor vehicle seat belts, Vulcan[5] reported that many investigators in the field of crash injury protection had the opinion that upper torso restraints were superior. They stated that no *direct* conclusive statistics were available.

There are many types of restraints other than the single lap, diagonal, or lap and diagonal combination. These include the full harness, the three point, the lap, and the diagonal as two independent belts. The last three systems are found on only a small percentage of vehicles involved in accidents and therefore only a limited amount of statistical information is available.

In 1963, Lister and Milson[6] reported a comparison of seat belts in a series of accident investigations. According to them, the overall reduction in injuries resulting from the wearing of seat belts was 51 per cent with a greater reduction in the serious injuries than in the slight injuries. The percentage of persons not injured when wearing seat belts was about the same for each of the four different types of belts. These included full harness, lap and diagonal (pillar attachment), lap and diagonal (floor attachment), and diagonal only. They concluded that upper restraint systems yielded fewer head and neck injuries but more chest injuries including bruising caused by the seat belt assembly.

Through August 1962, only 7 per cent of all cars were equipped with seat belts and almost 30 per cent of the drivers were *not* wearing them.

Huelke and Gikas[7] reported in 1966 that 38 of 48, or 79 per cent, ejected occupants would have survived had they been wearing only a lap belt and another 2 per cent would have been saved if a shoulder and seat belt combination had been used. In attesting to the effectiveness of restraining devices for all victims irrespective of their seating position, type or severity of collision, or the objects impacted, they claimed that 40 per cent of all victims would have been saved had they been wearing a lap belt, 13 percent more if a seat and shoulder harness were used and another 7 per cent if a seat and double shoulder (full harness) belt had been used.

In 1962 and 1963, Campbell investigated thirty-three fatal auto crashes in Colorado[8] in which at least one person was wearing a seat belt. He reported that twenty-three wearing seat belts were fatally injured and twenty-six survived. Fifteen of the fatalities were drivers and eight were passengers. Eight passengers were fatally injured and eight survived. Campbell further reported that twenty-eight unbelted occupants were fatally injured and fifty-two survived. Of the drivers, eight were fatalities and eighteen survived. Of the passengers, twenty were fatally injured and thirty-four survived. Twenty-three of those fatally injured wearing seat belts died from steering assembly displacements, roll-overs, or crushing of car interiors. One belted passenger struck the instrument panel and suffered a fatal head injury.

Thus far the seat belt has proven its effectiveness in the ejection type situation. In an effort to determine the seat belt effectiveness in the nonejection situation, a comparison of 232 pairs of belted and unbelted occupants was made by Campbell and Kihlberg.[9] This comparison was made on the basis of the following: (a) no difference in injury severity (b) belted occupant *more* severely injured than unbelted (c) belted occupant *less* severely injured than unbelted (Table 21–III).

TABLE 21-III

Car Collision	Stiff (Solid) Column Medical Injury	Energy Absorbing Hub Car Index	Med. Index	Remarks	Collapsible Column Car Index	Med. Index	Remarks	Collapsed Length
10 Moderate	2–Minor 2–Moderate 4–Dangerous 2–Fatal	3–Minor	1–None 2–Minor 2–None	1–W.L.B. 1–W.L.B. 2–W.L.B.	3–Minor	1–None 2–Minor 3–None 9–Minor 7–Mod. 2–Dang.	1–L.B. 2–L.B. 3–L.B. 1–L.B.	0–1/2"
2–Severe	1–Dangerous 1–Fatal	5–Mod.	3–Minor	1–W.L.B.	21–Mod.			1/4"–4"
3–Critical 1 Person Lap Belted	3–Dangerous	1–Crit.	1–Minor		3–Crit.	3–Minor		1 1/2"–5 1/2"

(*Courtesy of I. Laskey from "Automotive Cardio-Thoracic Injuries."*)

They concluded that there is very little difference in the use of a lap belt in the reduction of injuries. Campbell and Kihlberg[9] suggested that an additional 5,000 lives per year could be saved if efforts for an improved restraint system would be extended to include upper torso restraints, and *built-in* anchorages for three-point belts.

The largest single source of information regarding the effectiveness of the three-point belts has come from Sweden. The AB Volvo Company[10] offers a 5-year guarantee against collision for every car sold in the Scandinavian market. This includes collision repair and where the car is totally demolished, the factory replaces it with a new one. As part of the program Volvo prepared a two page questionnaire which every car owner involved in an accident and covered by the guarantee had to complete. The data compiled from the results of the poll indicated that three-point restraining belts were effective in reducing injuries. An equal number of cases are described where the occupants were *not* wearing the three-point belts. In every accident in which belts were not worn, at least one occupant received a severe, if not fatal injury.

In determining the effectiveness of any system to reduce injury, the investigator must always check to be certain that *the system* did not produce the injury.

In the United States, the majority of seat belt installations before the 1968 model cars were of the lap belt type only. In almost every case, the injury which has been reportedly caused by the belt was due to improper placement. The belts were usually placed high on the abdomen above or near an imaginary line connecting the pelvic iliac crests. Upon impact, the body was forced against the belt. No longer having the hard bony pelvic structure to distribute the load the body was being subjected to, the belt may have ruptured and sheared the soft abdominal viscera.

A report by Le Mire, Early, and Hanley[11] stated twenty-three cases of abdominal injuries were due to seat belts. Proper placement of the seat belts would have decreased the chance of injury. By their snubbing, jerking, or shearing action seat belts cause internal injuries which may not be initially manifested. Types of intra-abdominal injuries most frequently seen include the following: (1) Rupture of the pancreas and the duodenum, (2) Splenic rupture, (3) Perforation of the proximal part of the jejunum, (4) Hepatic vessels torn from the vena-cava, (5) Rupture of the left kidney and spleen and left renal artery torn from aorta, (6) Laceration of the mesentery, and (7) Tear in the duodenum and the mesosigmoid colon.

Recently, LeMire, Early, and Hanley[11] reported two cases in which the seat belts were worn very high on the abdomen resulting in large hernias. In one instance in which the seat belt broke, there was a 4 cm perforation of the proximal end of the victim's small intestine. Initial examinations did not show the injury on roentgenograms but several hours later, repeat abdominal films showed a trace of free air which confirmed evidence of severe intra-abdominal injury.

With thousands of people saved each day from permanently disabling or fatal injuries, no one can claim that these reported injuries constitute sufficient evidence to warrant not using the lap belt.

In Europe, many cars are fitted with a diagonal belt only. Saldeen[12] (Sweden) described three cases of fatal neck injuries incurred by occupants wearing that type of belt. He concluded that the injury was probably caused when the lower jaw was temporarily caught under the belt as the occupant slipped out of the belt and was ejected from the car.

This information only adds data to the mounting evidence that the diagonal belt *cannot* control the "submarining" action of occupants, especially in the angular type collision where a torque is applied to the vehicle and the occupant has the greatest chance of being ejected.

Since most occupants have not been using seat belts as shown in the preceding studies, and the use of seat belts appears to cause an increase in the frequency with which the occupant strikes the *steering assembly* and the *instrument panel*, it has become necessary for the automotive engineer to redesign them to make them less dangerous to the occupant.

Steering Assemblies

In 1967, two safety features were added to the steering assembly. Some manufacturers provided an energy-absorbing hub attached to the steering wheel and others installed a collapsible column. A report[13] comparing these two safety features with the old solid column as a function of cardiovascular injury due to frontal force accidents established the importance of these devices.

In a series of accidents studied, the solid *shaft* produced three fatal and seven serious type of injuries while the energy-absorbing hub and collapsible column taken together showed only two serious type injuries. This data shows the effectiveness of the collapsible column and energy-absorbing hub (Table 21-IV).

TABLE 21-IV

	Total Number Of Head Injuries	Dangerous Or Fatal	% Of Dangerous Or Fatal
Not Ejected	339	15	4.4
Ejected	41	6	14.6
Totals	380	21	5.5

(*Courtesy* of J. K. Kihlberg & H. K. Gensler from "Head Injury in Automobile Accidents Related to Seated Position and Age.")

The fact that no single device can completely reduce injuries is illustrated in the following two examples[14]:

An 18-year-old male was driving a 1967 Cougar on an expressway exit ramp. A 1961 Ford was stopped on the ramp. The Cougar struck the Ford in the rear at approximately 70 mph. The Cougar slid 125 feet. The Ford continued on for another 120 feet. The driver of the Ford jackknifed over the steering wheel impacting the energy-absorbing hub between his diaphragm and his umbilicus. He suffered a massive laceration of his liver, a partial avulsion of his gall bladder, a right renal contusion, and a massive intra-abdominal hemorrhage. The driver survived and has completely recovered. If the vehicle had not been equipped with the energy-absorbing hub he might not have survived the accident.

A 63-year-old male was driving a 1967 Chrysler on an expressway exit ramp. A 1966 Buick tried to pass and forced the Chrysler into a light pole. The approximate impact speed was 60 mph. The contact was on the left front side causing the driver to impact the steering wheel on the left side more than the right. The column collapse was less than ¼ inch due to the off-center impact. The driver suffered three fractured ribs. Without the energy-absorbing column the driver could have incurred a *very* serious injury.

In both of these cases, the driver was not wearing any restraint.

Windshields

All cars produced after 1966 have the new 30 mil HI laminated windshields. The new laminate with its optimum moisture content bulges or "pockets" when impacted by the human head. The plastic is weakened to the point where it separates from the glass at the broken glass edge effectively increasing the length of the plastic which can stretch. This absorbs much higher levels of energy.

In 1964, a comparison study was made between the standard 15 mil laminate glass and the new 30 mil HI laminate at Wayne State University by Patrick and Daniel.[15] The first penetration of the 15 mil glass occurred at 12.9 mph. The same experiments were run using the 30 mil windshields but the results were strikingly different. The 30 mil HI laminate did not penetrate until a velocity of 29.3 mph was attained.

Although the windshield ranks as the number one cause of all injuries to the driver and his right front passenger,[16] the severity of injury is greatly reduced by the improved windshield. Table 21–V shows a comparison of head injuries of ejected and nonejected occupants.[17]

The best method to show the windshield's effectiveness is to observe its performance under accident conditions. Nahum has reported two wind-

TABLE 21-V

	Overall	Head	Neck	Thorax	Abdomen	Arm	Leg
Padded Car Occupants							
Injuries Less Severe	249	232	35	118	53	140	206
Tie	321	386	722	558	693	513	386
Padded Car Occupants							
Injuries More Severe	220	171	32	114	42	137	201

(*Courtesy* R. Wolf from ACIR Report VJ-1823-R2.)

shield injury cases in great detail.[18] "A 1966 Buick collided almost head-on with a 1962 Chevrolet. The right front passenger moved forward until his legs contacted the lower portion of the glove box, causing a fracture of the right upper leg. His chest impacted the leading edge of the instrument panel, causing three fractured ribs on the right side. His head continued forward until his face contacted the windshield. He received a large curved laceration of the right side of his head and a small wound across his forehead. The corner of the hood broke through the windshield and inflicted the large laceration, the windshield caused the small wound. The vehicle's effective impact velocity was approximately 35 mph."

In the second case, a 1966 Plymouth struck the front of a parked 1957 Chevrolet. The driver impacted the steering wheel, bending it. She continued up along its plane until she contacted the windshield. "The glass was bowed out about 2 to 4 inches and was fractured and ruptured sufficiently to leave strands of hair but no tissue in the glass. Both inner and outer layers were fractured but the midliner remained intact. The driver sustained a tiny laceration of the left side of the face. The vehicle velocity was approximately 17 to 22 mph."

To show the effect of a pre-1966 windshield, Dr. Nahum has cited this case. "A 1961 Valiant struck a parked vehicle at approximately 15 to 20 mph. The driver sustained multiple deep facial lacerations."

Another example of the post-1966 windshield is an accident in which a 1967 Ambassador[19] traveling between 50 to 60 mph impacted the rear end of a semitrailer and "submarined" under the rear of the truck. The lower edge of the truck caught part of the hood and pulled it and the windshield back into the vehicle. The windshield almost completely enveloped the driver's face, causing many superficial lacerations. The attending plastic surgeon stated, "Had the windshield been of the pre-1966 car model design, the lacerations would undoubtedly have been very deep and greatly disfiguring."

Instrument Panels

Since about 1956, American cars have had various types of padding available on the forward areas of vehicle. Until 1967, it was an option at extra cost except on higher priced models.

A report released in 1963 by ACIR compares instrument panel injuries to the right front passenger (RFP) and center front passenger (CFP) in matched accidents between cars with and without padding.[20] Only frontal force accidents and closely matched cars, occupants, and injuries were compared. The report included 792 matched accidents. Table 21-VI shows

TABLE 21-VI

Padded Car:	None	Minor	Nondangerous	Dangerous To Fatal	Not Reported	Total
Number	383	316	77	16	0	792
%	48.4	39.9	9.7	2.0	—	100
Unpadded Car:	332	337	103	17	3	792
Number	42.1	42.7	13.1	2.1	—	100
%						

(*Courtesy* R. Wolf & B. J. Campbell From ACIR Report VJ-1823-R2.)

the comparison between padded and unpadded instrument panels with respect to several body area injuries.

The greatest effect obtained from the padded panel is in the minor and nondangerous category of injuries. There appears to be little or no effect from the padding in the fatal and dangerous injuries. This can be attributed to the fact that the padding reaches its limit of energy absorption and "bottoms out." If the panel is not of the deformable energy-absorbing type, the force will be transferred to the human body producing the dangerous to fatal class of injuries such as skull fractures and brain damage.

It is evident from the ACIR report that the padded instrument panel has been very effective in reducing injuries but more consideration to design should be given in the future since more seat belts are now available and more occupants will be wearing them. The frequency with which the center front and right front passenger will impact the instrument panel will greatly increase.

Experimental

The previous discussion has been concerned with standard items found on production motor vehicles. These standard devices were developed by the research facilities of many companies. New devices and systems are being developed and tested in the hope of further reducing the injury potential to automobile occupants.

Inflatable Devices

Complete immobilization of an occupant during the "second collision" has been the basic idea behind this device. The device basically consists of a plastic type bag which is stored inconspicuously and on command from a crash sensor or manual trigger, is inflated in less than .04 seconds to a volume of 5 to 10 feet^3 per occupant.[21]

A complete airstop restraint system has been proposed by Clark.[22] It would consist of inflatable seats and sections of instrument panels and door coverings which would inflate under impact and then deform without metal failure. The system would automatically inflate when the car reaches an acceleration of 3 g in any direction. Additional protection is obtained by inflation of an airbag over the steering wheel hub and all side windows. The occupant airbag would receive additional pressure proportional to the car speed to prevent "bottoming."

In the Spring of 1966 at UCLA-ITTE, tests were carried out using some parts of the proposed Clark restraint system. Their comments were as follows: "The dummies in an air-seat rebounded vigorously when lap belted. The unrestrained dummy also rebounded vigorously from just the use of a chest airbag."

An improvement on this basic idea was tested by Chute and Haas[21] with promising results. Their airbag system contains orifices by which the energy transferred from the occupant to the gas is dissipated, thereby reducing the amount of rebound. Results of forty-two crash simulator tests and one barrier test gave the following conclusions:

1. Seat belt loads were reduced 50 to 70 per cent in comparable 30 mph crashes.
2. 40 to 50 per cent reduction in head and chest decelerations were recorded.
3. A need for a bag pressure relief system to reduce spring rate was demonstrated.
4. That additional development of airbag configuration was necessary.
5. Determination of best gas release method.

Some problems still exist such as the denotating system, the packaging problems, the post-crash visibility, the effects of various size people on impact performance, the acceptable noise level, the pressure rise, the environmental exposure, and the quality control.

In this phase of development, the gas bag concept has demonstrated a good potential as an upper torso restraint.

Combination Upper Torso Restraint System

A new type restraint system has been tested using primates to determine physiological responses to impact.[23] The inertia-locking reel with inverted-Y yoke torso harness was compared with the single-lap belt, single diagonal belt, and the three-point harness. The inertia-locking reel allows upper torso motion during normal driving activities but instant automatic locking during panic braking or impact. The only cars currently using this harness and reel are the specially modified Shelby Mustang GT 350 and GT 500's. There have been no reported accidents involving vehicles of this type.

Snyder's study of belt restraint systems has suggested the following conclusions:

1. The lap belt combined with a yoke harness is the most effective belt restraint system of those evaluated.
2. The forward-facing position tests were survivable (with reversible injury) at 43 g, but marginal at 49 g. Marked contusions from webbing were observed.
3. In two tests, the inertia reel locked satisfactorily at impact but the mechanism was so damaged that the reel could not be used again without repair.
4. 0.3 g activation without initial bracing allowed the subject to slump forward in the seat rendering useless the restraint feature for the upper torso.
5. Impact loads were fairly equally distributed between the lap and torso belts.

The yoke harness allows the occupant to withstand greater "g" loadings with a minimum of trauma in comparison to the lap and shoulder belt combination.

Seats and Seat Backs

The automotive seat must function as part of a system with the other restraining devices. Bobbs and Hilton[24] propose a package safety seat which will support the body up to 30 g in a forward direction. The seat proper and anchorages within the body shell must be strong enough to withstand a forward load of 4,950 pounds and a downward vertical load of 3,505 pounds. The neck should be supported and protected to guard against whiplash type injuries and safety belts should be an integral part of the seat. Finally, the seat must be comfortable, adjustable, and attractively styled.

The seat itself should act as the major component in a system used to protect the occupant in any type of crash conditions. Two other proposals for integral safety seats include all crash conditions. The Liberty Mutual Survival Car[25] has a capsule type chair with armrests as an extension of the seat and wings which wrap around at the shoulder level to protect the occupant in side impacts. Each chair will withstand a 5,000 pound impact from the front, either side, and rear. The restraint system is an integral part of the seat and a special latch will release all connections.

The New York State Safety Car[26] uses a slightly different principle in that the seat frame of tubular construction is attached to the "B" pillar transverse bulkhead. The structure of the bulkhead will yield at 30 g. This deformation will be sufficient to keep occupant-loading within tolerable physiological limits. The upper restraints are again an integral part of the seat and are connected to multi-axial rate-sensitive inertia reels. The lap belts are push-button recoil-mounted at the seat juncture. This will allow a neat appearance when not in use. Since the restraints are attached to the seat directly they must only resist the loads of the occupant not the seat, while the anchorage points are strong enough to resist any loads developed in the design collision conditions.

Design parameters have been very difficult to obtain for seats and seat backs. Severy, Brink, and Baird[27] have proposed the following:

1. Seat back height for all passenger vehicles should be at least 28 inches. (Seat back strength over 16,000 but not 33,000 inch-pounds will provide satisfactory protection against the injury-producing forces of most rear-end collisions.)
2. The 28-inch seat back should have a deformable or energy-absorbing top edge to conform to neck arch during the rear-end loading.
3. Increasing seat-back rigidity reduces rebound following peak acceleration and reduces head and torso displacement up the plane of the seat.

A mathematical simulation for a controlled seat back rotation with and without a headrest has been prepared by Mertz.[28] With a constant seat back torque level of 600 foot-pounds the seat back rotates 12 degrees for a stiffness of −250 pounds while a 29 degree rotation occurs with a −50 pound stiffness. These values occurred for a simulated 23 mph rear-end impact. For any given level of seat back torque the head load is greater when there is initial separation. The head load also increases as the seat back torque level increases. Therefore, from a standpoint of interference with rear seat occupants and mitigation of injury during more severe rear collisions, the smaller change in seat back angle offered by the stiffer seat back is most desirable. This stiffness should be of the structure-cushion combination type.

Headrests

Experimental work is being done to develop a head rest to minimize injury to the neck. Two separate approaches have been undertaken by the industry. They are the separate add-on type which is supported by a tubular frame and the second type is part of the seat back.

The New York State Safety car[26] has a headrest which is an extension of the bulkhead and not the seat back but is not adjustable since the seat itself is vertically adjustable. It is padded in all directions to provide protection.

Severy, Brink, and Baird[27] offer the following conclusions based on "controlled collisions" at UCLA:

1. Head restraint for front seats should be designed as an extension of the seat back and preferably not as an attachment or an adjustable unit. It should not be attached to the roof structure, independent of the seat back, since it is regarded as compromising the motorist's protection.
2. The closer the head restraint to the motorist, the better his protection. Head offsets as much as 6 inches do not greatly increase the exposure to injury.
3. The head restraint should not be weaker than the seat back.
4. Head restraints should be an integral part of the vehicle.
5. The restraint, be it integral extension or tack-on unit, should be 15 inches wide but not less than 10 inches wide.

Since many vehicles are not fitted with headrests, there are not too many accident statistics available regarding their effectiveness. Gissane[29] reported two group studies of neck injuries stated that of 315 car occupants examined, thirty-nine had severe neck injuries, thirty-five were cervical fractures or fracture dislocations, four with complete cord transections. The majority were frontal collisions, only one was a rear impact, although overturning was commonplace.

The second group consisted of two well-documented impacts:

1. The driver of a car hit the rear of a truck with a large overhang. During the first impact the driver's neck was hyperextended, and as the car was forced under the overhang, the roof deformed downward impacting the driver's chin, increasing hyperextension of his neck. All deep neck structures were divided and both C_7 and T_1 vertebrae were fractured, and cervical cord damage resulted with avulsion of his right brachial plexus.
2. The second accident was one in which a small parked sports car was impacted by a much larger, heavier car traveling 40 mph. Both the driver and right front passenger experienced very severe impacts. The moving vehicle had rigid seat backs incorporating built-in head supports with shoulder and lap belts. The mild steel pillows which supported the headrests were deformed, one 22 degrees and the other

27½ degrees. This suggests an impact force of about 150 pounds. The driver, a young girl, suffered a tenderness of the neck for six months. The right front passenger was not injured.

Based solely on this evidence, one could easily recommend a retro-fit headrest without much hesitation.

Special Uses of Restraining Systems

This category covers only a small percentage of the population but to many investigators they are most important: women and children.

Restraints for pregnant women are often a topic for much discussion, but not much work is being done at the present time. A report by Snyder, et al. has shown some promising results. They used pregnant baboons in their study. Snyder states that there are only thirty *reported* cases of pregnant women wearing seat belts who were involved in accidents. Almost half had a partial or a complete separation of their placenta with subsequent death of the fetus.

A suitable restraining device for children from the pre-toddler stage to the young adolescent age has always been a problem for automotive engineers, not only from the standpoint of comfort and safety for the children but ease of entrance and egress for the parent who must put the children into the device.

Figures released in 1960 by ACIR[30] showed that only 8.8 per cent of persons involved in injury-producing accidents were children under 11 years old and only 11 per cent in the 12 to 18 year group. The report goes on to show that the frequency and severity of injury of children and adolescents was always markedly less than the adult groups examined.

Present child restraints are now divided into pre- and post-toddler types. The young adolescent can usually use the lap belt and a modified shoulder belt system. The pre-toddler devices consist of a bucket type seat with a restraining bar which hangs over the front of the front seat. This contraption is usually catapulted about the car during the accident, resulting in injury to the child.

The second system for the post-toddler stage is a harness type vest made of seat belt webbing. The vest is such that it distributes the load across the entire torso of the child. The vest has attachments at the top, sides, and crotch allowing the child to stand. When this occurs, the device has lost most of its effectiveness because the child will again be flailed about within the car impacting various structures.

A new device called Tot-guard℗ for post-toddler children has been made a production item. The device consists of a plastic form which is padded on the upper interior surface and is placed over and around the seated child. He is strapped in by the standard safety lap belt. Controlled collisions performed by Ford Motor Company have shown some promising results. These tests were runs up to 30 mph for frontal force and roll-over type accidents. Head accelerations were much lower than those under similar conditions for the lap-belted child.

DISCUSSION AND CONCLUSIONS

Many facts, figures, and statistics have been presented showing what occurs during an automobile accident, what safety devices and equipment are available to the occupants of motor vehicles, and how effective they are. The purpose of this paper is to be as objective as possible when evaluating these devices; therefore, flaws were pointed out when necessary.

Each device and piece of equipment is discussed and evaluated on its own merits in reducing injury to the occupants. This is the way it should be done, but it is only a preliminary review since a system, like a chain, is only as strong as its weakest link.

The automobile is a system of devices which when taken together form a safety package. The whole system when in use will give the occupant a much better chance to survive an automobile accident. Therefore, a concentrated effort to increase the effectiveness of a single component such as the windshield, seat belt or energy-absorbing column is not the complete answer. The research should evaluate each component but its effectiveness should not be judged until it is returned to the system where the entire safety package can be evaluated.

As an example, examine the average driver. The new energy-absorbing steering column is all that he needs, but add the lap belt then a shoulder harness and even consider prepositioning before impact and the driver has increased his chances of reduced severity of injury by as much as 60 per cent.

The automotive safety engineer must apply the principles of systems engineering to his complex safety package.

REFERENCES

1. Tourin, B., and Garrett, J.W.: Safety belt effectiveness in rural California automobile accidents. *ACIR Report*, 1960.
2. Tourin, B., and Garrett, J.W.: Report of safety belts to the California legislature. *ACIR Report*, Feb. 1960.
3. Robertson, J.S.; McLean, A.J., and Ryan, G.A.: Traffic accidents in Adelaide, South Australia. *Australian Road Research Board Special Report No. 1*, July 1966.
4. Lister, R.D., and Neilson, I.D.: The effectiveness of safety belts. *RRL Report No. 16*, 1966.

5. VULCAN, A.P.: Review of the relative merits of various types of motor vehicle seat belts. *J Aust Road Res Board*, 2(8):33–40, June, 1966.
6. LISTER, R.D., and MILSON, I.: Car seat belts—an analysis of the injuries sustained by car occupants. *Practitioner*, 191:332–340, Sept. 1963.
7. HUELKE, D.F., and GIKAS, P.W.: Causes of deaths in automobile accidents. *ORA Report #06749*, April 1966.
8. CAMPBELL, H.E.: Thirty-three fatal crashes with seat belts. *Rocky Mountain Med J*, 61(8), August 1964.
9. CAMPBELL, B.J., and KIHLBERG, J.K.: Seat belt effectiveness on the non-ejection situation. *Proceedings of the Seventh Stapp Car Crash Conference*. 1963.
10. SHARP, J.E.; CAMPBELL, H.E., and UTANS, P.: Analysis of lap shoulder belt effectiveness in accidents. *Proceedings of the Ninth Stapp Car Crash Conference*. 1965.
11. LE MIRE, J.; EARLY, D., and HAWLEY, CHAPLIN: Intra-abdominal injuries caused by automobile seat belts. *JAMA*, 210(10), Sept. 1967.
12. SALDEEN, T.: Fatal neck injuries caused by use of diagonal safety belts. *J Trauma*, 7(6). Nov. 1966, 21–23.
13. LASKEY, I.I.; SIEGAL, A.W., and NAHUM, A.M.: Automotive cardio-thoracic injuries: a medical-engineering analysis. *SAE Paper #680052*, 1968 SAE Congress.
14. Unpublished Data from Wayne State University files.
15. PATRICK, L.M., and DANIEL, R.P.: Comparison of standard and experimental windshields. *Proceedings of the Eighth Stapp Car Crash Conference*, 1964.
16. KIHLBERG, J.: Driver and his right front passenger in automobile accidents. *ACIR Report No. VJ-1823-R16*, Nov. 1965.
17. KIHLBERG, J., and GENSLER, H.K.: Head injury in automobile accidents related to seated position and age. *Cal. Report No. VJ-1823-R26*, July 1967.
18. NAHUM, A.; SIEGEL, A., and TRACHTENBERG, S.B.: Causes of significant injuries in nonfatal traffic accidents. *Proceedings of the Tenth Stapp Car Crash Conference*, 1966.
19. SKEELS, P.: The General Motors energy-absorbing steering column. *SAE Paper #660785*. 1966 SAE Congress.
20. A study of injuries related to padding on instrument panels. *ACIR Report No. VJ-1823-R2*, August 1963.
21. KEMMERER, R.M.; CHUTE, R.; HASS, D.P., and SLACK, W.K.: Automotive inflatable occupant restraint system. *SAE Paper #680033*, Jan. 1968, SAE Congress.
22. CLARK, CARL C.: Airbag restraints and air litter systems for the alleviation of highway injury. In Selzer, M.L.; Gikas, P.W., and Huelke, D.F. (Eds.): *The Prevention of Highway Injury*, April 19–21, 1967, pp. 221–237. Highway Safety Research Institute, Ann Arbor, Mich.
23. SNYDER, R.G.; YOUNG, J.W., and SNOW, C.C.: Experimental impact protection with advanced automotive restraint systems. *Proceedings of the Eleventh Stapp Car Crash Conference*. Oct. 1967.
24. HILTON, B.C., and BOBBS, F.W.: The packaging of car occcupants—a British approach to seat design. *Proceeding of the Seventh Stapp Car Crash Conference*. 1963.
25. CRANDALL, F.J.: The Liberty Mutual survival car II. In Curran, W.J., and Chayet, N.L. (Eds.): *Trauma and the Automobile*.
26. The safety sedan—summary of final report, the New York State safety car. Fairchild Hiller, Republic Aviation Division. August, 1966.

27. SEVERY, D.M.; BRINK, H.M., and BAIRD, J.D.: Backrest and head restraint design for rear-end collision protection. *SAE Paper #680079*, Jan. 1968. SAE Congress.
28. MERTZ, H.J., JR.: The kinematics and kinetics of whiplash. A Dissertion, Oct. 1967.
29. GISSANE, N.: The causes and the prevention of car occupant neck injuries. In Selzer, M.L.; Gikas, P.N., and Huelke, D.F. (Eds.): *Prevention of Highway Injury*. April 1967, pp. 216–217. Highway Safety Research Institute, Ann Arbor, Mich.
30. MOORE, J.W.; TOURIN, B.; GARRETT, J.W., and LILIENFELD, R.: Child injuries in automobile accidents. *ACIR Report*, Feb. 1960.

BIBLIOGRAPHY

1. ASHAR, VIJAY: Seat belt sales survey. *ACIR Bulletin #1*, June 1, 1962.
2. BRECK, L.A., and PALAFOX, M.: Automobile seat belts. *Texas J Med*, 58:395–396, June 1962.
3. Auto seat Harness. *Consumer Union Report*, Oct. 1962, pp. 484–487.
4. Safety belts would curb mass highway injuries. *Med Tribune*, 2(27), July 3, 1961.
5. BASTIAANSE, J.C.: Confidential preliminary report. *Rai-Tno-Instituut Voor Wertransport Middelen*, Sept. 24, 1965.
6. BASTIAANSE, J.C.: Test directions for seat belts. *Rai-Tno-Instituut Voor Wertransport Middelen*, Oct. 11, 1960.
7. ROSE, CLARENCE: A safety engineering approach to child restraining devices. *Proceedings of the Seventh Stapp Car Crash Conference*. 1963.
8. APPOLDT, F.A.: Dynamic tests of restraints for children. *Proceedings of the Eighth Stapp Car Crash Conference*. 1964.
9. ALDMAN, BERTIL: A protective seat for children—experiments with a safety seat for children between one and six. *Proceedings of the Eighth Stapp Car Crash Conference*. 1964.
10. Shattering. *The Auto Car*, Dec. 18, 1959.
11. Transport safety. *The Auto Car*, Jan. 13, 1959.
12. RODLOFF, G., and BREITENBURGER, G.: Conditions of the perfect windshield. *SAE Paper #670191*, 1967 SAE Conference.
13. NAHUM, A.M., and CANTY, T.: Case study investigation of human injury patterns and the relation to vehicular design. *Proceedings of the Seventh Stapp Car Crash Conference*. 1963.
14. PATRICK, L.M.; LANGE, W.A., and HODGSON, V.R.: Facial injuries—causes and prevention. *Proceedings of the Seventh Stapp Car Crash Conference*. 1963.
15. DANIEL, R., and PATRICK, L.M.: Instrument panel impact study. *Proceedings of the Ninth Stapp Car Crash Conference*. 1965.
16. PATRICK, L.M.: Prevention of instrument panel and windshield head injuries. *Prevention of Highway Injury*, 1967, pp. 169–181. Highway Safety Research Institute, Ann Arbor, Mich.
17. MARQUIS, D.P.; SKEELS, P.C., and HANSON, H.L.: Drivers chances of survival in head-on crashes improved with energy absorbing steering column. *SAE Journal*, Oct. 1967.
18. SCHWIMMER, S., and WOLF, R.: Leading causes of injury in automobile accidents. *Automotive Crash Injury Research Report*, June 1962.
19. ALDMAN, BERTIL: Biodynamic studies on impact protection. *Acta Physiol Scand*, 1962.

20. CAMBELL, H.E.: The automobile seat belt and abdominal injury. *Surg Gynec Obstet, 119*:591–592, Sept. 1964.
21. GRIME, G.: The effectiveness of car seat belts. *International Road Safety and Traffic Review, XI* (3), 1963.
22. DuBOIS, E.F.: Seatbelts are not dangerous, *Brit Med J,* Sept. 27, 1952..
23. SNYDER, R.G.; CROSBY, W.M.; SNOW, C.C.; YOUNG, J.W., and HANSON, P.: Seat belt injuries in impact. *The Prevention of Highway Injury.* pp. 188–210. Highway Safety Research Institute, Ann Arbor, Mich.
24. STAPP, J.P.; MOSELY, J.D.; LOMBARD, C.F.; NELSON, G.A.; NICHOLS, G., and LARMIE, F.: *Analysis of Biodynamics of Selected Rocket-Sled Experiments.* U.S.A.F. School of Aerospace Medicine, Aerospace Medical Division, (AFSC), Brooks Air Force Base, Texas. July, 1964.
25. STETSON, C.H., JR.; PARKS, W.G.; GENEST, R., and KATZ, F.: Seat belt webbing service life. *NASA Document #N65, 19795,* Sept. 1964.
26. LISTER, R.D.: Safety glass for windscreens. *Automobile Engineer,* Sept. 1961.
27. EGLI, A.: Stopping the occupant of a crashing vehicle—a fundamental study. *SAE Paper #670038,* Jan. 1967, SAE Congress.
28. PETTRY, D.K.: A survey of the problem of protecting the passenger in the event of a collision. *American Society of Body Engineers Convention.* Oct. 1954.
29. HAYNES, A.L.: Studies of barrier and car to car impact. Presented before the Harvey Cushing Society, April 1957.
30. MARTIN, D.E., and KROELL, C.K.: Vehicle crush and occupant behavior. *SAE Paper #670034,* 1967 SAE Congress.

DISCUSSION

Richard G. Snyder

Dr. Lange and Mr. Van Kirk have very competently surveyed current protective methods in automotive vehicles, and carefully assessed the contributions of each in preventing or attenuating trauma in collisions. Their emphasis upon the effectiveness of the *system* concept, as a number of components designed into the safety package is important. Too often, individual devices are considered separately, as an entity rather than in the ecological anlaga of the total package.

Accident studies serve to make most valuable contributions in both pointing out initial problem areas and in eventually providing the statistics to demonstrate the effectiveness of various protective devices. I should like to point out, however, that such methods are usually introduced primarily as a direct result of substantial experimental research and development by the manufacturer *before* it is put into production vehicles. This involves not only the use of prior accident information, but a combination of experimental sled tests and highly instrumented full-scale automotive crash tests on the proving ground under carefully controlled conditions. In fact, the vivid explanation presented by Dr. Lange for each injury potential in the time capsule of occupant impact kinematics is typical of documentation obtained only by instrumented experimental tests. Since while the clinician can speculate, he cannot know, the precise causation for each injury in each case.

A system approach should not overlook the probability that emphasis of improvement of some components of the total safety package can perhaps offer greater dividends than others. For example, in an automobile collision, the original purpose was to prevent ejection from the vehicle. But now that doors are provided with improved safety latches to resist opening during an accident, a more important function is to limit injurious contact with the interior of the vehicle. If an effective restraint can be provided, therefore, the occupant will not be as likely to strike other portion of the interior, and thus their importance may diminish. However, the degree of restraint crash protection depends in large part upon the total environment. In some high velocity impacts, passenger compartment integrity can become a greater problem than restraint because of compartment collapse and intrusion. Our experimental FAA studies, with various restraint systems conducted with subhuman primates on the Holloman Daisy Track, have also indicated that abdominal and thoracic trauma may be attributed to restraint systems and closely correlate with clinical observations made by Dr. Walt yesterday. Furthermore, that the likelihood of most such injuries are greatly increased when the particular restraint system is incorrectly or too loosely worn. The preliminary experimental studies of fetal and maternal protection will be continued by Dr. Crosby of the University of Oklahoma, and some two hundred cases of restrained and unrestrained pregnant women involved in automobile accidents have been collected to date, although data are incomplete to comment more fully at this time. One small correction—there is no "requirement" concerning the energy absorbing steering wheel. This should be credited to company research and development, not government edict.

Evidence to date certainly suggests that the energy-absorbing hub and deformable column, the 30 mil laminated windshield, and instrument panel and interior padding have provided improved occupant protection. Future vehicles may be anticipated to provide even more improved protection as, and if, greater biomedical-engineering emphasis is concentrated on these problems.

Chapter XXII

OCCUPANT RESTRAINT SYSTEMS OF AUTOMOTIVE, AIRCRAFT, AND MANNED SPACE VEHICLES:
An Evaluation of the State-of-the-Art and Future Concepts

RICHARD G. SNYDER

It is probable that no single device has contributed as effectively to the protection and survival of vehicle occupants involved in crash impacts as has the occupant restraint system. The most familiar of such restraints is the simple webbed lap belt used in automobiles and general aviation aircraft, and by passengers in air transport and most military aircraft. But in severe crash environments, the effective protective limits of the single belt restraint may be exceeded. Greater protection of the vehicle occupant, therefore, will depend upon development of more advanced restraint systems.

In aviation, the advent of new ultra-high-speed military aircraft has made the environmental problems of ejection loading, windblast, and tumbling more crucial, resulting in a need for improved aircrew restraint systems. New problems and the complex functional requirements of extraterrestrial exploration vehicles and hypervelocity manned spacecraft have required the design of relatively sophisticated restraint systems incorporating some entirely new functions. Projecting into the future, one can safely speculate that even greater innovations will be necessary for all modes of tomorrow's transportation.

In the accident situation, the interaction of the vehicle and the struck object represents the initial or primary collision. A "secondary collision" occurs between the vehicle interior and the occupant, who continues at the same velocity as the vehicle prior to impact (Huelke 1967). Recently, interest has been focused on the "tertiary collision," as used by Snyder et al. (1968a), and Lasky et al. (1968) to describe the impingement of the body upon the restraint system itself. While there is now more universal acceptance of the dictum that a restraint system properly installed and worn offers the single best protection for a vehicle occupant during an impact, there is growing recognition that some systems can offer substantially greater protection than others. The initial evidence for this conclusion has been obtained through sled or crash-barrier proving ground tests with anthropomorphic dummies, experiments with human volunteers at low, noninjurious g-levels, and tests at higher levels with anesthetized animals under carefully controlled conditions. The final performance of restraint systems in automobiles, however, cannot be measured except by the careful investigation and analysis of actual accidents. Until adequate accident evidence is obtained, which may take a considerable amount of time after introduction of a new restraint system, comparisons of different systems must be made by experimental research studies.

Since each type of specialized vehicle to be considered in this chapter has particularly unique characteristics, the somewhat different requirements of the respective occupant restraint for each will be discussed. That there should be differences, and the reason for them, is not always clearly understood. Why, for example, the more sophisticated systems developed for aerospace technology cannot simply be adapted to the automotive vehicle as so many people assume, will be discussed. To understand the necessary differences between the restraint systems for each segment of transportation, one must also understand the differing operational environments as well as the impact conditions which are a consequence of them. In addition, one must also understand the occupant packaging constraints imposed by the intended consumer population. While pregnant women, the infirm, and elderly, do not drive nuclear or solar powered interplanetary vehicles, astronauts do drive cars. Ironically, one astronaut and two U.S. jet aces have recently been fatally injured in automobile accidents. No restraints were reported worn.

There are, therefore, some distinct variations in the purposes of occupant restraint systems. In an automobile collision, the primary purpose originally was to prevent ejection from the vehicle, but now that doors are provided with improved safety latches to resist opening during an accident, a more important function is to limit injurious contact with the interior of the vehicle. Conversely, in a military aircraft, ejection may be desirable, but the restraint system must now protect against severe seat-to-head acceleration and provide more complex protection. In space vehicles, the occupant must be protected against severe forces on his capsule both in flight acceleration profiles and in landing impact, or during ejection. But in either instance, the main purpose of the restraint system is to retain the occupant in the most protective manner in his seat. He is in a "seat" in the module.

Modern technology has spawned the systems engineering approach. Thus, the simple lap belt now must be considered by the design engineer as only part of the total "system," which also may include any restraint attachments or tie-down, the seat and its occupant, and the larger environment into which the system must be integrated. The seat itself, with side or head restraints, thigh roll-up, seat pan dishing, lateral wings, built-in back support, or pedestal flexion or energy absorption devices, often becomes an integral part of the restraint protection. It is quite possible that in the future automobile, the entire interior of the compartment may be considered part of the restraint system if trends toward passive retention and protection of occupants continue.

Since other chapters in this book have discussed various aspects of restraint protection in detail, the objective of this study has been to examine current state-of-the-art of restraint systems in air, space and ground transportation vehicles and briefly consider directions of some projected concepts. Particular attention will be focused on the unique automobile requirements and a summary of recent pertinent research findings.

AUTOMOTIVE VEHICLES

The earliest version of the Ford automobile, built in 1896, simply employed a bicycle saddle mounted over a 3-gallon gasoline tank, although this was soon replaced by a standard buggy seat. Seats have since improved, with the development of many versions of the bench seat, and an increasing trend toward the bucket seat (which may lead to greater "wrap-around" with individual occupant side and head protection).

Restraints themselves have been used by automobile occupants only during the past decade, except for racing vehicles, whose drivers most clearly understand their value. Some early automobiles (1885 to 1905) used "belts" in some instances to prevent passengers from bouncing out of vehicles on rough, rutted roads. In 1922, Barney Oldfield introduced seat belts to racing cars (Schrum, 1968). Although both upper and lower torso restraints have been used for over 50 years in aircraft (an upper torso harness was used prior to 1917 in the Spad III see Fig. 22–1, making its use nearly as old as the lap belt itself), emphasis until World War II was on the lap belt system. Restraints were not used in any U.S. production vehicles until 1955 (although a form of lap belt was provided in some models of the 1949 Nash reclining right-front seat to retain occupants while sleeping). Both Ford and Chrysler first offered "safety belts" as optional equipment in late 1955, but public acceptance was limited. Anchorages for lap belts were required as of January 1, 1962, in all new automobiles sold in New York State, although by 1964, when most automotive manufacturers installed two lap belts in the front seat as standard equipment, only half the states had anchorage requirements for belt installation. In 1966, automotive manufacturers installed four lap belts per

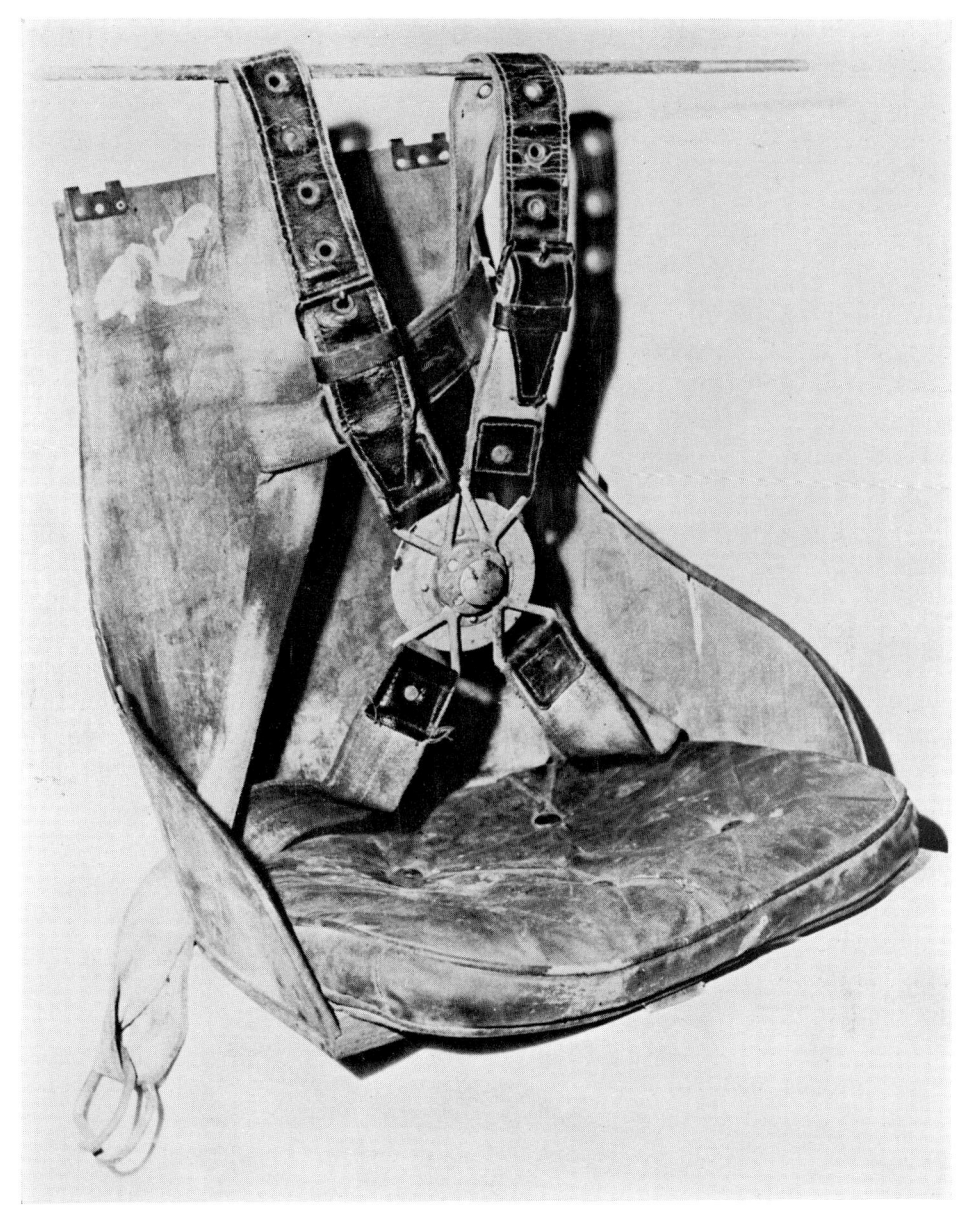

FIGURE 22–1. Spad III fighter aircraft upper torso restraint of 1917 (*from* National Air Museum, Smithsonian Institute, Washington, D.C.).

car, voluntarily preceding by two years Federal legislation requiring restraints. Restraint systems are presently not required for trucks, multipurpose passenger vehicles, and buses, but are under consideration (Nield, 1968).

Various "standards" pertaining to occupant restraint systems for adults (seat belts, anchorages, assemblies, restraint devices, harnesses) known to the author have been summarized in tabular form in Appendices 22–I and 22–II for the reader's reference, with sources for more specific information. Child restraint "standards" will be discussed in a separate paper (Snyder 1968c).

Current Type 2 Restraint Systems

The Type 2 (or 2a) restraint system (having both a lap belt and upper torso restraint) is required to be installed in the outboard front seat positions in all new cars, except convertibles, manufactured for sale in the United States since January 1, 1968. Except for the Shelby-American double-shoulder Y-yoke with inertia reel (Fig. 22–2E), all manufacturers have installed three-point harnesses (Fig. 22–2C).

Although there are a number of variations, at present most American so-called three-point restraints are actually four-point in that both ends of the lap belts and the single shoulder belt are separately anchored. This differs from the European style three-point, in which the shoulder belt slips through a slip joint and forms half of the lap belt, and in which there are only three attachment points. The European three-point system has one major disadvantage when compared to the American, in that the pelvic or lap belt is more difficult to correctly adjust and often in an impact will not retain its position over the pelvic area. It can, in effect, be raised up by the shoulder belt attached to it and, thus, may allow submarining under the lap portion to occur. However, no restraint system is of any value unless it is used, and most studies conducted in the United States have indicated lap belt usage varying between 17 to 30 per cent. Increased usage is thus going to be necessary before any substantial reduction in the accident trauma statistics may be expected.

Since Type 2 restraints were not installed in American production cars prior to 1967, accident experience with this system in American vehicles has been limited to racing accidents (States, 1967), or accidents in the U.S. involving European type vehicles and European type three-point harness (Fisher, 1965; Fletcher and Bragdon, 1967; Ebbetts, 1962). These and other European studies of the three-point restraint system are discussed in detail in Snyder et al. (1967b).

To evaluate and compare the relative protection offered by various restraint systems, a series of sixty tests was conducted by the Federal Aviation Administration on the Holloman AFB Daisy Decelerator, utilizing anesthetized baboon subjects. (Snyder et al., 1967a; 1967b; 1967c; Crosby, 1967). A major objective of these tests of six current and experimental restraints was to determine experimentally the relationship between body

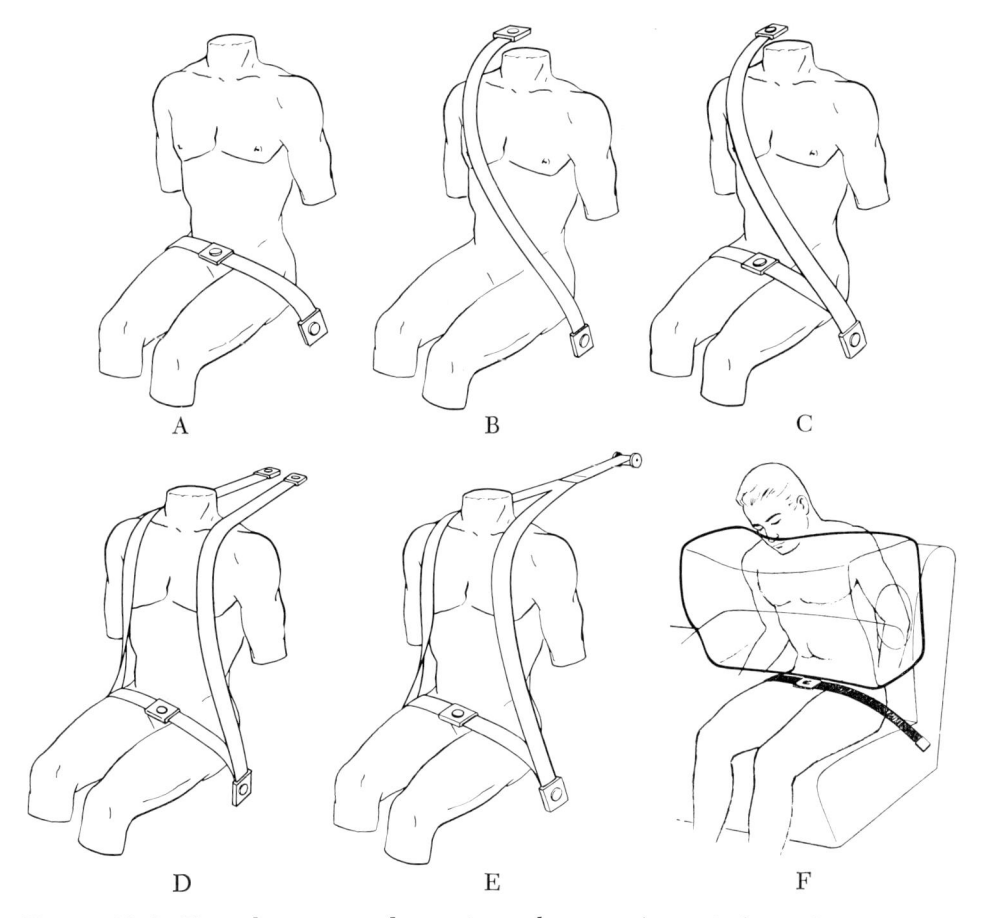

FIGURE 22–2. Typical current and experimental automotive restraint systems.
A. Lap belt restraint.
B. Bandolier European single torso harness.
C. Type 2 combination lap belt and single diagonal torso belt (three-point) available on most late 1967 automobiles and required on all automobiles manufactured since January 1, 1968 for sale in the United States.
D. Double shoulder harness used in racing vehicles. Often of 3 inch wide aircraft type webbing.
E. Inverted "V" double shoulder harness with lap belt with Hamill inertia reel. Used in Shelby-American GT500 and GT350.
F. Experimental airbag concept.

and seat orientation, force patterns, and the effectiveness of various restraint configurations. Five tests were conducted with the three-point harness configuration. Two were forward-facing at 22 and 30 g; two were rearward-facing at 20 and 30 g; and one was conducted in the 90 degree side-facing position at 30 g. Impact velocities ranged from 60 to 84 feet per second, onset rates from 2500 to 5500 g per second, and total time durations from 77 to 108 milliseconds. No trauma other than minor belt contusions was found in either the forward-facing or rearward-facing impacts under these deceleration conditions, and this system appeared to offer much greater protection than either the single diagonal (found to be nonsurvivable in our tests) or the lap belt only. However, in the 90 degree left side impact ("driver" wearing a Type 2 [American three-point] restraint) the impingement of the torso harness on the neck was sufficient in the absence of any structure to restrain sideward movements to cause fatal injury (total dislocation of occipital-atlantoid joint and intramuscular hemorrhage extending from the 1–6 cervical areas). However, since no automobile door or side panel was simulated, this seat may not be representative of hazards in side collisions where an occupant would be prevented from extreme neck impingement by striking the side structure. Additional tests simulating many angles of impact forces will have to be conducted to fully explore torso belt/occupant loading relationships. Further, in a right-side impact the driver would not be restrained laterally and could slip out of the upper torso belt. The possibility that torso belts may be mechanically involved in injury to the wearer, or provide no upper torso restraint in some impacts, even under the best conditions of adjustment, demonstrates the need to pursue improvements which can offer more comprehensive protection.

These experiments and observation of dummy kinematics reemphasize the criticality of restraint positioning. Even the best restraint system may provide ineffective protection if it is improperly positioned on the body. High priority should be given to a means of adjusting the Type 2 (European or American "3-point") outboard upper torso attachment to allow more flexible positioning for various occupants' shoulders. The combination of occupant size variation and seat adjustment range limits the positioning of the torso belt because both ends of the belt are rigidly attached. Thus, the present system cannot provide optimum restraint for all occupants. If, as in some European cars, the upper belt attachment is low or too far forward relative to the seated occupant, the resulting belt angle can be so low (off to the side of the upper arm), that in forward impact, the occupant could not only flex over it and slip out of the upper torso restraint entirely but could also be subjected to a simultaneous rotational torquing motion which may be particularly injurious. Similarly, an anchorage location too far to the rear, relative to the occupant's seated position, can cause the diagonal belt to impinge across the neck, causing discomfort even during normal driving. Should this create significant pressures upon the nerves and such blood vessels of the neck as the carotid artery, it could have a subtle but disastrous effect upon the occupant. In impact, a severe neck injury could occur should the torso belt impinge upon the neck. Perhaps just as unfortunate, uncomfortable fit may also be detrimental to occupant acceptance and future usage of the current Type 2 (three-point) restraint system if, upon first experience, it is uncomfortable, chafes and irritates the neck, and prevents adequate freedom to reach controls. In addition, improvements are being pursued to overcome the tendency of current belts to "twist." Presently, if the occupant does not straighten out his belts prior to adjusting, body contact area may be decreased and this can potentially greatly decrease restraint effectiveness. Here, outboard retractors may assist.

To many the most "obvious" improvement in current Type 2 (three-point) system would be the addition of attachment adjustment and an inertia-locking reel such as has been developed by independent researchers; but, as with so many other items, complex problems remain to be solved.

One might expect, for instance, that available aircraft inertia-locking reels could simply be installed in automobiles. But an aircraft inertia-locking reel is designed to lock at between 2 and 3 g, while the automotive reel must, by Federal regulation (Appendix I), lock at .5 g, a much more sensitive level, because of braking decelerations not common in the aircraft. In fact, to be sure of meeting this requirement, reels may have to be set as low as .35 g. Consequently, a reel designed for the automotive environment, with associated hardware providing improved adjustment ranges, seems to be the most feasible route for future improvements in upper torso restraint systems. For despite its problems, the Type 2 or three-point, harness configuration, when properly positioned on the body can offer a substantial increase in protection over the use of a lap belt alone. Recent tests conducted at Holloman AFB on the Daisy Decelerator with volunteer male subjects by the National Bureau of Standards indicated good protection resulted up to 17 g, the highest voluntary level of deceleration run (Armstrong 1967).

Inverted-Y Double Harness

The most advanced system in road use, and one which seems to offer the most effective protection in survivable accidents for adults, is the Y-yoke double torso harness with inertia reel, which is standard equipment in the low volume Shelby-American GT 350 and GT 500 automobiles (Fig. 22–2E). The inertia-locking reel (attached to the roll bar) allows completely free upper torso movement but automatic positive restraint by locking upon initiation of sudden braking or impact forces of .5 g. Since the upper torso restraint goes over the shoulders and down to each side in front, it fits women comfortably and does not bind clothing. In addition, the yoke, coming to a "Y" behind the head, has proven to be an effective head extension restraint in at least one rear-end accident, although it would probably not be effective without further modification for off-center impact since the head might easily miss the yoke.

In the series of over sixty impact tests, conducted by the Federal Aviation Administration on the Holloman AFB Daisy Decelerator, comparing six different automotive restraint systems, four experiments involved the yoke harness equipped with a Hamill inertia-locking reel (Snyder et al. 1967c). Anesthetized adult baboons were placed in a scaled-down sled seat with the belts properly adjusted (lap belt to static tension of 1.5 kg). Tests consisted of three runs in the forward-facing body orientation at 30, 43, and 49 peak g, and one side-facing (lateral 90 degree) test at 32 peak g. Entrance velocities ranged from 73.6 to 94.4 feet per second, onset rates from 2700 to 6100 g per second, and time plateaus from 45 to 60 milliseconds. These severe tests were initiated at the loads where conventional harness systems failed to provide adequate protection and proceeded to 49 g (sled), far higher than was found survivable for baboons in restrained torso systems. Belt forces were measured, and both gross and microscopic necropsies were conducted. Lap and torso belt loads were found to be about equal. The forward-facing position was probably survivable (with reversible injury) at 43 g, but appeared marginal for survival at 49 g. Myocardial fragmentation (transverse rupture of muscle fibers), as well as tearing of the pectoralis major chest muscles occurred at the 49 g level. In summary, the Y-yoke harness system with inertia reel offered greater body protection under these test conditions than either the lap or three-point harness systems, and had distinct practical advantages over the fixed double shoulder harness.

Tot-Guard "Child Restraint"

A second unique current system, which has only been on the market a few months, is the Ford Tot-Guard child restraint which employs a totally new concept (Fig. 22–3) (Heap, 1968). The Tot-Guard is designed for children with sitting heights between 18 and 25 inches (about 1 to 5½ years) or up to 40 pounds weight. It forms a cushioned protective "shield" about the child, and is attached to the seat by any standard lap belt, which goes around the shield. The child is free to move to some extent within his seat, but during sudden braking or impact he will be cushioned against the gently sloping forward portion. The important difference between this and more common webbing systems is that the full impact force is more evenly distributed over the body surface and the head and neck are protected. In contrast, many widely offered child restraints have offered

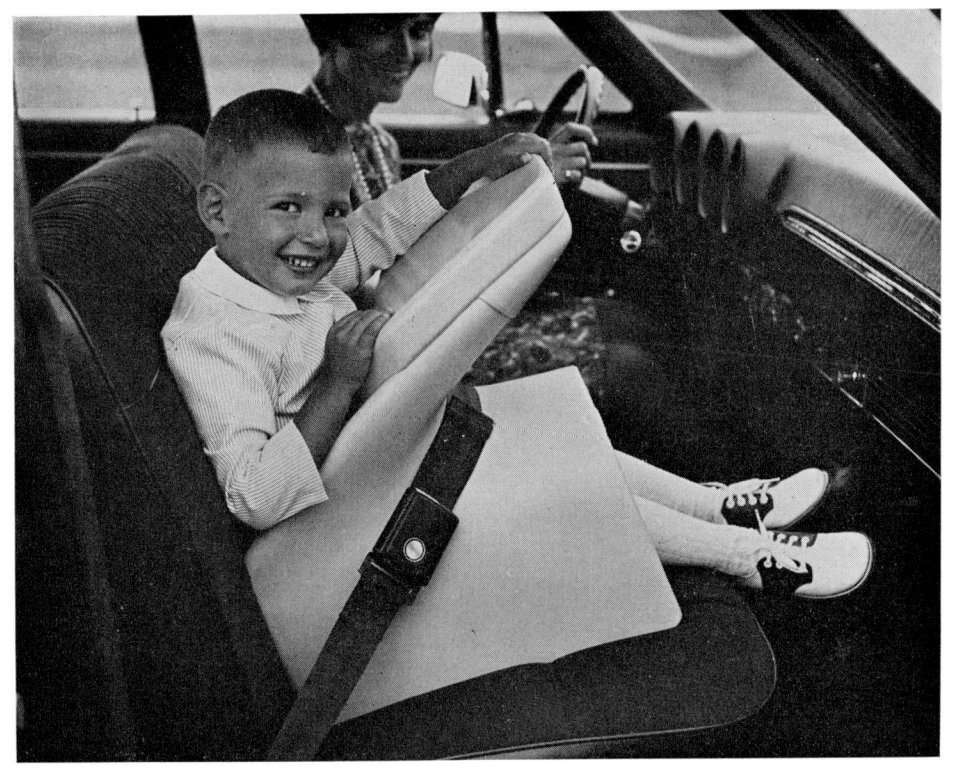

FIGURE 22-3. Ford Tot-Guard restraint concept for children of 15 to 25 inches sitting height (about 1 to 5½ years). In impact forces are distributed over entire body and head.

dangerously poor protection. Most of the "over the seat" attachment types provide a seating platform, but they can become a missile in even a low-speed accident. Other systems have not recognized that the child's structure differs from the adult's, and potentially dangerous injuries may be inflicted by misinformed placement of webbing, etc. (Snyder 1968b). It is vital that a child not be tightly restrained by his shoulders, since with the proportionately larger mass of the head and the much weaker cervical structure of the neck serious neurological injury could be caused by the head "snapping" forward on the restrained upper torso. Experimental evidence indicates the Ford Tot-Guard system provides restraint protection far superior to that provided by any other child restraint system. In tests this system also provided protection in 45 degree side impact to 35 g (Young 1967a). Such a system might be used for child passengers in aircraft, and although it might be a hazard to evacuation, is currently being evaluated for possible use by commercial airlines. It is possible that the concept could be used to develop "capsule" protection for adults in future vehicles.

Among experimental systems the seats illustrated in Fig. 4 have been acclaimed as offering potentially superior collision safety although some of them have yet to be tested in actual impacts.

New York Safety Car

The New York State Safety Sedan, designed by the Republic Aviation Division of Fairchild-Hiller Corporation, is the result of five different concepts derived from the Phase I feasibility study. One (Fig. 22–4A), of several restraint concepts considered, provides a double torso harness joining in front in a "V," and attached over the shoulders to the seat. A single point quick-release attachment is used for the lap belt, shoulder harness and a crotch strap. While crotch straps are used in some military configurations (and in the Pacific Scientific Company five-point aircraft harness), they are uncomfortable for women wearing clothing other than slacks. Also, the crotch strap is not needed to the same extent in the automobile because "submarining" is not as likely as it is in the aircraft's higher relative impact angle. However, low placement of the upper torso attachment may itself produce a downward force over the shoulders increasing the possibility of submarining, and indicating a possible need for a crotch strap.

In the final "optimal" New York State Safety Sedan design, four "individual contour seats" (bucket seats) are incorporated, each with an integral restraint system, including head support, shoulder harness, and lap belts (Fig. 22–4B). The seat is attached to bulkhead structure designed to yield at 30 g. The driver's head support is rigidly attached to the transverse bulkhead of the B pillar, and has two inertia reels and shoulder harnesses stored within it. The reels used differ from those in other automotive restraint systems as they do not lock until 2 g or more. An "X" upper torso webbing harness is used with a separate lap belt. Either upper belt, or both, can be used (The Safety Sedan 1968).

Cox Seat

The Cox seat, developed by Cox of Watford, Ltd., England, incorporates a strengthened frame, special anchorages, a headrest, and absorbable mounting in its latest development. In the original version, a full double-shoulder retractable harness was used (Fig. 22–4C), (Babbs & Hilton, 1965; Hilton, 1963), but in the latest modification this has been simplified to a "one-piece" lap and diagonal belt (Fig. 22–4D). In the original unique arrangement, the shoulder and lap belt for each side were one continuous piece, which allowed the entire harness to be donned by inserting the

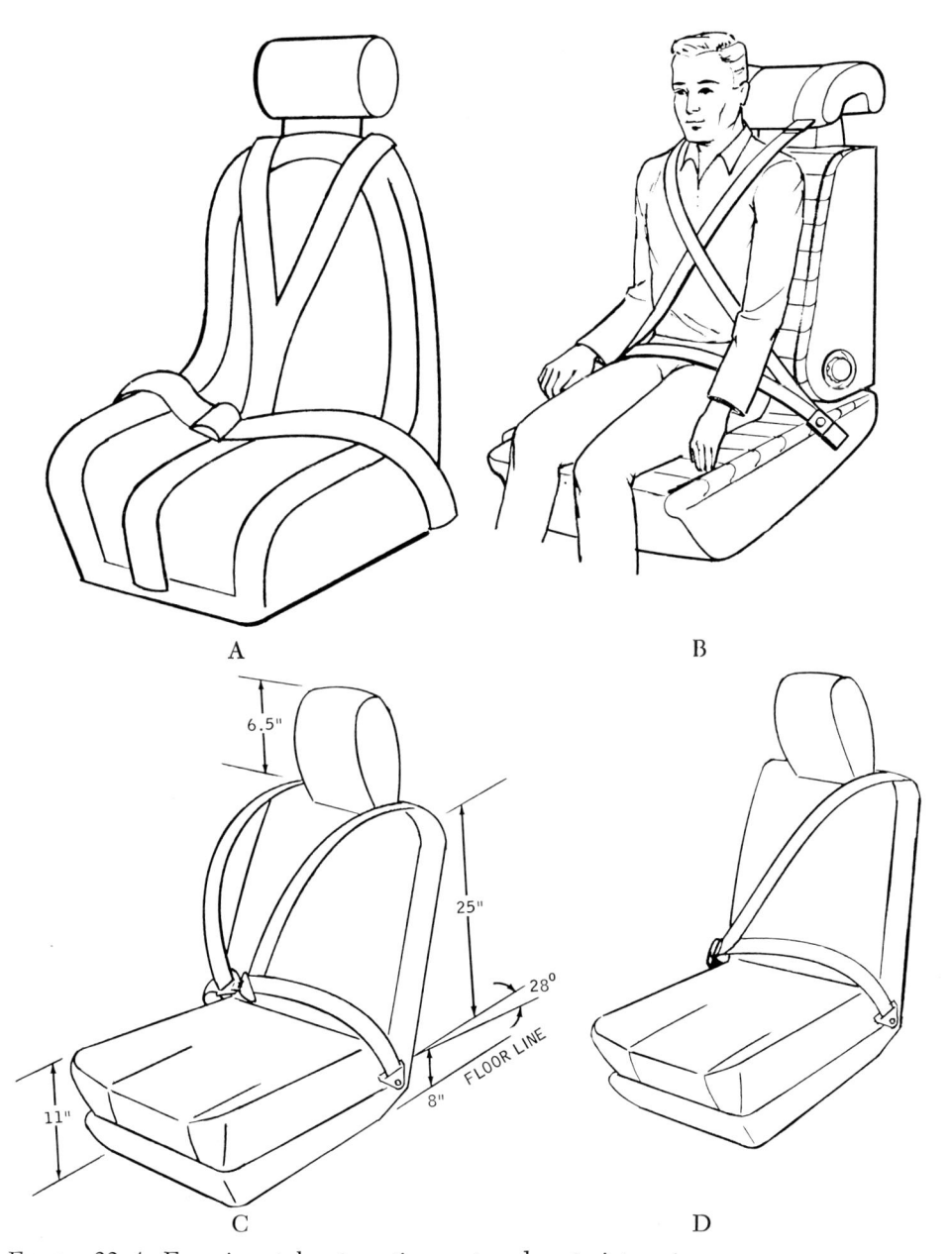

Occupant Restraint Systems of Manned Vehicles 507

FIGURE 22–4. Experimental automotive seat and restraint systems.
A. An early New York safety car restraint concept of Fairchild-Hiller Corporation. Note crotch strap, headrest and "Y" shoulder harness.
B. "Optimal" New York State safety sedan contour seat, using integral upper restraint belts in an "X" configuration with lap belt. Either or both shoulder belts can be used.
C. Early version of cox seat. Utilized unique single piece lap and shoulder belt combination.
D. Late version of cox seat uses one-piece lap and diagonal shoulder belt.

508   *Impact Injury and Crash Protection*

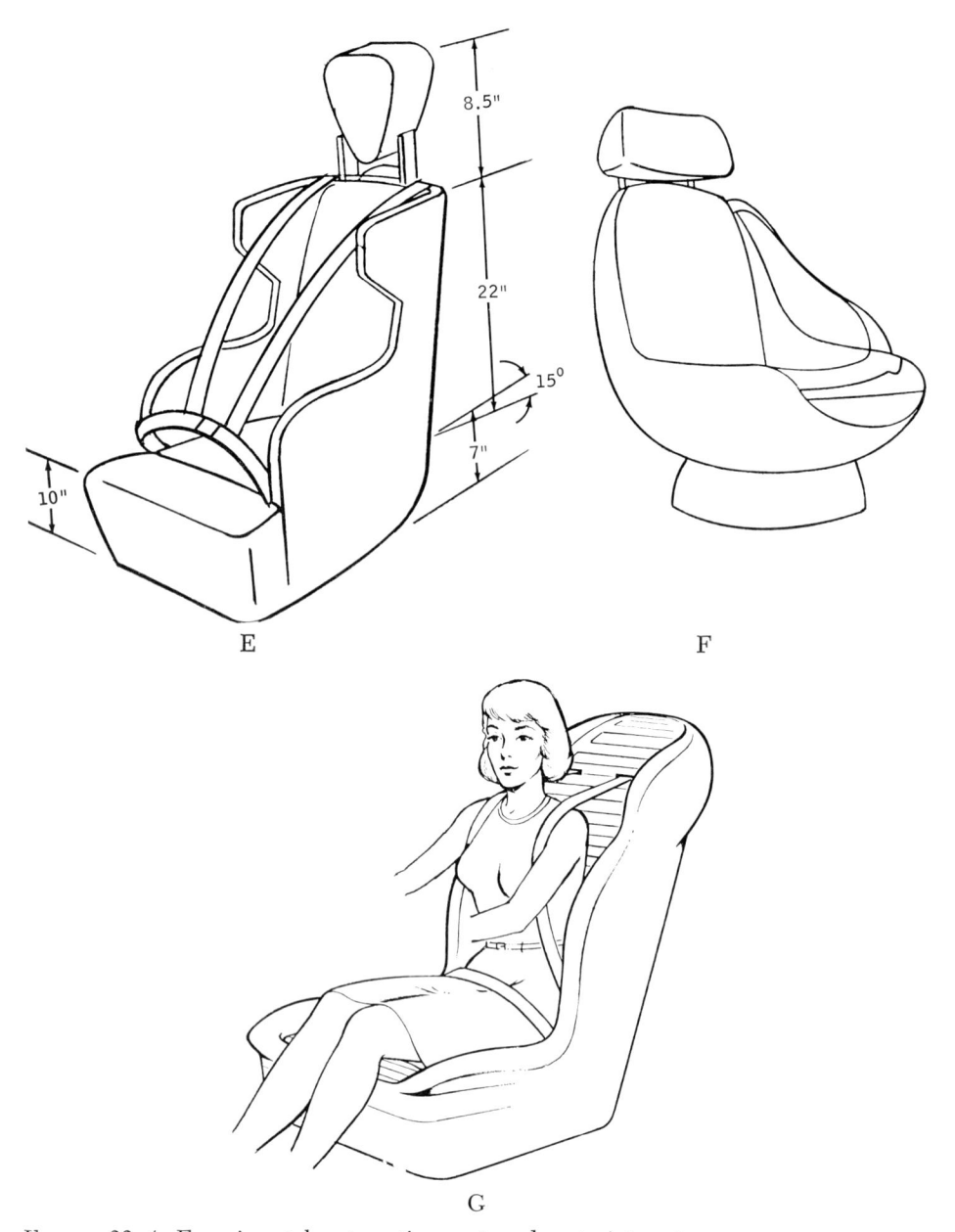

FIGURE 22–4. Experimental automotive seat and restraint systems.
E. Liberty Mutual capsule seat. High sides intended to offer lateral impact protection.
F. Winebrenner (Dow Chemical–Cranbrook Institute) design. Note lateral protection. Restraint is designed to be "in the way" unless worn by occupant.
G. Author's concept of an integrated seat-restraint system. Note head restraint (cushioned for rear occupant impact), side protection, deep-dish seat, and double-shoulder harness with integral automatic locking inertia reels in the seat. Shoulder harness allows free motion and is easily slid into by female occupants.

FOR ENTRANCE AND EXIT
SEAT TURNS 90°

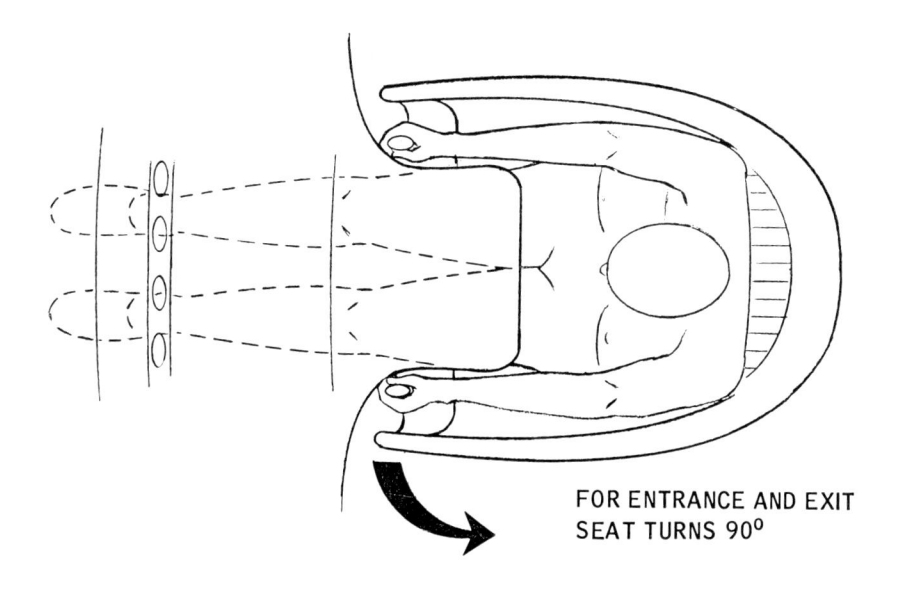

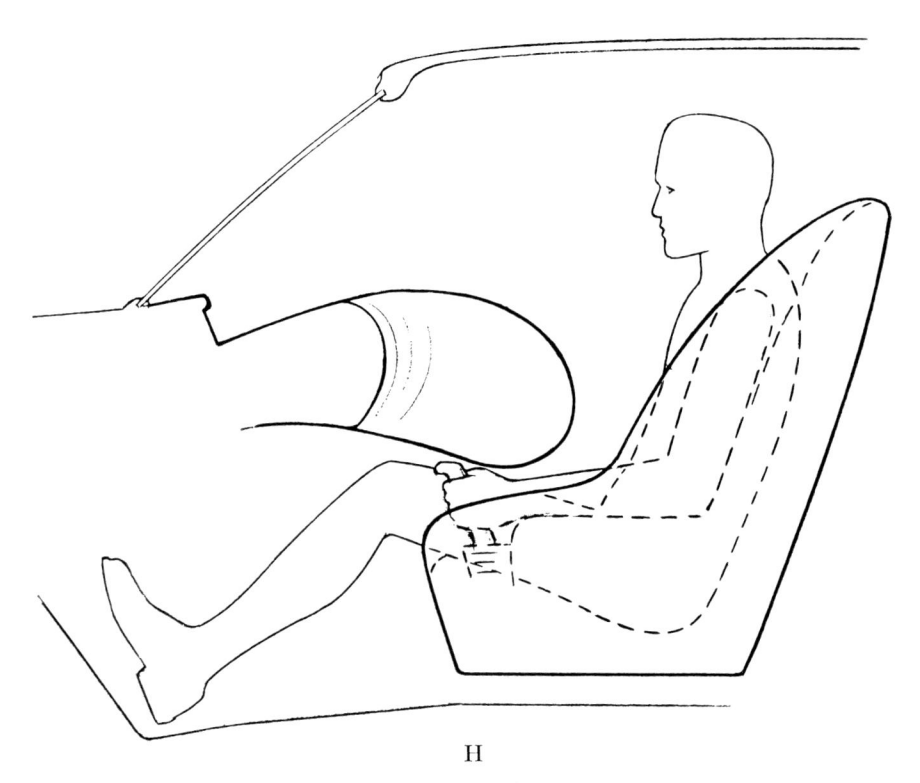

H

FIGURE 22–4. Experimental automotive seat and restraint systems.
H. Author's concept of seating capsule with protective energy-absorbing forward panel. Removal of steering assy. would allow use of passive restraint concept with no occupant belt system necessary. High sides of capsule offer side impact protection and head protection. Capsule could swivel to enter, or outboard section could be integrated with door.

arms and then snapping both sides together at the central attachment. However, this was found to be "unsuitable" for women (Hilton, 1967). As with the earlier versions of the New York Safety Car seat, the upper torso harness in both the original double shoulder harness and present three-point harness is attached low on the seat top below the head rest, which allows a downward slope. This could contribute to submarining action in impact, particularly if the lap belt portions are not snugged tight, and can create uncomfortable loading. The recommended bioengineering shoulder angle is generally about 30° above the horizontal (Young, 1966). While the New York design attached the lap and torso portions with a single-point upper torso "V," in the original Cox arrangement, both shoulder straps were continuous with the lap straps, coming together in front in the shape of ╲╱. In both of these systems, the restraint was designed as an integral part of the bucket seat, thereby avoiding the multiple (as many as twenty-four separate straps in a 1968 station wagon with bench seats) strap mess of the 1968 Type 2 installations, and further assuring reasonable fit for each occupant. The most recent Cox modification, however, employs only a single diagonal torso strap, joining the lap belt in a single continuous piece when the buckle is fastened. Since the buckle fastens to the inboard side of the occupant, it is located anterior to the superior iliac crest, and could result in bruising upon impingement, unless it were moved lower to the side. In the latest three-point arrangement, the belt is fastened by a simple plug and socket device. This 20 pound seat and restraint system has proved effective in four actual accidents involving seven belted individuals in crashes estimated to be 10 to 20 g (Hilton 1967), and has been favorably evaluated by Severy in crash tests (Severy et al., 1967).

Liberty Mutual Capsule Seat (Fig. 22–4E)

The Liberty Mutual capsule seat was designed to protect the occupant from both the sides and rear, and also featured an integral full harness restraint for frontal collision forces, as well as a head support. This design appears to offer much greater protection against lateral displacement of the occupant, and greater side impact protection than either the Cox seat or earlier New York State (Fairchild-Hiller) safety seat designs. One feature of this capsule seat is that it can be swiveled to the side to facilitate entrance and egress, and also has fore and aft adjustment. The pedestal base allows flexion at the junction with the floor pan, allowing the entire seat to flex as a unit during an impact.

Both the Cox seat and the Liberty Mutual seats and restraint systems have been studied in impact tests (Severy et al., 1967), involving two 30 mph rear-end, and two 40 mph intersection-type collisions. Severy concluded that the "Cox safety seat embodies many of the advances in motorist protection afforded by the Liberty Mutual capsule chair (e.g., shoulder and lap retractable inertial reel units attached to a strong, firmly anchored, contoured seat frame, full backrest with head support) but does not provide as much lateral support or resistance from collision intrusion as does the Liberty Mutual chair. The diagonal chest strap of the Cox seat can slip from the shoulders, but the Liberty Mutual harness remains correctly placed during the following collision." (See Severy, Brink, and Baird, 1968b.)

The Irvin Safety Seat

Another concept for future seating, not illustrated, is the Irvin Safety Seat which features a pressed-steel framework, side-impact deep-dish seat, built-in three-point harness with 0.3 g inertia reels, and suspended upholstery (Baker, 1965).

The Winebrenner Concepts (Dow Chemical)

The Liberty Mutual, New York Safety Sedan, and Cox, seat designs have provided valuable contributions to improved occupant protection over that presently available. However, it should be noted that further "second generation" improvements of even these designs are apparent in advanced concepts studies for future vehicles being conducted by automotive and seat manufacturers and especially by independent research organizations. Typical of advanced design concepts for future seating in the tradition above are several designs by James Winebrenner, in studies performed cooperatively by Cranbrook Academy and Dow Chemical Company. One features a deep-dish bucket seat, head restraint, pedestal mounting, and improved lateral restraint afforded by the flaring sides. In another design (Fig. 22–4F) high and low-density polystyrene foams and Ethafoam® polyethylene foam are utilized along with lateral flaring for side protection, and the back is highly padded for rear occupant head protection. This design also incorporates a unique restraint system in that the belts are anchored to inertia reels with a preformed plastic portion located so that it is in the way of the occupant if not buckled, in an attempt to force the occupant to utilize the restraint.

Rearward-Facing Seats

Rearward-facing seating has been proposed for two positions in the New York State (Fairchild-Hiller) Safety Car (Design Concept No. IIB 4+3

Passenger, 4-door sedan) (Fig. 22–5), and is a feature of the Volvo child restraint seat. This would provide greater protection by distributing of force over a larger body area in impact. The only production vehicles to currently utilize rearward-facing seating are station wagons having a third rearward-facing seat. The seat back is not high enough to prevent an adult from being exposed to "whiplash" type of extension-flexion trauma in a frontal collision in such seats. If they were higher, the driver would have no rearward vision. However, these are mainly used by children, and sitting height is often less than the height of the seat back, so that effective head protection is offered for forward impacts.

The protective advantage of facing rearward in a crash has been well demonstrated (Stapp, 1949; 1951; 1953; Pinkel and Rosenberg, 1956; Quimby and Hasbrook, 1956; Ruff, 1950; Fryer, 1959; Snyder et al., 1967a; Pesman and Eiband, 1956; and others). Rearward full body restraint offers considerably greater distribution of force over the body surface than can be provided in forward facing impacts of identical force. In forward-facing impacts with a single 2 inch lap belt, a contact area of about 40 inches squared is provided, while a three inch lap belt provides about 60 inches squared contact area. In contrast, the rearward facing seat provides approximately 208 inches squared (Ruff, 1950) to 262 inches squared (Stapp, 1951) for young male adults. The relative loading is thus greatly decreased with the greater restraint area. One other, minor, consideration is that in lateral impact, the additional friction between the body and the seat back would help retain the occupant in a better restraint position, assuming the vehicle had forward acceleration at impact. It should be noted however, that a rear-facing seat must be stressed to take greater loads than a forward facing seat because the occupant will load the seat rather than the belt and floor pan. There is some evidence that acceptance of rearward-facing positions in automobiles might be poor, especially at night, facing the headlights of following cars. Another drawback to rear facing seats in an automobile for adults and some children, might be the reported "car sickness" and general uncomfortable feeling of an adult passenger in not seeing what's coming but rather "where he has been" (Haynes, 1968). Note that the Federal Aviation Administration does not require aft facing passenger seats for civil aircraft, although the Air Force (MATS) has installed them in all Air Force transports.

Head Restraints

Effective January 1, 1969, all new automobiles manufactured for sale in the United States will be required to include head restraint protection for occupants at each outboard front seating position. FMVS Standard 202

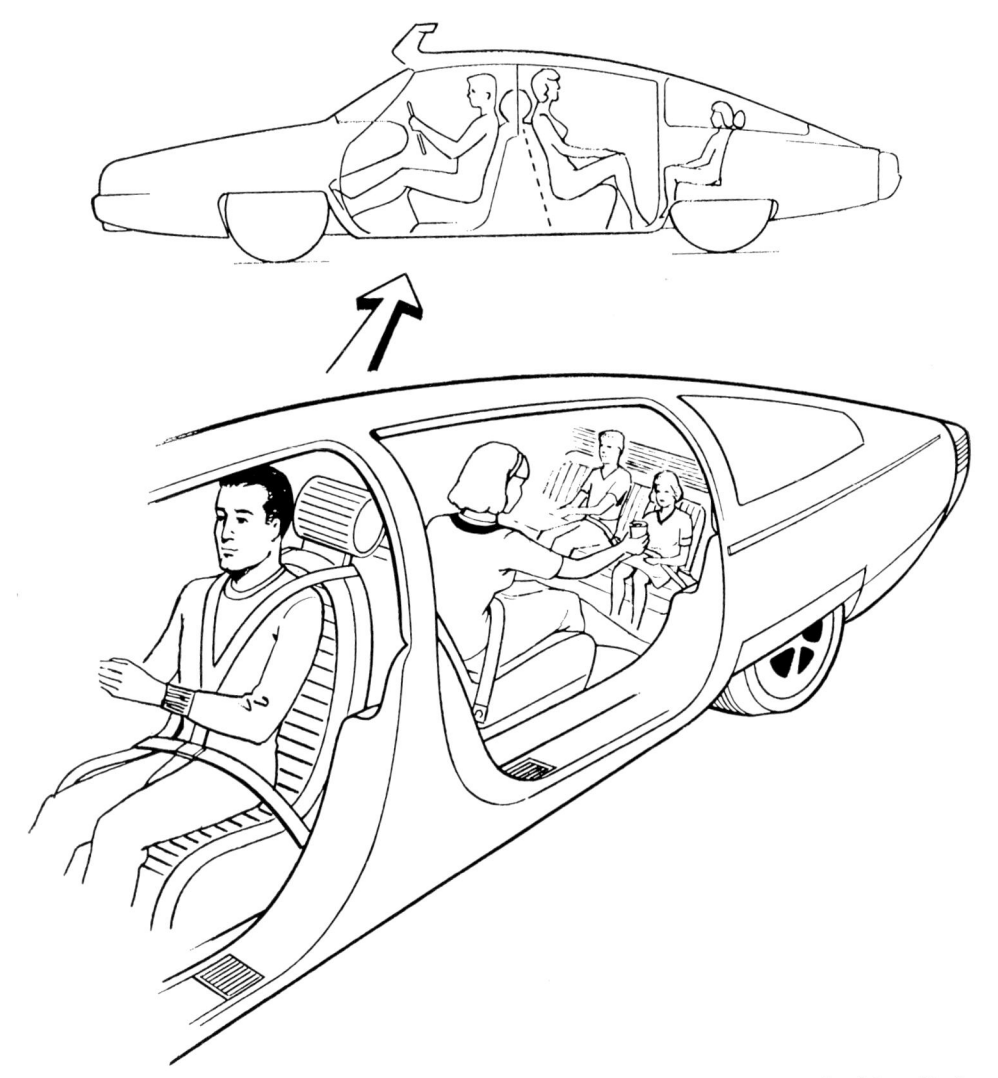

FIGURE 22–5. Rearward facing seating as proposed for two positions in the New York state (Fairchild Hiller) safety car (design concept no. 11B 4+3 passenger, 4-door sedan).

specifies that during a specified acceleration, the rotation of the head relative to the torso shall be limited to 45 degrees, on/or when adjusted to its fully extended position 25.5 inches or more above the SRP, the head restraint shall not allow displacement of the head from more than 4 inches rearward of the displaced torso line during application of the specified load. (Head Restraints—Passenger Cars, *Federal Register* 28 December 1967 [32 F.R. 20865] Amendment 2/68).

Despite considerable literature on clinical aspects of cranial-cervical extension-flexion trauma, the specific mechanisms still remain in doubt. Recent preliminary electromyographic studies sponsored by Ford at Michigan State University, for example, suggest combinations of clinical and laboratory techniques to provide objective and new diagnostic criteria for determining degrees of myotendonal damage (Adams, 1968). Recent studies of rear-end crashes of 1968 automobiles with anthropomorphic dummies have been carried out by Severy and colleagues at UCLA under Ford grant (Severy 1968a), and additional studies on the effect of seat-back height by Berton (1968). Experimental work is also being conducted currently by Young (1968), by the U.S. Army and U.S. Navy and led by Dr. C.L. Ewing, using facilities at Wayne State University and Army volunteer subjects (wearing helmets) (Patrick, 1968), at Wayne State University (Mertz & Patrick, 1967), by Ommaya, Hirsch and Martinez (1967) at Tulane University, and others. Too great a seat-back height can adversely affect another critical safety consideration, that of vision (Meldrum, 1965). Although there is little doubt that raising seat-back heights should help reduce the potential for "whiplash" injuries, there are numerous other factors involved—such as distance of head from head-restraint at impact, angle of restraint, etc.—to be resolved and it is hoped that overly rigid specifications will not be imposed until adequate scientific evidence is available. In this connection, there are other methods and designs to reduce whiplash (three of which are shown in Fig. 22–6A,B,C), which may be as effective as a higher seat-back.

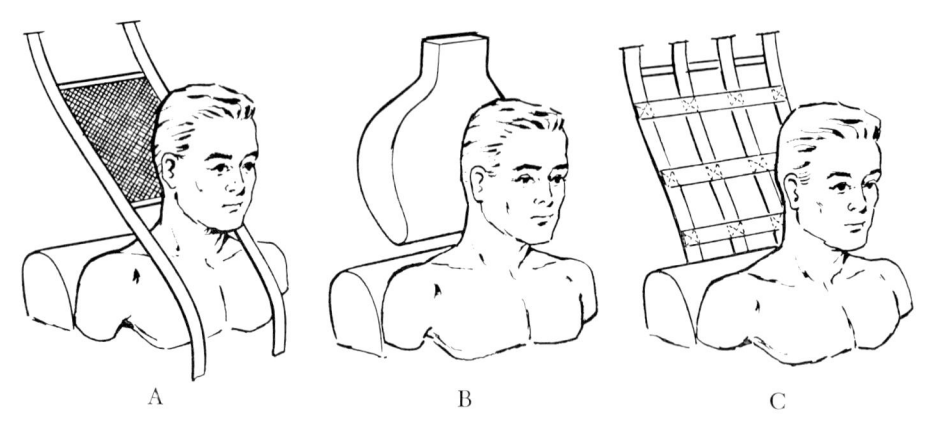

FIGURE 22–6. Typical head restraints not integral with the seat.
A. Headrest net integral with shoulder restraint system. The Shelby American-Hamill inverted Y-yoke (Fig. 4E) harness in limited use has been effective in one rear end impact collision to date.
B. Ceiling mounted headrest concept.
C. Experimental Liberty Mutual head support net (Severy, exp. 88, 1967).

Rotating Seats (Sabena and Other Systems)

The Belgian airline, Sabena, designed and used briefly (1958 to 1959) a seat which automatically rotated the seat at a pre-set level of impact, positioning the occupant to best protect against both longitudinal and vertical g forces (Braun 1958). However, this seat required a 57 inch width to function adequately, and there is no evidence whether this seat could be activated rapidly enough to be effective in an automobile crash in which the impact durations are considerably shorter than in aircraft crashes. Its use was discontinued due to various problems, including the difficulty of evacuating passengers from a semireclining position. Similar devices have been suggested for automobiles, some concepts adding the feature of rotating the seat to face the acceleration direction.

It should be noted, however, that a tilted seat will direct the deceleration force parallel to the long axis of the body, which will result in a lower tolerance level when compared to forces perpendicular to the long axis. Seats in racing cars, which may approach a 45 degree back angle in order to reduce vertical height of the vehicle, also position the occupant so that upper torso restraint may become a liability, by contributing to "submarining" potential (States, 1968). The astronaut couch, on the other hand, orients the body so that it is optimally perpendicular to the direction of loading.

Passive Restraint Systems—The Air Bag

The air bag restraint concept, which is still in experimental research and development evaluation, represents a transition between current restraining devices dependent upon webbing adjusted to the body (prior to any impact), and a future ultimate true "passive" restraint system in which the occupant wears no restraint at all and is fully protected by automatically initiated environmental devices.

The airbag system consists of a flexible bag device which may be stored out of sight in the instrument panel, seat back, header, side of the seat, or other location forward of the occupant (Fig. 22–2F). During an impact, a sensor releases compressed gas which instantaneously inflates the bags. Such devices can inflate a 7 cubic-foot bag in less than 40 milliseconds, thus providing the occupant a cushion to distribute the impact force. As the occupant's upper torso moves into the bag, the gas is simultaneously released through ports or orifices in the side of the bag, thus allowing a regulated deceleration, and preventing a rebound. The system still requires that the occupant wear a lap belt so that it is not yet a true passive restraint. However, should the airbag fail for any reason, the lap belt would still provide secondary protection from ejection, if not jack-knifing. Recent airbag development has been directed at system reliability (Kemmerer, 1968; Slack, 1968), since the reliability of the system components, particularly under conditions of long storage without use, heat, deterioration, and lack of maintenance is unknown as yet. In addition, the possibility of explosive air blast pressure and noise at actuation in a closed vehicle compartment causing injury to the occupants is being further explored. Possible inadvertent activation also is an obvious problem since it could cause the driver to lose control of the vehicle.

To determine the relative merits of this system as a protective device, 13 impact tests were conducted by the Federal Aviation Administration, using 11 anesthetized adult baboons seated on a F-111 test frame modified for a baboon seat and mounted on the Holloman AFB Daisy Decelerator Omnidirectional Sled (Snyder et al. 1967c). All tests were in the forward facing body orientation, with a seat pan angle 13 degrees below the horizontal and seat back angle of 28 degrees. Paired subjects survived impacts from 33 to 57 peak g (64 mph impact velocity) at an onset rate of 5900 g per second for 79 milliseconds total duration. Although microscopic evidence of lung, pancreatic, and adrenal hemorrhage appeared in one subject impacted at 47 g, and a bladder hemorrhage and rupture in a second subject after three successive impacts of 46, 46, and 50 peak g, a third 47 g impact resulted in no evidence of clinical trauma whatever. Post-impact observation for 4 to 12 weeks, followed by microscopic and gross autopsy of three animals apparently not injured, indicated that biochemical changes consistent with stress and tissue cellular trauma occurred but these findings were not remarkable. At 57 g, using the airbag restraint, the injury tolerance level was still not reached for these subjects. The overall evaluation of the airbag concept suggests that it offers potentially far greater protection than that provided by other systems tested. However, no tests were made of air blast pressure or noise effects in a closed environment, and this might be a problem, particularly to infants.

Special Vehicle Restraints

Due to unusual requirements of vehicle operation or configurations, more specialized systems of restraint may be necessary.

POST OFFICE VEHICLES: A good example of such problems is demonstrated by the mailman who may have to mount and dismount from his vehicle several hundred times a day. In this case, ordinary restraint systems are too time consuming, may be too awkward to use, and may not adequately protect the occupant. In addition, the postman may

Occupant Restraint Systems of Manned Vehicles 517

operate either a ½ ton right-hand drive vehicle, a 1-ton parcel delivery, or a ¼ ton three-wheel cycle vehicle, and in some combinations must be able to drive from either a standing or seated position. In recognition of the unique problems these factors present, the U.S. Post Office Department has contracted with All-American Engineering Company of Wilmington, Delaware to study advanced restraint concepts for the U.S. Post Office vehicles. In their study, over a dozen different system concepts were designed and evaluated, most of which involved radically different systems. Several examples showing the variety of systems considered are illustrated in Figure 22–7A,B,C,D. In the sit or stand hinged-

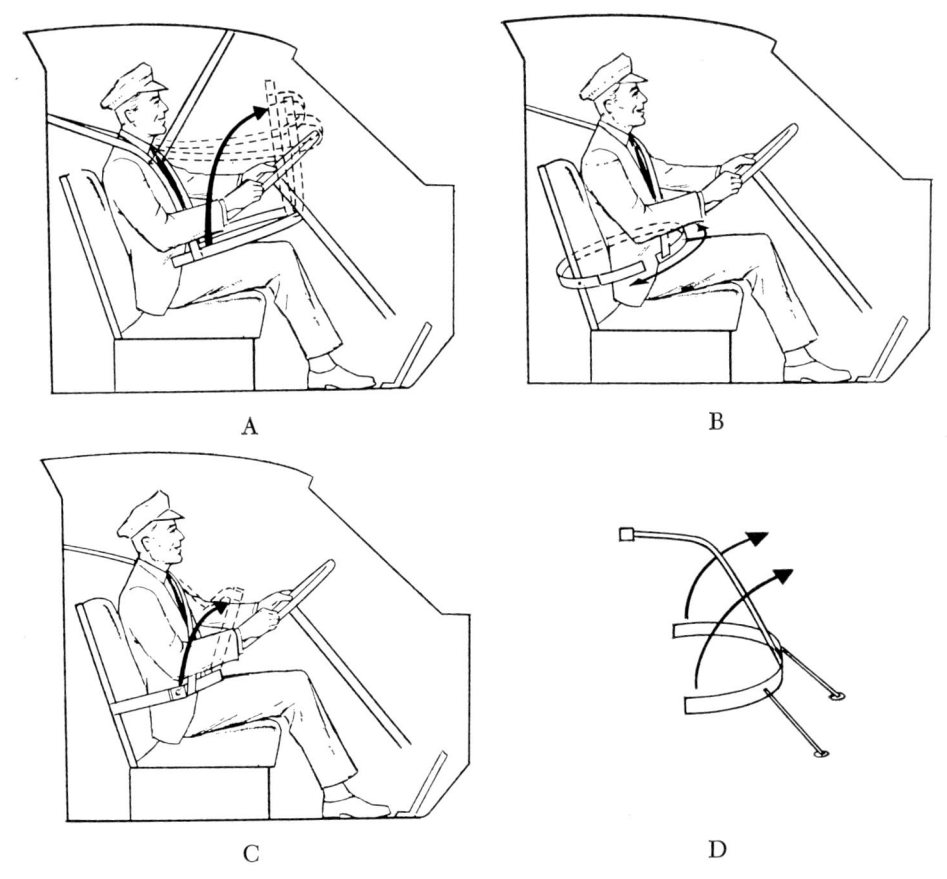

A

B

C

D

FIGURE 22–7. Typical examples of advanced concepts for post-office special vehicles.
A. Sit-or-stand hinged-arm restraint concept, designed for driver of ½ tone right-hand drive vehicle.
B. Ring gate/shoulder strap system, considered for one ton parcel delivery trucks.
C. Swing-arm/full harness type of restraint system for use in a ¼ ton three-wheeler vehicle. This swings into position from a single attachment on the steering column.
D. Restraint system is pivoted from single point on steering column.

arm restraint designed for a ½ ton right-hand drive vehicle (A), the system is activated when the driver gets into the seat, or stands in position and pulls the restraint bar down in a single action. This automatically positions a Y-belt joined at the midchest in a yoke, which is attached over the left seat back by an inertia-locking reel. In concept (B), a ring gate/shoulder strap device considered for one ton parcel delivery trucks, the one-handed operation positions both the circular lap restraint and a diagonal shoulder harness attached to an inertia reel. Concept (C) is a swing arm/full harness type of restraint for use in a ¼ ton three wheeler. The system can be positioned or removed easily and is stored by overhead bands, allowing it to swing easily into position. Concept D features a lap plus diagonal restraint which swings into position from a single point attachment to the steering column. In addition, numerous other concepts are being investigated, including automatic magnetic restraint locks built into clothing. Ease of use, reliability, impact protection, and convertibility to either a standing or seated occupant obviously present unique problems in the design of restraint systems for these vehicles, and it would seem reasonable that from such specialized concept studies, better restraint application to other vehicles may result.

Racing Vehicles: Probably no other segment of the automotive driver population has as great an appreciation of the value of good restraint for protection as does the racing driver. As a result, lap belts were first "standard" in racing cars, and shoulder harnesses were required by most racing associations (USAC, NASCAR, NHA) as long ago as 1960, with the Sports Car Club of America making shoulder harnesses mandatory in 1967 (States 1967). (Figure 22–2D,E) However, in many of these specialized vehicles, the restraint is considered as part of a total system and, occupant seating patterns differ radically from those of the more orthodox "family sedans." Thus, the National Association of Stock Car Automobile Racing requires modified stock cars to have special deep bucket seats extending to the sides of the driver's chest for lateral displacement protection and also requires groin straps similar to parachute harnesses anchored to the seat and to the lap and shoulder belt buckle. Similarly, the United States Auto Club requires single seat vehicles with very narrow bodies which also provide side protection, and in addition, to prevent submarining under the lap belt, recommends the use of a deep trough for the buttocks and a hop-up for the thighs to prevent forward movement in a head-on collision.

In racing cars having modified seat pans and extreme seat back angles, the impact forces in an impact more closely approach the aircraft crash situation and provide more potential for "submarining" than occurs in the normal automobile. The use of deep bucket seats with trough and "hop-up" and lateral protection are of great value here. For racing, the Sports Car Club of America does not allow use of the three-point harness, although it is permitted for rallys. A single point release must be used (Fig. 22-2D). in addition, in racing automobiles having semi-reclining seats (approaching 45 degree back angles), the SCCA requires an upper torso harness, but warns drivers it might contribute to submarining (States, 1968). A foam block in seat is also advised to reduce risk of compression vertebral fractures in an impact. The experience of these racing associations in restraint protection may be very valuable in considering effective protection for all automobile occupants.

Passive Restraint Systems: Protective Shield

Another technique which has been proposed is the design of the instrument panel to form a protective cushion during an impact. This might also utilize a lap belt, as with the airbag system, but in some variations even this might not be needed. Winebrenner, following earlier consideration by automotive designers, proposes moving the windshield forward and de-

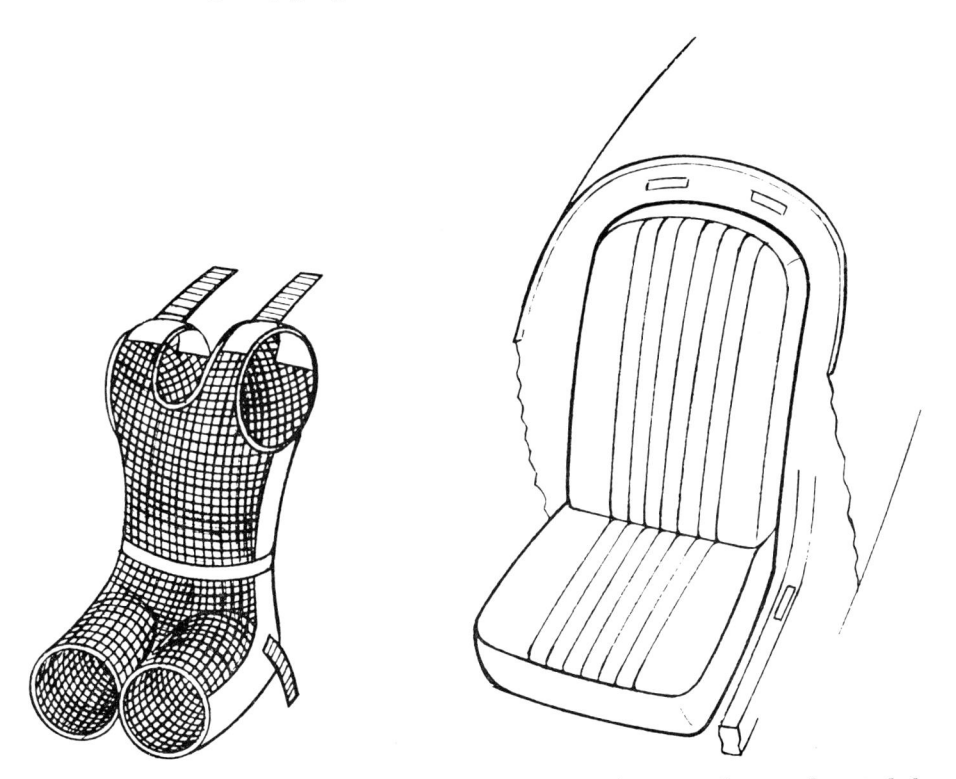

FIGURE 22-8. Experimental restraint system concept for race drivers designed by J. W. Young. System is integrated with form fitting driver's clothing.

signing protective panels using multiple layers of energy-absorbing materials to allow the body to flex forward and distribute the force in a controlled deceleration. As mentioned earlier in this section, modification of the Ford Tot-Guard child restraint for adults could conceivably include either a large shield integration, or a step further, redesign of the instrument panel as a continuous energy absorbing shield, designed to smoothly decelerate the body and equally distribute the force on the energy absorbing construction. Used together with deep bucket seats with lateral and head protection such panels might make effective passive restraint. Two concepts offering improved occupant protection are proposed by the author in Figure 22–4G and H.

However, in the future as now, no one design will probably be universally appropriate for all vehicles. The heavy truck driver or operator of a 60-ton earth mover subjected to vertical accelerations of 2 g at 1½ to 7 cps frequency (Marsh, 1966), have environmental problems quite different from those experienced by the occupant of the semireclined sports car seat. Seating and restraint are dependent upon the variable "package" limitations and the unique features of each particular vehicle type. Thus the total system must be considered. The present sedan, for example, can accommodate different restraint systems than a soft-topped sports car; similarly some of the restraint systems used in smaller European cars would be considerably less effective in large-size American vehicles (see evaluation of experimental restraint tests, European single diagonal belt, Snyder, 1967). Further, development of new special vehicles such as the electric car, "flivver-bug," or the Ground Effects Machine (GEM). Muller's suggestion that future heavy trucks could incorporate a practical ejection seat is not as "James Bondish" as it would initially appear (Muller, 1967). Also, I believe that advanced transportation forms will involve some vehicles which are quite omnidextrous—as able to fly vertically as skim over, or under, the water or hook onto a high-speed transcontinental automatic highway system. At that point, the FAA, NHSB, and USCG may have some interesting jurisdictional and licensing considerations.

AIRCRAFT VEHICLES

Today it is axiomatic that no pilot, and few passengers, would think of flying in an aircraft without first fastening his "safety belt"—even the neophyte air carrier transport passenger automatically obeys the seat belt instructions. However, this was not always so. As originally employed in the aeroplane or free air balloon, a restraint device was simply designed to keep the occupant from falling out. Since in the earlier days of flight, prior to World War I, parachutes were not worn (it was not until 1922 that the first life was saved by use of a parachute), failure to observe this simple precaution of using some attachment between the occupant and the structure could be disastrous. Similarly, lap belts were not considered necessary in early aeroplanes despite the fatal crash of Lieutenant Selfridge in 1909, followed shortly by fatal crashes of other national aero-pioneers such as the Honorable C. S. Rolls in England, and Chile's national air hero Jorge Chavez, both in 1910. In some respects, the Chavez and Rolls crashes were similar. In reconstructing and analyzing the crash forces some 53 years later (Fig. 22–9), it seems probable that had even a lap belt

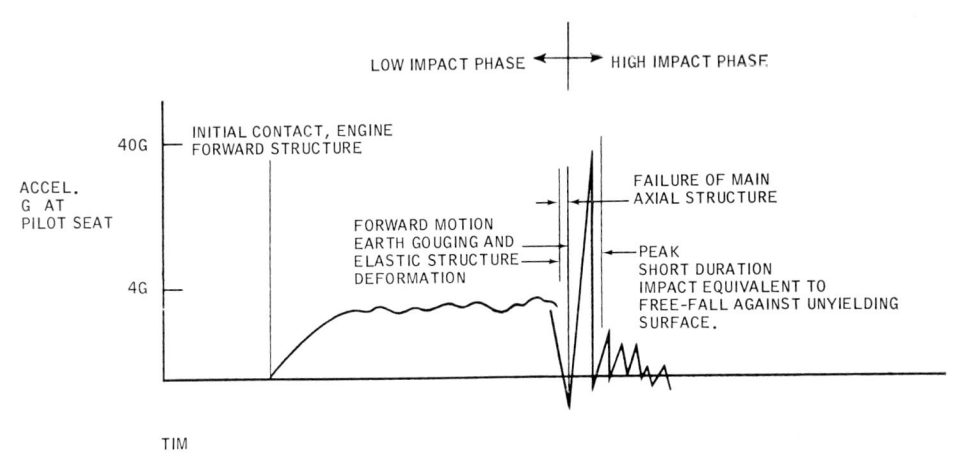

FIGURE 22–9. Reconstruction of impact forces in 1910 aeroplane crash of Jorge Chavez in Bleirot-XI Monoplane. The pilot was unrestrained and subsequently died from his injuries although impact forces were minimal. The pilot wore no restraint.

restraint been used at least Chavez might have survived, since calculated forces were only 4 g at 15.2 to 34.5 feet per second change of velocity (Snyder, 1962). His only protection was a leather helmet. In comparison, in recent National Bureau of Standards tests of male subjects wearing lap belts only on the Daisy Decelerator at Holloman AFB, forces to 17 g (measured on the sled) were tolerated without injury (Armstrong et al. 1967). Aviation's first "safety belt" was probably that modified for Lieutenant (now Maj. Gen., Ret.) Foulois in 1910 by a Field Artillery saddle maker who modified a trunk strap for U.S. Army aeroplane No. 1 (Foulois, 1960).

World War I Restraints

Seating in World War I aircraft was simple, most using wicker seats (R.E. 8, Sopwith Camel, Dolphin, Snipe and D.H. 9), but some (Westland Wagtail) using an aluminum bucket seat, and at least one (S.E. 5) "was turned out with simply a board to sit on and a straight three-ply back, with no reference at all to anatomical requirements, except the fact that *the board was slightly tilted* so as to allow the pilot to lean back a little" (Hill, 1918). This may well have been the origin of the seat pan angle of today's automobiles and aircraft! Note that the seat weight of the typical WWI fighter was 3 pounds 12 pounces (R.E. 9). In contrast, today's airline seats are often over 100 pounds and fighter seats may be over 134 pounds.

By World War I, the need for some sort of restraint became evident as fighter pilots of the era participated in aerial dogfights, and in fact originated most of the aerial combat maneuvers used for some 40 years until the advent of the jet fighter (which is often restricted from violent maneuvers by the limitations of the ultrasensitive electronic gear utilized). It may be surprising to note that the shoulder harness was developed almost contemporaneously with the simple lap belt. Figure 22–1 shows the seat and upper torso restraint used in the English Spad III fighter of 1917. In this version, a continuous webbed belt from a central sternal attachment extended down on each side through a hole in the back of the seat to a floor ring fitting, and continued back up through the same opening up the back and over the shoulder, attaching again in front of the chest in a quick release device. Adjustment was by belt-type eyelets of both shoulder harnesses. There was no lap belt or pelvic protection. Such a restraint system undoubtedly provided some stability and courage to the 1917 fighter pilot, although it could have provided little crash protection and seemed designed to contribute to downward shoulder forces and "submarining." On the other hand, crash forces in such aircraft were often not as high as commonly experienced today.

World War II Restraints

For the next 20 years, there were few real advances in the state-of-the-art of restraining the aircraft occupant, although the lap belt became standard equipment. In the Army Air Corps, safety belts ranged from those for gunners such as the A-1 (0–25A airplanes) pedestal mounted belt, to the A-4 of 1942, which fastened behind the gunner's shoulders across the door of a ball turret. The B-series belts for pilots consisted of either lap belts or shoulder types and were standard from 1929 through the B-15 of 1944. "C" safety belts were for troop and turret gunner's positions of 1945 aircraft. Figure 22–10 shows examples of European experimental restraints of this period.

During World War II, new aircraft developments spurred restraint studies, the work of Col. Stapp at Holloman AFB during 1945 to 1946 marking the initiation of modern biomedical studies. While shoulder harnesses remained standard in fighter aircraft and were provided for pilots of transport and bomber types, they were seldom worn by the latter since they were often uncomfortable and cumbersome on long missions. On the other hand, the fighter pilot was restricted in movement anyhow and was often subjected to deceleration forces requiring upper torso restraint. At this time, the 40 g cockpit became a reality, with the Republic P-47 Thunderbolt, the North American P-51 Mustang, and other Warld War II fighters. Emphasis during this period was on improving the webbing and attachment, and introduction of the inertial reel for the shoulder harness. The 3 inch lap belt webbing was standard protection for the occupant.

Net Restraints

Net devices have been used for restraint as well as in seating since the inception of the aeroplane. Octave Gilbert, for example, used a prone net seat in his 1903 model (Bacon, 1967). Experimental work during World War II was done for pilot restraints in the prone position utilizing a net restraint and "seat" (Hertzberg, 1948). The net concept, which provides wide distribution of force on the body, was also used for a B-36 crew

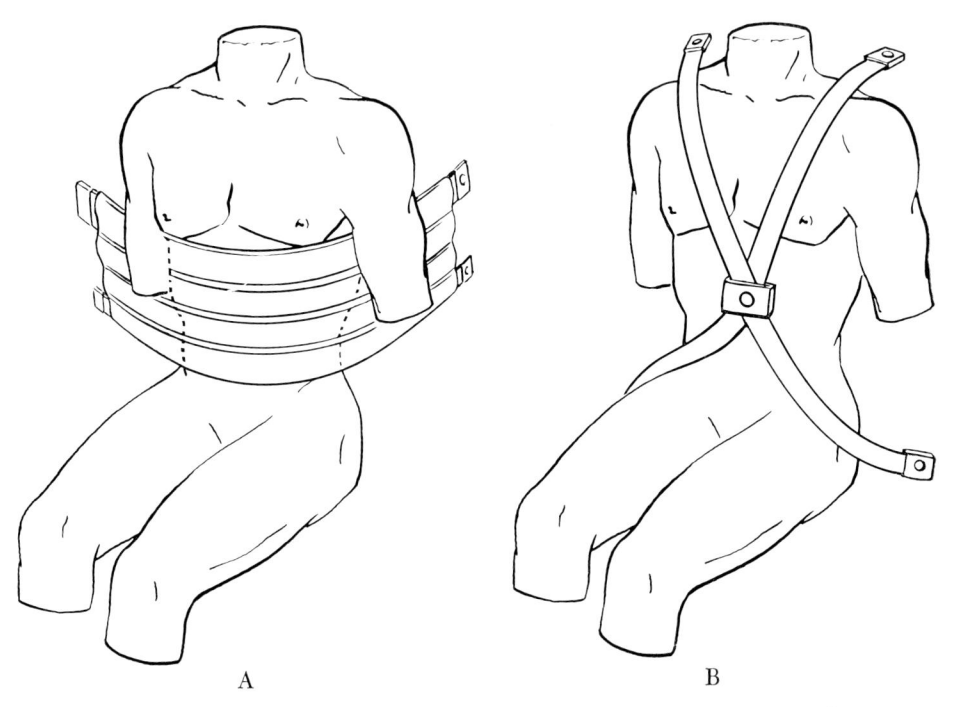

FIGURE 22–10. Some examples of early experimental restraint harness configurations.
A. Ruff 16 inch wide abdominal belt (Germany, 1938).
B. Schaparelli Belt.

sleeping hammock (Hertzberg 1949), and in the RB-57 aircraft for cramped quarters (Hertzberg, 1961.) Supine seating and restraints have also been used, and such a system was developed for high-stress tests of primates in 1959 by Eisen & Zeigen. Crash tests of the Liberty Mutual automotive restraint included a net-type head restraint reported to be very effective (Severy). This, and another type, integral with the shoulder

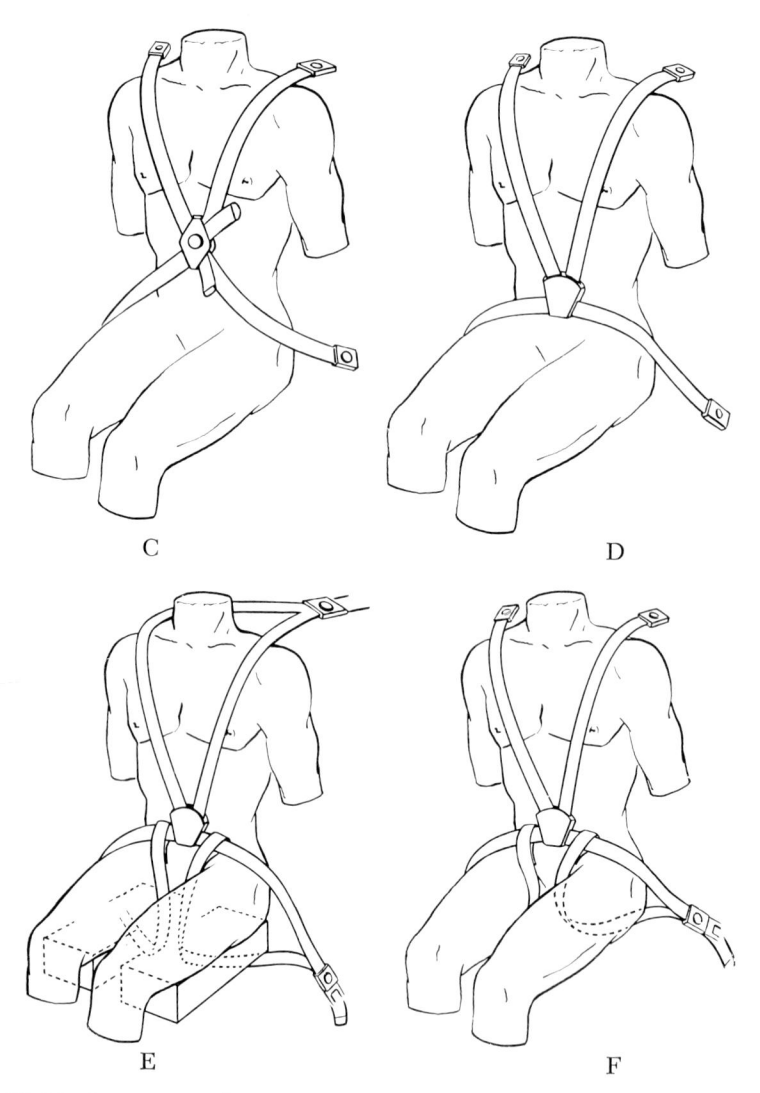

FIGURE 22–10. Some examples of early experimental restraint harness configurations.
C. Sutton Harness (1939).
D. Z-Harness (Stewart, England, 1943).
E. Combination Harness (England, post-World War II).
F. Combination Harness (England).

harness, is shown in Figure 22–6C. The dynamics of safety nets have been analyzed by Payne (1961, 1965). More recently, a new crew seat concept for space vehicles has been designed, consisting of a bonded aluminum honeycomb back rest and welded tubular steel truss seat pan and leg rest covered with Nylon Raschel Knit Cloth as the seating surface (USAF 1962). Net restraints, depending upon the characteristics of the materials used, offer advantages of comfort and potentially good distribution of forces.

Light Aircraft

All U.S. general aviation aircraft use a simple lap belt, conforming to Federal Air Regulation 23, requiring a seat strength of 1.5 g sideward, 3.0 g upward, 9.0 g forward, and 6.6 g downward, and minimum belt strength of 2250 pounds (Table 22–I).

In a study of eighty-two accidents reported in 1951, DeHaven and Hasbrook had found that so long as the cabin structures remained relatively intact in a crash, the shoulder harness effectively decreased the probability of dangerous head injury in severe accidents (DeHaven and Hasbrook, 1951). Young, comparing a number of basic light aircraft restraint systems

TABLE 22-I
FEDERAL AVIATION ADMINISTRATION
Seat g Load Factors For Civil Aircraft

Direction of Force Applied	Utility Aircraft Far 23.561 To 23.785	TSO C39 Additional Requirements	Transport Aircraft Far 25.561 To 25.785	TSO C39 Additional Requirements	SST (Proposed) Crew	Passengers
Forward	9 g	9 g*	9 g	9 g*	16 g	9 g
Sideward	1½ g	3 g	1½ g	3 g	16 g	3 g* (within 20° of long axis)
Upward	0 g	3 g	2 g	2 g	7.5 g	4.5 g
Downward	0 g	7 g	4½ g	6 g	13 g	7.5 g

* Fitting factor of 1.33 for additional load requirement on a particular component on system, such as a bolt ("These load values shall be multiplied by 1.33 for design of seat and safety belt attachment") thus 9 g forward = 12 g, etc.

in Federal Aviation Administration deceleration track tests, concluded that the complete restraint harness, with torso as well as lap belts, provided far superior protection to occupants (1967). In contrast to Federal regulation of automobiles, however, the lap belt is still the only FAA requirement. Currently, U.S. general aviation aircraft exported to England are required by British regulations to have shoulder harnesses installed if they are to be used for aerobatics (Stewart, 1967).

Similarly, since August, 1967, Australia requires upper torso restraint on all light aircraft newly certified after that date. Ironically, Australia had fifteen types of aircraft prior to building its first automobile in 1947. Some manufacturers offer a combined shoulder harness-lap belt as optional equipment, as in the Beech Bonanza. The Beech safety harness was developed using 1500# webbing in 1951 for the Model 35 aircraft, and first protective value in a crash occurred in 1953 (Sprinkle, 1951; Miller, 1953). Both the Helioplane Courier (1953) and a two-place Myers 145 (1953) offered a combination three-point "must-be-worn" type safety belt (4,275 lb.) as standard equipment, but the upper harness anchorage was placed so low in the bulkhead behind the seats that extreme down loadings could result on the shoulders (see Fig. 22–19, DeHaven, 1953). Similarly, in some models of Army light aircraft, where shoulder harnesses are required, the shoulder harness is attached over the seat back, but there is no lock, as in automobiles, to prevent the seat back from moving.

A recent FAA advisory specifies acceptable installation methods for shoulder harness attachment, based upon work by Young (1966). Hasbrook and Snow found shoulder slope of 67.5 degrees (±5 degrees) in a sample of young males (1965). In recent work conducted to determine optimum restraint for Army aircraft, the concept selected was a modification of the conventional lap belt and shoulder harness by effecting the following: (1) adding a center tiedown to the lap belt to prevent submarining, (2) addition of a single tiedown to the lap belt to assist in lateral restraint as well as to further prevent submarining, and (3) addition of a single line head/helmet restraint attached to the shoulder harness inertia reel (AVSER, 1967).

Civil Airlines

About 90 per cent of all airline passenger seats are manufactured by four major manufactures: Aerotherm Transportation Equipment Division of the Universal Oil Products Co., Bantam, Connecticut; Fairchild-Hiller's Burns Aero Seat Co., Burbank, California; Dayco Corp's Hardman Tool & Engineering Co., Los Angeles, California; and Weber Aircraft Division of Walter Kidde & Co., Inc., Burbank, Calif. New lighter models of seats are now being made ranging from 52 pounds to 78 pounds (Hunter, 1955). For future aircraft such as the Boeing 747, Douglas DC-10, airbus, and SST, this trend would increase range or payload by several tons per airplane. Side-facing seats, such as those in the lounge area, must have both seat and shoulder belt for lateral protection by October 1, 1969 under new FAA regulations. The SAE aeronautical recommended practice (ARP) discourages side-facing seats.

ENERGY ABSORBER SEAT DEFORMATION: Many of these seats are now designed for controlled structural deformation as a means of energy absorption to protect the occupant during the impact of a crash. In these, the front legs collapse as load is applied. Note that FAA regulations specify that seats must be structurally capable of withstanding loads of 9 g forward, 3 g sideward, 2 g rearward, and 6 g downward. Energy could be absorbed in various deceleration devices built into the seat system. Many would have cost, reliability (Fryer, 1959), or other problems which would not make them practical.

While seats, energy absorbers, and hardware may seem peripheral to the scope of this chapter, the seat is often an integral part of the restraint and several components will be briefly noted. Such devices absorb part of the energy of impact by allowing controlled forward displacement of the seat when subjected to load. Early work was done by Pinkel and Rosenberg (1956), and Hart (1958) which showed the potential effectiveness of these devices. The "piccolo tube" decelerator is a linear hydraulic energy absorber which dissipates energy by the displacement of water through multiple, sharp-edge orifices in the tube wall. By varying the orifice hole sizes along the length of the tube, a constant pressure, and thus a constant retarding force, can be achieved throughout the arresting stroke. Another energy absorber is the stainless steel strap decelerator which absorbs energy in straining the material. The lengths depend upon the magnitude of deceleration and pulse-time duration desired. The Kroell or invert tube (1962), absorbs energy simply by turning a thin-walled ductile metal tube inside out. Another system, the load-limiting (all-over) type of energy absorber, is based upon extrusions of wire-bending devices. These are recommended for cargo restraints (Russo, 1966) and take three major configurations. The two-spool, single-platen unit has two spools attached to one end of the platen, one of which stores all wires woven through the top side of the end hole in the platen, while the bottom spool stores wires woven out of the bottom side of the same hole. A variation of this is the two-spool, double-platen unit, utilizing two platens functioning as a single unit. A third type involves wires stored like a ball of twine in a canister. Another form of load-limiter uses the shock-tube controlled collapse principle of some airline seats. Because of dissatisfaction with the performance of stainless steel straps, mechanical springs and hydraulic energy absorber units, a unique energy absorption system was devised for the rear supporting legs of the Aerotherm passenger seats for air transport aircraft (45 pounds double, 59 pounds triple). The sheet metal seats deform, instead of fracturing as an extrusion or tube might, and the rear legs *extend* when a 9 g load is exceeded. This extension is produced by metal deformation functioning as the energy absorber, allowing the seat to pivot forward. Such a design can take a load of 30 g for 0.04 seconds, or 20 g for 0.065 seconds, allowing the seat and tie-downs to remain more intact in an impact (Hawthorne, 1958). An earlier Aerotherm concept called the Bennett Hammock-Type Aircraft Seat consisted of two large springs, between which the seat was suspended freely, designed to absorb the shock of turbulence. The passenger's seat position is controlled by his shift of weight, since his CG would always be below the hammock's pivot point (Bennett, 1951) (Fig. 22–11). Other types, designed for cargo, but possible for seat packaging as well, would utilize a net system, a net attached to load limiters (attenuators), or an inextensible net attached to load limiters (Avery, 1965). One problem with a shock-absorbing or energy-absorbing devices is that they are usually one-shot devices. Thus in cases of multiple deceleration peaks, no protection may be offered in the second jolt and the occupant may also be in a disadvantageous forward tilt at second impact.

Various cargo delivery systems have been developed, and one demonstrating the feasibility of truck drops repeated in a second phase with "people pallets" was not continued due to excessively high vertical acceleration on the dummies.

The Supersonic Transport (SST)

The Boeing B-2707–100 SST, which should be in service by early 1971,

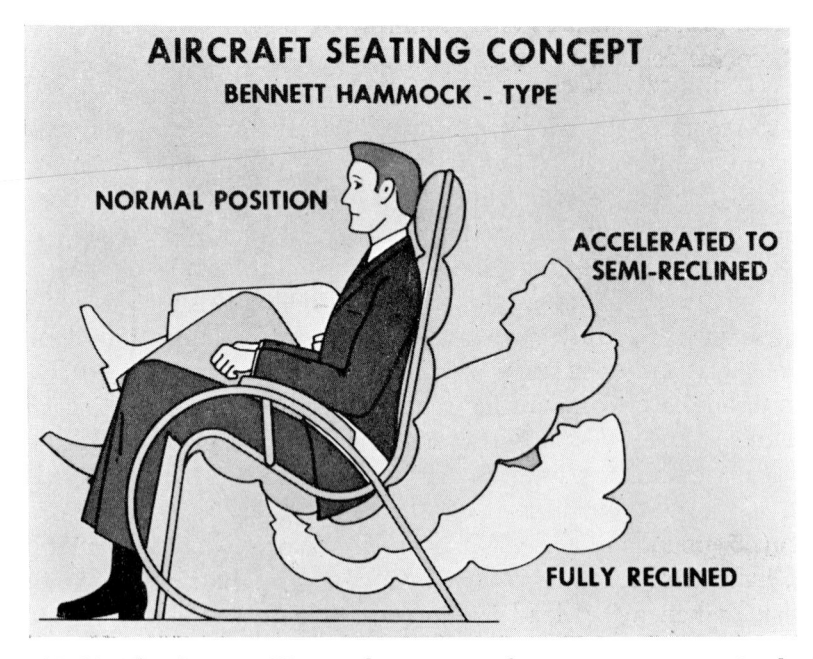

FIGURE 22–11. The Bennett Hammock-type aircraft seat concept consisted of two large springs between which the seat suspended freely. The seat position is controlled by the passenger's shift of weight.

is designed to carry from 280 passengers (international version) up to a maximum of 350 in its most efficient seating arrangement and to travel at 1780 mph (2.7 mach). The English-French Concorde (1450 mph, 2.1 mach) carrying 124 passengers should be flying by late 1968.

A unique feature of the Boeing SST, due to its length of 306 feet and resulting bending moment, is that some seats may have to be designed to comply with FAA load factors of 9 g forward, 7.5 g downward, 4.5 g upward and 3 g sideward, times a factor of 1.33 (Table 22–I.) Those toward the ends of the cabin will be subjected to greater bending moment and greater load factors than at stations toward the center. Crew stations will require ultimate seat load factors of 16 g forward, acting within 20 degrees to either side, compared to 12 g for passengers. Crew members will wear shoulder restraints at least during takeoff and landing as do flight deck crews of present commercial jet transports. These are not presently required for passengers. Since any turbulence can create severe vertical loadings on passengers, upper torso restraint should be mandatory. In two cases within the past year, restrained airline passengers have been so violently slammed upward and then forward that they have received major injuries.

Although the SST presented an excellent opportunity to evaluate the concept of passenger protection and evacuation as an integral part of the total air-frame design and to test the application of advanced restraint systems concepts, apparently during its development, little thought was given to such considerations by either the FAA or air-frame manufacturers. As a result, the seats and restraints to date for the SST do not vary greatly from conventional systems in current transport aircraft. Until the systems approach is actually utilized and designers and human-factors scientists are encouraged to use advanced concepts, it seems unlikely that any great changes in the area of passenger safety will be demonstrated by SST-type commercial aircraft. The restraint system in commercial air transportation is still designed more as an afterthought than as an integral part of the aircraft system. This situation was also reported by the earliest medical and human factors scientists; Hill, in a 1918 RAE report stating that, "The aeroplane has been designed and the pilot fitted in afterward." (p. 1).

Similarly, in-flight passenger evacuation has not been seriously considered although some scientists, including the author, believe that it could be accomplished. Note that in 1962, one passenger survived the impact of a 32,000 foot free-fall lying across his seat, when the jet airliner in which he was riding exploded in flight although he subsequently died.

If one were to speculate regarding occupant restraint for aircraft without regard to factors of reliability, consumer acceptance and cost/benefit ratios, as is so fashionable a pastime with respect to automobiles, a number of fascinating and apparently technically feasible ideas might be considered. Why couldn't seats be designed, for example, with a simple drogue chute packed in the back for automatic deployment in a mid-air disintegration. There are a number of other techniques which might be evaluated. The final restraint configuration for the SST should consider upper torso protection because of the potentially greater loadings passengers may be subjected to in a crash-landing impact, or exposed to during extreme inflight turbulence. Due to the high seat backs in air transport aircraft, upper torso restraints which retract into the back of the seat should be relatively simple to design, although the higher seat back mass might necessitate stronger tie-downs. Similarly as advances in airbag restraints are realized, good protection could be afforded by installing these restraints, to be initiated at a present force level, in seat backs. Much greater seat strength and additional restraint protection, could be had by completely redesigning the seat, possibly as an individual container, or by gimbaling it to rotate into the most advantageous position.

While radically new off-ground vehicles, high-speed and with large capacity, continue to be developed, no radically new restraint systems have been proposed for such aircraft, which will probably continue to have lap belts as the sole means of passenger restraint.

Water Vehicles

Restraint systems in water vehicles (exclusive of amphibians) have been confined to a few specialized crew needs in submarines and deep-submersibles. The slow deceleration of water vehicles and the lack of impact exposure limit the necessity of restraint systems in this environment. However, new craft, able to skim over the water at speeds in excess of 100 mph, may change this picture. The British SR-N4 Hovercraft, for example, a 165-ton vehicle, can carry five-hundred passengers or 166 passengers and thirty automobiles at speeds up to 70 knots. While specialized forms of restraint systems may be developed as new requirements arise, none have yet been publically proposed.

Current Military Aircraft Restraint

As military aircraft achieve greater performance, restraint problems become more complex than those in either civil aircraft or ground vehicles because of the requirement for in-flight emergency escape. Emergency egress from high performance aircraft may result in simple uni-axial (catapult) or complex multi-axial accelerations, and in this environment, every part of a system designed for restraint becomes critical. Restraint and positioning subsystems of ejection seats such as the A3J-1 Supersonic Escape System (Carter 1959) or Douglas ESCAPAC II, were designed to minimize vertebral injuries during emergency escape. Spinal injuries resulting from complex acceleration environments can occur from 17 g to 22 g (Chandler, 1967). Restraint systems in current fighter type aircraft must be designed to protect the occupant from upward ejection accelerations of 200 to 300 g per second onset 12 to 22 g peak, 70 ± 10 feet per second terminal velocity, and 0.01 to 0.08 seconds of peak g exposure. (Henzel et al., 1968) Two experimental systems developed since WW II specifically to protect from such forces are the Douglas "D" prototype harness, and the Navy "Model C" vest restraint.

DOUGLAS "D" HARNESS (EXPERIMENTAL PROTOTYPE): After analzing the distribution of mass of the upper body, and finding that 90 per cent of the upper body mass is above the fifth thoracic vertebra (level or armpits), Poppel (1958) designed the Douglas Model D prototype harness (Fig. 22-12). This is one of the few harnesses designed by a physician on the basis of anatomical function and support required for $+g_z$ ejection accelerations. This has embodied the principles of support under the arms, crossing over the sternum, extension along lines following the resultant of anticipated forces, and ending in two points for attachment to the seat structure. This was found to relieve compressive spinal loading.

VEST HARNESS (MODEL "C" EXPERIMENTAL): Bierman utilized the principles of distributing impact force over a large area and to parts of the body best able to withstand high impact forces, gradual rate of application, damping of small irregularities during impact, small distances of movement in the same direction of impact during the period in which the force would exceed the injury threshold, and maintaining the force below the injury threshold at all times (1947). His design resulted in a vest restraint harness of undrawn nylon. Tests indicated this would protect humans from forces equivalent to 10,000 pounds on a dummy with the conventional harness. This material has effectively reduced accelerations of 5.4 g to 6 g and human volunteers exposed to 15 feet free-falls were decelerated in less than 0.2 seconds at only 6 g (Fig. 22–12B).

Two major problems in ejection are that at airspeeds in excess of 0.85 mach, acceleration profiles necessary to clear the aircraft tail structure may exceed human tolerance limits, and the abrupt exposure to windblast at such velocities may also exceed these limits. Downward ejection and capsule escape systems have been developed as partial solutions. However, acceleration trauma in the caudalcranial and cranial-caudal ($\pm g_z$) axis remains as great a problem today as 30 years ago when German scientists first developed the ejection seat for high performance aircraft.

A

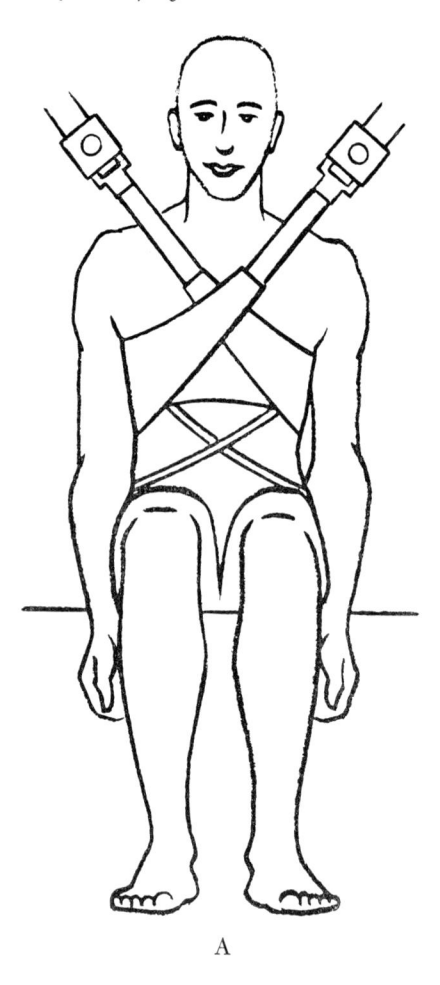

Various studies have shown that the current incidence of vertebral fracture is about 25 per cent in nonfatal ejections. As pointed out by Henzel, this should be of great concern. He found that structural failure of the vertebral column, seat-to-head spinal acceleration, may occur as a result of unsymmetrical vertebra-disc load distribution and anterior lip compression when the pilot slumps to grasp poorly positioned D-rings and poorly designed armrests. Yanking on the D-ring can also cause preloading and contribute to spinal flexion and anterior lip overloading. Proper armrest supports can assist in taking some of the load from the body structure by minimizing flexion. Henzel found two other restraint factors which cause injury. An individual with a high percentile sitting height or seated on a thick seat pack can incur severe downward loading from the harness, and improperly designed face curtains may cause considerable upper body flexion changing voluntary tolerance from 20 to 12 g. Kazarian, Mohr,

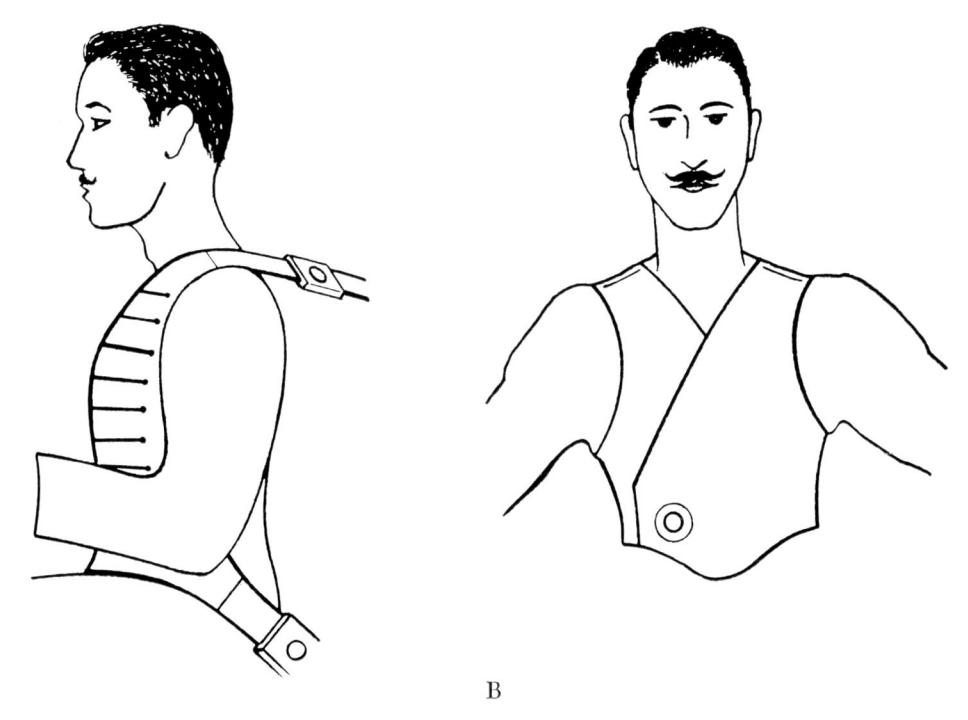

FIGURE 22–12. Experimental aircraft restraint systems.
A. Douglas Model D restraint harness designed by Poppen, 1958, to offer maximum protection in upward ejection from aircraft.
B. U.S. Navy experimental "Model C" vest restraint, constructed of undrawn nylon material woven to resist a 2300# draw load and protecting human subjects to maximal loads of 10,000 impact pounds. (Bierman, 1947).

and von Gierke have recently described a new mechanism of vertebral body injury in which they found the initial stress affected the vertebral body itself through compressive force (1968). Impact in seat-to-head direction can also result in severe cardiovascular injury (Snow et al., 1968).

Henzel, in a recent review of past studies concerning the dynamic response characteristics of the human vertebral column during accelerative loading in the $+g_z$ axis notes, "Design capability continues to be limited by biologic breaking points. The challenge is to precisely define and utilize these end points to their maximum benefit." His statement, I feel certain, is echoed by biomechanical scientists concerned with the problem of human tolerance in all areas of restraint, impact and deceleration.

F-11A RESTRAINT SYSTEM: Among the new military aircraft, the Lockheed YF-12A prototype interceptor, the North American X-15 (which flew 4534 mph, October 9, 1967) and the XB-70 Valkyre demonstrate increased performance capabilities; however, the most advanced military restraint system is that of the the General Dynamics F-111 fighter aircraft. The F-111A crew module (made by McDonnell Douglas) is shown in Figure 22–13.

As an integrated part of the forward fuselage, the module is a pressurized emergency escape vehicle which can be activated even at zero speed and altitude. The two pilots carry out their mission in a "shirt-sleeve" environment, with no parachutes or survival gear worn. The present General Dynamics restraint system employes two harnesses (Fig. 22–14). The upper harness provides shoulder restraint, with lateral support being given by two side straps attached to the seat on each side of the pilot's thorax. A separate system, consisting of a lap belt with crotch strap for each leg, protects the pelvic area. However, due to test findings of severe upper chest and back discomfort when the shoulder straps were tensioned to simulate firing of the power inertia locking reel, reports of some collar bone, groin, and throat discomfort, and the need for pilot access to forward controls is prevented by the chest straps being tight, and contributed little to chest support, later versions have been developed. The RAF IAM F-111 harness did away with the lateral chest straps and combined the upper and lower harnesses into a single restraint. A contour back was also tried but discarded in the RAF fourth version (fifth modification of this harness), and this (still experimental) restraint will possibly also be used by future F-111 pilots (Fig. 22–14). Note the large abdominal pad with

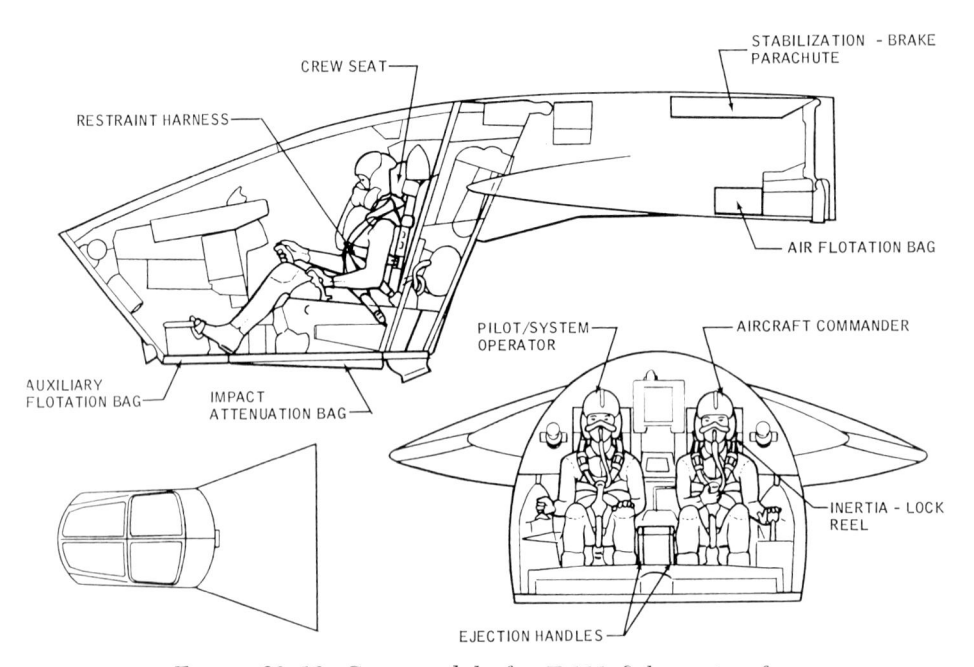

FIGURE 22–13. Crew module for F-111 fighter aircraft.

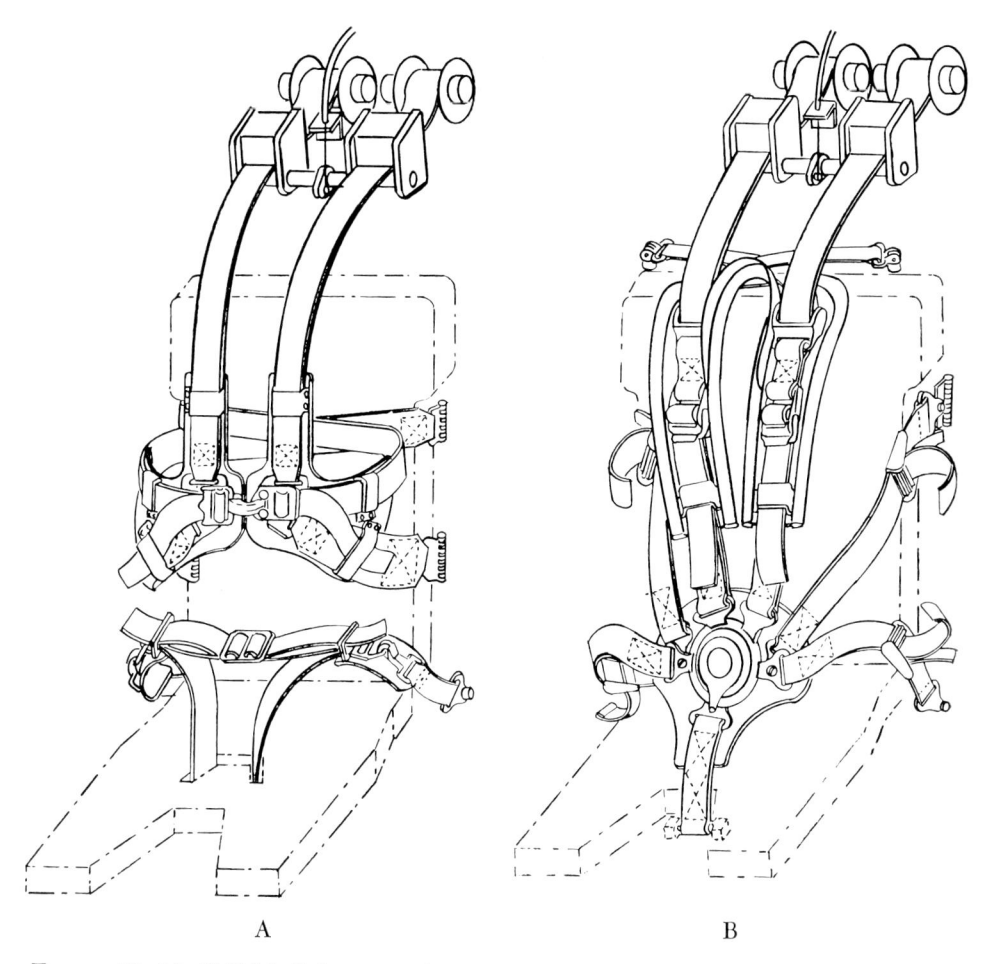

Occupant Restraint Systems of Manned Vehicles 535

FIGURE 22–14. F-111A figher restraint systems.
A. Current U.S.A.F. (General Dynamics) F-111A restraint harness. Note upper torso harness is separate from lower restraint.
B. Experimental RAF F-111 Harness which may be adopted by U.S.A.F. Note single point release, lateral chest support, and unique shoulder configuration. In most recent U.S.A.F. version both lateral belts have been removed.

quick release and the use of seven belts, including a single crotch belt of 4000 pound Terylene® webbing, which are heavily padded and connected to the top of the seat by a unique attachment which provides lateral motion restraint. Tests with human volunteers have been conducted on the RAF IAM F-111A restraint up to 17.7 g in the lateral plane (g_y) at 390 g per second onset rate; 14 g and 215 g per second in the forward (g_x) axis, and 8.2 g and 184 g per second in the 45 degree left-forward orientation.

In a test flight of an F-111A on 19 October 1967, an emergency necessitated crew ejection at mach .87 over Texas; the only injury occurred when one of the crew scratched his finger on a nearby barbed wire fence after landing and leaving the capsule. The F-111 restraint system undoubtedly represents the most sophisticated operational state-of-the-art.

AEROSPACE

Efforts to further develop advanced restraint system concepts for manned space flight have recently been decreased by NASA. However, a new related study is now being initiated. This will involve plans for earth-orbital emergency escape devices for a space station laboratory in the 1970 to 1978 era. These will include 1 and 3 nonbailout systems and a reentry vehicle (Golovin, 1967).

NASA's seating and restraint system developed for the extended lunar surface exploration program will probably be adapted for a variety of highly mobile lunar surface vehicles. However, despite the unusual environmental conditions which man can be subjected to in space flight, normal deceleration forces may ironically be less than that of a typical low-velocity automobile "fender-bender" accident. For example, in January 1968, NASA's Surveyor 7, after a 225,000 mile flight, was braked by retrorockets from 6000 to less than 7 mph, striking a rocky ridge of the Moon's Tycho crater with a jolt equal to a 13 foot free fall.

Apollo Restraint System

The Apollo Command Module (first manned mission, October, 1968) has been developed for a three-man lunar mission, terminating in an earth landing by parachute. To date, Mercury, Gemini, and unmanned Apollo 5 and 6 landings have been in water, but since it is desirable to have an earth-environment landing capability as well, several of these have been tested for Apollo. Since "passive" landing systems (not requiring braking rockets or heat-shield deployment) can exceed human acceleration tolerance levels: two "active" systems were developed for Apollo. One consists of 6 vertically oriented hydraulic struts and 8 horizontally oriented honeycomb struts, and the other of 4 vertical struts and 6 lightweight strain straps.

Manned U.S. spacecraft missions to date have all terminated in water impact landings, which provide greater attenuation and less chance of exceeding human tolerance limits than land impacts (Snyder, 1966). In vehicles such as Dynasoar or the Gemini type paraglider, which touch down at a relatively high horizontal and a low vertical velocity, either a conventional runway or level hard-packed surface must be utilized. Paraglider-type systems may produce horizontal landing velocities of 60 to 100 feet per second and vertical velocities of 0 to 5 feet per second. Parachute landing systems are designed to produce descent rates of 20 to 30 feet per second, resulting in 20 to 50 g impact forces on the vehicle under favorable conditions. (p. 328 Manned Spacecraft) Apollo's "normal landing" is designed not to exceed 1000 g per second onset rate and not to exceed 20 g at 28 feet per second (Brinkley et al., 1963).

The most favorable position for the occupants during landing impact of the Apollo Capsule is backward facing, 45 degrees from the vertical (Stapp and Taylor, 1959). This minimizes relative motion between the occupant and seat and, by compressing the body into the form fitting couch, the seat and not the harness webbing restrains the occupant and provides optimum support. The Apollo Capsule is designed for a landing attitude with the bottom parallel to the impact surface. This places the astronauts in the optimum body position (Fig. 22–15).

Isovolumetric Systems

As previously noted, maximum protection by a restraint system has been experimentally accomplished by fluid environment. However, results approaching this ideal have also been obtained from a system being studied by Lombard (Lombard et al., 1964, 1966a, b) which restricts the torso in a flexible but essentially isovolmetric support-restraint. Work to date has involved guinea pigs and small primates in the SARS I (Support-restraint System I) and SARS III. SARS I consists of a body contoured enclosure completely surrounding the subject (epoxy plastic lined with ⅛ inch ensolite, reinforced with fiberglass cloth, and heavy steel frame members welded to steel pivots). SARS III is designed as a soft nylon webbing restraint for the full torso, the knees, and a full-face web net head restraint. (Fig. 22–16). With such systems, guinea pigs have survived up to 240 g for 3 milliseconds at 100,000 g per second onset rate. Further research is in progress with a view toward space program applications.

Lenticular Vehicle Seat Rotation

Recently several aerospace designers have proposed disc-shaped aerospace vehicles. Fischer, for example, in an SAE paper in 1961, discussed utilization of the most optimum human body orientations to withstand MAV maneuvering loads and suggested a lenticular (disc) shaped vehicle as most practical. Rather than use a double-gimbal seat to provide the proper seating change sequences, which would provide a high weight penalty, he would control body orientation by rotating about a vertical axis through the center of the disc, resulting in rotation about an axis

538   *Impact Injury and Crash Protection*

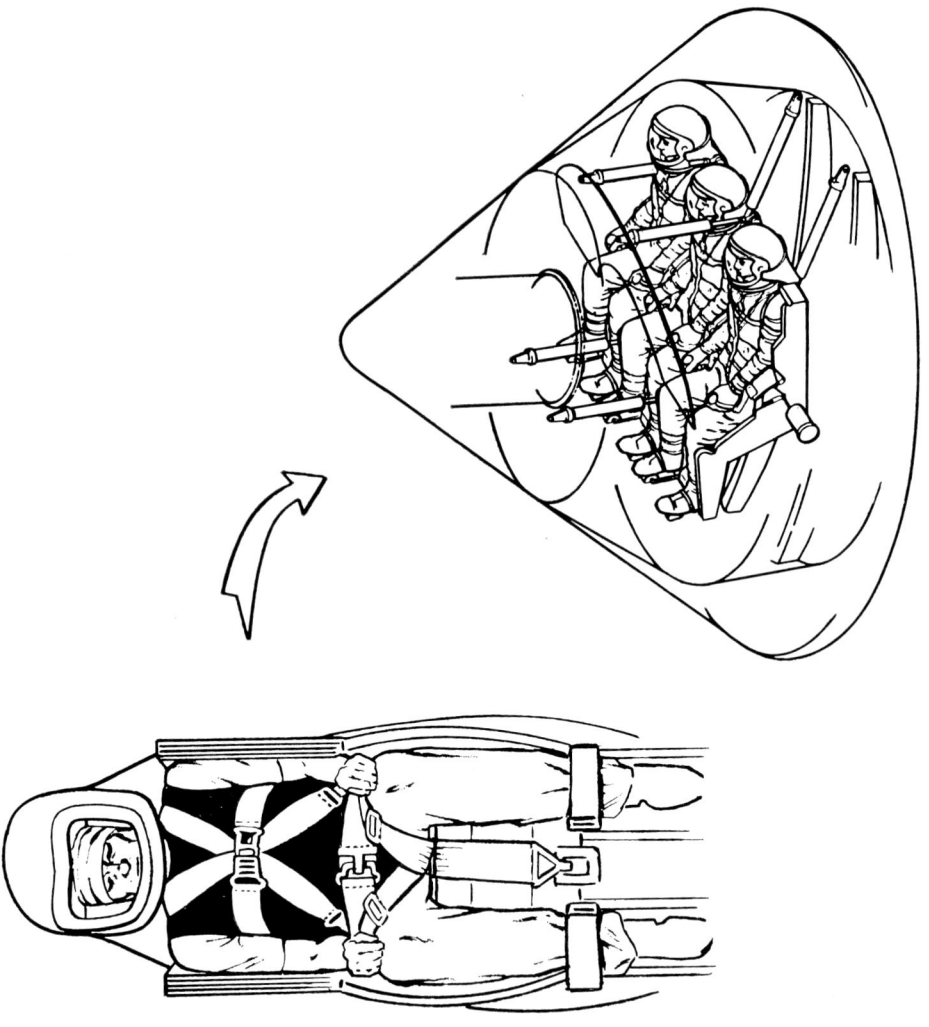

FIGURE 22–15. Apollo spacecraft restraint system (North American Rockwell, Los Angeles).

parallel to the passenger's spine. Unfortunately, in this nonconventional system no restraint needs were considered.

During the past few years a number of restraint systems for space flight have been proposed and evaluated. Figure 22–17 illustrates some of these concepts.

Conley (1952) proposed lightweight zippered supporters made of webbed cotton fabric worn beneath the underclothing as a "second skin" to restrain and protect the body against space accelerations. The author (1960) proposed a mechanical cable restraint system employing inertia reels or powered pulley devices with electro-hydraulically activated links

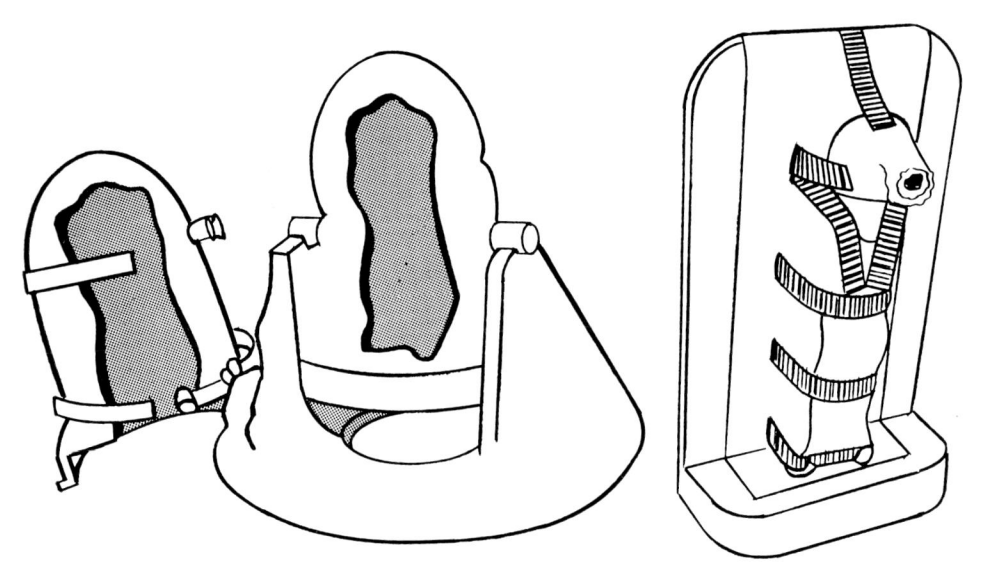

Figure 22-16. Two examples of advanced experimental restraint systems offering protection to extreme impact forces (designed by Lombard).

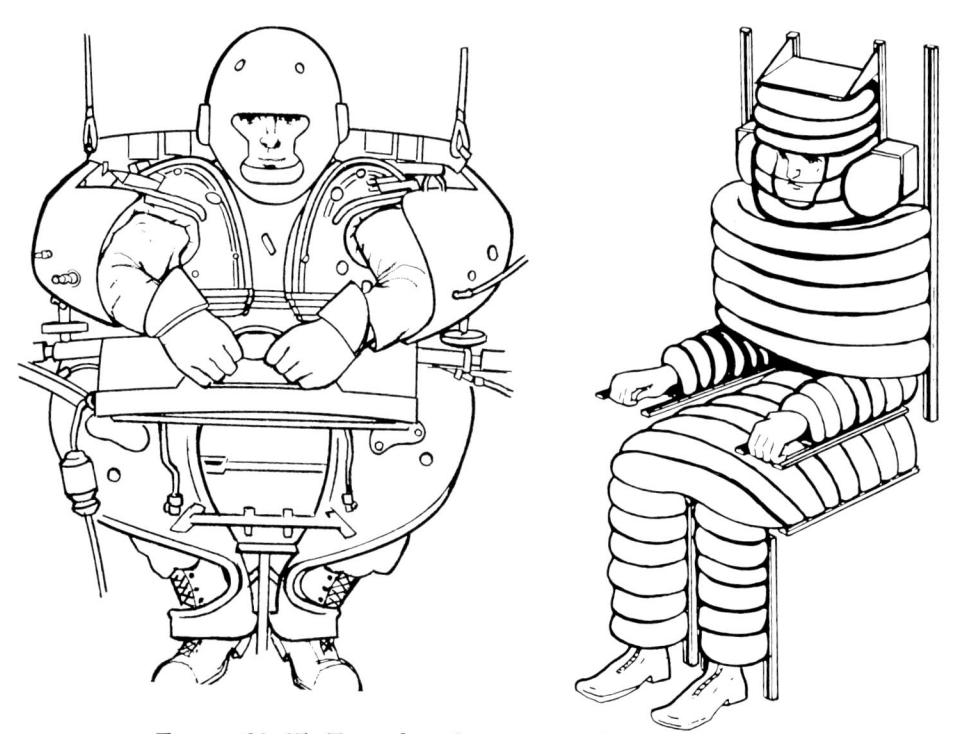

Figure 22-17. Examples of experimental restraint systems.
A. "Clamshell" restraint system.　　　　　　B. Caterpillar restraint system.

for the head and arms. A second concept proposed was an inflatable plastic torso restraint consisting of an inflatable bladder between the webbing and torso. A third design for use under flight clothing was an internal bracing system consisting of a back brace with abdominal and thoracic support. Design requirements for a 60 g omnidirectional personnel restraint system for space flight were investigated by Boyce and Freeman, 1961; and later by Ripley, 1966; who evaluated and discarded concepts for an *integrated garment,* and *caterpillar, clamshell,* and *hardshell* systems to withstand 60 g in $\pm g_y$ directions, 30 g in the $+g_z$ and 20 g in the $-g_z$ directions. Unit pressures ranged from 45 psi at 60 g on the forehead and chin, 9 to 30 psi on the rest of the body, except for 113 psi on the kneecaps.

The caterpillar concept was designed to provide minimum encumbrance, utilizing inflatable bladders supported by semicircular metal forms. The bladders can be stowed by means of track slides attached to the forms. After the occupant is positioned, the bladders can be inflated to provide restraint, pressing the body and limbs down and into the the seat (Fig. 22–17B).

To provide wide, low unit pressure restraint a universal fit-soft harness was designed. The occupant wears an integrated nylon net restraint suit. The seat is lined with microballoons, while the seat back pivots about a floating point on the seat pan (Fig. 22–17D).

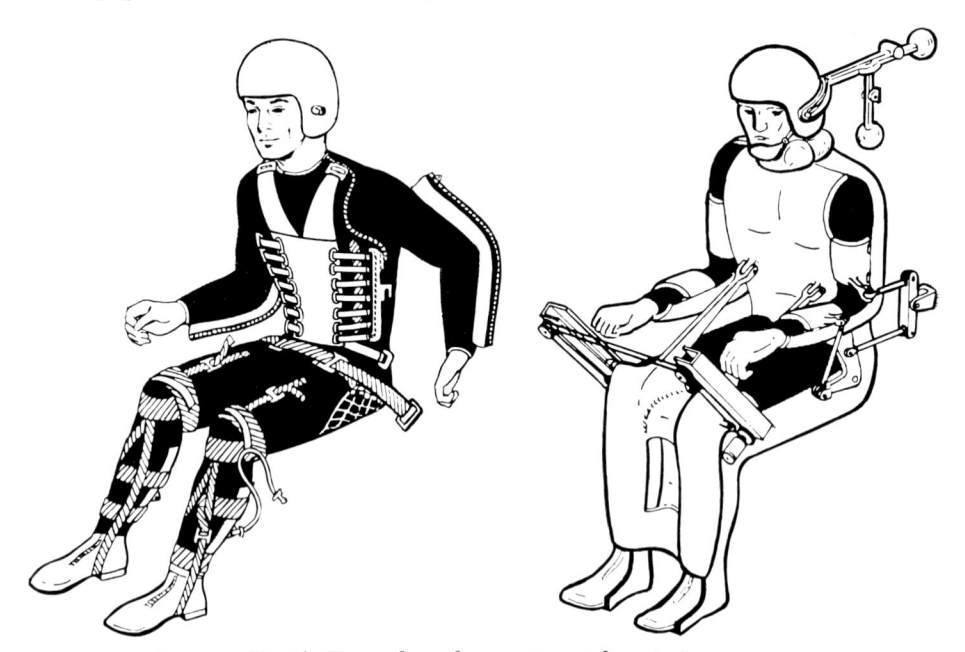

FIGURE 22–17. Examples of experimental restraint systems.

C. Integrated soft harness restraint concept.

D. Universal integrated couch restraint concept.

The integrated soft harness restraint system consisted of an integrated suit and harness reinforced with dacron net and a form-fitted helmet (Fig. 22–17C).

The clamshell restraint system was designed to provide maximum protection and mobility for a man in a flight system not requiring crew rotation. This system consists of a Mercury couch molded to fit the occupant. The occupant wears a form-fitted helmet, a sacroiliac corset and lap belt, an anterior thorax shell and leg shells (Fig. 22–17A).

An interesting design was the microballoon body support-restraint concept. This consisted of a laminated fiberglass back and seat pan supported by a welded assembly made from 4130 chrome-molybdenum steel tube and plate. Support within the shell is provided by a contoured pad, which is filled with hollow plastic spheres (microballoons). When differential pressure is zero, the spheres permit the pad to contour to the body shape, but when the air is removed the pressure leaves the spheres and the rigid contour is retained (USAF 1961).

The Boling hammock full body restraint system is a net system suspended on cables. The cables form a "V" yoke which straddles the arms. The torso is restrained by a net vest attached to the "V" cables. The zippered vest uses ensolite for shoulder pads (Boling). Another type of zippered restraint is being considered for the Douglas S4B Saturn Work Shop and Space Stations.

Several couch designs have been developed. One universal couch consists of a steel framework with a one-piece of epoxy fiberglass. A wax shell mold is made for each occupant. The mold is covered with a 2 inch layer of soft urethane, a 2 inch layer of firm urethane, and a 2 inch layer of polyethylene, bonded together, and sprayed with hypalon for a tough but smooth surface (USAF n.d.).

Probably the most comprehensive study ever published on space restraint systems was conducted by Ripley for the Air Force Systems Command (1966). Besides evaluating many of the systems noted above, he recommended the following: a *mobile hardshell* seat back for optimum torso protection, dacron webbing retained by a soft helmet and padded chin strap for head restraint, the arm sleeve zippered to the armrest, a zippered tube leg restraint and a liquid foam universal seat pan with lateral thigh pads and lap belt.

ULTIMATE PROTECTION

Fluid Restraint Systems

Several systems offering considerably greater protection against acceleration forces have been devised for space flight. In order to gain maximum protection, other factors must be sacrificed so that most of these systems are impractical, at present, for aircraft or automotive adaptation, and some even for spacecraft.

On a theoretical basis, complete immersion in fluid offers the greatest increase in significant g tolerance. A number of studies have explored this potential. Notable are the works of Margarita (1958), Morris et al., (1958), Bondurant (1958), and Webb and Gray (1958, 1959), and more recently by NASA researchers. Margarita has demonstrated that rats when immersed in water could survive 1000 g impacts, a number one hundred times the normal survival tolerance. He concluded that a limit to the acceleration tolerance of terrestrial animals is imposed by the large difference in density between the lung tissue which is filled with air and the rest of the body. He showed that when pregnant rats were impacted, the fetuses (without air in their lungs) survived impacts of 10,000 g (0.14 seconds duration) without injury (1958).

Webb and Gray noted that fluid restraint protection balanced fluid pressure within the blood vessels by the gradient of pressures developed in the water, preventing blood vessel distension and maintaining circulation. By adding a solute to the water, the specific gravity could be adjusted to that of the arms and legs, theoretically preventing tissue deformation or fractures. Tests on humans (wearing masks) have been confined to long-term acceleration type studies, although impact studies with human subjects have been considered (Zaborowski, 1959).

Drugs to Increase Tolerances

It is believed that for space flight stresses, Russian scientists have employed anabiosis, and the artificial deceleration of the physical processes of the human organism (Yegorov, 1967), developed from animal experiments which showed that drugs could increase normal tolerance "many times over." Experiments in the United States with rats have also indicated that drugs such as the dimethyl-aminoethyl ester of parachlorophenoxyacetic acid (2-Dimethylaminoethyl P-Chlorophenoxy-Acetate Lucidril) significantly increased long-term acceleration survival time by three times at 20 g (Polis, 1962). To date there is no evidence, however, that drugs can increase impact tolerance. While such techniques may have space applications, it is doubtful that drugs would be a practical or even desirable means of protecting automobile occupants due to possible side effects, and since simpler, more effective restraints have been achieved for impact.

Exoskeletal Restraints

Although protective garments for manned space and high-performance aircraft are generally designed primarily to provide adequate pressurization, temperature, flexibility and other conditions necessary to survive in an environment hostile to the human organism, some protective devices may be incorporated. The g-suit is typical in that air pressure exerted on critical parts of the body increases acceleration tolerance. Modern extravehicular (EV) protective garments designed for astronauts contain mesh materials which provide acceleration protection and might conceivably be employed or adapted specifically to increase impact protection. Recent studies by Richardson (1967), and by Ripley (1966) have evaluated advanced EV restraint technology.

SUMMARY

Experimental evidence indicates that it is within the state of the art to provide increased protection to vehicle occupants in certain kinds of impacts in excess of 60 and, possibly, involving as 200 g. However, this could be accomplished with present and foreseeable concepts only at extreme expense in comfort, convenience, and practicality: Unlike the case of spacecraft, where a small, selected group of young male occupants in top physical condition can be personally form-fitted to a highly sophisticated protective system, the automobile population presents a wider range of sizes and tolerances and poses a more complex restraint problem, particularly since use of automotive restraint is still a highly *voluntary* action. And unless a car restraint is easy to use, comfortable, doesn't rumple clothing, stores readily, and allows sufficient freedom of motion, occupants are unlikely to wear them. Thus, a compromise between restraint protection on the one hand, and practicability and ease of use, on the other, will be required for the immediate future.

In our rapidly changing technology, it is important in considering advanced concepts to keep in mind technical innovations likely during the next 30 years. From such a "lead-time" perspective, it becomes apparent that occupant restraint system design will have to undergo considerable innovation in the future to keep up with the requirements of changing transportation. New forms of transportation, such as the air cushion vehicles capable of traveling off-highways and over water at speeds above 100 knots, and individual flying platforms already exist. By the year 2000, major use of rockets for commercial and private transportation, either terrestrial or extraterrestrial, is considered an "even-money bet" by the Hudson Institute. Such advanced vehicles suggest that a wide variety of new restraint system concepts will be necessary.

For the present, however, one thing seems certain: automotive occupant restraint systems will show the greatest relative advances over those for other modes of transportation. Even though experimental studies are under way and new concepts are under consideration by the industry, development times and reliability requirements suggest that dramatic changes will not occur overnight in automotive vehicles. Rather, gradual improvement of the current Type 2 restraint, through easier and better adjustment, and greater use of improved self-adjusting and locking webbing playout devices seem most imminent. The trend toward bucket rather than bench seating may allow such alternatives as double shoulder type harness with integral inertia reels stored in a higher seat back which also will provide head restraint. Lateral thigh and side protection, combined protection using a lap belt in combination with air bag systems or improved interior cushioning devices, and, possibly, eventually a totally passive restraint in which the occupant "wears" nothing, but is protected by devices positioned at the instant of entry or impact, or is packaged in a protective capsule are all long range possibilities. Still other methods, such as rear-facing seats, as proposed for some passengers in the New York Safety Car, also could offer increased occupant protection. For some specialized vehicles, even such exotic concepts as an ejectable capsule may provide the optimum solution.

Restraints integral with seats, as in the Cox seat and the Liberty Mutual or New York State Safety Car Design of a decade ago, offer advantages of protection for the occupant while eliminating the problem of what to do with all the present straps. Even better systems are theoretically within the state of the art.

Current three-point (Type II) systems offer improved protection over the single lap belt. However, fixed upper and lower torso attachment points sometimes produce discomfort and may even prove dangerous if fitted too high, along the occupant's neck, or too low and off the shoulder. In the first case, cervical injury could be attributed to the belt in lateral (left for driver, right for passenger) impact, and in the second case, the upper torso could flex and twist, setting up vertebral rotational trauma. Development of both a reliable inertia reel, to allow freedom of movement, and a suitable adjustable upper attachment point to allow proper positioning of the upper torso portion are critical requirements for improved functioning of this system.

To date, the greatest promise of increased effectiveness, among currently available automobile restraint systems, appears to lie in the inverted Y-yoke upper torso system with inertia reel attached to the roll bar in two-seater applications such as the Shelby GT's.

The most effective child restraint system tested by the author is the Ford "Tot-Guard," in which the force of an impact is distributed over the entire anterior surface of the body and head.

The degree of restraint crash protection depends in large part upon the total environment. In some impacts, passenger compartment integrity can become a greater problem than restraint because of compartment collapse and intrusion. The highest-performance aircraft, such as the F-111, utilize the capsule module to protect the occupants from the high speed ejection problems of wind blast, tumbling, and deceleration. Possibly, a capsule concept might someday increase protection against side intrusion of automobiles. An integrated restraint system, with the seat designed as a protective capsule in side impact, rollover, and rear impact should be considered part of any future "total impact" protection system.

Ironically, U.S. general aviation aircraft today offer less occupant restraint protection than post-1967 automotive vehicles, and have no restraints (with the exception of highly specialized agricultural aircraft) that were not available to the pilot of 50 years ago. Note that U.S. general aviation aircraft sold to England as well as to the U.S. Army must be modified to meet their respective torso harness requirements.

A major change in U.S. commercial transport aircraft restraint systems did not occur until 1963, when flight deck crews were required to wear shoulder harnesses on take-off and landing. By 1969, side-facing occupants (stewardesses, lounge passengers) will have additional side restraints. At present no device other than the lap belt is assured for any future transports such as the SST or air-bus type of vehicle.

Restraint use will probably spread to other advanced vehicles such as air cushion vehicles, high speed trains, and deep submersible vehicles.

Concentration of research on "maximum" restraint devices probably will continue to be confined to requirements for Mars and Lunar extra-terrestrial exploration vehicles, military hypersonic aircraft, and manned space craft.

ACKNOWLEDGMENTS

The author gratefully acknowledges the support and assistance of a number of organizations and individuals who contributed to the work reported in this chapter.

REFERENCES CITED

ADAMS, T.: *Research in Progress.* E. Lansing, Mich. State, 1968.
ALDMAN, B.: Biodynamic studies on impact protection. *Acta Physiol Scand* (Supple. 192) 1962, Vol. 56.
Anonymous.: Plain talk about 3-point safety belts. *Road and Track*, Jan. 1968, pp. 101–102.
Anonymous: SR-N4 Tether tests precede sea trials. *Aviation Week and Space Technology*, 88(6):52, Feb. 5, 1968.

APPOLDT, F.A.: Dynamic tests of restraints for children. In Patrick, L.M. (Ed.): *Eighth Stapp Car Crash and Field Demonstration Conference.* Detroit, Wayne, 1966. (Presented in 1964, published in 1966).

ARMSTRONG, R., et al.: *National Bureau of Standards Tests.* Holloman AFB, New Mexico, Briefing Conference, Gaithersburg, Virginia. Aug. 1967.

AVERY, J.P.: *Cargo Restraint Concepts for Crash Resistance.* Aviation Safety Engineering and Research. Phoenix. AVSER–64–13, USAAML–TR–65–30, 1965.

Aviation Crash Injury Research, Flight Safety Foundation, Inc., Phoenix: Personnel restraint systems study, basic concepts. U.S. Army Transportation Research Command, Virginia, *TEREC Tech. Rept. 62–94,* 1962.

Aviation Safety Engineering and Research, Division of Flight Safety Foundation, Inc. Phoenix, Arizona: Occupant restraint harness design study. *AVSER memo dept. M67–7.* Oct. 1967.

Aviation Safety Engineering and Research Division of Flight Safety Foundation, Inc.: Occupant restraint harness design study. U.S. Army Aviation Material Laboratories, *AVSER Memo. Dept. M67–7,* 1967.

BABBS, F.W., and HILTON, B.C.: The packaging of car occupants—a British approach to seat design. *Seventh Stapp Car Crash Conference,* 1965, pp. 456–464.

BACON, R.: Photograph of Octave Gilbert in early net aeroplane restraint. *Flight International,* Sept. 8, 1967, p. 546.

BAKER, A.: Is this the seating of the future? *Automotive Design Engineering,* 5(3): 56–57. March, 1965.

BENNETT, J.B.: Hammock-type plane seat may prove crash safety aid. *Technical Data Digest,* 16(3):11–12, 1951.

BERTON, R.: Whiplash: tests of the influential variables. *SAE Paper No. 680080.* Jan. 1968.

BIERMEN, H.R.: The protection of the human body from impact force of fatal magnitude. *Milit Surg, 100:*125–141, 1947.

Boeing Aircraft Co.: Technical report, hammock full body restraint system. No. D7–2449, Sept. (n.d.).

BOHLIN, N.I.: A statistical analysis of 28000 accident cases with emphasis on occupant restraint value. *1967 Stapp Car Crash Conference, Proceedings.* SAE Paper 670925, 1967.

BONDURANT, S.; BLANCHARD, W.G.; CLARKE, N.P., and MOORE, F.: Effect of water immersion on human tolerance to forward and backward acceleration. Wright Air Development Center. *Tech. Report NADC–MA–5708,* July 1958.

BOYCE, W.C. and FREEMAN, H.E.: Considerations affecting the design of a 60 G personal restraint system. *ARS Journal,* 32(6):939–942, June 1962.

BRAUN, F.: Introducing the rocking aircraft passenger seat. *Sabena Report XA–002,* 1958.

BRINKLEY, J.W.; WEIS, E.B.; CLARKE, N.P., and TEMPLE, W.E.: A study of the effect of five orientations of the acceleration vector on human response. *AMRL Memo M–28,* Feb. 1963.

CAMPBELL, B.J.: A review of ACIR findings. In Patrick, L.M. (Ed.): *Eighth Stapp Car Crash and Field Demonstration Conference.* Detroit, Wayne, 1966 (presented in 1964, published in 1966).

CARTER, R.L.: Human tolerance to automatic position and restraint systems for supersonic aircraft. Columbus, North American Aviation, Inc. *Report NA59H–220,* 1959.

CHAFFEE, J.W.: Anthropometric considerations for escape capsule design. Convair 1 General Dynamics Corporation, Fort Worth. *Internal Furnishings Report 302*, Jan. 18, 1960.

CHANDLER, R.: Impact acceleration limits. USAF Aerospace Medical Research Laboratories, 1967 (in preparation).

CHISMAN, S.W.: Restraint harnesses—a review. Royal Aircraft Establishment, Farnborough, England, *RAE TN ME375*, 1963.

CONLEY, M.: A method of supporting the human body structure during space flight. *J Space Flight*, 4(9):3–4, Nov. 1952.

CRANDELL, F.J., et al.: Packaging the passenger; design for collision project car. *American Society of Mechanical Engineers Annual Winter Meeting Paper No. 62–WA–287*, 1962, pts. I and II.

CROSBY, W.M.; SNYDER, R.G.; SNOW, C.C., and HANSON, P.: Automotive Injuries to Pregnant Women. Presented by Crosby, Civil Aviation Medical Association, Oklahoma City, Sept. 12, 1967.

CROSBY, W.M.; SNYDER, R.G.; HANSON, P.; SNOW, C.C., and PRICE, G.T.: Impact injuries in the pregnant female. I. Experimental studies. Presented, Annual Meeting, Central Region Association of Gynecologists and Obstetricians. 14 September, Detroit. *Amer J Gynec Obstet*, 101(1):100–110, 1967.

DEHAVEN, H., and HASBROOK, A.H.: Shoulder harness: its use and effectiveness. Aviation Crash Injury Research, Cornell University. *AF Tech Report 6461*, Wright-Patterson AFB, Dayton, Ohio, Feb. 1951.

DEHAVEN, H.: Development of Crash-Survival Design in Personal, Executive and Agricultural Aircraft. Crash Injury Research, Cornell University, New York, May, 1963.

DUDDY, J.H.: Light-weight seating: design research and development of a net seat for project man high. *WADC Technical Report 58–307*. Dec. 1958.

DYE, E.R.: Kinematics of the human body under crash conditions. *Clin Orthop*, Fall 1956, No. 8.

EBBETS, J.: Seat belts and cervical spondylosis. *Practitioner*, 188:802, 1962.

EISEN and ZEIGEN: A supine seat for high-stress testing of primates. Wright-Patterson AFB, Dayton, Ohio. *WADC TR 59–165*, 1959.

ERNSTING, J.: Aeromedical aspects of the F111 K Aircraft proposed VK seat harness for the F111. RAF Institute of Aviation Medicine. *Report No. 405*, May, 1967 a. Aeromedical aspects of the F111 escape system. RAF Institute of Aviation Medicine. *Report S 1004/47/88*, August, 1967b.

Fairchild Hiller, Republic Aviation Division, New York: Feasibility study of New York State safety car program. Final report. *FHR 3040–3*, August 31, 1966.

Fairchild Hiller, Republic Aviation Division, New York: The safety sedan. Summary of final report. FHR 3526 (Submitted to New York State Department of Motor Vehicles). Sept. 1967.

Federal Aviation Agency. Washington, D.C.: General aviation: a study and forecast of the fleet and its use in 1975. *DDC Report AD 649 338*, July, 1966.

Federal Aviation Agency: Advisory Circular Change. Chapter 9. Shoulder Harness Installation, for Effective Restraint Handles and Attachment Methods Pertinent to Installation of Shoulder Harness. AC: 43. 13–2 Effective 5–26–67.

FENTON, J.: Automotive seating. A proprietory trimmed seat and specialized equipment. A firm-by-firm review. *Automotive Design Engineering*, 5(2):42–59 Feb. 1966.

FISCHER, J.C., JR.: The exploitation of the maximum capabilities of the human body to withstand maneuvering loads in manned aerospace vehicle design. *SAE Paper 4248*, Oct. 1961.

FISHER, P.: Injury produced by seat belts: report of 2 cases. *J Occup Med*, 7:211–212, 1965.

FLETCHER, B.D., and BRAGDON, B.G.: Seat belt fractures of the spine and sternum. *JAMA*, 200(2):177–178, April 10, 1967.

FOULOIS, B.: And teach yourself to fly. *The Readers Digest*, 77:50–55. Oct. 1960.

FREEMAN, H.E.: Research program to develop a 60 "G" personnel restraint system in *Impact Acceleration Stress: Proceedings of a Symposium with a Comprehensive Chronological Bibliography*. National Academy of Sciences, National Research Council, Publication No. 977, 1962, pp. 259–264.

FREEMAN, H.E.; BOYCE, W.C., and GELL, C.F.: Investigations of a personnel restraint system for advanced manned flight vehicles. Chance Vought Corporation, *Report AMRL–TDR–62–128*, Wright-Patterson AFB, Dayton, Ohio, Dec. 1962.

FRYER, D.I.: Passenger survival in aircraft crashes. *Aeronautics*, April 1959, pp. 31–37.

GADD, C.W., and PATRICK, L.M.: System versus laboratory impact tests for eliminating injury hazard. *SAE Paper 680053*, Jan. 1969.

GADD, C.W.: Use of a weighted-impulse criterion for estimating injury hazard. *SDE Paper No. 660793*, 1968.

GARRIDO-LECCA FRIAS, G.: *El accidente de jorge chavez*. Institute Peruano de Fomento Educativo, Lima, 1963.

GELL, C.F.: Bio-Engineering of Protective Systems. Paper, 31st Annual Meeting of the Aerospace Medical Association, May 9–11, 1960.

GOLOMB, S.W.: Mathematical models—uses and limitations, *Astronautics and Aeronautics*. Jan. pp. 57–59.

HAIN, K. (Translated by D. R. Raichel): Acceleration in planar mechanisms. *Applied Kinematics*, 2nd ed. 1967, chapt. 6, pp. 148–149.

HALEY, J.L., JR.: Personnel restraint systems study—basic concepts. *TCREC Tech. Dept. 62–94*. U.S. Army Transportation Research Command, Fort Eustis, Virginia, 1962.

HART, G.: Designing aircraft seats to save lives. *American Aviation*, July 28, 1958, pp. 29–30.

HASBROOK, A.H., and SILLE, J.R.: Structural and medical analysis of a civil aircraft accident. *Aerospace Medicine*, 35(10):958–961, 1964.

HAWTHORNE, R.: Energy absorption applied to seat design. *Space/Aeronautics*. Oct. 1958.

HAYNES, A.L., Personal communication, 1968.

Head restraints—passenger cars. *Federal Register*, Dec. 28, 1967 (32 F.R. 20865. Amendment Feb. 1968).

HEADLEY, R.N. et al.: Human factors responses during ground impact. *WADD TR 60–590*, Nov. 1960.

HEAP, S.A., and GRENIER, E.P.: The design and development of a more effective child restraint concept. *SAE Paper 680002*, Jan. 1960.

HENZEL, J.H.; MOHR, G.C., and VONGIERKE, H.E.: Reappraisal of biodynamic implications in human ejections. *Aerospace Med*, 39(3):329, March, 1968.

HENZEL, J.H.: The human spinal column and upward ejection acceleration: an appraisal of biodynamic implications. Aerospace Medical Research Laboratories, Wright-Patterson Air Force Base, Ohio, *Tech. Report 66–233*, 1967.

HERTZBERG, E., and COLGAN: A prone position bed for pilots. Wright-Patterson AFB, Dayton, Ohio, *MR MCREXD–695–71D*, June, 1948.

HERTZBERG, E.: Hammock for the B-36 Aircraft. Wright-Patterson AFB, Dayton, Ohio, *MCREXD–720–143*, Oct. 1949.

HERTZBERG, E.: Nylon net seat for a modified RB-57 Aircraft. Wright-Patterson AFB, Dayton, Ohio, *ASD TR 61–206*, 1961.

HILL, R.M.: Comparison of pilot seating in military aircraft. *Royal Aircraft Establishment Report K 1330*, 1918 (Smithsonian Institution).

HILTON, B.C.: *Car Seat of the Future*. 1963.

HILTON, B.C.: The development of vehicle safety seating for injury prevention. *Proceedings—American Association for Automotive Medicine*. Alamogordo, N. Mex., Nov. 10, 1966.

HILTON, B.C.: Design of low cost seating for effective packaging of vehicle occupants. *1967 Stapp Car Crash Conference*. Society of Automotive Engineers, New York, SAE Paper 660797, 1967.

HUELKE, D.F., and GIKAS, P.W.: Ejection—the leading cause of death in automobile accidents. *Tenth Stapp Car Crash Conference*. 1966, pp. 12 (SAE Reprint, 1967).

HUELKE, D.F.: The second collision reprint. *Traffic Safety Magazine*, National Safety Council, Chicago, Illinois, 1967.

HUNTER, H.: Conventional and New Type Flight Restraint Equipment, Evaluation of. Naval Air Development Center, Johnsville, Pennsylvania, Project TED ADC AE–6301, Dec. 1955.

ISADA, N.M., and SARKEES, Y.T.: Dynamic Response of Aircraft Seat and Restraint System. Research in Progress Under NIH Grant AC 00270, 1968.

KAHN, H., and WIENER, A.J.: One hundred technical innovations very likely in the last third of the twentieth century. *The Year 2000*. New York, Macmillan, 1967.

KAZARIAN, L.E.; MOHR, G.C., and vonGIERKE, H.E.: Mechanics of Vertebral Body Injury in Monkeys as a Result of Spinal (Z) Impact. Paper presented—Aerospace Medical Association Meeting, Bal Harbour, Fla., May 6, 1968.

KEMMERER, R.M., CHUTE, R., and HASS, D.P.: Automotive inflatable occupant restraint system. *SAE Paper 680033*, Jan. 1968, pt. I.

KROELL, C.K.: A simple, efficient, one-shot energy absorber. *Bulletin #30, Shock, Vibration and Associated Environments*, Feb. 1962, pt. III.

LASKY, I.I.; SIEGEL, A.W., and NAHUM, A.M.: Automotive cardio-thoracic injuries: a medical-engineering analysis. *SAE Paper No. 680052*, 1968.

LEGUEN, G., and JOLYS, J.: Dynamic testing of a safety harness—equations of the movement of the occupant. *Aspects Techniques de la Securite Routiere*. Brussels, 30:3:1–3, 58, June, 1967 (in French).

LITTLE, ARTHUR D., Inc.: The State of the Art of Traffic Safety: A Critical Review and Analysis of the Technical Information on Factors Affecting Traffic Safety. June 1966, pp. 24–25.

LOMBARD, C.F. and ADVANI, S.H.: Impact protection by isovolumetric containment of the torso. *Tenth Stapp Car Crash Conference*. New York, Society of Automotive Engineers, 1966, pp. 196–206. Also *SAE Paper No. 660796*, 1966a.

LOMBARD, C.F.; ROY, A.; BEATTIE, J.M., and ADVANI, S.H.: *The Influence of Orientation and Support—Restraint upon Survival from Impact Acceleration*. Northrop Space Laboratories, Dept. ARL–TR–66–20, 6571st Aeromedical Research Laboratory, Holloman AFB, New Mexico, 1966b.

LOMBARD, C.F., BRONSON, S.D.; THIEDE, F.C.; CLOSE, P., and LARMIE, F.M.: Pathology and physiology of guinea pigs under selected conditions of impact and support-restraint. *Aerospace Med*, Sept. 1964.

MARGARITA, R.; GUALTIEROTTI, T. and SPINELLI, D.: Protection against acceleration forces in animals by immersion in water. *J Aviation Med*, 29(6):433–437, June 1958.

MARSH, J.A.: Case for suspension seating. *Automotive Design Engineering*, 5(2):54–55, Feb. 1966.

MELDRUM, J.: Automobile driver eye position. SAE Paper No. 650464, May, 1965.

MERTZ, H.J., and PATRICK, L.M.: Investigation of the kinematics and kinetics of whiplash. *SAE Paper No. 670919*, 1967.

MOORE, J.O.: Feasibility study of New York State safety car program—a preliminary report. *SAE Paper 660345*, 1966.

MORRIS, D.P.; BEISCHER, D.E., and ZARRIELLO, J.J.: Studies on the G tolerance of invertebrates and small vertebrates while immersed. *J Aviation Med*, 29(6):438–443, June, 1958.

MULLER, G.: Why a second collision? *The Prevention of Highway Injury*. Highway Safety Research Institute The Univ. of Mich. pp. 272–284. 1967 (oral version).

NEFF, R.J.: Federal seat-belt regulation—a progress report. In Patrick, L.M. (Ed.): *Eighth Stapp Car Crash and Field Demonstration Conference*. Detroit, Wayne, 1966, pp. 72–78.

NEILSON, I.D.: Notes on the British Standards Institution dynamic test rig for seat belt assemblies. Dept. of Scientific and Industrial Research, Road Research Laboratory, *Lab. Note No. LN/160. IDN*, 1962.

NICKERSON, J.L.; DRAZIC, M.; JOHNSON, R.; UDENSEN, H., and Turner, K.: A study of internal movements of the body occurring on impact. *Tenth Stapp Car Crash Conference Proceedings*. Also SAE Paper No. 670915, 1967.

OMMAYA, A.K.; HIRSCH, A., and MARTINEZ, J.L.: The role of whiplash in cerebral concussion. *SAE Paper No. 660804*, 1967.

PATRICK, L.M., Personal communication, 1968.

PATRICK, L.M.; MERTZ, H.J., and KROELL, C.K.: Impact dynamics of unrestrained, lap belted and lap and diagonal chest belted vehicle occupants. *Proceedings, Tenth Stapp Car Crash Conference*. Holloman AFB, New Mexico, No. 8–9, 1966, pp. 22–53.

PATT, D.I. Comfort evaluation of the hammock-type fighter seat. Wright-Patterson Air Force Base, Ohio, *WADC TR No. TSEAL 3–65–32EE*, 1945.

PAYNE, P.R.: The Dynamics of Human Restraint Systems, Paper presented at the National Academy of Sciences Symposium on Impact Acceleration Stress. San Antonio, Nov. 27, 1961.

PAYNE, P.R.: Dynamics of human restraint system. Washington, D.C., *NAS–NRC Pub. 977*, 1962, pp. 195.

PAYNE, P.R.: Personal restraint and support system dynamics. Wright-Patterson AFB, *Report AMRL–TR–65–127*, Oct. 1965.

PESMAN, G.J., and EIBOND, A.M.: Crash Injury, in NACA Conference on Crash Impact Loads, Crash Injuries and Principles of Seat Design for Crash Worthiness. Lewis Flight Propulsion Lab., Cleveland, 1956.

PHILLIPS, N.I.: Future seat restraint seen as passive system. *Automotive News*, Nov. 1967, p. 36.

PINCE, B.W.; BRIAN, M.; LIFE, J.S.; HEBERLEIN, P.J., and GESINK, J.W.: Comparative responses of live-anesthetized and dead embalmed monkeys exposed to impact stress. Space/Defense TR 66–107, dated Sept. 16, 1966. (Submitted to *Science* as Comparative Pathology of Live and Embalmed Monkeys Exposed to Impacts.)

PINKEL, I., ROSENBURG, E.G.: Seat design for crash worthiness. NCAA Report on Conference on Crash Impact Loads, Crash Injuries and Principles of Seat Design for Crash Worthiness. Lewis Flight Propulsion Lab., Cleveland, 1956.

POLIS, B.D.: Increase in acceleration tolerance of the rat by 2-dimethylamine ethyl P-chlorophenoxy-acetate (1 ucidril). *Aerospace Med*, 33:930–934, August, 1962.

POPPEN, J.R.: Support of upper body against accelerative forces in aircraft. *J Aviation Med*, 29:76–84, Jan. 1958.

PURSER, P.E.; FAGET, M.A., and SMITH, N.F. (Eds.): *Manned Spacecraft: Engineering Design and Operation.* New York, Fairchild, 1964, pp. 327–328.

QUIMBY, F.H., and HASBROOK, A.H.: Prevention of injuries in 'unpreventable' aircraft accidents. *Res Rev*, August, 1956.

READER, D.C.: The Restraint Afforded by the USAF and Proposed RAF IAM Seat Harness for the F–111 under High Forward and Lateral Decelerations, 1967 (in preparation.

RICHARDSON, D.L.: Research to advance extravehicular protective technology. Arthur D. Little Co., Wright-Patterson AFB, Ohio, *Tech. Report AMRL–TR–66–258*, 1967.

RIPLEY, H.S. Investigation of a crew seating system for advanced aerospace vehicles. Northrop Corp., Norair Division, Air Force Flight Dynamics Laboratory, Wright-Patterson AFB, Ohio, *Tech. Report AFFDL–TR–66–214*, Nov. 1966.

ROBBINS, W.A.; POTTER, G.L.; and LOMBARD, C.F.: The influence of Support-Restraint in Survival from $\pm G_x$ and $+G_z$ Impacts Using an LD 50 Criterion with Guinea Pig Subjects. NASA and USAF sponsored research in progress, 1968.

ROTHSTEIN, and HANSON, P.: Cardiac rate changes in human after abrupt deceleration, *J Appl Physiol*, April 1967, vol. 22, No. 4.

Royal Aircraft Establishment: Report on pilot's seating accomodations. *Report No. K. 1330*, June 21, 1918.

RUFF, S.: Brief acceleration: less than one second: In Dept. of the Air Force, *German Aviation Medicine, World War II.* Washington, D.C.: U.S. Government Printing Office, 1950, Vol. I, Chapt. VI–C, pp 584–597.

RUSSO, A.: Aircraft cargo restraint system *USAAVLABS Tech. Report 66–50.* All American Engineering Co., Wilmington, Sept. 1966.

Safety belts—model designation. Type designation sheets. 1932–1944. Air Force Technical Services Division Reference Branch, Wright-Patterson AFB, Ohio.

Safety car program. Feasibility study. Fairchild Hiller Corporation, Farmingdale, New York, PB 173313, August, 1966.

Safety car program, Feasibility study—Summary of final report. Fairchild Hiller Corporation, Farmingdale, New York, PB 173312, 1966.

SAMUEL, G.D., and SMITH, E.M.B.: A comparison of seven anthropometric variables of American, British and Canadian pilots. RAF Institute of Aviation Medicine, *Report No. 322*, April 1965.

SCHNEIDER, R.C.; SMITH, W.S.; GRABB, W.C.; TURCOTTE, J.G., and HUELKE, D.F.: Lap seat belt injuries; the treatment of the fortunate survivor. *Mich Med*, 67(3):171–186, Feb. 1968.

SCHRUM, D.J., and PROVOST, E.J.: Dynamic research of passenger restraining devices. PATRICK, L.M. (Ed.): *Eighth Stapp Car Crash and Field Demonstration Conference.* Detroit, Wayne, 1966 (presented in 1964, published in 1966).

SEVERY, D.M.; BRINK, H.M., and BAIRD, J.D.: Collision performance, LM safety car SAE Paper No. 670458, 1967.

SEVERY, D.M.; BRINK, J.M., and BAIRD, J.D.: Backrest and head restraint design for rearend collision protection. SAE Paper No. 680079, 1968a.

SEVERY, D.M.; BRINK, H.M., and BAIRD, J.D.: Full-scale crash tests show liberty mutual capsule seat protects passengers best. SAE Journal, 76(3):56–61, March 1968b.

SLACK, W.K.: Automatic inflatable occupant restraint system. SAE Paper No. 680033, Jan. 1968, pt. II.

SMEDAL, H.A.; STINNETT, G.W., and INNESS, R.C.: A restraint system enabling pilot control under moderately high acceleration in a varied acceleration field. NASA, TN D–91, 1960.

SMEDAL, H.A.; VYKUKAL, H.C.; GALLONT, and STINNETT, G.W.: Crew physical support and restraint in advanced manned flight systems. American Rocket Society Journal, 31(11):1544–1548, Nov. 1961.

Society of Automotive Engineers, Inc. New York:

Aerospace Recommended Practice (ARP) 583B, Issued 3–1–60/1960 Cabin Attendant Stations.

SAE Recommended Practice (SAE J842). Restraining Devices for Children (8 months to 6 years) for use in Motor Vehicles—SAE J842. Report of Motor Vehicle Seat Belt Committee, approved Nov. 1962.

1965 Passenger Seat Design. Aerospace Recommended Practice (ARP) 750. Issued April 20, 1965.

Safety Lap Belts (for Civil Transport Aircraft). ARP 682A. Issued April 15, 1961, Revised August 31, 1967a.

Crew Restraint System. ARP 998. Issued Nov. 15, 1967b.

SAE Aerospace Recommended Practice (ARP 766) Issued Sept. 30, 1967. Restraint Device for Small Children. Prepared by Committee S–9, Cabin Safety Provisions, 1967c.

SAE Aerospace Recommended Practice (ARP 998) (Proposed Draft). Crew Restraint System. Prepared by Sub Committee S–7/S–9, Flight Deck Provisions, 1968a.

SAE Aerospace Recommended Practice (ARP 682A) Issued April 15,1960, Revised August 31, 1967. Safety Lap Belts (for Civil Transport Aircraft). Prepared by SAE Committee S–9, Cabin Safety Provisions, 1968b.

SAE Aerospace Recommended Practice (ARP 767) (Proposed Draft). Impact Protective Design of Occupant Environment—Transport Aircraft. Prepared by SAE Committee S–9, Cabin Safety Provisions, 1968c.

Occupant Restraint Systems. Performance levels. In draft preparation by SAE Occupant Restraint Systems Committee, SAE. Feb. 1968d.

Occupant Restraint System. General Aviation Aircraft. SAE Committee A23 Draft Aerospace Recommended Practice, 1968e (in preparation).

SLACK, W., Personal communication, 1968.

SNOW, C.C.; GEYER, J.R.; SHIRES, T.K.; ROWLAN, D.E.; ALLGOOD, M.A., and PARRY, W.L.: Physiological and Pathological Findings in Primates Subjected to $-G_z$ Deceleration. Paper presented Aerospace Medical Association Annual Meeting Bal Harbour, Florida May 6, 1968.

SNOW, C.C., and HASBROOK, A.H.: The angle of shoulder slope in normal males as a factor in shoulder-harness design. Federal Aviation Administration, Report AM 65–14, 1965.

SNYDER, R.G.: Design and fabrication of a restraint system for advanced manned flight. Proposal to the AMC Aeronautical Systems Center, WADC. PR 96126, Applied Research Laboratory, *University of Arizona Report 60–Q–8,* 1960.

SNYDER, R.G.: Calculation of Crash Impact Forces and Opinion of Injuries and Survival Potential with Assistance of J. Earley, Impact Dynamics Lab. and S. Mohler, Director, CAMI, FAA. Communication of 2 August to Dr. Gmo. Garrido Lecca, Lima, Peru for Inclusion in Report of Accident, 1962.

SNYDER, R.G.: Physiological effects of impact: man and other mammals. ALTMAN, P.L., and DITTMER, D.S. (Eds.): *Environmental Biology.* Federation of American Societies for Experimental Biology, Bethesda, 1966, pp. 231–242.

SNYDER, R.G.; SNOW, C.C.; YOUNG, J.W.; PRICE, G.T., and HANSON, P.: Experimental comparison of trauma in lateral ($+G_Y$), rearward facing ($+G_X$) and forward facing ($-G_Z$) body orientations when restrained by lap belt only. Aerospace Med, 38(9):889–894, 1967a.

SNYDER, R.G.; CROSBY, W.M.; SNOW, C.C.; YOUNG, J.W. and HANSON, P: Seat belt injuries in impact. In SELZER, M.L.; GIKAS, P.W., and HUELKE, D.F. (Eds.): *The Prevention of Highway Injury.* Ann Arbor, U. of Mich., 1967b, pp. 188–210. (Presented at Sesquicentennial Symposium of the Prevention of Highway Injury, University of Michigan Medical School, Highway Safety Institute, Ann Arbor, 21 April.)

SNYDER, R.G.; SNOW, C.C., YOUNG, J.W.: Experimental impact protection with advanced automotive restraint systems: preliminary primate tests with air bag and inertia reel/inverted-Y yoke torso harness. Proceedings, *Eleventh Stapp Car Crash Conference,* Anaheim, California, SAE Paper, 1967c (hardback, in press)

SNYDER, R.G.; SNOW, C.C.; YOUNG, J.W.; CROSBY, W.H., and PRICE, G.T.: Pathology of trauma attributed to restraint systems in crash impacts. Presented, Joint Committee on Aviation Pathology, Toronto, Canada, Sept. 12, 1967. *Aerospace Med.* 39(8):812–829. 1968a.

SNYDER, R.G.; SNOW, C.C.; YOUNG, J.; CROSBY, C., and PRICE, T.: Pathomechanics of Automotive Restraint System Injuries. Presented, International Meeting on Accident Pathology, Washington, D.C., June 1968b.

SNYDER, R.G.: Biomechanical considerations in child restraint system design. For presentation, *Twelfth Stapp Car Crash Conference.* Detroit, Oct. 22–24, 1968c (in preparation).

Sports Car Club of America: 1968 harness specifications.

STAPP, J.P.: Human exposures to linear deceleration. Preliminary survey of aft-facing seated position. *Tech. Report 5915,* Wright-Patterson AFB, Ohio, 1949, pt. 1.

STAPP, J.P.: Human exposures to linear deceleration. The forward-facing position and the development of a crash harness. WADC Tech. Report 5915, 1951, pt. 2.

STAPP, J.P.: Crash protection in air transports. Aero. Engineering Review, 12(4):71–78, April, 1953.

STAPP, J.P., Personal communication, (Kurt Schversler, Heinkel Aircraft Co., Made first ejection seat tests. 1937–38.) 1965.

STAPP, J.P.: Human Factors and Design Aspects of Transportation Safety. Presented American Association for the Advancement of Science, New York, Dec. 30, 1967.

STAPP, J.P., and TAYLOR, E.R.; Space cabin landing impact vector effects on human physiology. Aerospace Med, 35(4):1117–1133, 1964.

STAPP, J.P.; TAYLOR, E., and CHANDLER, R.: *Apollo Landing Impact Tests NASA–TR,* 1967.

STAPP, J.P.: Whole Body Tolerance to Impact. Effects of Seat Belts. ALTMAN, P.L., and DITTIMER, D.S., (Eds.) *Environmental Biology*. Federation of American Societies for Experimental Biology, Bethesda, 1966, p. 229.

STAPP, J.P., and TAYLOR, E.R.: Space cabin landing impact vector effect on human physiology. *Aerospace Med*, 35(12):1117–1133, Dec. 1959.

STAPP, J.P.: Human Factors and Design Aspects of Transportation Safety. Paper Presented at American Association for the Advancement of Science, 134th Meeting, New York, Dec. 30, 1967.

STATES, J.D.: Case studies of racing accidents. Patrick, L.M. (Ed.): *Eighth Stapp Car Crash and Demonstration Conference*. Detroit, Wayne, 1964. pp. 251–257.

STATES, J.D., and BENEDICT, J.F.: Safe and unsafe upper torso restraints for occupant protection in motor vehicles. *Seventh Stapp Car Crash Conference*. 1965, pp. 312–323.

STATES, J.D.: *Restraint System Effectiveness in Racing Accidents*. Paper Presented at Annual Meeting of the American Association for Automotive Medicine, Oct. 21, Philadelphia. Springfield, Thomas, 1967.

STATES, J.D., Personal communication, 1968.

STEWART, W.C.: Fatal Accidents Involving Light Aircraft, a Review of U.K. Experience 1955–1966. Paper presented at Sixth Scientific Session, Joint Committee on Aviation Pathology, Ottawa, Sept. 12, 1967.

STUBBS, S.M.: Landing characteristics of the Apollo spacecraft with deployed heat shield impact attenuation systems. *NASA Tech. Note TND–3059*, 1966.

THOMAS, B.K.: NASA may jump to manned Apollo flight. *Aviation Week and Space Technology*, 88(5):25. Jan. 29, 1968.

TITUS, J.: Shelby Mustang GT 350 and GT 500. *Sports Car Graphic*, March 1967, pp. 32–55.

TURNBOW, J.W.; CARROLL, D.F.; HALEY, J.L., JR.; REED, W.H.; ROBERTSON, S.H., and WEINBERG, L.W.T.: Crash survival design guide. AV-SER, Flight Safety Foundation, Phoenix, *USAALABS Tech. Report 67–22*, July, 1967.

ULSAMER, E.E., and HUNTER, G.S.: Seat makers emphasize reduced weight. *Aviation Week and Space Technology*, Dec. 18, 1967, pp. 39–41.

ULSAMER, E.E.: Who will build the airbus? *Air Force*, Jan. 1968, pp. 76–82.

USAF: Investigation of a new crew seat concept for advanced flight vehicles. *ASD Tech. Report 61–546*, June, 1962.

USAF: Design and fabrication of microballoon body support restraint system. *Contract AF 33(616)–8429*, Dec. 1961.

USAF: Development of a pilot universal couch for acceleration, vibration and shock. *Contract No. HG 2269–2759* (n.d.).

VON GIERKE, H.E.: Biodynamic response of the human body. *Appl Mechanics Rev*, 17(2):951–958, Dec. 1964.

VYKUKAL, H.D., and LYMAN, E.G.: Human restraint systems development for use in acceleration research. *NASA Report TM–X54780*, 1965.

VYKUKAL, H.C.; GALLANT, R.P., and STINNETT, G.W.: An interchangeable, mobile pilot-restraint system, designed for use in a moderately high acceleration field. *J Aerospace Med*, 33(3):279–285, March 1962.

WEAVER, J.; RUBENSTEIN, M.; CLARK, C.C., and GRAY, R.F.: Encapsulation of humans in rigid polyurethane foam for use as a restraint system in high acceleration environment. *Report NADC–MA–6147*, U.S. Naval Air Development Center, Johnsville, May 1962.

WEBB, M.G., and GRAY, R.F.: Human tolerance to high acceleration stress (Mayo

Tank). U.S. Naval Air Development Center, Johnsville, *Tech. Report TED ADCAE-1411,* May 1958.

WEBB, M.G. and GRAY, R.F.: Protection against acceleration by water immersion. *American Rocket Society Reprint 805-59,* June 1959.

WINQUIST, P.G.; STUMAN, P.W., and HANSEN, R.: Crash injury experiments with the monorail decelerator. Air Force Flight Test Center, Edwards, Calif., *AF Tech. Report AFFTC 53-7,* April 27, 1953.

YEGOROV, B.: Experiments in anabiosis, Aviats a S. Kosmonavtika. In *Flight International,* Sept. 21, 1967.

YOUNG, J.: Unpublished test data. Ford Motor Company, Dearborn, 1968.

YOUNG, J.W., and SNYDER, R.G.: Unpublished test data. Ford Motor Company, Dearborn, 1967a.

YOUNG, J.W.: A functional comparison of basic restraint systems. OAM Report AM 67-13, Federal Aviation Administration, June 1967b.

YOUNG, J.W.: Recommendations for restraint installation in general aviation aircraft. *OAM Report 66-33,* Federal Aviation Administration, Washington, 1966.

ZABOROWSKI, A.: Personal communication, 1959.

APPENDIX 22-I
AUTOMOTIVE STANDARDS FOR ADULT OCCUPANT RESTRAINT SYSTEMS. BELT STRENGTH.

Vehicle Type	Organization	Belt Type	Webbing Breaking Strength (in lbs) Upper	Webbing Breaking Strength (in lbs) Lap	Requirement Reference
Automobiles	DOT(FMVSS)[1]	Type 1 (lap belt for pelvic restraint)	(1.8 inch min)[4]	6000	Dept. of Commerce, National Bureau of Standards, Standards for Seat Belts for use in Motor Vehicles (15 CRF 9) (31F. R.11528).
		Type 2 and 2A (pelvic and upper torso combination)	4000	5000	Dept. of Commerce, National Traffic Safety Agency, Federal Motor Vehicle Safety Standards. No. 209 Title 23 Part 255. 31 January, 1967. (FMV 209-seat belt assembly. FMV 210-seat belt anchorage).
		Type 3 (child under 50 lbs) seat back webbing connecting webbing	4000 3000		
	SAE (Rec. Practice)			6000[5] (2 inch)	Society of Automotive Engineers Inc., New York, N.Y. SAE J4C 1967 Handbook
				6700	Federal Register 31 August.

Occupant Restraint Systems of Manned Vehicles 557

Automobiles	SAE (Rec. Practice) (Continued)		SAE J4b "Motor Vehicle Seat Belt Assemblies."
			SAE J854 "Harness Type Restraint Assemblies for use in Motor Vehicles."
		6700	SAE J842 "Restraint Devices for Children (8 Months to 6 Years) for Use in Motor Vehicles."
			SAE J787 "Motor Vehicle Seat Belt Anchorages."
Competition	SCCA	Must conform with SAE J4A[7] 5000 (2 inch belt)	Sports Car Club of America, Specifications, Ch.3. Shoulder Harness. Parts 300.1 to 300.3.
	USAC	8 (3 inch width favored)	United States Automobile Club.
	NASCAR	9	National Association of Stock Car Automobile Racing.
	NHA	10	National Hot Rod Associaton.
Automobiles Sweden		11	Swedish Standard SIS 88 28 SIE Safety Belts for Motor Cars.
		(1.8 inches wide)	SMS2470–1967.08.15–Issue 1 "Seat Belt Anchorages."
		306.9 (1500 kgf)	

APPENDIX 22-I
AUTOMOTIVE STANDARDS FOR ADULT OCCUPANT RESTRAINT SYSTEMS. BELT STRENGTH.

Vehicle Type	Organization	Belt Type	Webbing Breaking Strength (in lbs) Upper	Webbing Breaking Strength (in lbs) Lap	Requirement Reference
England			2250 (1⅜ inches wide)	3000 (1⅞ inches wide)	British Standards Institution. Specification for Seat Belt Assemblies for Motor Vehicles. BS.3254:1960 The Motor Vehicles (Construction and Use) Regulations. 1966[12].
Canada					Canadian Government Specifications Board STANDARD FOR RESTRAINING DEVICES ANCHORAGES FOR AUTOMOTIVE VEHICLES, Ottawa, Canada.
					Canadian Standards Association MOTOR VEHICLE SEAT BELTS CSA Standard D159.1 1963.
Australia					Standards Association of Australia, Australian Standard Specification for Seat Belt Anchorage Points. AS D11 1967. Seat Belts. ASE35.

Italy	None			
France	None			
Russia	Interested, but none yet.			
Germany	Similar to 15CFR9 U.S. Nat. Bureau of Standards.	2866[13] (1.88 inches wide)	3968[14] (1.78 inches wide)	Pp. 534–536 Strebenverkehrs-Zulassungs—Ordnung.
International Standards 150			3300 (1 13/16 inches wide)	International Organization for Standardization, London. Draft ISO recommendation no. 1142. Seat Belt Assemblies for Motorists.

1. Applies to all automotive vehicles manufactured after certain dates for sale in U.S.
2. Width not less than 1.8 inches.
3. Attachment bolts must withstand 5000 pound force for one pelvic restraint belt, 9000 pound force for two or more pelvic belt attachments.
4. Elongation 20 per cent at 2500 pounds.
5. 2 inch belt.
6. Shoulder harness mandatory (Jan. 67) except in semireclining seat. In cars with semireclining seat, shoulder harness not required, but seat should have deep trough for buttocks and roll-up (sides) for thighs. Proposed revisions in rules for 1968 include: three-point harness should not be permitted in racing; all installations should meet 40 degree upper belt anchor angle.
7. Recommends deep trough to seat for buttocks, and hop-up for thighs.
8. Requires crotch straps anchored to seat and to lap and shoulder belt buckle. Use modified stock cars with special deep bucket seats with side protection.
9. Shoulder harness mandatory, 1960.
10. 46 mm (1.81 inches) wide under kgf load. Breaking load of at least 1500 kgf (3,306.9 pound).
11. British Standard for Seat Belt Assemblies for Motor Vehicles (B.S. 3254:1960) part 51 applies to every motor car registered on or after 1 April, 1967. Anchorage points are now required although restraints are not. A Type 2 restraint system is expected to be required soon.
12. 48 mm (1.88 inches) wide lap belt, 1300 kg (2,865.98 pound) load strength.
13. 45 mm (1.78 inches) wide shoulder belt, 1800 kg (3,968.28 pound) load strength.

APPENDIX 22-II
AIRCRAFT STANDARDS FOR OCCUPANT RESTRAINT SYSTEMS. BELT STRENGTH.

Vehicle Type	Organization	Belt Type	Webbing Breaking Strength (in lbs) Upper	Webbing Breaking Strength (in lbs) Lap	Requirement Reference
Civil Transport Aircraft.	SAE (ARP's)				Society of Automotive Engineers, Inc. SAE ARP 682A, Revised 8-31-67. SAE Committee S-9 "Safety Lap Belts (for Civil Transport Aircraft)." SAE ARP 767 "Impact Protective Design of Occupant Environment-Transport Aircraft." SAE ARP 998 "Crew Restraint System" ref. to: ARP 682, FAA TSO-C22. SAE ARP 583B "Cabin Attendant Stations." SAE ARP 750 "Passenger Seat Design."
Civil General Aviation Aircraft (United States).		Lap Belt Single Occupant Double Occupant		2250 4500	Federal Aviation Administration.[1] Technical Standard Order (ISO) C22E 3.1.1.
Requirements for mfg. or license.		Single rate strength for whole belt assembly.		1500	FAA Advisory Circular Change.[2] AC no. 43.13-2 effective 5-26-67. See also,
		Double rate strength for whole belt assembly.		3000 (5000)	SAE A-23. "Occupant Restraint System. General Aviation Aircraft." (In preparation) (See also, Young, 1966)

Occupant Restraint Systems of Manned Vehicles 561

(England)		Type 2, lap belt with upper torso restraint required.		Royal Aeronautical Establishment.
Aircraft, Military	USAF		(2000) (2250) 5500	(AF Tech Order 13A1-1-2).[4] Mil W4088 E Revision
	US Army Aviation	Lap Belt Upper Torso	6000 4000	USAF HIAD AF SCM80-1 2.6.1.3. Safety Belts & Harness. Part C. Ch. 6 pp. C.6-28A.
	US Naval Air		5500	MIL W4088 F Revision

1. FAA TSO Requirements should be considered as minimum only; belt strength should exceed strength of seat-floor attachment; elongation should be held to minimum; belt-floor-hip angle should be to (±) degrees.
2. Double over shoulder ceiling mounted harness 5 degrees down to 30 degrees up from horizontal. Double or single type shoulder harnesses, which use a continuous strap through a slip or "D" ring arrangement are *not* recommended. Double shoulder harness should be attached as far to side as possible, not at center buckle.
3. Shoulder belt upper attachment angle should not exceed 30 degrees from horizontal plane. Loaded resultant angle of lap belt 45 to 55 degrees. Side-facing seats are not recommended for use in aircraft.
4. USAF and USN now both use MIL W4088 E Revision or F Revision Type 24 for safety seat belts 5500 lbs. minimum tensile requirement 2 inches (11 11/16 inches overall) width, which is generally 6500 to 6800 pound tensile strength. USN used MIL W8630 until recently. However, in practice, USAF still operationally equipped for most part under AF Tech Order 13A1-1-2, requiring only 2000 (2250) pound strength of webbing.

DISCUSSION

John P. Stapp

Dr. Snyder is to be commended on preparing a comprehensive review and evaluation of aircraft and automotive crash restraint systems.

From the historical standpoint, the only significant omission has been the work of Pekarek, Gilson and Stewart at the Institute of Aviation Medicine, Farnborough, during World War II. This work was mainly written in internal publications of limited distribution. Pekarek was a Polish Resistance Flight Surgeon and Pilot who work with the Royal Air Force in 1941 to 1945, whose principal contribution was the Pakarek Safety Cell, a fabric restraint for crashing and ditching positions of bomber crewmen, based on biomechanical analysis of crash forces.

The historical perspective of crash restraints upholds the concept that safety, like religion, becomes a special subject in times of stress. Most recently, this has been demonstrated in the manned space flight project of the past 10 years. The astronauts were actually selected before the design of the Mercury Space Capsule was completed. The couch and restraints were custom fitted to the mold of each astronaut. For the first time in engineering history, a vehicle was actually designed and built around the occupant. Energy absorption in the expanded polyurethane couch lining was optimized, and the couch was mounted on crushable aluminum honeycomb metal supports. Restraint straps were faithful copies of the optimum design for maximum protection developed from human volunteer experiments on crash sleds. No sooner had the first successful manned flights taken place than straps began to be peeled off as confidence grew among the astronauts.

The Gemini flights began with less effective protection than that of the last Mercury flight, and during one violent reentry commotion of the Gemini Capsule, an astronaut sustained a severe blow to the head against the interior wall, although he was wearing a helmet. Apollo couches are no longer molded to fit a single occupant on the premise because space pilots might want to change places during prolonged flight; and the restraints were designed by engineers and submitted to crashworthiness testing, reversing the original order of development, which started with the requirements of the Mercury astronaut.

More recently, the designs of future long duration space flight vehicles have been developed to the point of looking for places to put the crew, in the best tradition of aircraft designers. Those concerned with the human factors have been told in how many cubic inches and in what configuration the pilot astronaut will be fitted into the nose of the spacecraft. The design requires that the pilot lie on his back with legs up in seated position, the long axis of his back only 2 degrees above the horizontal plane, for a 90 minute count down before launch. In the event of an abort just before or just after launch, the retro-rockets on the space cabin would serve as propulsion for escape, and subject the pilot to 20 seconds of thirteen times gravity acceleration, at the end of which the ballistic trajectory would quickly go into several seconds of weightlessness. The pilot would then be compelled to fly the spacecraft to a glide landing at a lift to drag ratio of 1.3, approximating the performance of a brick with aerodynamic hallucinations. The final landing maneuver would consist in pitching the nose straight up, letting the craft come down on its retro-rocket nozzles for a crunch landing. The question put to the human factors experts is, how can the astronaut be made equal to this task, even though three out of four who tried the legs-up reclining position for 90 minutes complained of headaches? This of course gives human factors experts headache number 40. In 10 short years, full cycle, from tailoring the space craft to fit the astronaut, to cramming him into an uninhabitable corner for an unendurable experience, has been run by former aircraft engineers turned into spacecraft designers.

A little confidence is a dangerous thing when dealing with margins of human safety which can determine the margin of mission success. In this regard, Dr. Snyder is ever mindful of human frailties in assessing the value of protective design. He is the first to give serious consideration to special requirements for protection of pregnant occupants in the automobile. His authoritative review of crash restraint development will be a valuable reference for safety design engineers, covering a multitude of technical notes and reports of intramural publications not readily accessible to library reference. Much repetition of work already done can thus be avoided.

INDEX

A

Abdomen, blunt injury to, 101
Abdominal injury
 physical factors in, 124
 radiology in, 110
 types of, 102
Acceleration in head injury, 34
Angular acceleration, subdural hematoma, 50
Anoxia in head injury, 100
Aorta, injury to, 89
Aortic rupture, 382

B

Biliary-pancreatic injuries, 119
Biomechanics
 bones and joints, 125
 spinal cord injury, 69
 spine injury, 66
Blood flow in spinal cord injury, 71
Blunt injury to, abdomen, 101
Bones and joints, biomechanics of, 125
Bowel laceration, 107
Brain, elasticity of, 294
Brain motion, natural frequency, 210, 354
Brain stem, 30
 shear stress in, 31
Bronchi, rupture of, 385
Bronchus, injury to, 94

C

Central hemorrhages in head injury, 46
Cerebral edema, 171
Chest injury, mechanics of, 86
Classification of head injury, 7
Colonic injuries, 121
Concussion
 cerebral, 27, 29, 43, 275
 medullary, 29
 physical factors in, 275, 285
 physiological factors in, 277
Conscious state, 28
Cortical bone, mechanical characteristics of, 136

D

Deformation in head injury, 32, 235
Deformation, skull, 243
Dentate ligament, 65, 70
Diaphragm, rupture of, 108
Disc, intravertebral, 67
Duodenal injuries, 119
Dynamic overshoot, 430

E

Elasticity of brain, 294
Encephalopathy, fine changes in, lead, 162
Endoradiosondes, 148
Energy absorbing
 devices, 452
 padding, 439
 steering column, 393
Epidemiology of injury, 5
Ergastoplasm, 163

F

Femoral
 head, forces about, 129
 neck fracture forces, 418
Fracture, experimental, skull, 235, 237
Frequency, natural, of brain, 354

G

Golgi apparatus, 163, 164, 165

H

Head injury
 acceleration in, 34
 anoxia in, 100
 classification of, 7
 deformation in, 32, 235
 mechanisms of, 27
 negative pressure in, 46
 pulmonary damage associated with, 95, 99
 varieties of, 27
Headrests, 487
Heart, injury to, 86

I

Inflating device, automatic, 438, 484, 515
Injury, multiplicity, 8
Injury prediction, mathematical model for, 214, 230
Injury reduction
 current methods of, 475
 kinetics and kinematics of, 423
Instrument panels, 483
Intracranial pressure, 32, 180, 186

K

Kinematics, whole body, 223
Kinetics and kilematics of injury reduction, 423

L

Lamellar bodies of capillary, 170
Ligament, tensile pattern of, 137
Liver
  fracture, 105
  rupture of, 374
Lung
  pneumothorax, 381
  pulmonary contusion, 381
  wet, 381

M

Mechanisms of head injury, 27
Medullary concussion, 29
Mitochondria, 163
Monitors, implanted, 180
Momentum exchange principle, 426
Multiplicity of injury, 8

N

Natural frequency, brain motion, 210
Negative pressure in head injury, 46

P

Padding, energy absorbing, 439
Pericytes, 161
Pressure gradients, intracranial, 32
Pulmonary damage associated with head injury, 95, 99

R

Relative motion, excessive, 450
Restraint
  child, 504
  head, 487, 512
  inverted-Y double harness, 503
  lap and shoulder, 435, 478, 496
  lapbelt, 432, 476, 496
  passive, 438, 484, 515, 519
Restraint systems, 458
  aircraft, 520
  Type 2, 500

S

Seat
  Cox, 506
  Liberty Mutual Capsule, 510
  rearward-facing, 511
Severity of injury, 14
Shear stress in brain stem, 31
Skull, experimental fracture, 235, 237
Skull volume, 33
Spinal cord, 64
  plastic deformation, 69
Spinal cord injury, 63
  biomechanics of, 69
  blood flow in, 71
  cooling, 78
  experimental, 73
Spinal vascular unit, 65
Spine injury, 63
  biomechanics of, 66
Spleen, rupture of, 107
Steering
  assemblies, 481
  column, energy absorbing, 393
Stresscoat, 235
Structure of cerebral damage, fine, 160
Subdural hematoma, angular acceleration, 50

T

Telemetry, 145, 157, 180, 186
Tolerance
  long bones, impact, 402, 408
  pelvis, impact, 402 403
  subhuman primate brain to cerebral concussion, 352
  thorax and abdomen, 372
  to impact, human, 448
  voluntary human, 308
Tolerance data, application of, 445

V

Varieties of head injury, 27
Ventricular rupture, 384
Vertebral column, 64

W

Whiplash, 354, 359
Whiplash injury to primates, 361
Windshields, 482
Work-energy principle, 424

X

X-ray
  cinematography, 197, 199, 211
  flash, 201
  high speed, 196

RD96.6
I5